Ear, Nose, and Throat Diseases

A Pocket Reference

Walter Becker, Hans Heinz Naumann, and Carl Rudolf Pfaltz

With the cooperation of
Claus Herberhold and Ernst Kastenbauer

Edited by Richard A. Buckingham

497 Illustrations by Rudolf Brammer
39 color plates

Second, revised edition

1994
Georg Thieme Verlag   Thieme Medical Publishers, Inc.
Stuttgart · New York   New York

II

Library of Congress Cataloging-in-Publication Data

Becker, Walter, 1920—
  [Hals-Nasen-Ohren-Heilkunde. English]
  Ear, nose and throat diseases : a pocket reference / Walter
Becker, Hans Heinz Naumann, and Carl Rudolf Pfaltz : With the
cooperation of Claus Herberhold and Ernst Kastenbauer : edited by
Richard A. Buckingham ; illustrated by Rudolf Brammer, — 2nd rev.
ed.
    p. cm.
  Includes bibliographical references and index.
  ISBN 3-13-671202-1 (G. Thieme Verlag). — ISBN 0-86577-536-2
(Thieme Medical Publishers)
    1. Otolaryngology—Handbooks, manuals, etc.   I. Naumann, H. H.
(Hans Heinz), 1919—   .   II. Pfaltz, C. R. (Carl Rudolf)
III. Title.
  [DNLM: 1. Otorhinolaryngologic Diseases—handbooks.   WV 39 B396h
1994a]
RF56.B4313   1994
617.5′ 1—dc20
DNLM/DLC
for Library of Congress   93-47536
                                               CIP

Important Note: Medicine is an ever-changing science undergoing continual development. Research and clinical experience are continually expanding our knowledge, in particular our knowledge of proper treatment and drug therapy. Insofar as this book mentions any dosage or application, readers may rest assured that the authors, editors and publishers have made every effort to ensure that such references are in accordance with the state of knowledge at the time of production of the book. Nevertheless this does not involve, imply, or express any guarantee or responsibility on the part of the publishers in respect of any dosage instructions and forms of application stated in the book. Every user is requested to examine carefully the manufacturers' leaflets accompanying each drug and to check, if necessary in consultation with a physician or specialist, whether the dosage schedules mentioned therein or the contraindications stated by the manufacturers differ from the statements made in the present book. Such examination is particularly important with drugs that are either rarely used or have been newly released on the market. Every dosage schedule or every form of application used is entirely at the user's own risk and responsibility. The authors and publishers request every user to report to the publishers any discrepancies or inaccuracies noticed.

1st German edition 1982   1st French edition 1986
2nd German edition 1983   1st Spanish edition 1986
3rd German edition 1986   1st Italian edition 1988
4th German edition 1989   1st English edition 1989

This book is an authorized and updated translation from the 4th German edition published and copyrighted 1982, 1989 by Georg Thieme Verlag, Stuttgart, Germany. Title of the German edition: Hals-Nasen-Ohren-Heilkunde.

Some of the product names, patents and registered designs referred to in this book are in fact registered trademarks or proprietary names even though specific reference to this fact is not always made in the text. Therefore, the appearance of a name without designation as proprietary is not to be construed as a representation by the publishers that it is in the public domain.

© 1994 Georg Thieme Verlag, Rüdigerstrasse 14, D-70469 Stuttgart, FRG
Thieme Medical Publishers, Inc., 381 Park Avenue South, New York, N. Y. 10016
Typesetting by Druckhaus Götz GmbH, D-71636 Ludwigsburg
Printed in Germany by Appl, D-86650 Wemding

ISBN 3-13-671202-1 (Georg Thieme Verlag, Stuttgart)
ISBN 0-86577-536-2 (Thieme Medical Publishers, Inc., New York)   4   5   6

Preface to the Second Edition

Since the first edition of this pocket reference on ear, nose, and throat diseases, Otorhinolaryngology has shown the same progressive development as many other medical specialties, both with respect to diagnostic and therapeutic procedures, and also with regard to a new understanding of pathophysiologic mechanisms underlying some ear, nose, and throat disorders. For those reasons we have found it necessary to revise both text and illustrations in order to bring this textbook up to the present standard of scientific and technical knowledge. Again we were aiming at presenting the essentials of ORL to medical students in the first place, but also at providing residents and interested practioners with further information, which would allow a better understanding of the diagnostic and therapeutic problems of our specialty and its borderlands. We should like to thank Prof. Dr. C. Herberhold, Bonn and Prof. Dr. E. Kastenbauer Munich, for their cooperation, particularly for the revision of the section of color plates, and last but not least we wish to thank Dr. med. h. c. G. Hauff and his colleagues at Georg Thieme Verlag for their assistance and advice.

Fall 1993

H. H. Naumann, Munich   C. R. Pfaltz, Basel

Preface to the First Edition

Otorhinolaryngology has undergone rapid and impressive development both as regards diagnosis and treatment in recent years. In previous years the main interest of our specialty was infection of the ear and the upper airways and its complications. However, the surgical spectrum of our specialty has now been extended by inclusion of trauma and tumor surgery, bringing with it the closely allied techniques of corrective and reconstructive surgery of the head, neck, and face, so that the specialty is now more appropriately called otorhinolaryngology and head and neck surgery. Moreover, four main sensory functions (hearing, balance, smell, and taste) fall within the province of otorhinolarygology, and significant advances in sensory physiology have recently led to considerable improvements in diagnosis. This pocket-sized book is intended to present the basic essentials of ear, nose and throat diseases and surgery to the student, and also to provide him with further information so that he may better understand the diagnostic and therapeutic problems of our specialty, and also the important relations of the ear, nose and throat with neighboring organs. It is hoped that this book will also serve as a reference source for colleagues who are already in practice. The material is therefore presented in different forms of type:

basic information is given in normal type,
and supplementary information is given in small print.

Particular importance has been attached to supplementing the text by numerous figures. Tables are provided to simplify differential diagnosis.

For the practicing otorhinolaryngologist the visual findings are often the key to diagnosis once the history has been taken, but not every student has the opportunity to see for himself the important clinical findings in patients. Furthermore, the normal general practice a relatively high proportion of patients with symptoms referable to the ear, nose and throat. We have therefore provided about 100 color plates to illustrate typical ear, nose and throat diseases. These illustrations have been taken from the second edition of Dr. Becker's book *Atlas of Ear, Nose and Throat Diseases Including Bronchoesophagology,* published by W. B. Saunders in 1984.

The authors wish to thank the staff of their three clinics who took part in the preparation of this book. They also wish to thank Professors Karin Schorn (Munich), H. Eichner (Munich), C. Herberhold (Bonn), F. Martin (Munich), H. J. Opitz (Bonn), H. Scherer (Berlin), W. Wey (Basel).

Rudolf Brammer prepared the graphic illustrations with great skill and sensitivity. Finally, we wish to thank Dr. med. h. c. G. Hauff and his colleagues at Georg Thieme Verlag for their constant help and advice.

Fall 1988

W. Becker, Bonn   H. H. Naumann, Munich   C. R. Pfaltz, Basel

Addresses

Prof. W. Becker, M.D. †
(1920–1990)

Prof. H. H. Naumann, M.D.
Chairman emeritus, Dept. of Otorhinolaryngology
University Hospital, Klinikum Großhadern
Marchioninistr. 15
81377 Munich, Germany

Prof. C. R. Pfaltz, M.D.
Chairman emeritus, Dept. Otorhinolaryngology
University of Basel
Winterhalde 9
CH-4102 Binningen, Switzerland

Prof. C. Herberhold, M.D.
Chairman, Dept. of Otorhinolaryngology
University Hospital
Sigmund-Freud-Str. 25
53127 Bonn, Germany

Prof. E. Kastenbauer, M.D.
Chairman, Dept. of Otorhinolaryngology
University Hospital, Klinikum Großhadern
Marchioninistr. 15
81377 Munich, Germany

Richard A. Buckingham, M.D.
145 S. Northwest Highway
Park Ridge, Illinois 60068
USA

Contents

1. Ear 1

**Applied Anatomy and
Physiology** 1
Basic Anatomy 1
External Ear 3
Middle Ear and Pneumatic
System 4
Inner Ear, Peripheral Hear-
ing, and Balance Organs . . 10
Central Connections of the
Organ of Corti 17
Central Connections of the
Balance Mechanism 17
Facial Nerve 18
Physiology and Pathophysiol-
ogy of Hearing and Balance . . 20
Physiology of Hearing:
Middle and Internal Ear . . 20
Physiology of Hearing:
Retrocochlear Analysis of
Acoustic Information 23
Pathophysiologic Basis of
Hearing Disorders 25
Physiology of the Balance
System 26
Pathophysiologic Basis of
Functional Vestibular Dis-
orders 30

Methods of Investigation 33
Inspection, Palpation, Otosco-
py, Microscopy 33
Inspection of the External
Ear 33
Radiography 38
Functional Assessment of the
Eustachian Tube 40
Qualitative Assessment of
Tubal Function 40

Quantitative Measures of
Tubal Function 41
Audiometry 41
Testing the Hearing Without
an Audiometer 41
Audiometry 43
Fundamental Physical and
Acoustic Concepts 43
Pure-Tone Audiometry 43
Speech Audiometry 52
Electric Response Audio-
metry 57
Hearing Tests in Infants and
Young Children 59
Vestibular Function Tests . . . 60
Vestibulospinal Reflexes . . 60
Tests for Spontaneous and
Provoked Nystagmus 63
Experimental Tests of the
Vestibular System 67
Optokinetic Function and
Pursuit Tracking 68
Fistula Test 69
Investigation of the Facial
Nerve 69

**Clinical Aspects of Diseases of
the External Ear** 71
Nonspecific Inflammation of
the External Ear 71
Specific Forms 73
Otomycosis and Eczema . . 74
Specific Chronic Inflamma-
tion 75
Trauma 75
Wax and Foreign Bodies 77
Tumors 78
Benign Tumors 78

Precancerous and Malignant
Tumors   78
Congenital Anomalies   81
Reconstructive Operations
on the Auricle   82

**Clinical Aspects of Diseases of
the Middle and Internal Ear** . .   82
Disorders of Ventilation and
Drainage of the Middle Ear
Spaces   82
Acute Tubal Occlusion
(Serotympanum)   84
Chronic Seromucinous
Otitis Media   85
Syndrome of the Patulous
Eustachian Tube   86
Nonspecific Inflammation of
the Middle Ear and the Mas-
toid   87
Acute Otitis Media   87
Specific Types   90
Mastoiditis   91
Chronic Otitis Media   94
Congenital Cholesteatoma
of the Temporal Bone   105
Course of Specific Forms of
Cholesteatoma   105
Adhesive Otitis (Middle Ear
Fibrosis)   105
Otogenic Infective Complica-
tions   106
Labyrinthitis   106
Epidural Empyema   107
Otogenic Meningitis   108
Otogenic Sinus Thrombosis   109
Otitic Hydrocephalus   110
Otogenic Brain Abscess . . .   111
Petrositis   113
Specific Inflammatory Disease
of the Middle Ear and the Mas-
toid Process   113
Tuberculosis   113

Syphilis   113
Noninflammatory Diseases of
the Labyrinthine Capsule . . .   114
Otosclerosis   114
Otologic Manifestations of
Generalized Skeletal Dis-
orders   117
Trauma of the Middle and
Inner Ear   117
Temporal Bone Fracture . .   118
Labyrinthine Concussion . .   121
Direct Injuries to the Middle
and Internal Ear   122
Barotrauma   123
Caisson Disease and Diving
Accidents   124
Acute Acoustic Trauma . . .   124
Tumors of the Middle and In-
ternal Ear, the Vestibulo-
cochlear Nerve, and the Facial
Nerve   127
Nonchromaffin Paragangli-
oma (Glomus Tumor)   127
Bony Tumors   129
Middle Ear Carcinoma . . .   129
Acoustic Neuroma or
Schwannoma   130
Facial Nerve Neuroma . . .   133
Histiocytosis (Reticulo-
endotheliosis)   134
True Congenital Cholestea-
toma   134
Congenital Anomalies of the
Middle and Internal Ear . . .   134
Combined Anomalies of the
External and Middle Ear . .   134
Congenital Anomalies of the
Internal Ear   136

**Clinical Aspects of
Cochleovestibular Disorders** .   136
Toxic Damage to the Hearing
and Balance Apparatus   136
Aminoglycoside Antibiotics   136

Ototoxic Occupational
Toxins 137
Inflammatory Lesions of the
Hearing and Balance Appa-
ratus 138
  Herpes Zoster Otitis (Ram-
  say-Hunt Syndrome) 138
  Other Viral Infections . . . 139
  Serous Labyrinthitis 139
Trauma 139
Ménière's Disease 139
Acute Vestibular Paralysis
(Vestibular Neuronitis) 144
Sudden Deafness 145
Symptomatic Cochleovestibu-
lar Disorders 146
Presbycusis 147
Sensorineural Deafness Due to
Other Causes 153
  Deafness in Children
  (Pediaudiology) 153
  Clinical Aspects of Central
  Deafness 153

Basis of Rehabilitation of
Deafness in Children and
Adults 155
Classification of Deafness
Depending on the Degree of
Severity 155
The Completely Deaf Child . . 157
The Cochlear Implant 157
  Hearing Aids 157

Clinical Aspects of Central
Balance Disorders 160

Clinical Aspects of Disorders
of the Facial Nerve 163
  Inflammatory of Otogenic
  Facial Paralysis 163
  Idiopathic Facial Paralysis
  (Bell's Palsy) 163
  Traumatic Facial Paralysis . 165
  Reconstructive Surgery Af-
  ter Facial Paralysis 165

Synopsis of Ear Symptoms . . . 168

2. Nose, Nasal Sinuses, and Face

. . . . 170

Applied Anatomy and
Physiology 170
Basic Anatomy 170
  External Nose 170
  Nasal Cavity 171
  Nasal Sinuses 174
Basic Physiology and Patho-
physiology 180
  The Nose as an Olfactory
  Organ 180
  The Nose as a Respiratory
  Organ 182
  The Nasal Mucosa as a Pro-
  tective Organ 184
  The Nose as a Reflex Organ 184

Influence of the Nose on
Speech 185
Function of the Nasal
Sinuses 185

Methods of Investigation of
the Nose, Paranasal Sinuses,
and Face 186
External Inspection and Palpa-
tion 186
Anterior Rhinoscopy 187
Posterior Rhinoscopy 189
  Indirect Examination 189
Assessment of Nasal Patency . 193
Olfactometry 194

Radiology of the Nose and
Sinuses 196
Lavage of the Sinuses 199
Nasal Endoscopy 202
Specific Diagnostic Methods . . 202

**Clinical Aspects of Diseases of
the Nose, Sinuses and Face** . . 203
Inflammatory Diseases of the
Nose and Paranasal Sinuses . . 203
Inflammations Confined
Mainly to the External
Nose 203
Inflammations Localized
Mainly in the Nasal Cavity . 207
Basics of Local Conservative
Treatment of the Upper
Respiratory and Digestive
Tract 222
Inflammation of the Sinuses   224

Complications of Sinus In-
fections 245
Orbital Phlegmon 247
Epistaxis 253
Diseases of the Septum 260
Trauma to the Nose, Paranasal
Sinuses, and Facial Skeleton . . 263
Trauma to the Nose 263
Trauma of the Middle Third
of the Face and the Sinuses . 265
Congenital Anomalies and
Deformities of the Nose 279
Congential Anomalies of the
Nose 279
Disorders of Shape of the
External Nose 281
Tumors of the Nose and
Sinuses 289
Benign Tumors 289
Malignant Tumors 290

3. Mouth and Pharynx 299

**Applied Anatomy and
Physiology** 299
Basic Anatomy 299
Oral Cavity 299
Naso-, Oro- and Hypo-
pharynx 304
Lymphoepithelial System of
the Pharynx 307
Physiologic and Pathophysio-
logic Principles 309
Eating, Preparation of
Food, and Swallowing 309
Taste 311
Immune-Specific Functions
of Waldeyer's Ring 312
Formation of Sound and
Speech 315

Methods of Investigation 315
Inspection, Palpation, and Examination with the Mirror . . . 315

Endoscopy 318
Radiography 318
Gustometry 319
Specific Diagnostic Proce-
dures 319

**Clinical Aspects of Diseases of
the Mouth and Pharynx** 320
Hyperplasia of the Lympho-
epithelial Organs 320
Adenoid Hyperplasia 320
Tonsillar Hyperplasia 322
Inflammatory Diseases 324
Labial, Oral, and Pharyn-
geal Mucosa 324
Tongue 335
Waldeyer's Ring 344
Other Pharyngeal Inflam-
mations 361
Other Diseases Simulating
Infections 364

Basics of Conservative
Treatment of Disease of the
Mouth and Pharynx 369
Trauma of the Mouth and
Pharynx 369
Alkali and Acid Burns and
Scalds 369
Foreign Bodies 370
Mucosal Injuries of the
Mouth and Pharynx due to
Foreign Bodies and Trauma. 370
Neurogenic Disorders 371
Hypopharyngeal Diverticulum
(Synonyms: Zenker's Divertic-
ulum, Pharyngeal Pouch) . . . 372
Congenital Anomalies of the
Mouth and Pharynx 373
Median Cervical Cysts and
Fistulae 374

Clefts of the Lip, Jaw, and
Palate 374
Tumors of the Mouth and
Pharynx 376
Benign Tumors of the Oral
Cavity Including the Tongue
and the Oropharynx 376
Malignant Tumors of the
Oral Cavity (Including the
Lip and Tongue) and the
Oropharynx 377
Benign Tumors of the Naso-
pharynx 385
Malignant Tumors of the
Nasopharynx 386
Tumors of the Hypo-
pharynx 387

4. Larynx, Hypopharynx, and Trachea 388

Larynx 388

**Applied Anatomy and
Physiology** 388
Basic Anatomy and
Physiology 388
Embryology 388
Anatomy 388
Physiology 393

Methods of Investigation 395
Inspection 395
Palpation 395
Indirect Laryngoscopy 395
Telescopic Laryngoscopy . . . 397
Direct Laryngoscopy 397
Microlaryngoscopy 398
Radiography 399

Clinical Aspects 399
Congenital Anomalies 399

Laryngomalacia 399
Neurogenic Disorders 400
Atresias and Webs 401
Laryngoceles 401
Subglottic Stenoses 401
Hemangioma 401
Functional Disorders 402
Recurrent Laryngeal Nerve
Paralysis (Unilateral or
Bilateral) 405
Unilateral or Bilateral Para-
lysis of the Superior Laryn-
geal Nerve 407
Combined Lesions of the
Laryngeal Nerves 407
Traumatology 409
Vocal Abuse 409
Contact Ulcer 410
Intubation Injury 410
External Trauma 411

Inhalational Trauma by
Chemical Toxins 413
Foreign Bodies 414

Inflammation 414
Acute Laryngitis 414
Croup Syndromes 415
Chronic Laryngitis 417
Tumors 420
Benign Tumors 420
Leukoplakia, Dysplasia, and
Carcinoma In Situ of the La-
ryngeal Mucosa 422
Malignant Tumors 423
Hypopharynx 432

Tracheobronchial Tree 434

**Applied Anatomy and
Physiology** 434

Basic Anatomy 434
Basic Physiology 436

Methods of Investigation . . . 436
Bronchoscopy 436

Clinical Aspects 437
Stenoses 437
Tracheotomy, Laryngot-
omy, and Intubation 446
Foreign Bodies and Trauma . . 452
Foreign Bodies 452
Trauma 453
Infections 453
Congenital and Hereditary
Anomalies 454
Tumors 455
Malignant Tracheal Tumors   455

5. Esophagus 457

Applied Anatomy 457

**Physiology and
Pathophysiology** 458

Methods of Investigation . . . 458
Clinical Examination 458
Radiography 459
Esophagoscopy 459
Manometry 462

Clinical Aspects 463
Traumatology 463
Burns by Acid or Lye 463

Foreign Bodies 465
Blunt and Penetrating Inju-
ries, Perforations, and the
Mallory-Weiss Syndrome . . 466
Esophageal Diverticulum . . . 467
Inflammations and Inflamma-
tory Stenoses 468
Motility Disorders of the
Esophagus 469
Esophageal Varices 470
Congential Anomalies and
Fistulae 471
Tumors of the Esophagus . . . 472
Malignant Tumors 473

6. Neck (Including the Thyroid Gland) 474

**Applied Anatomy and
Physiology** 474

Basic Anatomy and
Physiology 475

Regions 475
Fascia 476
Spaces 478
Blood Vessels 479
Cervical Lymphatic System 484
Nerves 487
Basic Physiology 490

Methods of Investigation 490
Inspection 490
Palpation 491
Technical Methods of Investi-
gation 493

Clinical Aspects 493
Inflammation of the Cervical
Soft Tissues 493
Superficial Infections 494
Abscesses 494
Mediastinitis 494
Inflammatory Cervical
Lymphadenopathy 495
Nonspecific Lymphadenitis 495
Specific Lymphadenopathy 496
Trauma 500

Congenital Anomalies 501
Lateral Branchial Fistulae
and Cysts 501
Thyroglossal Duct Cysts and
Fistulae 504
Musculoskeletal Defects . . 504
Tumors 505
Vascular Tumors 505
Neurogenic Tumors 507
Torticollis 508
Cervical Lipoma 508
Neoplastic
Lymphadenopathy 510
Principles of Surgery 517
Prescalene Node Biopsy . . 517
Mediastinoscopy 518
Neck Dissection 519
Thyroid Gland and Otorhino-
laryngology 521
Goiter 523
Hypothyroidism 524
Hyperthyroidism 524
Infections of the Thyroid
Gland 525
Thyroid Malignancy 526

7. Salivary Glands

. . . . 529

Embryology, Structure, Con-
genital Anomalies 529
Anatomy and Physiology of
the Major and Minor Salivary
Glands 531
Parotid Gland 531
Submandibular Gland 532
Sublingual Gland 532
Minor Salivary Glands 533
Formation and Function of
Saliva 533

Methods of Investigation 536
Radiographic Diagnosis 537
Biopsy 538

Clinical Findings 539
Inflammatory Diseases 539
Acute Bacterial Infections . 539
Viral Infections 540
Chronic Inflammation 542
Sialolithiasis 545
Sialadenosis 547
Trauma 547
Injury to the Nerves or
Ducts and Salivary Fistulae . 547
Salivary Tumors 548
Benign Tumors 548
Malignant Tumors 550
Basic Principles of Treatment
of Salivary Tumors 554

8. Emergency and First Aid Procedures 558

9. Further Reading 559

Index 560

Color Plates following Index

1. Ear

Applied Anatomy and Physiology

Basic Anatomy

The hearing and balance systems comprise the *peripheral receptor apparatus* (i.e., the ear in its strict sense), the *nervous pathways,* and the *centers* within the central nervous system. Two main subdivisions can thus be distinguished:

Peripheral Part
- External, middle, and inner ear
- Auditory nerve with its two parts, the cochlear and the vestibular divisions

Central Part
- Central hearing pathways
- Subcortical and cortical auditory centers
- Central balance mechanism

The *anatomic boundary* between the *peripheral* and *central* parts is the point of entry of the VIIIth cranial nerve into the brain stem (the cerebellopontine angle) at which point the *peripheral* part of the auditory nerve passes into the *central* part interspersed with glial cells. In *functional* terms, however, the peripheral neurons end in the primary centers.

The sensory organs for hearing and balance develop from ectoderm. From this is formed the *membranous labyrinth* which initially is surrounded by *embryonal mesenchymal tissue.* This is converted partly into cartilage whose outer layer forms the *labyrinthine capsule* and partly, by vacuolization, into a fine reticular network which forms the inner layer of the *perilymphatic space.* The eustachian tube and the mucosa of the middle ear arise from a diverticulum of the first pharyngeal pouch (endoderm). The malleus and incus develop from Meckel's cartilage which arises from the first branchial arch and is supplied by the trigeminal nerve. The stapes arises from Reichert's cartilage which arises from the second branchial arch and is supplied by the facial nerve (see Table 6.**3**).

The external meatus and the tympanic membrane develop from an ectodermal diverticulum between the first and second branchial arches. *Developmental disorders* cause deformities of the external and middle ears. Bilateral lesions causing severe conductive deafness or a psychologically unacceptable deformity must be corrected for both esthetic and functional reasons (see pp. 81 and 134) (Figs. 1.**1a** and **b** and 1.**2a–d**).

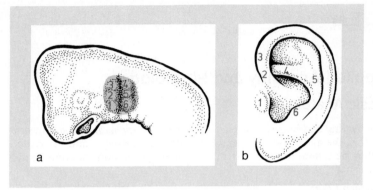

Fig. 1.**1a** and **b**   Development of the external ear. **(a)** 11 mm embryo, from the side. Outer ear development from 6 hillocks arising from the 1st and 2nd branchial arches. **(b)** 1, tragus; 2 crus helicis; 3, helix; 4, crus anthelicis; 5, anthelix; 6, antitragus.

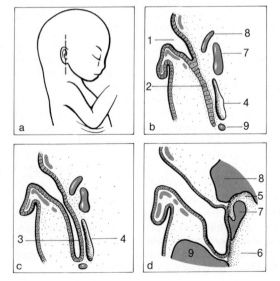

Fig. 1.**2a–d**   Diagram of development of the middle ear. The first ectodermal branchial arch forms the primary anlage of the cartilaginous part of the external auditory meatus. The funnel-shaped tube is shown by b1. A string of epithelial cells grows mediocaudally toward the pharyngeal pouch (b2). The tympanic membrane (c3), the bony part of the external auditory meatus, the primitive middle ear cavity (b4 and c4), and the anlage of the tympanic plate (b9 and d9) develop later. The parts of the middle ear then begin to develop: the epitympanum (d5), the mesotympanum (d6), the malleus (b and d7), and the squamous part of the temporal bone (b and d8). (Modified from Nager.)

External Ear

The *auricle* consists of a framework of elastic cartilage covered by skin, lying between the temporomandibular joint anteriorly and the mastoid process posteriorly. The skin adheres tightly to the perichondrium on the anterior surface but is more loosely attached posteriorly. For this reason contusions of the anterior surface often lead to detachment of the skin-perichondrial layer and to the formation of a *hematoma* (see p. 76).

The *external meatus* is about 3 cm long and consists of an outer cartilaginous part and an inner bony part. The cartilaginous meatus is curved and lies at an angle to the bony part. The tympanic membrane and the middle ear lying beyond it are thus protected from direct trauma.

> *Note:* The curved cartilaginous mobile part of the external auditory meatus must be drawn upward and posteriorly to bring it into the same axis as the bony part, to allow an otoscope to be introduced accurately.

The cartilaginous part is attached firmly to the rim of the *bony meatus* (os tympanicum) by connective tissue and is covered by a thin layer of skin which adheres to the periosteum. It contains no accessory structures, in contrast to the cartilaginous part of the meatus which demonstrates numerous hair follicles and ceruminous glands which form wax (epidermis scale, sebaceous matter, pigment) (see p. 71).

The external meatus narrows medially so that *foreign bodies* often become impacted at the junction of the cartilaginous and bony meatus. The meatal cartilage does not form a closed tube but rather a channel closed superiorly by fibrous tissue. The cartilage contains a number of dehiscences (Santorini's clefts) which provide a pathway for spread of severe bacterial infection to the parotid space, the infratemporal fossa, and the base of the skull. The so-called *malignant otitis externa* is often lethal (see p. 74)

The auricle and the cartilaginous meatus have a very rich *lymphatic drainage* to an extensive regional lymphatic network consisting of parotid, retroauricular, infraauricular, and superior deep cervical nodes. *Infections* of the external meatus with regional lymphadenitis can thus cause extensive swelling in these areas.

The *sensory innervation* is supplied by the trigeminal, great auricular, and vagus nerves and the sensory fibers of the facial nerve. The latter two branches respectively explain the cough reflex which can be elicited from the posterior meatal wall and the hypoesthesia of the posterosuperior meatal wall in a patient with an acoustic neuroma (see discussion of Hitselberger's sign, p. 18 and Table 1.**14**: p. 132).

Relations (Fig. 1.**3**). The cartilaginous meatus abuts on the parotid gland, thus allowing extension of infections or malignant tumors. The posterosuperior wall of the bony meatus forms a part of *the lateral attic wall (the partition between external auditory meatus and attic),* the mastoid antrum, and

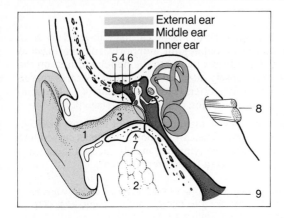

Fig. 1.3 Relations of the external auditory meatus: 1, cartilaginous part; 2, parotid gland; 3, bony meatus; 4, lateral attic wall; 5, mastoid antrum; 6, attic; 7, temporomandibular joint; 8, facial, vestibular and auditory nerves; 9, Eustachian tube.

the adjacent pneumatic system of the mastoid process. A middle ear infection can thus break through into the external auditory meatus causing *sagging of the posterosuperior wall* or fistula in *acute mastoiditis*. Equally, *destruction of the lateral attic wall* by *cholesteatoma* may form an open communication between the external auditory meatus and the attic or mastoid antrum. The anterior wall of the bony meatus forms part of the temporomandibular joint. There is thus a risk of *fracture as a result of a blow to the chin*.

Middle Ear and Pneumatic System

The *middle ear cavity* consists of an extensive *pneumatic system* aerated by the eustachian tube. Its parts are:

- Eustachian tube
- Tympanic cavity
- Mastoid antrum
- Pneumatic system of the temporal bone

The *eustachian tube* consists of a mobile, cartilaginous portion ($\frac{2}{3}$) suspended from the skull base, and a bony portion ($\frac{1}{3}$). The bony portion together with the tensor tympani muscle forms the musculotubal canal in the temporal bone.

This canal lies adjacent to the internal carotid artery. The funnel-shaped pharyngeal ostium of the cartilaginous part (torus tubarius) lies in the nasopharynx. The bony end opens into the middle ear.

The junction between the two parts of the tube is very narrow. This *isthmus* is the site of predilection for inflammatory stenosis of the tube. The

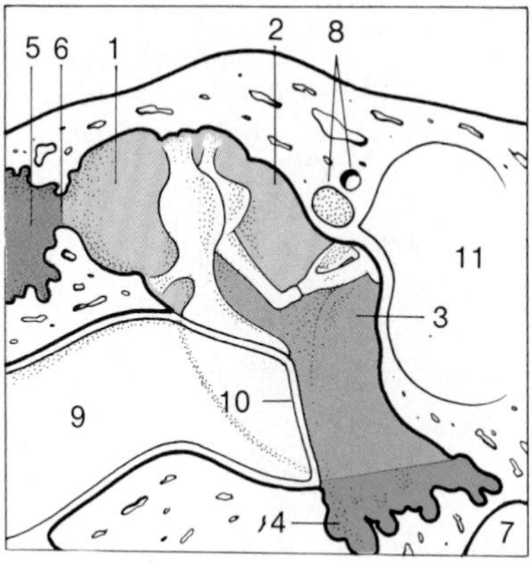

Fig. 1.4 Anatomy of the middle ear cavity: 1 and 2, epitympanum; 3, mesotympanum; 4, hypotympanum; 5, mastoid antrum; 6, entrance to the antrum; 7, internal jugular vein. The lower part of the attic (2) is markedly narrowed by the facial nerve and the horizontal semicircular canal (8). External meatus (9), tympanic membrane (10), and inner ear (11).

tube serves to equalize the pressure between the middle ear and the nasopharynx, and thus to equalize the pressure on each side of the tympanic membrane (see pp. 50, 82). An increase in pressure in the tympanic cavity is usually compensated for passively via the eustachian tube to the nasopharynx, whereas a decrease in pressure usually requires active ventilation from the nasopharynx along the tube to the middle ear cavity. The tube opens and closes in response to movements of the neighboring muscles and differences of air pressure between the nasopharynx and the middle ear cavity which tend to equalize spontaneously. The principal closing mechanism is the elastic recoil of the cartilage of the tube and the valvular action of the pharyngeal ostium of the tube. The tube is opened by contraction of the tensor palati and levator palati muscles. The mechanism is partially under the control of voluntary muscle, but the reflex movements on yawning and swallowing and the muscle tone are under autonomic control. Tension on the opening muscles is provided by the elastic recoil of the tubal cartilage and the pressure of the peritubal tissues, i.e., the pterygoid muscles, Ostmann's fatty bodies, the venous and lymphatic plexus of the tubal mucosa, and the pterygoid venous plexus.

The *middle ear cavity* is an air-containing space lying between the external ear and the inner ear. It is divided into three parts (Fig. 1.4):

- Epitympanic recess or attic
- Mesotympanum
- Hypotympanic recess

Between the epi- and mesotympanum there is an anatomic constriction which can lead to retention of secretions in inflammation and to deficient aeration of the attic. This is due to the considerable narrowing of this area

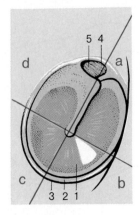

Fig. 1.5 Macroscopic appearance of the right tympanic membrane: 1, pars tensa; 2, anulus fibrosus; 3, bony tympanic anulus; 4, tympanic notch; 5, pars flaccida. The visible part of the surface of the tympanic membrane is divided into four quadrants: anterosuperior **(a)**, anteroinferior **(b)**, posteroinferior **(c)**, and posterosuperior **(d)** in order of investigation.

caused by the head of the malleus, the body of the incus, numerous ligaments, nerves (the chorda tympani), and mucosal folds and pockets. This is one of the causes for the chronic inflammation of the epitympanum *(chronic epitympanitis)* which is one of the causative factors of epitympanic cholesteatoma (see p. 98). A further narrow zone lies at the junction of the attic and the mastoid antrum *(the aditus ad atrum)* which may be closed by granulation tissue in chronic inflammation leading to deficient aeration or drainage of the mastoid cell system. The lateral wall of the middle ear cavity is formed by the tympanic membrane. The hypotympanum is closely related to the bulb of the internal jugular vein.

The *tympanic membrane* consists of the pars tensa and the pars flaccida. The *pars tensa* forms the stiff vibrating surface of the membrane and is attached to a fibrous ring *(the anulus fibrosus)* lying in the tympanic sulcus of the tympanic part of the temporal bone. The *pars flaccida* is that part of the membrane in the area of the tympanic notch (of Rivini), where the anulus fibrosus is discontinued (Fig. 1.5).

The *microscopic appearances* of the tympanic membrane are shown in Figure 1.6. The epithelial or cuticular layer (stratum corneum) is similar in structure to the skin of the external auditory meatus, but the marginal zone bordering on the tympanic anulus shows extremely active proliferation due to papillary ingrowths into the stratum germinativum. This is a further important factor in the genesis of cholesteatoma (see pp. 96–105).

The keratinizing squamous epithelium does not regenerate by superficial desquamation, as does the remaining part of the skin, but by migration of the epidermis from the center of the tympanic membrane to the periphery. Clinically, this can be traced by the migration of a blood clot from the

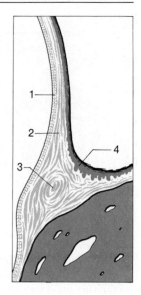

Fig. 1.**6** Microscopic appearance of a sagittal section through the posteroinferior quadrant of the tympanic membrane: 1, middle ear mucosa; 2, middle fibrous layer; 3, anulus fibrosus; 4, epidermis layer with papillary downgrowths similar to the meatal skin bordering the tympanic membrane.

tympanic membrane to the external meatus. This migration of the outer epidermal layer forms an important part of the self-cleaning mechanism of the external meatus.

The *lamina propria* has an external radial layer of fibers and an internal circular layer. The anulus fibrosus forms a thickening of the edge of the tympanic membrane and is formed by both layers of fibers. A lamina propria can also be seen in the *pars flaccida,* but it lacks the characteristic radial-circular structure described above which provides the normal pars tensa with the necessary functional tension.

The *medial wall of the middle ear* also forms the lateral wall of the labyrinthine capsule (Fig. 1.7).

The *mucosa* that lines the middle ear space consists of pseudostratified ciliated epithelium around the mouth of the eustachian tube, becoming flattened peripherally to a stratified cuboidal epithelium. A few goblet cells and submucosal glands are normally present. The submucosa is very thin so that the mucosa lies directly on the periosteum to form a tightly bound unit, the *mucoperiosteum*. In pathologic conditions such as tubal occlusion or chronic otitis media, the structure of the mucosa changes considerably to show hyperplasia of the glands, proliferation of the goblet cells, edema of the submucosa, vascular buds, and transformation of the flattened cuboidal epithelium to a columnar epithelium.

The middle ear mucosa forms several pouches and folds *(Prussak's space, Troeltsch's pouch)* which are responsible for narrowing the junction between the

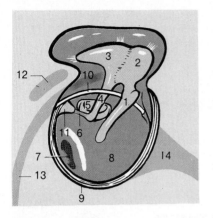

Fig. 1.7   Medial wall of the middle ear: promontory (8) at the basal turn of the cochlea. Above is the oval window niche with the stapes (5) whose footplate is held loosely in the oval window by the annular ligament. The long process of the incus (4) forms a joint by its lenticular process with the head of the stapes. The body of the incus (3) forms the joint surface for the head of the malleus (2). The malleus and incus vibrate as one body in the middle part of the frequency range. The round window (7) lies below the pyramidal eminence (11) with the stapedius muscle whose tendon (6) runs to the head of the stapes. The bony facial canal (13) runs inferior to the horizontal semicircular canal (12). The handle and short process of the malleus (1) lie lateral to the chorda tympani (10). The pars tensa is anchored by the anulus fibrosus (9) in the bony niche of the anulus tympanicus. The middle ear cavity is aerated via the eustachian tube (14).

attic and the rest of the middle ear and between the attic and the antrum. Myxomatous embryonic connective tissue lies between the ectodermal and endodermal ingrowths and makes a preformed middle ear cavity. If this myxomatous tissue does not involute properly after birth, the epitympanic recess remains as a narrow cleft. This "mesenchyme" can completely obliterate the epitympanum if a chronic hyperplastic inflammation follows an infection. The ventilation and drainage of the attic is then impeded by thickened masses of inflammatory tissue, despite normal tubal function. Deficient aeration and drainage of this small space favors the development of chronic *epitympanitis* and plays a considerable role in the *pathogenesis of chronic otitis media* (see p. 95–105), especially attic cholesteatoma.

The *arterial blood supply* originates from the basilar artery (the labyrinthine artery), the maxillary artery (the middle meningeal and tympanic arteries), and the stylomastoid artery. The venous drainage is partly into the middle meningeal veins, partly into the venous plexus of the internal carotid artery and of the pharynx, and partly into the bulb of the internal jugular vein.

The *nerve supply* of the mucosa is provided in part by the tympanic branch of the glossopharyngeal nerve and partly by the auriculotemporal branch of the trigeminal nerve.

Note: This joint sensory supply of the oral and aural regions explains pain referred to the ear in diseases of the teeth and the jaws, and of the larynx and the pharynx.

Pneumatic System of the Temporal Bones

The air-containing cells of the mastoid process are in continuity with the air in the middle ear. These multiple interconnecting spaces arise from the

Fig. 1.8 Pneumatic system of the temporal bone: 1, transverse sinus; 2, mastoid process with tip cells; 3, mastoid antrum; 4, eustachian tube; 5, zygomatic cells; 6, cells of the squamous part of the temporal bone; 7, sinodural angle; 8, retrosinus cells.

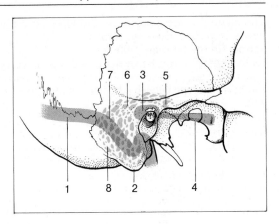

Fig. 1.9 Topographic relations of the middle ear cavity: 1, facial nerve: inflammation and trauma often affect the mastoid segment; 2, tegmen tympani which is the site of predilection for a rupture of a mastoiditis into the middle cranial fossa; 3, bulb of the internal jugular vein which is the site of predilection for extension of a glomus tumor into the middle ear cavity (see p. 127); 4, internal carotid artery [in petrositis, (see p. 113), the inflammation can extend in the venous plexus around the carotid artery to set up a cavernous sinus thrombosis]; 5, cavernous sinus; 6, apical cells [purulent infection of cells in petrositis (see p. 113) causes Gradenigo's syndrome]; 7, pneumatic system of the mastoid process.

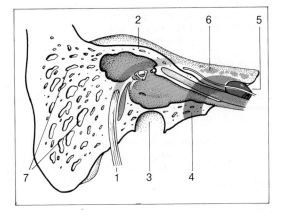

mastoid antrum and show great variability in their degree of *pneumatization*. On the one hand, *pneumatization* may be well developed, extending to the temporal and occipital bones and the origin of the zygomatic arch. Acute infections of the mastoid may cause inflammatory swellings in these regions. On the other hand, the mastoid process may consist exclusively of compact bone if it is *poorly pneumatized* and the pneumatized cells are restricted to those in the immediate neighborhood of the antrum.

The mastoid process begins to develop after birth as a small tuberosity which is pneumatized synchronously with the growth of the mastoid antrum. In the 1st year of life it consists of spongy bone so that true mastoiditis cannot occur. Between the 2nd and 5th years of life as pneumatization proceeds it consists of mixed spongy and pneumatic bone. Pneumatization is complete between the 6th and the 12th years of life (Figs. 1.8 and 1.9).

Principle of pneumatization. Bone is destroyed by an enzymatic lacunar osteoclastic process. The resulting bony spaces are lined by continuous ingrowth of mucoperiosteum from the antrum. A system of hollow cavities results, consisting of numerous spaces lined by mucosa and communicating with each other.

It is obvious that the process of pneumatization can be related to the biological competence of the middle ear mucosa. The mucosa may be described as *biologically normal* or *inferior* depending on the degree of pneumatization. *Good pneumatization* indicates a biologically competent middle ear mucosa, whereas *restricted pneumatization* indicates biological incompetence of the middle ear mucosa which can partially be explained by immunology. A biologically incompetent middle ear mucosa may indicate a defective enzyme system which does not allow pneumatization to proceed satisfactorily. Equally, the local immune system of the respiratory mucosa and of the mucoperiosteum may be so incompetent that chronic recurrent otitis can occur. *Normal tubal function* is a prerequisite for a biologically active healthy middle ear mucosa, and thus for the normal process of pneumatization.

> *Note:* Characteristically, pneumatization of the temporal bone is absent or restricted in chronic otitis media.

The better the temporal bone is pneumatized the easier it is for infection to break through the thin cortical bone. In poor pneumatization (the so-called dangerous mastoid process), the inflammatory process may be concealed in the depths and lead to unexpected complications.

Inner Ear, Peripheral Hearing, and Balance Organs

The inner ear or labyrinth embedded in the temporal bone is divided into two functionally separate receptor mechanisms:

- *Vestibule and semicircular canals* (the vestibular end organ)
- *Cochlea* (the acoustic end organ)

The labyrinth can also be divided morphologically into a *bony* and *membranous* part. The first is formed by the *labyrinthine capsule* which arises by periosteal and enchondral ossification.

It shows characteristic histopathologic and chemical abnormalities in systemic bone diseases (e.g., Paget's disease and osteodystrophy) and in localized diseases (e.g., otosclerosis). Both of these demonstrate continuous remodeling of bone.

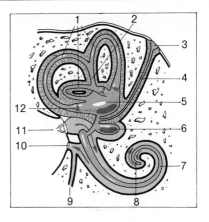

Fig. 1.**10** Diagram of the inner ear: 1, membranous semicircular canals (horizontal, superior, and posterior); 2, crus commune of the posterior and superior canal; 3, saccus endolymphaticus on the posterior surface of the pyramid; 4, ductus endolymphaticus; 5, utricle; 6, saccule; 7, cochlear duct; 8, helicotrema; 9, perilymphatic duct; 10, round window; 11, oval window; 12, ampulla of the posterior semicircular canal with a cupula.

The round and oval windows form the bony and membranous openings to the labyrinth from the middle ear cavity, closed, respectively, by the stapes footplate and round window membrane (see p. 114).

Membranous labyrinth and inner ear fluids (Fig. 1.**10**):

The *membranous labyrinth* develops from the ectodermal otic placode. It encloses a hollow system filled with *endolymph*. This passes via the endolymphatic duct to end in a blind sac, the *saccus endolymphaticus,* lying in the epidural space on the posterior surface of the petrous pyramid close to the sigmoid sinus. The *perilymphatic system* forms a hollow space consisting of intercommunicating intercellular clefts communicating directly with the subarachnoid space via the cochlear aqueduct. Perilymph separates the membranous labyrinth from the internal layer of the labyrinthine capsule surrounding the various spaces. Furthermore, the perilymphatic system communicates with the lymphatic clefts of the middle ear mucoperichondrium so that exchange of metabolites and fluid can occur between the middle and internal ear due to a hydrostatic pressure gradient. The *cochlear aqueduct* and *endolymphatic ducts* end in the jugular foramen and the posterior cranial fossa, respectively.

The *perilymph* is the immediate *substrate* of the *cochlear* and *vestibular sensory cells*. It is formed partly by *filtration* from the *blood* and partly by *diffusion of cerebrospinal fluid*. The *endolymph* is a filtrate of perilymph, but its concentration of sodium and potassium is completely different. The latter is kept constant by the epithelium of the *stria vascularis* (see Fig. 1.**17a**). The *electrolyte composition of the endolymph* regulates the volume of the fluid circulating in the endolymphatic system. The basis of the electrolyte exchange system for the maintenance of a constant ion concentration is the *cellular potassium-sodium exchange pump* found in the stria vascularis, the utricle, and the saccule. Furthermore, there is *passive diffusion* between the endo- and perilymphatic spaces with potassium-sodium ion exchange in the saccus endolymphaticus. Functional disturbances of this electrolyte regulation system lead to a disorder of the middle ear known as *Ménière's disease* (see p. 139).

Vestibular-Semicircular Canal System

The balance mechanism is shown in Figures 1.**11** to 1.**15**. It consists of the *utricle* and *saccule* enclosing the *static maculae* with the sensory end organs for the reception of linear acceleratory stimulation. They consist of *supporting cells* and *hair cells* whose *cilia* are embedded in a gelatinous mass consisting of sulfomucopolysaccharides. On their surface lie the *otoliths* (or statoconia) which consist of rhomboid calcium carbonate crystals. Linear acceleration changes the otolith pressure and thus deflects the sensory hairs. This stimulates the sensory cell by alteration of *resting potential*.

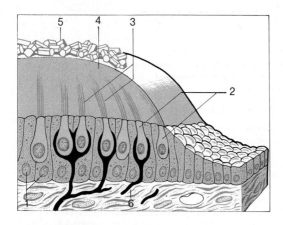

Fig. 1.**11**   Diagram of a static macula: 1, supporting cells; 2, sensory cells; 3, cilia; 4, statolith membrane; 5, statoliths: 6, afferent nerve fibers.

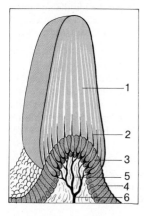

Fig. 1.**12**   Diagram of a receptor in the semicircular canal: 1, cupula; 2, cilia; 3, sensory cells; 4, supporting cells; 5, crista ampullaris; 6, afferent nerve fibers.

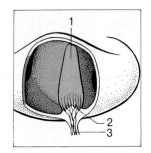

Fig. 1.**13** Diagram of the ampulla of a semicircular canal: 1, cupula; 2, crista ampullaris; 3, afferent nerve fibers.

Fig. 1.**14** Diagram of polarization of a vestibular sensory cell in the cupula: each sensory cell possesses one kinocilia (black fingerlike shape) and about 60 stereocilia (light). Displacement of the cupula and with it the cilia toward the kinocilia causes a nerve stimulation by an increase of receptor potential. Each displacement in the opposite direction inhibits the spontaneous receptor potential. In the horizontal semicircular canal polarization is toward the utricle, but in the vertical canal polarization is in the opposite direction toward the semicircular canal.

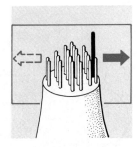

Fig. 1.**15a–d** The principle of function of the mechanoreceptors of the horizontal semicircular canal (see Figs. 1.**27a–c** and 1.**28**). Positive acceleration in a clockwise direction causes endolymph flow in the opposite direction due to inertia, and utriculopetal deflection of the cupula in the right horizontal semicircular canal (**b**) and utriculofugal deflection in the left horizontal semicircular canal (**a**). The receptor potential thus increases on the right side and falls on the left side. Deceleration in a clockwise direction induces the opposite reaction: utriculopetal deflection on the left side (**c**) and utriculofugal deflection on the right side (**d**) with corresponding change in the receptor potentials (1 = Cupula).

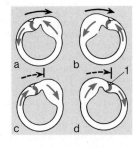

The three semicircular canals arise from the utricle and have a pear-shaped expansion at one end called the *pars ampullaris*. They enclose the sensory cells which are stimulated by angular acceleration. They consist of the *crista ampullaris* on which *sensory hair cells* are so arranged that their cilia extend to the *cupula* which reaches to the roof of the ampulla. The cupula acts as a mobile partition which closes off the pars ampullaris and is relatively impervious to endolymph (Fig. 1.**13**.) The structure and function of the vestibular sensory cells are shown in Figures 1.**14** and 1.**15a–d**.

Note: The hair cells of the maculae and cristae ampullares have similar structural principles. They are mechanoreceptors which respond to a tangential bending of their cilia.

Cochlea (Acoustic End Organ)

The macro- and microscopic structure of the bony and membranous cochlea are shown in Figure 1.**16a** and **b** and Figure 1.**17a** and **b**.

Functional structure of the organ of Corti. The cilia of the sensory cells are in contact with the tectorial membrane. Radial forces occur between the

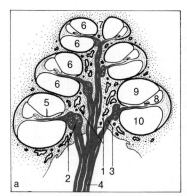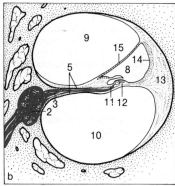

Fig. 1.**16a** and **b**   Axial cross-section through the cochlea, **(a)** and cochlear duct **(b)**. The cochlea is spirally wound ($2\frac{1}{2}$ windings) around the central modiolus (1) lying horizontally. Its base lies against the lateral end of the internal acoustic meatus and its apex is directed anterolaterally toward the medial wall of the middle ear. The spiral ganglion, i. e. the ganglion of the cochlear nerve (2) is located within the modiolus and its nerve fibers (3) join to form the stem of the cochlear nerve, the pars cochlearis nervi vestibulocochlearis (4). The lamina spiralis ossea, called also bony spiral lamina or spiral plate (5) is a bony plate running spirally from the base to the apex (7). Nerve fibers pass through the channels of the spiral lamina to the organum spirale, or organ of Corti (12). The cochlear duct **(b)** contains the ductus cochlearis (8) filled with endolymph, and lying between the scala vestibuli (9) above and the scala tympani (10) below, both of which contain perilymph. The lamina spiralis ossea (5) and the lamina basilaris (11) form the separating wall between the scala tympani on the one hand and the scala vestibuli as well as ductus cochlearis on the other. Reissner's membrane (15) separates the scala vestibuli and the ductus cochlearis. The stria vascularis (14) forms the lateral wall of the ductus cochlearis and has numerous vessels. This layer of fibrous vascular tissue is the site of production of the endolymph. Laterally it borders on the ligamentum spirale cochleae (13). The perilymphatic spaces of the cochlea, the scala tympani and scala vestibuli, communicate with each other at the apex of the cochlea (**a**, 7) at the helicotrema (see Fig. 1.**10**, 8) and are also connected with the perilymphatic space of the membranous labyrinth of the vestibule which contains both the utriculus and the sacculus (see Fig. 1.**10** 5 and 6).

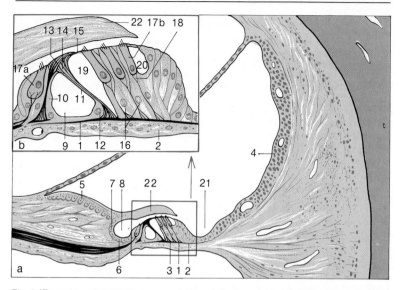

Fig. 1.**17a** and **b**   Schematic representation of ductus cochlearis **(a)** and the organ of Corti **(b)**. The organ of Corti **(b)** rests on the basilar membrane (1 and 2) in the cochlear duct. Medially, at the free edge of the lamina spiralis ossea is the limbus spiralis (5) with two labia (6 and 7) and enclosing the sulcus spiralis internus (8). The highly vascularized stria vascularis (4) with intraepithelial capillaries lies laterally. The organ of Corti **(b)** consists of inner (10) and outer (11 and 12) supporting or pillar cells constituting the borders of the inner tunnel (perilymph – 9). Above (13 to 15) is the top part of the supporting structure, the tonofibrils, below the supporting bodies (18) of the phalangeal cells (16) carrying the sensory cells (17). Between the outer pillars (11, 12) and Deiter's or outer phalangeal cells (16), acting as supporting cells of the organ of Corti, is Nuel's space with perilymph (19). In the extreme lateral position we have the outer tunnel (20) which borders on the sulcus spiralis externus (21) and the stria vascularis (4), respectively. Above the hair cells (inner and outer, 17a and 17b) is the membrana tectoria (22), a gelatinous mass extending from the limbus spiralis (5). The intercellular spaces of the organum spirale (9, 19, 20) contain perilymph also known as cortilymph.

tectorial membrane and the basilar membrane when the latter vibrates. This exerts a shearing force on the cilia of the hair cells and distorts them tangentially. The *shearing of the cilia* is the sensory stimulus for the *hair cells*. The mechanical stimulation is converted in the receptor organ to a neuronal stimulus. The *inner hair cells* form only one row whose single elements connect to afferent individual fibers. According to Spoendlin these constitute 95% of all fibers in the acoustic nerve, whereas the *outer hair cells,* although they form three rows, converge in groups onto single afferent nerve fibers and form only 5% of the fibers of the auditory nerve.

These cells are believed to generate the otoacoustic emissions (see pp. 23 and p. 59).

> *Note:* The entire frequency spectrum of 18 to 20,000 Hz is represented in the hair cells of the organ of Corti over the entire basilar membrane. The highest frequencies are localized to the most basal segment of the cochlea and the lowest frequencies near the helicotrema in the apical turn. This arrangement forms the morphologic basis of the "tonotopic" organization of the cochlea, i.e., the point-to-point connection between the sound wave receptors and the signal-converting central neurons of the auditory system.

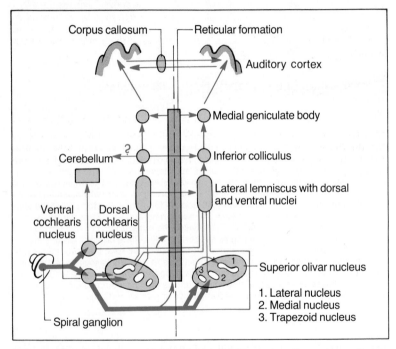

Fig. 1.**18** Simplified diagram of the afferent hearing pathways. The pathways for one cochlea only are shown for the sake of simplicity. The fibers at the commissures at the level of the lateral lemniscus and the inferior colliculus are shown in one direction only, because it is generally accepted that fibers that have crossed to the opposite side do not cross back again. That does not exclude the possibility of connection to the side of origin after synaptic transmission to neurons arising from the opposite side. By means of the horseradish peroxidase technique, it has recently been demonstrated that there are further afferent connections to the inferior colliculus, e.g., from the ipsilateral and contralateral nucleus of the trapezoid body, and to the contralateral ventral cochlear nucleus.

Central Connections of the Organ of Corti

The cochlear division of the VIIIth nerve (pars cochlearis) is formed from the bipolar neurons of the spiral cochlear ganglion. It runs through the internal auditory meatus, unites with the vestibular division, crosses the cerebellopontine angle, and enters the brainstem at the lower border of the pons, at which point the central auditory pathway begins (Fig. 1.**18**).

The central auditory radiation incorporates the strict tonotopic arrangement, as does the *auditory cortex*. Thus, the cochlea is represented, as it were, unrolled, from the basal turn to the helicotrema. The *auditory cortex* is considerably larger than the area of Heschl's transverse striations since these represent only the *primary auditory field* (AI) in which the auditory radiation ends. The secondary acoustic field (AII) and the posterior ectosylvian gyrus, like the visual cortex, include secondary integration areas, such as *Wernicke's speech center*. Numerous commissural systems allow an exchange of fibers between the two halves of the brain. These are very important in directional hearing.

Central Connections of the Balance Mechanism
(Fig. 1.**19**)

The bipolar neurons of the vestibular ganglion send their peripheral processes as two divided bundles of fibers to the sensory cells in the macula of the utricle, to the lateral and superior semicircular canals (superior division), and to the posterior semicircular canal and the macula of the saccule (inferior division).

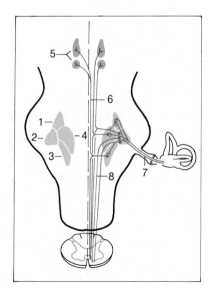

Fig. 1.**19** Diagram of the central vestibular connections in the brain stem. 1, Superior vestibular nucleus of Bechterew; 2, lateral vestibular nucleus of Deiters; 3, inferior vestibular nucleus; 4, medial vestibular nucleus of Schwalbe; 5, centers for the eye muscles; 6, medial longitudinal bundle; 7, vestibular nerve; 8, vestibulospinal tract.

The central processes combine to form the vestibular division of the VIIIth nerve which unites in the internal auditory meatus with the cochlear division to form the vestibulocochlear nerve which has a common nerve sheath. The vestibular division sends ascending fibers to the vestibular centers after it has entered the medulla oblongata. The *secondary vestibular pathway* is connected to the spinal cord by the *vestibulospinal tract*. Its fibers end on the spinal intermediate neurons and activate the motor alpha- and gamma-neurons of the extensor muscles. They are thus the antagonists of the pyramidal pathway and produce principally flexor inhibition and activation of extensors. They are thus part of a phylogenetically old antigravity system serving to maintain balance. In addition, there are important ascending pathways to the cerebellum, the reticular formation (a multisensory integration center), and the centers for the eye muscles (where the oculomotor muscles are coordinated) via the *medial longitudinal bundle*.

A *vestibulocortical connection* is provided via the thalamus. Vestibular stimulation is projected to a small area in the *ventral postcentral* somatosensory *region* near the visual area. This region is said to represent a primary vestibular cortical area.

Note: Connections between the vestibular centers, the centers for the ocular muscles, and the cervical musculature together with the cerebellum form the morphologic basis for the extremely precise coordination of the three functional systems. This allows the visual fixation of an object even during movement of the head. Control of the synchronized coordination of the ocular and cervical muscles is achieved through the vestibular apparatus via the gamma-neurons.

Facial Nerve

The VIIth cranial nerve carries *motor fibers* for the mimic muscles of the face and *taste fibers* and *visceroefferent secretory neurons* in a separate nerve bundle, the nervus intermedius.

It must also now be accepted that the nerve contains the *sensory fibers* that supply the posterior wall of the external auditory meatus. This explains the reduced sensation of this area of skin in patients with acoustic neuroma *(Hitselberger's sign)* (Figs. 1.**20** and 1.**21**).

The *motor* fibers originate from the facial motor nucleus in the floor of the fourth ventricle, run round the abducens nucleus (the internal "genu"), and leave at the lower border of the pons together with the *visceroefferent* fibers of the nervus intermedius arising from the superior salivatory nucleus. The *gustatory* fibers arise from the subcortical taste centers in the nucleus of the solitary tract. These branches now form the *nervus intermediofacialis* which first runs in the internal auditory meatus *(the meatal seg-*

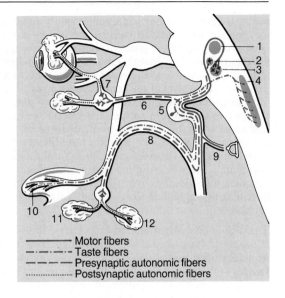

Fig. 1.**20** Course of fibers in the facial nerve: 1, abducens nucleus; 2, secretory nucleus of the nervus intermedius; 3, motornuclei of the facial nerve; 4, nucleus of the solitary tract; 5, geniculate ganglion; 6, greater superficial petrosal nerve; 7, pterygopalatine ganglion with the lacrimal anastomosis; 8, chorda tympani; 9, stapedius nerve; 10, taste fibers to the anterior two thirds of the tongue; 11, sublingual gland; 12, submandibular gland.

——————— Motor fibers
—·—·—·— Taste fibers
— — — — Presynaptic autonomic fibers
················· Postsynaptic autonomic fibers

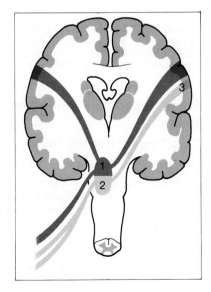

Fig. 1.**21** Diagram of the bilateral corticobulbar innervation of the facial nucleus. This is important in the differential diagnosis of peripheral and central facial paralyses. The branch for the forehead i.e. frontal derives its fibers from the rostral facial nucleus (1) which is innervated by both cortices. The caudal nucleus (2), however, only receives fibers from the contralateral motor center (3). Therefore the function of the fibers of the facial nerve for the forehead remains mainly intact in central paralysis since it receives motor impulses from the intact homolateral cortical centers. In *peripheral and nuclear* facial paralyses all the fibers are paralyzed.

ment). It enters the bony canal immediately adjacent to the labyrinth *(the labyrinthine segment)* and runs to the hiatus in the canal for the facial nerve. At this point the greater superficial petrosal nerve divides off from the main trunk. This branch goes to the lacrimal gland and also supplies fibers to the glands of the nasal mucosa. The first "genu" of the facial nerve lies at the level of the geniculate ganglion. The nerve then turns into the horizontal *tympanic segment* and then passes at the level of the entrance to the mastoid antrum, the second "genu," into the vertical *mastoid segment.* In this area it gives off fibers to the stapedius muscle and to the chorda tympani which contains taste fibers for the anterior two-thirds of the tongue and visceroefferent fibers for the sublingual and submandibular glands. After leaving the mastoid process through the stylomastoid foramen, it divides into five extratemporal branches: temporal, zygomatic, buccal, marginal mandibular, and cervical to the platysma. There is a great variability of these branches (see Fig. 1.77).

The facial nerve is surrounded in its course through the temporal bone by a tough fibrous sheath. Its individual fascicles are embedded in a well-developed *epineurium* of loose connective tissue which encloses the vessels and nerves. The fiber bundles are enclosed in *perineurium.* In repairing an injury of the nerve, the epineurium must be resected from the stump, and a perineural suture must be used so that the site of anastomosis can be adapted exactly, to prevent the formation of a scar tissue neuroma resulting from connective tissue infiltration of the anastomosis (see p. 166).

> *Note:* Knowledge of the topographic-anatomic details of the facial nerve is a prerequisite for understanding the neurologic diagnosis of a facial paralysis (the differential diagnosis of central and peripheral paralyses and the topographic diagnosis of the lesion; see p. 163).

Physiology and Pathophysiology of Hearing and Balance

Physiology of Hearing: Middle and Internal Ear

The functions of the various parts of the ear are as follows:

- The external and middle ear transport the stimulus.
- The cochlea distributes the stimulus.
- The inner hair cells transform the stimulus.
- The outer hair cells function as a frequency-specific cochlear amplifier.

Stimulus Transport

In the *external auditory meatus,* the resonance effect lowers the hearing threshold to between 2,000 and 3,000 Hz, the main range of the speech frequencies.

The *tympanic membrane* is a sound pressure receptor and transformer.

The *ossicular chain* is responsible for impedance adaptation between the middle ear in which the medium is air and the inner ear in a fluid medium, and *pressure transformation*. The enhancement in pressure is 1:17 due to the ratio between the surface of the tympanic membrane and the stapes footplate. The ratio due to the mechanical advantage of the incudomalleolar joint is 1:1.3. The total pressure on the stapes footplate is therefore enhanced 22 times.

The physical molecular movements which we perceive as sound set the tympanic membrane in motion. The frequency of the motion is the same as that of the vibrations of the air, and its amplitude is proportional. The transmission of the sound waves from the air medium to the fluid medium of the peri- and endolymphatic space demands a relative increase in power because of an increase of density, i.e., *impedance adaptation by sound pressure transformation* (impedance = acoustic resistance).

The prerequisite for normal transmission of sound to the inner ear is a tympanic membrane of normal position and mobility and a similar air pressure in the outer and middle ears. Impedance measurements at the tympanic membrane provide information about the function of the sound transmission apparatus, and this is used as a clinical method of investigation called *impedance audiometry* (see p. 50). Sound energy reaches the cochlea first via the sound transmission apparatus of the middle ear *(air conduction)* and second through the bone of the skull which is set in motion in a sound field. The sound energy is thus transmitted directly to the cochlea via the labyrinthine capsule *(bone conduction)*.

Audiometry is used to measure the hearing threshold for both air and bone conduction (see p. 45).

Stimulus Distribution

The main function of the cochlea is *mechanical frequency analysis* which depends on its *hydrodynamics*. Periodic movements at the stapes are converted into aperiodic movements to produce a traveling wave on the basilar membrane (Fig. 1.**22a** and **b**). Since the inner ear fluids are incompressible, a volume displacement on the stapes footplate leads to an equal volume displacement at the round window, and this produces a bulging of the round window membrane equal in extent to the depression of the stapes footplate. This volume displacement produced by *periodic vibrations* of the stapes footplate leads to a displacement of the *scala media* (the space surrounded by the basilar membrane and Reissner's membrane between the scala vestibuli and scala tympani) (see Fig. 1.**16a** and **b**). A wave motion is formed by this initial displacement which proceeds along the partition to the helicotrema. This is an *aperiodic vibration* or traveling wave. The wavelength becomes shorter as the wave approaches the helicotrema, but the

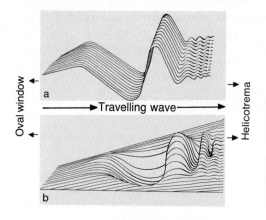

Oval window ← → Helicotrema

a
→ Travelling wave →
b

Fig. 1.**22a** and **b**   Three-dimensional diagram of the vibration of the basilar membrane, as described by Tonndorf. The traveling wave runs from left to right. Both diagrams clearly show the formation of a frequency-dependent maximal amplitude.

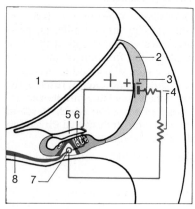

Fig. 1.**23**   Diagram of stimulation of the sensory cells in the organ of Corti, and the production of the nerve impulse (Keidel). 1, Reissner's membrane; 2, stria vascularis; 3, Keidel's battery model; 4, changeable resistance in the tissues; 5, tectorial membrane; 6, hair cells the "microphone", 7, polarized relay between hair cells and nerve fibers which produces the nerve impulse; 8, afferent nerve fibers.

amplitude becomes greater. The amplitude reaches a maximum at one specific point and then immediately begins to fall sharply and dies away toward the helicotrema. The traveling wave causes a displacement between the tectorial membrane and the basilar membrane at its point of maximal amplitude so that the cilia of the hair cells are displaced at this point, forming the sensory stimulus for these mechanoreceptors (Fig. 1.**23**).

The frequency-dependent development of the maximal amplitude on the traveling wave induces a corresponding *frequency-dependent localized stimulus* on the basilar membrane in those sensory cells of the organ of Corti lying at the point of maximal amplitude. A *first analysis* of the sound is thus achieved in accurately defined *frequency stimulus patterns* (Békésy's dispersion or traveling wave theory).

The maximum displacement of the traveling wave lies at a different point for each frequency: it is nearer the helicotrema for the lower frequencies and nearer the stapes footplate for the higher. Every frequency is thus represented at a particular point of the basilar membrane. Since the distribution of the maximal amplitude across the basilar membrane determines the point of excitation of the organ of Corti and thus of the activity of the afferent nerve fibers in the cochlear nerve, the traveling wave hypothesis is also a "one-point" hypothesis as suggested by von Helmholtz, i.e., each point on the basilar membrane corresponds to a specific frequency.

Stimulus Transformation

The inner hair cells in the organ of Corti convert the mechanical energy of the sound waves into bioelectrical energy. The energy required for the conversion process is provided by the metabolism of the sensory cells (see Fig. 1.**23**).

The stria vascularis works by charging the endolymph positively as a source of energy. In electrical terms this represents a battery. Vibrations of the basilar membrane cause synchronous shearing of the cilia by the tectorial membrane, leading to depolarization of the hair cells due to a change of electrical resistance of the cell membrane. The hair cells may thus be compared to the variable resistance of a carbon microphone. Depolarization of the hair cells leads to a change of their receptor potential. As soon as this exceeds a certain threshold, an action potential is released in the afferent nerve fiber at the junction of the hair cells and the initial segment of the afferent neuron. This is an "all-or-none" response (Davis and Keidel). Stronger excitation of the hair cells causes more frequent discharge (the more frequent response of the relay is the basis of frequency modulation in the coding of sound intensity).

Frequency-Specific Cochlear Amplifier

Active contractions of the actin and myosin in the outer hair cells evoked by acoustic stimuli are believed to generate the "otoacoustic emissions" (see p. 59). This unique property of the outer hair cells was only recently discovered and is interpreted as a frequency-specific cochlear amplifier mechanism.

Physiology of Hearing: Retrocochlear Analysis of Acoustic Information

The electric stimulus pattern of the sensory cells in the organ of Corti is converted in the peripheral cochlear neuron into the action potential pattern of the auditory nerve. The many parameters of the sound stimulus such as frequency, intensity, temporal pattern, and periodicity of the action potentials must be encoded to allow information analysis in the central nervous system.

Sound frequency and *sound intensity coding* play a very important role in the central analysis of the acoustic signal.

Sound intensity coding by means of frequency modulation. With increasing sound intensity, the number of spikes in the sensory cell discharge increases.

Sound frequency coding. Specific sensory cell groups in the organ of Corti are stimulated depending on the sound frequency. *Tonotopy* (see below) allows these locally circumscribed *stimulus patterns* produced on the basilar membrane to be conducted without distortion by the auditory nerve to the higher centers.

Tonotopy. This is a point-to-point connection between the sound receptors and the neurons analyzing the signal. Each cochlear neuron has a so-called *best frequency,* i.e., it responds only to an acoustic stimulus whose frequency is identical with the frequency assigned to it (tonotopy).

The acoustic system can process the duration, intensity, and frequency parameters of the acoustic signal in the following ways:

With *increasing intensity* and *constant frequency* the action potential rate in the nerve fibers increases, and the number of stimulated afferent neurons also increases corresponding to the extent of the deflected area of the basilar membrane.

At *constant intensity* and *variable frequency,* the deflected area of the basilar membrane is displaced into the appropriate segment of the organ of Corti within the cochlea so that frequency is determined by *point analysis.* Furthermore, changes occur in the periodicity of the action potential series within the individual nerve fibers, which are analyzed by means of *periodicity analysis.* This provides another means of frequency determination.

A further means of differentiation is provided by the *temporal stimulus pattern* using long nerve fibers. The *sound frequency-adjustment* is based on the relation of several frequency-sensitive neurons. These are characterized by a *tuning curve* that encompasses the entire stimulus range of the neurons. The lowest point of the curve is the actual threshold, and it indicates the best sound frequency of the appropriate neuron (Fig. 1.**24**). This *neuronal tuning curve* is not to be confused with the *mechanical tuning curve,* which shows how the stimulus intensity must be changed relative to frequency so that a particular point on the basilar membrane always has the same deflection amplitude (Fig. 1.**24**).

Frequency analysis by means of local pattern scanning, *appreciation of intensity* by frequency modulation, and *time-periodicity analysis* by combined time and place pattern evaluation also proceed in the higher hearing centers thanks to tonotopy.

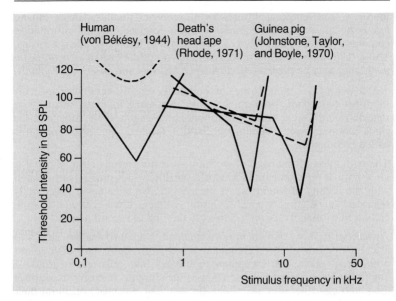

Fig. 1.**24** Comparison between the mechanical tuning curves of the basilar membrane (broken lines) and the corresponding tuning curves of individual nerve fibers (solid lines). The curves are recorded for the actual measured intensity area (from Keidel).

Pathophysiologic Basis of Hearing Disorders

Conductive or middle ear deafness is caused by lesions of the stimulus transport organ. A characteristic symptom of this type of hearing loss is that bone conduction functions better than the air conduction. The depression of the hearing threshold for air conduction is associated with an increase of acoustic impedance, e.g., as a result of stapes fixation due to otosclerosis.

Sensory deafness is caused by lesions in the stimulus transformation organ and/or in the auditory nerves and is therefore better known as *sensorineural deafness*.

Disorders of sound perception are caused by lesions in the subcortical or cortical auditory centers and by pathologic processes involving the central auditory pathway. As a result, the acoustic signals are falsely coded, stimulus patterns are wrongly analyzed, and acoustic information can no longer be integrated. The patient can then hear but not understand.

Central hearing disorders are characterized by a loss of integrative functions of the hearing centers. Differences in level of tone, differences in loudness, and temporal differences of acoustic stimulus pattern can no longer be analyzed. The *redundance* is also reduced, i.e., the information content is reduced due to loss of secondary and tertiary cochlear neurons. These disorders affect the understanding of *speech* (whereas *hearing for pure tones* may be preserved), *directional hearing,* and *speech intelligibility.*

Recruitment. In certain forms of unilateral sensorineural deafness, the loudness perception rises quickly with increasing loudness intensity so that despite different hearing thresholds both ears hear the tone with the same loudness once a certain threshold is reached. This phenomenon is called *recruitment.*

The pathophysiologic basis of recruitment is not entirely clear. Since it is an abnormal phenomenon of loudness sensitivity, it is probably associated with the coding of loudness. At present *positive recruitment* is generally regarded as a sign of a cochlear lesion, whereas *absent recruitment* indicates a retrocochlear lesion localized to the first or second neuron.

Hypothesis for the explanation of recruitment. Damaged sensory cells and afferent neurons of lower-frequency selectivity require very high sound pressure for excitation compared to healthy hair cells and neurons of higher-frequency selectivity. As soon as the stimulus intensity rises above the pathologically raised threshold, the number of sensory cells and their associated afferent neurons that are stimulated increases due to spread of the stimulus to neighboring neurons with a similar best frequency (the summation principle). Subjectively, this declares itself by a disproportionately rapid increase of sound sensitivity once the pathologically raised hearing threshold has been exceeded. Very loud sounds are uncomfortable for the deaf patient because he experiences distortion and even pain since the *dynamic hearing range* (i.e., the *difference* between the *threshold of hearing* and *that for pain*) is reduced (see pp. 48, 158, and Figs. 1.**25** and 1.**76a** and **b**).

Physiology of the Balance System

Balance is maintained by coordination of visual kinesthetic and vestibular regulatory mechanisms. These subserve *spatial orientation, upright posture,* and *gait:* control of all the static and motor muscle groups allows the body to counteract the influence of weight and centrifugal force (Fig. 1.**26**).

The main functions of the vestibular system are to:

1. *Provide information to the central nervous system* about the action of linear and angular acceleratory forces.
2. Coordinate function: movement is coordinated by continuous control of the tone of the skeletal muscles. Information from the vestibular sensory receptors is coordinated and integrated with information from the visual system. Spatial orientation is also subserved.

Fig. 1.**25**   Human auditory field. The sound pressure level (in decibels) and the loudness in phons are shown together in a coordinate system with the spectrum of human hearing in hertz. The abscissa shows frequencies, the ordinate decibels and phons. The isophons are curves of equal loudness. The curves for decibels and phons coincide only at 1,000 Hz, and deviate from each other above and below this frequency.

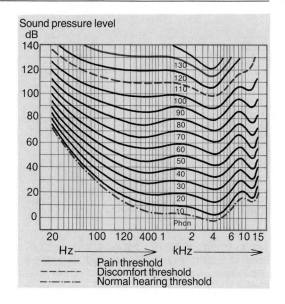

Fig. 1.**26**   Diagram illustrating the maintenance of balance. 1, visual information; 2, kinesthetic information from the superficial and deep receptors in the skin, muscles, tendon, and joints which react to pressure and traction forces caused by the force of gravity and inertia; 3, vestibular information from the semicircular canals and otolith apparatus.

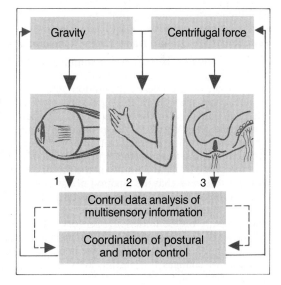

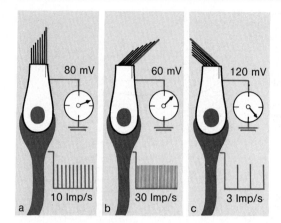

Fig. 1.**27a–c**   Diagram of the bioelectrical activity of the vestibular sensory cells at rest, and in response to stimulation (Jongkees). At rest **(a)**. Deflection of the sensory hair cells toward the kinocilium **(b)** causes depolarization and increase of the discharge frequency of the action potential. Bending in the opposite direction **(c)** causes hyperpolarization and inhibition of the resting activity (see Fig. 1.**14**).

The potential difference between the sensory cells and the extracellular fluid forms the *physiologic basis of the normal function of the vestibular sense organ*. A constant discharge of action potentials passes along the vestibular nerve fibers even if the end organs are at rest *(resting activity)*. Deflection of the sensory hair cells alters the resting activity by an increase of discharge frequency *(depolarization)* or by inhibition *(hyperpolarization)* (Fig. 1.**27a–c**). Modulation of resting activity thus enables the body to sense movement both in one direction and also in the opposite direction with the use of a single receptor.

Function of the Otolith Organ: Linear Acceleration Measurement

Linear acceleration is the sensory stimulus for the horizontally orientated macula of the utricle and the vertical macula of the saccule. Shearing forces occur during linear acceleration which shift the otoliths from their base, causing shearing of the hair cells (see Fig. 1.**11**) and providing an adequate stimulus for the sensory cells. The resulting neuronal impulses release the *maculoocular reflex* producing compensatory eye movements which ensure optimal static position of the eyes during linear movement. Furthermore, the *maculospinal reflex* is evoked, which influences the musculature of the trunk and limbs via the motor anterior horn cells in the spinal cord to ensure that the position of the body remains stable during linear movement. The otolith apparatus also fulfills the following important function: due to the continuous effect of gravity, the otoliths exert a constant pressure on the underlying sensory cells, even at rest. This pressure influences the resting activity of these mechanoreceptors. Linear acceleration, e.g., a fall, rapid lowering of the head, air travel, or fast movement in an elevator, changes this resting activity, thus guaranteeing continuous spatial orientation during vertical movement.

Fig. 1.**28**   Diagram of the vestibuloocular reflex. Angular acceleration from right to left (A) causes flow of the endolymph to the right because of the inertia of the inner ear fluid (B). Deflection of the cupula causes depolarization on the left side and hyperpolarization on the right.

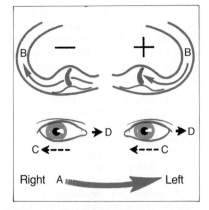

Increase of bioelectrical activity in the left vestibular sensory organ and the ipsilateral vestibular centers. Innervation of the left oculomotor nerve and the right abducens nerve via the medial longitudinal bundle (see Fig. 1.**19**). This induces a slow conjugated eye movement to the right in the direction opposite to the direction of rotation. This is the slow component of nystagmus (C).

Once maximal ocular deviation has been achieved there is a fast eye movement in the same direction as that of the rotation (D), i.e., the fast component of nystagmus. The eyes are thus returned to the neutral position. *The direction of nystagmus is always defined by that of the fast component.*

Function of the Semicircular Canals: Angular Acceleration Measurement

A positive or a negative angular acceleration causes endolymphatic movement within the semicircular canals lying in the plane of the centrifugal force. The stimulus always affects the semicircular canals of both sides: the cupula on one side is displaced toward the utricle *(ampullopetal stimulation)* and on the other side in the opposite direction *(ampullofugal stimulation)*. As a result, the resting activity of the semicircular canal whose cupula is deflected in an ampullopetal direction increases (depolarization effect), whereas the activity decreases in the opposite canal (hyperpolarization effect). This rule applies only to the horizontal canals since ampullofugal deflection causes depolarization in the vertical semicircular canals. This is the neurophysiologic basis for the stimulating mechanism of the *vestibuloocular reflex* (see Fig. 1.**15a–d** and Fig. 1.**28**).

The *vestibuloocular reflex* serves also for spatial orientation. It also assists in stabilizing the retinal image of the visual environment and induces vestibular nystagmus.

Note: The direction of the nystagmus is defined as that of the fast component.

Every movement of the head induces a slow conjugated movement of the eyes in the opposite direction to stabilize the field of vision on the retina for as long as possible during the movement. Two modifiable parameters determine the progress of the vestibuloocular reflex: the position of the head and the position of the eyes. The difference between these is the angle of vision. If the position of the head and of the eyes change at the same time but in the opposite direction and to the same degree, the angle of vision does not change and the field of vision remains focused sharply on the retina. In neurophysiologic terms, this is achieved by a two-fold integration:

1. Integration of the *acceleration indicators* in the cupula which indicates the speed of the head movement, which is transmitted to the vestibular centers. The latter form an important center for higher reflex coordination pathways. Vestibular information is collected, processed, and stored in these centers and is furthermore continually compared with visual and proprioceptive signals.
2. Integration of these *velocity signals* in the cerebellum and the reticular formation. This produces an equivalent velocity signal for the compensatory eye movements which determines their extent so that the movements of the eye parallel those of the head.

> *Note:* The vestibuloocular reflex coordinates the speed of the reflex eye movements (the slow component of nystagmus) to the speed of the head movement. In this way, clear visual control of the environment is ensured during movement. Fast return of the eyes is achieved by a reflex, the fast component of nystagmus.
> The conjugated eye movements due to the vestibuloocular reflex with typical slow and fast components is classified as vestibular nystagmus (see p. 63).

The intervertebral joints of the cervical spine and the deep muscles of the neck contain *mechanoreceptors* connected with the reticular formation by afferent fibers and from there to the vestibular and oculomotor centers. The *function* of these receptors is to provide continuous information about the position and movements of the head and to allow coordination of the eye movements by the *cervicoocular pathway.*

The *central vestibular system* embraces the cerebellum and the reticular formation of the brainstem, i.e., it is integrated in the *centers for multisensory data analysis.* This allows multisensory controlled coordination of posture, movement, and oculomotor functions.

Pathophysiologic Basis of Functional Vestibular Disorders

A vestibular disorder manifests itself by:

1. *Vertigo,* i.e., partial or complete loss of spatial orientation, e.g., an apparent movement of the environment as a result of spontaneous vestibular nystagmus (Fig. 1.**29a** and **b**) and/or
2. *A disturbance of balance,* with inability to maintain balance, to stand upright, or to walk properly (ataxia) (Fig. 1.**30**).

Vestibular disorders may be *peripheral,* caused by sudden unilateral failure of one labyrinth or by a unilateral lesion of the vestibular nerve. They may

Fig. 1.**29a** and **b** Diagram of production of apparent movement of the visual field during nystagmus and induction of rotatory dizziness. **a.** If the visual field moves on the retina with fixed gaze (Ax–xA') the environment appears to move in the direction of displacement of the visual field, as a result of displacement of the image on the retina in the opposite direction (A•x–xA'). **b.** If the visual field is stationary and the eyes move in conjugation (nystagmus), a subjective impression of

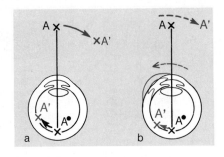

movement of the environment also occurs caused by displacement of the visual image on the retina (A'x–A¹). This is accompanied by a subjective sensation of rotatory vertigo in the same direction as the fast phase of the nystagmus (A–A').

Fig. 1.**30** Pathogenesis of disorders of orientation and balance. *Disorders of proprioceptive information:* loss of control over the ability to stand upright and walk straight causes a disorder of balance. *Disorders of visual information:* loss of the optical control of the visual field leads occasionally to *dizziness* due to discrepancy between the visual and vestibular information, causing disorientation. *Disorders of vestibular information* are due to involvement of spatial orientation and stabilization of the gaze axis leading to contradictory vestibular visual and kinesthetic information and *dizziness.* If central compensation of the loss of vestibular function is also absent there is an additional *disorder of balance* (see pp. 30–33).

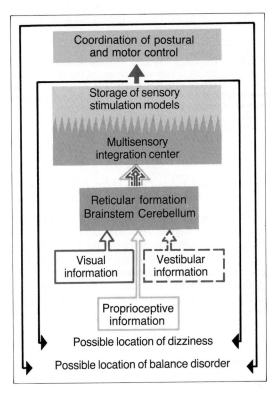

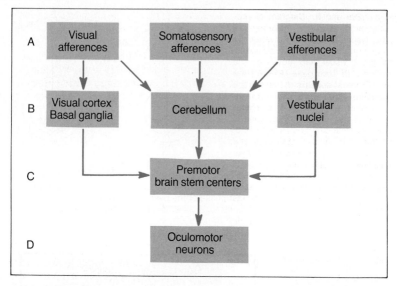

Fig. 1.**31** Oculomotor system. All three sensory systems **(A)** send their afferences via relay stations **(B)** in premotor centers of the reticular formation of the brain stem **(C)**. The motor neurons **(D)** which innervate the eye muscles begin at that point.

The cerebellum is the key to coordination: visual, somatosensory, and vestibular signals are continually compared with one another. If this structure receives contradictory information which could lead to disorientation and dizziness the vestibular signal is modified or, if necessary, completely suppressed.

also be *central,* caused by a lesion of the vestibular centers or their central connections to the cerebellum and reticular formation.

Every functional disturbance in a vestibular end organ causes an unequal activity in the higher vestibular centers. This central imbalance produces initially a disturbance of vestibular information. The multisensory spatial orientation can thus no longer function since vestibular information on the one hand, and visual somatosensory information on the other hand, contradict each other. This causes disturbance of orientation which in turn causes dizziness. If the central imbalance in the two vestibular centers influences the main neighboring coordination centers for eye movements in the reticular formation of the brainstem, spontaneous abnormal eye movements occur that have the characteristics of nystagmus (Fig. 1.**31**).

The direction of the sense of rotation is almost always the same as that of the fast phase of the nystagmus (see Fig. 1.**29a** and **b**).

Peripheral functional failure is compensated centrally by adjustment of the difference in neuronal activity in the vestibular centers and by substitution of visual and somatosensory regulatory mechanisms for the loss of peripheral vestibular function. This process is called *central vestibular compensation*. *Central vestibular disorders* are only incompletely compensated by the above mechanisms (or not at all) since the multisensory connections to the vestibular centers are damaged.

Methods of Investigation

Inspection, Palpation, Otoscopy, Microscopy

Inspection of the External Ear

The physician should look for redness, swelling, ulceration, tumors, malformations, fistula, or retroauricular scars.

Palpation

The mastoid process should be palpated with both hands, looking for swelling and for sensitivity to pressure of the surface of the mastoid process and its apex. The auricle is examined for pain on pressure on the tragus and pulling on the auricle. Finally, the regional lymph nodes in the pre- and postauricular areas and the upper deep cervical chain are examined.

Otoscopy

The external auditory meatus and the tympanic membrane are examined, and if a perforation is present the middle ear is also examined.

Indirect illumination with a head mirror is a difficult method of investigation for the nonspecialist since the correct adjustment of the light source and the head mirror require time and practice, especially when examining patients in bed (see Fig. 2.**14a–c**).

The electric *otoscope* is more widely used since it is easier to handle. It consists of a combination of a changeable *ear speculum* with a small but strong, built-in low-voltage *light source* and a *magnification attachment* providing a magnification of 1.5 to 2 (Fig. 1.**32a** and **b**). The specialist, however, will prefer to use the otomicroscope, which provides a magnification of 6 to 12× and is indispensable for an accurate examination of the tympanic membrane.

Technique of otoscopy. The cartilaginous part of the external meatus is stretched by pulling the auricle upward and backward. The speculum is then introduced into the long axis of the bony meatus; the instrument is held with the left hand so that the right hand remains free for handling instruments such as cotton wool probes, hooks, an aspirator, and aural forceps (Fig. 1.**33**).

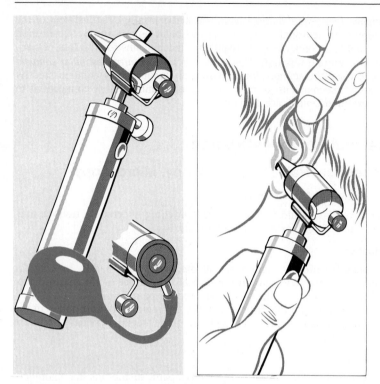

Fig. 1.**32 a.**   Otoscope with a pneumatic Siegle's speculum and Bruening's loupe.
b. Correct position of the otoscope during examination of the ear.

The speculum must be introduced carefully, and its end should not be moved abruptly since its opening has relatively sharp edges. The wall of the bony meatus is particularly sensitive and easy to injure, and contact with it should therefore be avoided. The speculum must not be pushed in and out unnecessarily.

In *infants* and *young children,* the auricle is pulled downward and backward to allow the speculum to be introduced. The short cartilaginous part of the external meatus is reduced to a cleft and will only admit a narrow speculum whose small lumen makes otoscopy difficult. The head must be fixed, either by an assistant or by a headrest on the patient's chair, to prevent unnecessary movements which can cause pain.

Wax and other material hindering the view in the external auditory meatus must be removed:

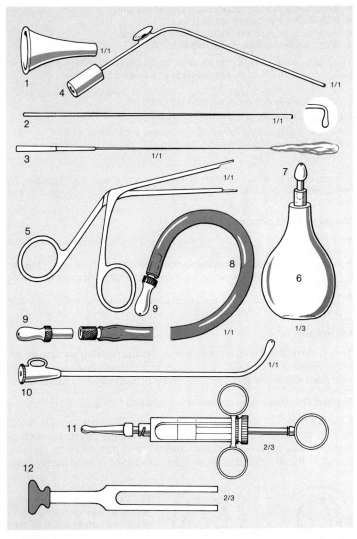

Fig. 1.**33** Important ear instruments. 1, Speculum; 2, hook; 3, cotton applicator; 4, aural aspirator with valve; 5, aural forceps; 6, Politzer balloon with metal olive; 7, olive; 8, hearing tube with changeable metal earpieces; 9, earpiece; 10, eustachian catheter; 11, irrigation syringe with bayonet closure; 12, tuning fork $A_1 = 440$ Hz or $c' = 512$ Hz.

- By syringing for foreign bodies, wax, and exudate
- With the hook or curette for hard wax
- With the aural aspirator for exudate or fluid wax
- With a cotton wool probe for exudate

The ear is *syringed* with tap water at body temperature. Hard wax is softened beforehand with 3% hydrogen peroxide or a commercial preparation.

Note: Syringing the ear is contraindicated in

- Dry perforations of the tympanic membrane
- Fresh injuries of the tympanic membrane and meatus
- Longitudinal and transverse fractures of the petrous pyramid with meatal trauma

It is important to obtain a history of previous perforation since syringing may rupture a thin scar. Failure to take a history in the U.S. today will result in a malpractice suit.

Mistakes to be avoided:

- A speculum that is too narrow and that penetrates too deeply into the sensitive bony meatus
- Introducing the speculum in the wrong direction, e.g., from above downward
- Not introducing the speculum far enough causing its opening to be blocked by otic hairs
- Unsatisfactory cleaning of the external meatus so that a proper view of the tympanic membrane is not obtained

Microscopy

This is carried out with a speculum under the operating microscope with a magnification of 6 to 40x in all cases in which routine otoscopic examination does not allow reliable assessment of the tympanic membrane.

Normal Otoscopic Appearance (Fig. 1.**34** and Color Plate **5c**)

Characteristics of the tympanic membrane. The pars tensa is the color of mother-of-pearl, i.e., greyish-yellow. The cutis layer is often slightly injected. The surface is smooth and without any relieving features apart from the handle of the malleus. The membrane is moderately translucent

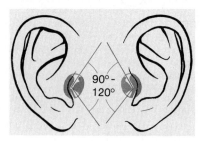

Fig. 1.**34** Only a small anteroinferior triangular part of the tympanic membrane lies perpendicular to the axis of the meatus due to the oblique position and funnel shape of the tympanic membrane. The incident light beam thus causes a triangular light reflex on the membrane. The reflex disappears or is broken up if the tympanic membrane is retracted.

but is only transparent in scarred areas. A tympanic membrane showing the properties described above is described as *normal.*

The *mobility of the tympanic membrane* is tested by a *Siegle's or Bruening's pneumatic otoscope* (see Fig. 1.**32a** and **b**).

The tympanic membrane is moved back and forth with positive and negative pressure while it is in the field of vision. Atrophic parts flutter, and the movement of the pars tensa may be limited by scar tissue. In the presence of a perforation, the remnants of the tympanic membrane are completely immobile.

Appearance of the Pathologic Tympanic Membrane
(Color Plates **5c, 6a−d, 7a−d, 8b−d, 9a, b and d**)

1. *Injection of the vessels and inflammation* are seen in otitis externa (occasionally), myringitis, and otitis media.
2. *Hemorrhage is red if fresh or brownish if old.* Blood vesicles are seen in influenzal otitis, and the hemotympanum is dark blue.
3. *Serous exudate.* A fluid level can be seen and there are air bubbles in the fluid. The tympanic membrane looks like oiled silk when there is a complete middle ear effusion. A blue tympanic membrane or "blue drum" is seen in advanced stages (see p. 85).
4. *Retraction of the tympanic membrane as a result of decreased pressure in the middle ear.* The short process of the malleus protrudes externally, and there is displacement of the manubrium of the malleus posteriorly and superiorly causing an apparent shortening of the malleus handle. The triangular light reflex is fragmented or disappears entirely.
5. *Bulging due to formation of exudate* behind the tympanic membrane, at times an irregular surface, which may be papillary with opacity of the surface.
6. *Atrophy of the tympanic membrane* with retraction pockets results from chronic inflammation and reduced pressure. The site of predilection is the posterosuperior quadrant.
7. *Thickening of the tympanic membrane* as a result of degenerative changes or as the result of inflammation results in a surface that is dark and lacking in luster.
8. *Scars of the tympanic membrane.* These may be thickened areas with or without calcium deposits or atrophic areas.
9. *Tympanic membrane perforations.* These may be either central or peripheral, meso- or epitympanic. Central or mesotympanic defects are the result of chronic mucosal inflammation (see p. 94), whereas peripheral or epitympanic perforations are usually associated with a cholesteatoma (p. 96).

Note: A tympanic membrane whose surface appears to be opaque and dull as a result of inflammatory infiltration of the pars tensa with hyperemia, edema, formation of bullae, and desquamation of the epidermal layer and distortion of the characteristic appearance of the handle of the malleus is designated as abnormal or pathologic.

Radiography

Because of the anatomic position of the temporal bone, it is overlapped by numerous other bony structures of the skull on the standard views. Therefore, the following special views must be taken for radiologic assessment of the temporal bone:

Schueller's View (Fig. 1.35a and b):

The cassette is placed on the diseased ear, and the beam is displaced 30° superiorly to avoid other superimposed bony structures. This demonstrates the pneumatic system especially of the mastoid process, the antrum, the squamous temporal bone, the sigmoid sinus, the mastoid emissary foramen, and the temporomandibular joint. Fracture lines are also shown if present.

The criteria to be assessed include the extent of pneumatization, the air content of the cells, and the structure of the intercellular septa, the sigmoid sinus, and the tegmen tympani.

Indications include disease of the middle ear such as mastoiditis, cholesteatoma, and longitudinal fracture of the petrous pyramid.

Stenvers' View (Fig. 1.36a–c):

The patient lies with the external border of the orbit of the diseased side at an angle of 45° to the cassette. The beam is displaced 10° superiorly.

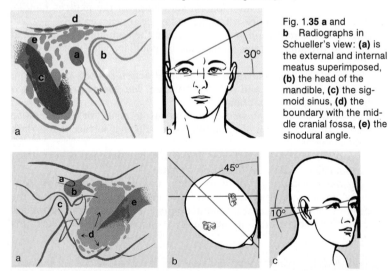

Fig. 1.**35 a** and **b** Radiographs in Schueller's view: **(a)** is the external and internal meatus superimposed, **(b)** the head of the mandible, **(c)** the sigmoid sinus, **(d)** the boundary with the middle cranial fossa, **(e)** the sinodural angle.

Fig. 1.**36a–c** Radiographs in Stenver's view. **a**, internal auditory meatus; **b**, vestibule with superior and horizontal semicircular canals; **c**, mandibular condyle; **d**, pneumatic system; **e**, sigmoid sinus.

This view demonstrates the apex of the petrous pyramid, the labyrinth, the internal auditory meatus, and the borders of the petrous pyramid.

The criteria to be assessed include the width of the internal auditory meatus, the bony structure of the labyrinthine capsule, the semicircular canals, the apex of the petrous bone, the surfaces of the petrous pyramid, and breaks in their contours due to fractures.

Indications include disease of the internal ear and the petrous pyramid, cerebellopontine angle tumors, acoustic neuromas, transverse fractures of the petrous pyramid, infection of the petrous pyramid, and occult cholesteatoma with invasion of the labyrinth and labyrinthitis.

Special views of the temporal bones such as those described by *Mayer, Chausseé, Guillen,* and others have now been largely replaced by tomography. *Tomograms* in the projections described by *Stenvers, Schueller, Towne,* and *Altschul-Uffenorder* are indicated for the *assessment of subtle changes* in the bony structures of the temporal bone. In addition to axial tomography to assess the skull base, the following supplementary *neuroradiologic investigations* are indicated for suspected neoplasms or space-occupying lesions of the middle or posterior cranial fossa:

- *Computed tomography:*

    The CT scan is a tomographic examination in which individual measurements of the intensity of the X-ray beam made through a fine screen are analyzed by a computer and reconstituted in one view. This modality not only demonstrates bony and calcified structures of the skull but can also define the soft-tissue elements of intracranial lesions by means of intravenous contrast enhancement.

- *Carotid angiography*
- *Vertebral angiography*
- *Magnetic resonance imaging (MRI)*

    Magnetic resonance imaging (MRI) differs from the currently available radiologic methods in the following way. In *classical radiology,* a part of the body, which is of course three-dimensional, is represented in a flat plane, or more accurately, the density distribution is projected on one plane transposed into shades of grey and reproduced as an image. The density distribution correlates well with the anatomic contours and the structure of the organs. *Computed tomography* produces a considerable improvement of soft tissue contrast in one layer. *MRI* improves the capability of tissue differentiation in the image and provides additional information about consistency and biochemical relationships.

Principle. A MRI signal is produced in the atomic nuclei of the tissues by an *electromagnetic high-frequency alternating field.* This produces information about the spin density, i. e., the inherent rotation of an electrically charged proton. Indirect information is thus provided about the *proton density,* i. e., the presence of hydrogen in the appropriate tissue. The MRI signal is measured point-by-point so that the coordinates in different projections within the tissue layers are plotted by a computer. The MRI apparatus is therefore in principle a computer-assisted *nuclear resonance spectrometer.* It is a noninvasive study that does not involve the use of ionizing radiation and has no known adverse biologic side effects.

Compared to radiology and ultrasound, MRI provides a higher-contrast image of the soft tissue structures. Views may be taken in all three planes without secondary reconstruction using a computer and without special positioning of the patient. Secondary effects due to the electromagnetic field have not yet been recorded. Normal tissues may be differentiated from pathologic tissues by the use of a contrast medium.

Functional Assessment of the Eustachian Tube

Tests of tubal function are always necessary in all patients with middle ear deafness, particularly before an operation to improve the hearing.

Qualitative Assessment of Tubal Function

Valsalva's test. The *principle* of this test is the demonstration of the normal tubal patency without external aids. Failure of this test does not prove pathologic occlusion of the tube, but further functional tests may be required.

After taking a deep breath, the patient pinches his nose and closes his mouth in an attempt to blow air into his ears.

Otoscopy shows bulging of the tympanic membrane, and auscultation reveals crackling.

Note: Inflation of air in patients with infection of the nose and nasopharynx carries the danger of transmission of infected secretions to the middle ear causing a tubogenic otitis media. In a patient with an atrophic scar of the pars tensa, there is also the possibility of rupture of the tympanic membrane, especially during air insufflation or catheterization of the tube.

Toynbee's test. The *principle* of this test is confirmation of the normal tubal air patency using a simple and safe method.

During swallowing the pressure in the middle ear falls if the nose is closed off. This can be seen by otoscopy as indrawing of the tympanic membrane and can be confirmed by auscultation using a tube to transmit the noise which occurs during this maneuver.

Politzer's test. The *principle* of this test is the physiologic process by which increased air pressure in the nasopharynx when the soft palate is elevated causes opening of the tube and increased pressure in the middle ear.

The doctor occludes one of the patient's nasal cavities with the olive of a rubber balloon and pinches the other nostril tightly. The patient elevates the palate actively by swallowing or saying "Kay, Kay, Kay." At the same time the air pressure in the closed nasal cavity is increased by compression of the Politzer balloon. The doctor can hear the rush of air into the middle ear by auscultation using a tube and can assess the degree of tubal patency from the noise produced. Optical assessment can also be used.

Tubal catheterization. The *principle* of this procedure is to introduce the end of a silver catheter angled 45° to 90° in the lower part of the nasal cavity into the pharyngeal tubal opening and to blow air into the tube with a rubber balloon. The noise produced by the influx of air is assessed through a tube.

The following complications may occur:

- Tubal otitis media due to transmitted organisms
- Rupture of an atrophic scar of the tympanic membrane
- Nasal bleeding arising from damage to the mucosa
- Submucosal surgical emphysema of the nasopharynx
- Damage to the tubal ostium

Quantitative Measures of Tubal Function

These include manometry, electroacoustic recording of tubal patency, sonomanometry, impedance audiometry, and tympanometry (see p. 50).

Audiometry

Testing the Hearing Without an Audiometer

This requires a quiet room of sufficient size (6 m long) since noise and poor acoustic properties such as a narrow room with smooth walls produce echoes which falsify the results.

Each ear is tested separately, the better ear being tested first. The opposite ear is masked by a moist plug of cotton wool pushed into the external auditory meatus with the index finger and moved in and out (Wagener's *vibration method of masking*).

The *hearing threshold for whispered voice* and *conversational speech* is determined as follows:

Two-syllable words are articulated at a decreasing distance from the patient until these test words can be correctly repeated. The distance is recorded in meters. When assessing severe unilateral deafness, and also when determining the *hearing distance for conversational speech,* vibration masking of the opposite ear is often not sufficient so that the *noise box* must be used. Two-syllable words are again used for the test.

Tuning fork tests. A C^1 fork with a frequency of 512 Hz is used:

Weber's test. The *principle* of this test rests on binaural comparison of bone conduction. The tuning fork is placed in the center of the skull at the hairline. The patient with normal hearing or with a symmetrical hearing loss localizes the tone either in the center of the head or equally in both ears. The patient with a unilateral conductive hearing loss (middle ear) localizes the tone in the diseased ear, whereas the patient with a unilateral inner ear deafness localizes the sound in the healthy ear.

This phenomenon rests on two factors: First, in middle ear disorders the mobility of the ossicular chain is reduced and it thus transmits less sound energy than under normal physiologic circumstances (Mach's sound wastage theory). Second, pathologic processes in the middle ear cause an increase in the mass of the sound conduction apparatus so that increased forces are caused at the oval window as a result of the inertia. This leads to greater stimulation of the inner ear (inertia theory).

Rinne's test. The *principle* of this test rests on monaural comparison of air to bone conduction.

If air conduction is better than bone conduction, *Rinne's test is positive*. This is the finding in normal hearing or sensorineural deafness (inner ear).

If bone conduction is better than air conduction, *Rinne's test is negative*. This is found in conductive or middle ear deafness.

The patient is asked whether the tuning fork placed in front of the ear is heard better than when it is placed behind the ear upon the mastoid process without striking it again. If the patient cannot decide with certainty, the decay period of the tuning fork is determined exactly for both air and bone conduction separately.

Schwabach's test depends on comparison of the bone conduction of the patient with that of the examiner, but is now seldom carried out since an audiogram is always obtained if inner ear deafness is suspected.

Gellé's test. The tuning fork is placed in the same position as for Weber's test. The external auditory meatus is compressed by a Politzer balloon. Excess pressure in the external auditory meatus produces stiffening of the ossicular chain and this reduces both air *and* bone conduction. Under the influence of increased pressure, the sound of the tuning fork fades as stiffening of the ossicular chain increases. In fixation of the footplate due to otosclerosis (see p. 114), the loudness of the tuning fork does not change (Gellé-negative) in contrast to the result in sensorineural deafness with a mobile footplate (Gellé-positive).

> *Note:* The determination of the hearing distance for whispered and conversational speech and tuning fork tests provide valuable information about the site of a hearing disorder. They remain the basic diagnostic methods of otologic examination (Table 1.1).

Audiometry

Fundamental Physical and Acoustic Concepts
(Tables 1.2 through 1.7)

Pure-Tone Audiometry

An *audiometer* is an electric tone generator used to determine the hearing threshold for pure tones, i.e., tones free of harmonics within a frequency range from 125 to 12,000 Hz.

The *hearing threshold* is measured for both air and bone conduction in decibel steps. The *normal hearing threshold* is indicated by a straight line of

Table 1.1 Evaluation of the Results of Clinical Hearing Tests.			
Test			
Test	Discrepancy Between Hearing Distance for Whispered and Conversational Speech	Lateralization test of Weber	Rinne test
Normal subject	None	Midline	Positive
Conductive deafness	Usually small	To the worse-hearing ear in unilateral deafness	Negative or equivocal
Sensorineural deafness	Usually large	To the better-hearing ear in unilateral deafness	Positive
Degree of deafness: Feldmann's classification:	Feldmann's classification hearing distance for conversational speech: Slight (>4m) Medium (<4m >1m) Severe (<1m–25cm) Almost total deafness (<25cm)	Luescher's classification of hearing for whispered speech: >4m <6m <4m >1m <1m Hearing is lost for conversational speech tested in a quiet room.	

0 dB. Hearing loss is measured in decibels relative to this threshold for all frequencies and is recorded on an audiograph (Fig. 1.**37a** and **b**).

The decibel (dB) is a *relative value* which compares one sound pressure to another. The reference point in audiometry is the human hearing threshold for 1,000 Hz. The sound pressure necessary to produce the subjective impression of hearing at a threshold of 1,000 Hz is 20 μPa (2×10^{-4} μbar) (see Table 1.**3**).

This is the average value for young subjects with normal hearing and is the reference point for the *physical* or *absolute* measurement of the *hearing threshold* in decibels [sound pressure level (SPL)]. The *relative hearing threshold* for pure tones is

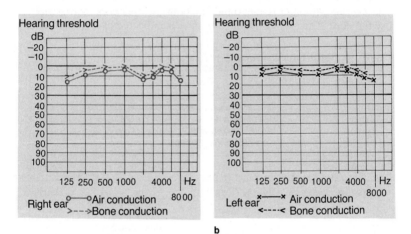

Fig. 1.**37a** and **b**   Diagram of a normal pure-tone audiogram.

Table 1.**2** Properties of Sound
Sound: A molecular vibration of an elastic medium propagated as a waveform (in air, water, bone, etc).
Speed of sound: 340 m/s in air, 1400 m/s in water
Sound pressure (P): This is the predominant change of pressure in a sound field. It is a function of time at any particular point. It is expressed in *pascals*.
Mass units: The old-fashioned unit was the microbar (μb), i.e., dynes/cm² The present unit of absolute sound pressure is the pascal (Pa) measured as newtons/m². 0.1 Pa = 1 μb.

Table 1.3 Hearing or Dynamic Range and Sound Pressure Level

Hearing range:

The lower limit,
which refers to the *hearing threshold* at 1 000 Hz,
is 20 μPa, previously 2×10^{-4} μb.

The upper limit
or pain threshold
is 20 Pa, previously 2×10^{2} μb.

Sound pressure level (SPL):

The *unit* is the decibel, logarithmic unit calculated as follows:

$$dB = 10 \log \frac{\text{Sound pressure I}}{\text{Reference sound pressure I}_o}$$

$$dB = 20 \log \frac{P}{P_o} = \frac{\text{Measure sound pressure}}{\text{Reference sound pressure}}$$

a simpler method for the demonstration and description of the hearing threshold. The reference point is no longer the absolute sound pressure but the just-audible threshold of hearing measured in dB [hearing level (HL)].

This allows the use of a coordinate system with a horizontal zero line. The *absolute hearing threshold* is curved compared to the *relative hearing threshold*. The reason for this is that a greater sound pressure is needed at high and low tones to produce a similar sensation of sound near the threshold than for the central part of the frequency range around 1,000 Hz (see Fig. 1.**25**).

A disorder of sound conduction may be ascertained by the difference between the hearing threshold for air and bone conduction, in a manner similar to the tuning fork tests.

Relationship Between Air Conduction and Bone Conduction

The normal conduction of sound to the inner ear via the sound-conducting apparatus is defined as *air conduction* (conduction via earphones). Sound is also conducted via the bones of the skull to the inner ear, either via the middle ear (*osteo- or craniotympanic bone conduction)* or by direct transmission via the labyrinthine capsule *(osteal or cranial bone conduction)* (conduction via vibrator).

Note: The audiometric characteristic of a conductive or middle ear deafness is that the threshold for air conduction is worse than that for bone conduction, producing an air-bone gap.

A conductive deafness results from an increase in impedance (Fig. 1.**38**). If the *elastic recoil* due to the air in the middle ear and mastoid process increases, the mobility in the middle and low tones decreases, at constant mass and tension. The resonance

Table 1.4 Hearing Range and Decibel dB Scale*		
Sound Source	Ratio of Intensity	dB
Jet engine	$1:10^{13}$	130
Riveting hammer	$1:10^{12}$	120
Drilling machine	$1:10^{11}$	110
Printing machine	$1:10^{10}$	100
Weaving machine	$1:10^{9}$	90
Machine workshop	$1:10^{8}$	80
Street traffic	$1:10^{7}$	70
Normal speech	$1:10^{6}$	60
Soft radio music	$1:10^{5}$	50
Soft speech	$1:10^{4}$	40
Whispering	$1:10^{3}$	30
Quiet livingroom	$1:10^{2}$	20
Rustling of leaves	$1:10$	10
Hearing threshold	$1:10^{0}$	0

* From Luepke.

Table 1.5 Sound Intensity, Sound Volume and Loudness

Scale of sound intensity

This is a physically defined decibel scale based on the square *amplitude value* of tones and not on subjective assessment of the loudness of the tone.

Volume of loudness level

is measured in phons which is a logarithmic unit. The tone is compared subjectively with a reference sound of 1 000 Hz. The sound pressure level (SPL) of the reference tone is adjusted so that the test tone and reference tone sound equally loud. The result in decibels SPL is expressed in phons. A sound of 50-phon loudness level produces the same sensation of loudness as a reference tone at 1 000 Hz at an SPL of 50 dB SPL.

Loudness

The unit is the sone which is a linear scale depending on subjective comparison to a determined value. The loudness of a test tone is compared with that of a reference tone of 1 000 Hz and a 40-dB SPL.

Isophon curves

(see Fig. 1.25) consist of curves of the same *loudness level* measured in phons but at different *frequencies* (in Hertz) and SPL (decibels).

Hearing range

is between the hearing threshold at 4 phons and the threshold of pain at 130 phons (see Fig. 1.25)

Table 1.6 Tone, Timbre, Noise

Tone	is a pure sinusoidal vibration in the audible range characterized by
Frequency,	which is vibrations per second, i. e., in Hertz.
Timbre:	a sound contains overtones in addition to the basic tone which determine the subjective *color* of the sound.
Noise:	sound whose pressure in the sound field is not a periodic function of time.
White noise	consists of equal components of all the audible frequencies from 18 to 20,000 Hz.
Loud noise	may be distressing or cause actual damage.

Table 1.7 Impedance

Acoustic impedance is resistance to the flow of sound pressure waves through a medium, proportional to:

- The mass of the vibrating system
- Its resistance
- Its restoring force

Resistance	is the frictional resistance in the joints, ligaments, and muscles of the sound-conducting apparatus.
Reactance	is an imaginary component determined by the stiffness and mass of the system.
Compliance	is the flexibility of the tympanic membrane.

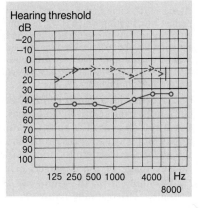

Fig. **1.38** Diagram of a pure-tone audiogram in a patient with a right-sided conductive deafness due to otosclerosis. The values for bone conduction are normal, but the hearing threshold for air conduction is depressed (35 to 50 dB).

point of the middle ear is displaced to the upper frequencies. A conductive deafness is characterized by a greater loss of hearing for air conduction in the lower frequencies, as seen, e.g., in ossification of the stapes anulus in *otosclerosis*. The conduction system is increasingly damped by the increase of *mass and tension,* and the resonance point of the middle ear is thus displaced into the lower tones. A hearing loss results which is greater for air conduction in the middle and higher tones, as occurs, e.g., in *glue ear exudate* in the middle ear and *impacted wax.*

A conductive deafness *in*dependent of frequency is caused by simultaneous elastic stiffening and dampening of the sound conduction apparatus. This may occur in advanced *otosclerosis,* in *middle ear cholesteatoma* with destruction of the ossicular chain, in *tympanosclerosis,* and in *congenital anomalies.* A flat air conduction curve is found in such cases.

Note: The bone conduction threshold curve is an expression of the function of the inner ear and to a limited extent of its central connections.

This rule applies with a few insignificant exceptions, e.g., bony closure of one or both windows. The audiometric characteristic of all forms of sensorineural deafness (inner ear and retrocochlear deafness) is that the thresholds for air and bone conduction coincide (see Figs. 1.**68**, 1.**69**, 1.**73**, and 1.**74**). Supplementary *suprathreshold tests* must be carried out to differentiate inner ear deafness from retrocochlear deafness.

Demonstration of Recruitment

The following tests are used:

- Fowler's test
- Luescher's test
- Short increment sensitivity index (SISI) test

Fowler's Test: This test is based on a subjective comparison of loudness between the right and left ear.

A tone of the same frequency and loudness is presented alternately to both ears of a patient with hearing which is worse in one side than the other. Because of the differences in hearing threshold between the healthy and diseased side, the loudness of the sound is unequal between the two sides. This difference disappears as the loudness of the test tone increases and appears to be *equally loud.* This phenomenon is described as *recruitment* (the pathophysiologic basis is described on p. 26). Fowler's test is shown in Figure 1.**39**.

The patient with an *inner ear deafness* showing recruitment often has difficulty in hearing relatively soft tones. In contrast, he hears loud conversational speech as well as subjects with normal hearing. Excessive loudness upsets him because of distortion and painful sensations as the *threshold of discomfort* is exceeded. In inner ear deafness, recruitment occurs in the frequency range of the damaged hair cells, which require a considerably higher sound pressure compared to the normal hair cells to produce a response. The resulting reduction of the dynamic hearing range has very

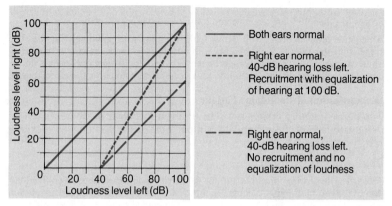

Fig. 1.**39** Fowler's loudness balance test on a patient with unilateral left-sided sensorineural deafness, with a 40 dB loss at 1,000 Hz.

deleterious effects so far as hearing of speech is concerned (see Fig. 1.**25** and pp. 155 ff.).

> *Note:* The demonstration of the recruitment phenomenon is currently accepted as indicating an inner ear or hair cell lesion, whereas this phenomenon is usually absent in retrocochlear neural hearing loss due, e.g., to an acoustic neuroma.

The *suprathreshold tests* in current use include the following:
Tone intensity-difference threshold as described by Luescher. This may also be used for bilateral symmetrical sensorineural deafness.

Principle. The ability to recognize small differences in intensity of a continuous tone *(amplitude increase)* depends on the signal strength, in subjects with normal hearing. At the threshold of normal hearing an increase of about 3.5 dB is necessary for a difference to be audible, but at 80 dB it is only about 0.35 dB. In a patient with recruitment, the subjective increase of loudness per decibel of increase in intensity, and the response to the difference in intensity, is considerably greater than in a normal subject. Recruitment is tested for by assessing whether amplitude increases in the deaf ear are recognized as well as in the good ear with sounds of increasing loudness. The threshold of intensity difference in decibels at the same distance above the hearing threshold is smaller in a diseased ear with recruitment than in the normal ear. However, it is greater in conductive or retrocochlear deafness in which recruitment is absent.

SISI test as described by Jerger:

A test tone is offered 20 dB above the patient's threshold and is increased by 1 dB every 5 s with a duration of 0.2 s. Twenty impulses are offered per test.

The results are expressed as a percentage so that 20% correct responses score 100%. Scores less than 20% are negative and those over 80% are positive.

A negative result is obtained in retrocochlear lesions with pathologic fatigue. The score is greater than 80% in patients with cochlear deafness showing recruitment. There is a large intermediate zone between 20% and 80% where the result is uncertain. The localizing diagnostic ability of this suprathreshold test is therefore limited.

Demonstration of Pathologic Fatigue

Pathologic auditory fatigue is a sign of a retrocochlear deafness. It can be demonstrated by the technically simple *tone decay test* and by *Békésy's test*.

Tone decay test (Carhart):

Principle. The hearing threshold and the sensitivity to loudness depend on the duration of the sound stimulus. Changes in threshold and loudness are called adaptation and auditory fatigue. Both parameters may influence the results of threshold audiometry and the measurement of recruitment. In the *tone decay test*, the increase of the hearing threshold due to pathologic fatigue in response to a continuous tone lasting 1 min is recorded.

Békésy audiometry:

Fatigueability of an ear is determined by measurement of the hearing threshold during exhibition of a continuous tone. Usually this produces a constant hearing threshold, but in pathologic fatigue the hearing threshold increases.

Nowadays, both methods have been largely replaced by electric response audiometry (ERA) (see p. 57) which allows considerably more accurate diagnosis of a retrocochlear hearing disorder.

Impedance Audiometry

This technique forms part of the functional diagnosis of the sound conduction apparatus. It includes the following two methods of investigation:

Tympanometry. This is the recording of the impedance (see p. 21) or an indirect measurement of the pressure in the middle ear when the tympanic membrane is intact, by means of pressure in the external meatus. This is an indirect test of tubal function.

Measurement of the stapedius reflex. The change in impedance caused by the acoustic stapedius reflex is measured.

Technique. The external auditory meatus is closed by an airtight plug through which pass three tubes. One tube carries the test tone; the second is connected to the pressure regulator which allows positive or negative pressure (± 400 mm H_2O) to be produced in the external auditory meatus. A microphone is connected to the third tube allowing measurement of the sound pressure of the test tone reflected from the tympanic membrane as the impedance changes.

Tympanometry. Normally, there is no pressure differential between the two sides of the tympanic membrane so that the acoustic resistance of the tympanic membrane

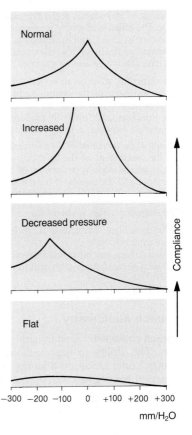

Fig. 1.**40** Summary of the four most important types of tympanogram (Lehnhardt). The curve shows the compliance of the tympanic membrane to changes in pressure of the external canal. *Normal:* the apex of the curve (mm H_2O) lies near to 0 on the pressure scale when the pressure in the meatus and the middle ear are equal. *Increased compliance:* if the tympanic membrane is abnormally compliant, e.g., due to atrophic scars of the pars tensa or interruption of the ossicular chain, the compliance is abnormally large and the apex of the curve appears to be abnormally high. *Decreased pressure in the middle ear:* the apex of the curve is displaced into the negative region below 100 mm H_2O. *Middle ear effusion:* a compliance peak can no longer be measured and the tympanogram appears to be flat if the tympanic membrane is damped due to a seromucinous exudate in the middle ear.

is minimal. A recording of the impedance of the tympanic membrane during a change in pressure in the external auditory meatus allows the pressure difference on the two sides of the tympanic membrane to be determined by measurement of its compliance. The greater the pressure differential, the greater is the impedance of the tympanic membrane. A recording of the impedance at pressures from –300 mm H_2O to +300 mm H_2O produces a curve with a peak at zero for a normally mobile tympanic membrane. It represents the maximal flexibility, i.e., compliance, of the tympanic membrane and thus minimal impedance. The apex of this curve is lower if the tympanic membrane is stiffened by scar tissue or damped by exudate in the middle ear. It becomes higher with increasing compliance due to atrophic scars of the pars tensa (Fig. 1.**40**).

Stapedius reflex. The *principle* of this test is that a sound stimulus greater than 70 dB above threshold induces a reflex concentration of the stapedius muscle. This causes a change of impedance at the tympanic membrane which can be recorded graphically. The effect is absent in immobility of the tympanic membrane, in disruption of the ossicular chain, and in fixation of the stapes in the oval window by otosclerosis. In simulated deafness this reflex is activated by loudness approaching the norm. In this case simulation can be assumed.

The stapedius reflex is an acousticofacial reflex. The afferent limb is the auditory nerve and parts of the central auditory pathway up to the auditory centers. The efferent limb is formed by the connections between the auditory centers and the facial nucleus, and finally by the facial nerve. Measurement of the stapedius reflex is therefore very useful in topical diagnosis of a facial paralysis.

Testing of the threshold of the stapedius reflex is of considerable diagnostic importance for the assessment of the following disorders of hearing: otosclerosis, recruitment (Metz recruitment is reduction of the difference between an elevated hearing threshold and the threshold for the stapedius reflex with increasing hearing loss for the high tones), retrocochlear deafness, and brain stem lesions.

The stapedius reflex is absent in:

- Retrocochlear sensorineural deafness as a result of auditory fatigue, i.e., in acoustic neuroma
- Otosclerosis and other middle ear diseases
- Facial nerve damage proximal to the point at which the stapedius nerve is given off
- Brainstem lesions with damage to the central reflex arc

Speech Audiometry

Speech audiometry is an integral part of audiometric methods of investigation. The ability to hear and understand speech is more important in human communication than the ability to hear pure tones. Speech audiometry therefore has both diagnostic and therapeutic significance.

The loudness of speech is perceived as an acoustic image whose frequency extends from 100 to 8,000 Hz. The *hearing loss for speech* is determined using two-syllable test words, and the *maximal discrimination* using one-syllable test words is also measured (see Fig. 1.**76a**; p. 159).

Speech audiometry is not carried out in the same way as the testing of the spoken voice (see p. 41), i.e., with an increasing distance between the patient and the sound source, but rather by varying the loudness strength measured in decibels, i.e., a *speech sound level* above 20 μPa (see p. 44, Table 1.**2**).

The speech or test material is recorded on a tape and is presented to the subject either by means of earphones or in a free field using a loudspeaker with varying loudness levels. The percentage of numbers, words, or sentences understood correctly at each loudness level is then assessed.

The dependence of comprehension of speech on the loudness level is tested by speech audiometry. In the standardized *Freiburg speech test* (DIN 45621) multisyllable numbers are first used. This allows a rapid rough estimate of the hearing loss.

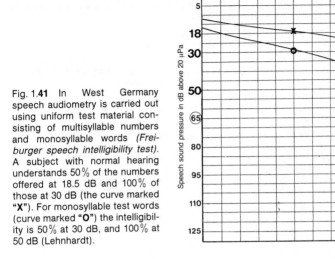

Fig. 1.**41** In West Germany speech audiometry is carried out using uniform test material consisting of multisyllable numbers and monosyllable words *(Freiburger speech intelligibility test)*. A subject with normal hearing understands 50% of the numbers offered at 18.5 dB and 100% of those at 30 dB (the curve marked **"X"**). For monosyllable test words (curve marked **"O"**) the intelligibility is 50% at 30 dB, and 100% at 50 dB (Lehnhardt).

A subject with normal hearing understands 50% of numbers presented at 18.5 dB. This normal value forms the basis of the hearing loss for numbers (Fig. 1.**41**). In addition, the ability of the subject to *comprehend monosyllable words* is tested. These words are considerably more difficult to understand than multisyllable numbers. The *purpose of this monosyllable test* is to assess a percentage comprehension and to ultimately achieve 100% comprehension values if possible by increasing the loudness level. The normal subject hears 100% of monosyllables at 65 dB, and in favorable circumstances at 50 dB, whereas 100% speech comprehension cannot be achieved even in normal subjects at a sound pressure level of less than 50 dB (Fig. 1.**42**).

Speech audiometry enables quantitative measurement of hearing. Determination of the *percentage hearing loss for speech comprehension* is achieved by ascertaining *the total word comprehension,* and determination of the *hearing loss for speech* is assessed from the speech audiogram (Fig. 1.**42**). The percentage comprehension values for monosyllables at 60, 80, and 100 dB are read off the speech audiogram and added up. This sum, whose maximum possible value is 300, is termed the *total word comprehension.* Second, hearing loss for speech may be determined by the number of decibels separating the number curve from the normal curve. These two values enable the *percentage hearing loss* to be determined from the accompanying table (Table 1.**8**). The curve for *number comprehension* is largely independent of the type of hearing disorder. With the exception of an almost complete HL of sensorineural type, and psychogenic hearing

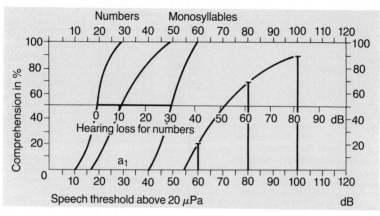

Fig. 1.42 Assessment of total word comprehension and hearing loss for speech from the speech audiogram (Feldmann).

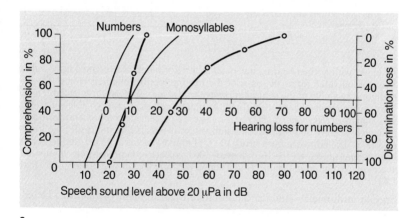

a

Fig. 1.43a–c Examples of various speech audiometer findings in noise-induced hearing loss (Feldmann).

disturbances, 100% comprehension can be achieved with sufficient loudness levels. The difference from the normal curve is expressed in decibels and is termed a *hearing loss for speech*. The curve for *one-syllable comprehension* is termed a *discrimination curve*, as it expresses the subject's *maximal comprehension*. The difference between the theoretical maximal comprehension (100%) and the effective maximum comprehension is termed

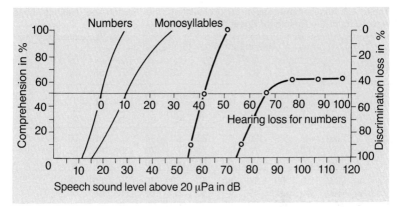

b

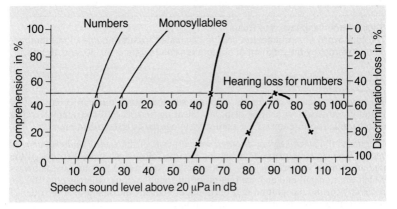

c

the *discrimination loss*. Unlike the curve for number comprehension, the discrimination curve changes with sensorineural deafness. It is flatter (Fig. 1.**43a**); in addition, it does not always achieve the maximum of 100% (Fig. 1.**43b**) or it assumes a bell shape (Fig. 1.**43c**), i.e., the curve achieves its maximum at a certain intensity, then falls with increasing intensity as lower levels of comprehension are reached.

Comparison of pure-tone and speech audiograms. The average hearing loss for speech within the main speech frequencies of 500, 1,000, 2,000, and 4,000 Hz (in decibels HL) corresponds overall to a 50% hearing loss for speech (in decibels HL).

Table 1.8 Assessment Table for Calculating the Percentage Hearing Loss According to the Results of Speech Audiometry

		Hearing Loss for Numbers in dB										
		< 20	≥ 20	≥ 25	≥ 30	≥ 35	≥ 40	≥ 45	≥ 50	≥ 55	≥ 60	≥ 65	≥ 70
comprehension	< 20	100	100	100	100	100	100	100	100	100	100	100	100
	≥ 20	95	95	95	95	95	95	95	95	95	95	95	100
	≥ 35	90	90	90	90	90	90	90	90	90	90	95	100
	≥ 50	80	80	80	80	80	80	80	80	80	90	95	100
	≥ 75	70	70	70	70	70	70	70	70	80	90	95	100
	≥ 100	60	60	60	60	60	60	60	70	80	90	95	
W_s = total word comprehension	≥ 125	50	50	50	50	50	50	60	70	80	90		
	≥ 150	40	40	40	40	40	50	60	70	80			
	≥ 175	30	30	30	30	40	50	60	70				
	≥ 200	20	20	20	30	40	50	60					
	≥ 225	10	10	20	30	40	50						
	≥ 250	0	10	20	30	40							

Source: Boenninghaus and Röser.
The total word comprehension (W_s) is calculated from the curve of comprehension of words, by the addition of comprehension results at 60, 80, and 100 dB.

Discrepancies between the results of pure-tone and speech audiometry are mainly found in retrocochlear hearing disorders. Hearing for speech is considerably worse than hearing for pure tones. The pathophysiologic basis is described on p. 25.

Diagnosis of *central hearing disorders* rests on tests of the *central understanding of speech*. The classical methods of testing hearing fail in such cases because of the phenomenon of *redundance*. This is the safety margin within the auditory pathways which can transmit and analyze billions of information units, whereas only 100 are necessary for the recognition and decoding of acoustic information. A disorder of the central summation and integration capacity can only be demonstrated under difficult circumstances such as distortion of speech by filtering out high frequencies and periodic interruptions of the speech signal or binaural application of garbled test words which reduce the information content of normal speech to a minimum (Feldmann's dichotic speech test).

Tests for simulated deafness. These are only mentioned briefly since ERA and impedance audiometry have largely taken their place.

1. *Stenger's test.* A tone of a certain intensity is offered to one ear. The opposite ear can only hear a tone of the same frequency if its intensity is higher. In unilateral deafness this influence of the opposite ear is absent, but it is preserved in simulated deafness.
2. *Doerfler-Stewart test.* The ability of a patient with an organic hearing loss to hear speech is influenced by a sound when the loudness of that sound exceeds the

speech intensity. In patients with psychogenic or simulated deafness, speech can no longer be understood when the sound level approximates the speech intensity or even before it exceeds this level.

3. *Lee's speech delay test.* The subject is disconcerted by playing back his own speech to him through earphones with a delay of 75 to 30 ms. This causes him to begin to stutter.

Note: Speech audiometry is indispensible for:

1. Determination of the remaining hearing for speech. This allows prediction of the probable benefit to be expected of a hearing aid. The loss of discrimination and the threshold of discomfort can be measured.
2. Assessment of hearing aids and of operations to improve hearing.
3. Investigation of a central deafness. It allows assessment of the integrative performance of the auditory centers.
4. Assessment of the loss of hearing for speech causing loss of earning capacity, for insurance purposes.

Electric Response Audiometry

Principle. The subject is exposed to an acoustic stimulus repeatedly, either regularly or irregularly, and an electroencephalogram (EEG) is used to assess whether there is any change in brain activity (see Fig. 1.**44**). The individual response is concealed on the EEG by the "noise" of brain activity. However, the specific response can be distinguished from the nonspecific brain activity on the EEG by mathematical analysis of numerous evoked individual potentials.

In contrast to the customary audiometric methods which test the hearing process as a complex phenomenon (an acoustic response analyzed by the central nervous system), ERA provides information which cannot be obtained in any other way about the physiologic processes in the end organ, the first neuron, and within the central auditory system. The auditory evoked potentials (AEP) that can be recorded by ERA include the following:

1. *Slow cortical potentials* (less than 50 ms). This is a cortically evoked potential by means of which a complete pure-tone threshold audiogram may be recorded.
2. *Late cortical potential* (contingent negative variation). This is an expression of generalized higher-order cortical function.
3. *Middle neurogenic potentials* (fast cortical potentials of 12 to 50 ms). These central vertex potentials correspond principally to the auditory tract system, including the primary cortical projection.
4. *Fast brain stem potentials:* (a) Brain stem auditory responses (ABR) (2 to 12 ms). These are important for the recognition of retrocochlear hearing disorders. The most important for diagnostic purposes is the latency of the individual potentials, particularly those between potential peaks I and V which are prolonged both relative to the hearing threshold and absolutely in neural functional disorders (see Fig. 1.**44**.)
   (b) Frequency-following responses (5 to 15 ms). The diagnostic significance of these responses has not yet been established.
5. *Electrocochleogram* (0 to 5 ms). This method is a particular type of ERA and provides the most reliable information about the presence of a functional disorder of the auditory nerves or the lower part of the brain stem. It is more

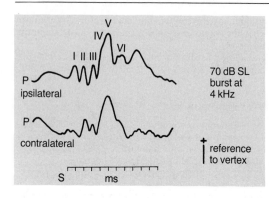

Fig. 1.**44** Fast brain stem potentials (brain stem electric responses).
P_I = action potential of the auditory nerve.
P_{II-IV} = brain stem potentials.

Table 1.**9** Checklist for Suspected Congenital or Early Acquired Deafness	
Family history:	hearing and speech disorders, psychiatric and neurologic diseases, congenital anomalies
History of pregnancy:	virus infection with rubella, measles, influenza, herpes zoster, coxsackie virus, or toxoplasma, drugs such as thalidomide or the aminoglycocides, diseases such as diabetes, neuropathy, or vaccination
Perinatal history:	Forceps or other mechanical damage, asphyxia, prematurity, kernicterus.
Postnatal history:	infectious disease, vaccination reaction, diseases of the central nervous system, trauma to the skull, intoxication, and drugs
Hearing:	Reaction to noise and speech, directional hearing, the time when the hearing disorder began, and the progress of the symptoms
Speech:	age at which the first sounds, words, and sentences were uttered

effective than ABR audiometry in the assessment of inner ear and auditory nerve function. The two most useful diagnostic parameters are the cochlear microphonics (CM) and the action potential of the auditory nerve (PI).

Measurement of the *evoked brain stem potential* (ABR) and *cochleography* are now two of the most important diagnostic methods for accurate differentiation of cochlear from retrocochlear deafness. The latter is due to an acoustic neuroma or a tumor of the posterior cranial fossa or multiple slerosis. Furthermore, ERA is very useful for investigating deafness in infants and young children. It also serves for the assessment of residual function of the central nervous system in patients with severe head injuries, coma, or other conditions marked by complete loss of consciousness. It does not, however, replace pure-tone audiometry or tympanometry (including the stapedius reflex), which still form the basis for audiometric evaluations.

Otoacoustic emissions (OEs) are sound signals emitted from the inner ear in response to acoustic stimulation. Although the clinical value of spontaneous otoacoustic emissions and their role in tinnitus are still debated, the recording of click-evoked OEs has become a routine diagnostic study. Click-evoked OEs cannot be recorded in ears with cochlear midfrequency hearing losses above 25 dB, but the use of sine tones as stimuli or distortion products (DP) provides reliable, reproducible frequency-specific results. DPs are intimately linked to outer hair cell function. Evoked OEs and DPs can be used to detect early discrete lesions of the outer hair cells, and they provide an important noninvasive screening method for cochlear impairment that can even be used in newborns.

Hearing Tests in Infants and Young Children

Note: Every child who does not respond normally to sound stimuli soon after birth, but at least after the first 6 months, must undergo otologic examination.

Since even a completely deaf child passes through a period of crying and babbling, a serious hearing loss only begins to be suspected when speech does not develop. Most children with hearing disorders are therefore presented to the general practitioner or otologist between the 1st and 3rd year of life. Even then there is a danger that the true cause of the delay in development of speech will be overlooked because of the lack of adequate methods of investigation. Therefore, the child may remain untreated for several more years. The following recommendations can be made:

- Early suspicion
- Early recognition
- Early treatment
- Early training

Note: The sense of hearing is a vitally important factor in the acquisition of speech. It is therefore essential that a hearing loss in a child should be recognized and treated. The earlier the treatment is instituted, the more successful it is. Treatment should be begun in the second half of the 1st year (Table 1.9, and Table 1.24).

Electric response audiometry and *impedance audiometry* are nowadays the workhorses of *pediatric audiometry*. These two methods have displaced previously common methods such as behavioral assessment, reflex and play audiometry, peep show tests, and so on.

Vestibular Function Tests

Investigation of the vestibular system consists of the following:

1. Testing of the vestibulospinal reflexes
2. Testing for spontaneous and provoked nystagmus
3. Experimental tests of vestibular and optokinetic systems

Vestibulospinal Reflexes

Romberg's test (Fig. 1.**45a** and **b**). In peripheral vestibular lesions, the body's center of gravity is usually displaced to the side of the labyrinthine lesion. In central disturbances of balance, the pattern of unsteadiness of gait and the direction of fall are irregular.

Blindfold gait and walking a straight line. Only gross abnormalities of gait are of diagnostic significance. The patient deviates to the same side as in Romberg's test.

Unterberger's stepping test. Stepping on one spot with the eyes closed: patients with peripheral disorders show a rotation of the body axis to the side of the labyrinthine lesion; in central disorders the deviation is irregular. Only deviations greater than 40° are of diagnostic significance.

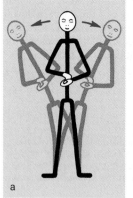
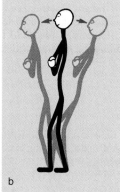

a   b

Fig. 1.**45a** and **b**   Romberg test. The patients stands upright with the feet parallel, the eyes closed, and the arms folded in front of the chest. The patient leans or tends to fall toward the diseased labyrinth.

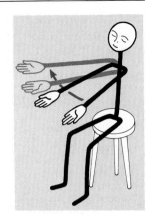

Fig. 1.**46**   Spontaneous deviation reaction. The arms are held horizontal in the supine position. Both upper extremities are displaced in parallel, usually to the side of the lesion.

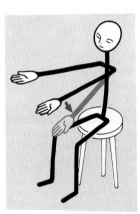

Fig. 1.**47**   Spontaneous arm–tonus reaction shows sinking of *one* arm on the side of the lesion due to cerebellar hypotonia.

Positional tests (Figs. 1.**46** and 1.**47**. Also see pp. 28 and 29):

Spontaneous deviation reaction, past pointing. Parallel displacement of *both* arms (in the supine position) occurs in accordance with the law stated above (Fig. 1.**46**).

Spontaneous tone reaction in the arms. The arm on the side of the cerebellar lesion sinks as a result of loss of tone of the muscles (Fig. 1.**47**).

Finger-nose pointing test. The index finger of the outstretched arm is brought to the point of the nose with the eyes closed. Ataxia and disorders of coordination (overshooting) indicate an ipsilateral cerebellar lesion or a disorder of the positional sense and deep sensation.

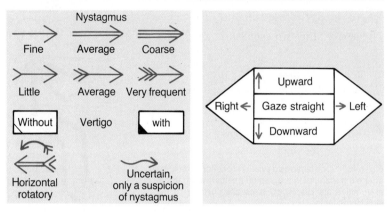

Fig. 1.**48** Diagram of eye movements.   Fig. 1.**49** Frenzel's diagram.

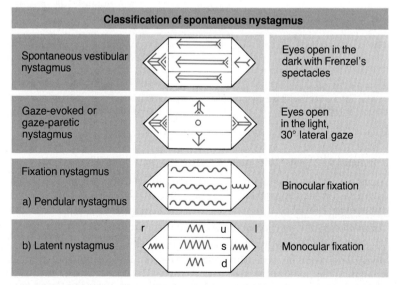

Fig. 1.**50** Classification of spontaneous nystagmus (u = upwards, s = straight, d = downwards).

Tests for Spontaneous and Provoked Nystagmus

Nystagmus. *This is a conjugated coordinated eye movement around a specific axis; this movement consists of rhythmic alternating slow and fast beating phases.* The direction of the fast component of the nystagmus determines the laterality of the nystagmus. Spontaneous vestibular nystagmus can be largely suppressed by visual fixation.

Observation with and without Frenzel's spectacles is used for the diagnosis of a *spontaneous nystagmus.* The patient is examined in a darkened room with + 15-diopter lenses which almost completely suppress optical fixation so that the visual fixation suppression of the vestibular nystagmus is abolished.

Direct gaze with and without fixation is used for the recognition of a *fixation nystagmus.* Lateral gaze and gaze upward and downward are used for the confirmation of a gaze-directional or gaze-paretic nystagmus.

The direction (←), frequency (≫—), and amplitude (=) of the eye movements observed are recorded on a Frenzel chart (Figs. 1.**48** to 1.**50**).

Electronystagmography (ENG)

Principle. The eye is a dipole in which the cornea is electropositive and the retina electronegative. Therefore, the periocular electrical field changes when the eyes move. This change of corneoretinal potential is proportional to the amplitude, frequency, and speed of the nystagmus. It can be picked up and recorded by electrodes and analyzed according to the above parameters. The direction of the eye movements recorded is given by the negative or positive sign of the corneoretinal potential (Fig. 1.**51a–c**).

Photoelectronystagmography (PENG):

The eye movements are recorded by a photoelectric cell instead of the corneoretinal potential. The change in intensity of the light reflected from the surface of the eye is measured by a photoelectric cell. These changes are proportional to the eye movements.

Spontaneous nystagmus. *This term includes all those eye movements that show the character of nystagmus and that are not induced by external stimulation of the vestibular and visual systems* (see Fig. 1.**50**). *The fast component usually beats toward the side of the functionally dominant vestibular center.*

This disorder may be due either to a peripheral vestibular disorder in which case the fast component of the nystagmus always beats toward the dominant labyrinth; or, it may be caused by a central vestibular disorder. The inhibitory impulses on the vestibular center are suppressed (see p. 32). The nystagmus beats on the side of the lesion.

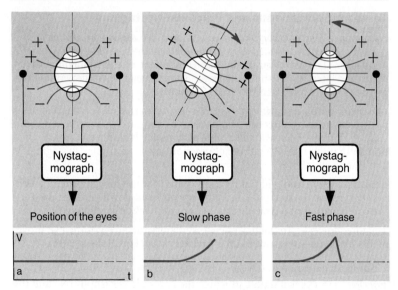

Fig. 1.**51a–c**   Principle of nystagmography. **a.** Gaze straight ahead. The nasal and temporal electrodes are positive, and the isoelectric baseline is horizontal. **b.** The bulb is turned slowly to the left. The nasal electrode is positive, the temporal electrode negative, and the baseline is displaced superiorly. **c.** The bulb returns quickly, the baseline returns to the neutral position, and both electrodes are positive.

Recovery nystagmus may be due either to a central compensatory process after a peripheral lesion or to the recovery of peripheral function. In both cases it is directed toward the side of the dominant vestibular center, i.e., in this case to the diseased ears.

Gaze-evoked and gaze-paretic nystagmus. This form of nystagmus is always induced by a central lesion. Often it beats to both sides and in both the horizontal and vertical planes. It only appears after deviation of the globe by more than 30° for at least 30 s.

An exceptional form of toxic gaze-evoked nystagmus may occur after barbiturate or alcohol poisoning due to release of the central inhibitory effect.

This form of nystagmus is due to a lesion of the voluntary motor control of gaze, which in serious cases is accompanied by paralysis of gaze. Transitions from gaze-evoked to gaze-paretic nystagmus are fluid. The latter is characterized by a nystagmus to the side of the gaze paresis.

This disorder is due to a congenital or acquired disorder (such as multiple sclerosis) of the gaze centers of the reticular formation of the pons (the center for horizontal gaze movement) and of the tegmentum of the midbrain (the center for vertical gaze movements). These centers subserve the central voluntary motor control of gaze (integration of voluntary gaze impulses and visual and vestibular afferents), binocular coordination via the medial longitudinal bundle (see Fig. 1.**19**), and the rhythm of nystagmus. Lesions in this area of the brainstem therefore lead to serious abnormalities of gaze movements and nystagmus, such as changes in rhythm and form of beat, dissociation of movements of the right and left eyes, extinction of the fast phase of nystagmus, unilateral or bilateral enhancement of optokinetic nystagmus, gaze-evoked and gaze-paretic nystagmus, and internuclear ophthalmoplegia.

Fixation nystagmus. This form of nystagmus has no typical fast and slow components but rather a pendular movement. It almost always occurs with binocular fixation but may rarely occur with monocular fixation. It is often congenital and may even be hereditary. Its synonyms include *congenital or hereditary pendular nystagmus.*

This disorder is usually due to a congenital lesion of the motor centers for gaze in the brain stem, though it may occasionally be due to acquired diseases such as syringobulbia. These disinhibit gaze movement causing gaze hyperkinesia: conjugated rhythmic eye movements therefore occur on every gaze intention, producing nystagmus in the plane of the direction of gaze. Unlike gaze-paretic nystagmus, it is usually not a symptom of a disease of the brain stem but of a congenital anomaly and often causes no symptoms (Fig. 1.**52**). It occurs quite commonly in *amblyopia.*

The three main forms of spontaneous eye movements with the typical characteristics of nystagmus must not be confused with the following:

End-point nystagmus, a short-lived, nonpathologic, rapidly decaying beat at the extremes of gaze, i.e., more than 50° deviation.

Differential diagnosis of spontaneous nystagmus						
	Eyes closed	Binocular fixation	View 30° r.	View 30° l.	Head shaking	Monocular fixation
Spontaneous vestibular nystagmus	NNNN	——	~~~~	——	MW ~~~~	——
Gaze-evoked or gaze-paretic nystagmus	——	——	NNNN	MMM	——	——
Fixation nystagmus (pendular nystagmus)	(~~)	~~~	~~~	uuu	——	~~
Latent fixation nystagmus	(NNNN)	——	(N~)	(~~)	——	~~~~

Fig. 1.**52** Differential diagnosis of spontaneous nystagmus (Kornhuber).

Fatigue nystagmus, which occurs during prolonged lateral gaze due to fatigue of the lateral rectus muscle, similar to tremor in skeletal muscles. It is also nonpathologic.

Adjustment nystagmus, which is due to adjustment of movements of a nystagmoid character when fixing on an object in the visual field. There is a rapid beat which fatigues quickly. It, too, is nonpathologic.

Provoked nystagmus. *Unlike spontaneous nystagmus, this is exclusively a vestibular-induced nystagmus which only appears after certain provoking measures such as change in the position of the body or of the head.*

Frenzel's spectacles are used to investigate this condition. The same *criteria* are used to assess provoked nystagmus as spontaneous nystagmus; however, the duration of eye movements is also taken into account. One of the following patterns of nystagmus may be seen:

- A *transitory* nystagmus which lasts less than 60 s.
- A continually beating *persistent* nystagmus.
- A *headshaking nystagmus,* i.e., a "release" spontaneous nystagmus of peripheral or central origin. It may be transitory or persistent.

Static positional nystagmus. This form of nystagmus is induced by a *specific position* of the head, and not by change of position. It is due to displacement of the contents of the skull, a change of cerebral circulation, of the cerebrospinal fluid (CSF) pressure, or of the pressure on the macula of the otolith organ.

Methods of examination. The patient is examined when he is lying in the following positions:

1. Horizontal on the examination couch
2. With the entire body turned on the right side
3. With the entire body turned on the left side

Types of positional nystagmus. After adoption of a particular position of the body, the following types of nystagmus can occur:

1. *Directionally determined positional nystagmus,* a "release" spontaneous nystagmus which is persistent and reproducible and which always beats in the same direction. It is induced peripherally or centrally.
2. *Regular direction-changing positional nystagmus* which is persistent and reproducible. It occurs in a particular position of the body and always beats to the same side. The direction of the nystagmus changes when the body position changes. It is usually induced centrally.
3. *Irregular direction-changing positional nystagmus* is always induced centrally. It is reproducible, irregular, and changing in direction in all positions, and usually persistent.

Dynamic positional nystagmus. The inducing factor is the kinetic action of *change of position.* It is due to mechanical stimulation of the joints of the cervical spine and especially to direct kinetic stimulation of the semicircular canals and otolith organs.

Method of examination:

1. The position of the body is changed rapidly from a sitting position to a supine one with the head hanging vertically.
2. Sitting up rapidly.
3. Rapid turning of the head to the right.
4. Sitting up rapidly.
5. and 6. Similar to 2 and 3 for the left side.

Classification:

1. *Paroxysmal positional nystagmus* (see p. 146). After rapid change of position, a nystagmus occurs with the following characteristics: a short latent period of 5 to 10 s; horizontal/rotatory beat toward the underlying ear, an increase in intensity which decreases 15 to 30 s later, and a marked subjective feeling of vertigo. Occasionally, a transitory nystagmus beating in the opposite direction occurs on sitting up. The *cause* of this nystagmus is probably a peripheral lesion, the so-called cupulolithiasis.
2. In addition *to paroxysmal positional nystagmus,* a persistent or transitory direction-determined nystagmus, a regular direction changing, and an irregular positional nystagmus may be observed. The latter is always of central origin, whereas the first two may be of peripheral or central origin.

Experimental Tests of the Vestibular System

These tests and their analysis should be carried out by a specialist.

Turning test. The rotatory or turning test uses *angular acceleration* as the stimulus for the investigation of the sensitivity of the horizontal semicircular canals. The principle of the technique is illustrated in Figure 1.**28** (see p. 29).

Caloric Labyrinthine Testing

The principle is shown in Figure 1.**53**. The horizontal semicircular canal is brought into a vertical position in the supine patient. The volume of the endolymph is changed by cooling or warming the labyrinthine capsule by irrigation with water at 30 °C or 44 °C for 30 to 40 s. This produces movement of the endolymph which deflects the cupula. Recent experience in European space laboratories shows that the deflection of the cupula is caused by alteration of volume of the endolymph rather than by a convection current. This process has exactly the same electrophysiologic effect as deflection of the cupula by angular acceleration (see Fig. 1.**28**), i.e., it induces a nystagmus via the vestibuloocular reflex.

The *extent of the caloric response* (the nystagmus and the subjective feeling of dizziness) gives some indication of the function of the stimulated labyrinth. *Reduced excitability* indicates partial functional loss, and *lack of*

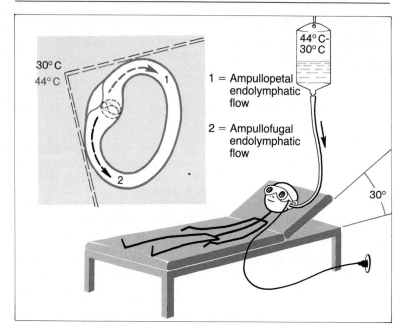

Fig. 1.**53**   Principle of caloric labyrinthine tests.

response indicates subtotal or complete loss of function. Directional prepon-derance indicates a difference in spontaneous activity in the higher pri-mary vestibular centers. The advantage of caloric tests is that the labyrinth of each side can be investigated separately.

Galvanic test. The principle of this method of investigation rests on the fact that galvanic current applied to the end organ and to the vestibular nerve induces a hyperpolarization and depolarization effect and thus a vestibular nystagmus. It also causes a vestibulospinal reaction of lateral displacement of the body's center of gravity or lateropulsion. *It is possible to test each vestibular organ and its nerve sepa-rately with this test and to differentiate a lesion of the end organ from one of the nerve.* The galvanic response is preserved after destruction of the vestibular sensory end organs, but disappears after degeneration of the nerve fibers.

Optokinetic Function and Pursuit Tracking

The optokinetic and eye-tracking tests are among the most sensitive methods available for the detection of central oculomotor lesions. They are indispensible for distinguishing a peripheral from a central disorder of balance since both systems are functionally very closely linked.

Principle: Observation of an object moving within a stationary visual field (foveal stimulation) or observation of the displacement of the entire visual field (foveoretinal stimulation). Only the latter induces the optokinetic reflex: a conjugated reflex eye movement which shows a slow movement in the direction of the displacement of the moving object or visual field (gaze following movement) and a fast phase (the central correction movement) in the opposite direction. This is described as *optokinetic nystagmus.*

Lesions of the brain stem, especially of the pons and cerebellum, produce changes of optokinetic nystagmus such as unilateral directional preponderance, disintegration of coordinated movement of the left and right eye, and complete unilateral or bidirectional disintegration of coordinated movement. *Gaze-evoked or -paretic nystagmus and simultaneous abnormalities of optokinetic nystagmus are characteristic early symptoms of multiple sclerosis.*

Fistula Test

In the presence of a fistula in the horizontal semicircular canal or elsewhere in the labyrinthine capsule (see p. 101), caused by an inflammatory osteolytic process such as cholesteatoma, a sudden increase in pressure in the external auditory meatus produces a subjective feeling of dizziness, objective nystagmus, and lateropulsion. The same phenomenon can also occur in the case of adhesions between the membranous labyrinth and the stapes footplate (fistula symptom without a labyrinthine fistula, see p. 114).

Technique. A Politzer balloon with a perforated olive is introduced into the meatus. Compression induces nystagmus toward the diseased ear and aspiration to the other side.

Pseudofistula symptom. Inflation or aspiration of air in a patient with a large defect in the tympanic membrane produces cooling of the horizontal semicircular canal which induces a caloric labyrinthine reaction and thus a nystagmus. However, this always beats toward the sound ear for both compression and aspiration.

Note: The fistula symptom must always be looked for if a cholesteatoma of the middle ear is suspected.

Investigation of the Facial Nerve

The first and most important investigation serves to differentiate a central from a peripheral paralysis.

In a central paralysis the function of the branches to the forehead is preserved (see Fig. 1.**21**).

In a peripheral paralysis all three branches are affected. The secretion of tears and the sensitivity for taste are affected, and hyperacusis may occur due to disruption of the stapedius reflex.

The *topographical diagnosis* of peripheral lesions of the facial nerve is shown in Figure 1.**20**.

Taste. The anterior two-thirds of the tongue is innervated by the chorda tympani. The test stimulus is 20% sugar, 10% saline, or 5% citric acid solution (see pp. 311, 319).

Gustometry. The peripheral taste fibers are stimulated electrically, and the threshold is measured in milliamperes (see p. 319).

Schirmer's test. The reduction of the secretion of tears due to interruption of the lacrimal anastomosis in the greater superficial petrosal nerve is measured on the paralyzed side (see Fig. 1.**20**).

The *stapedius reflex* is measured by impedance audiometry (see p. 50).

The severity and prognosis of a paralysis can only be determined by *electrodiagnosis.*

Note: Every facial paralysis of whatever cause must be investigated as early as possible by electrodiagnostic methods.
Three stages of a lesion can be distinguished:

Neurapraxia. There is complete absence of function but without interruption of the axon. This stage is reversible.

Axonotmesis. There is disruption of the axon with preservation of the connective tissue framework of the nerve (endo-, peri-, and epineurium). These lesions usually do not recover completely.

Neurotmesis. There is disruption of the axon and of the supporting tissues. It is irreversible without operative intervention.

The *purpose of electrodiagnosis* is to determine the proportion of blocked (neurapraxia) to degenerated (axonotmesis) nerve fibers.

Method:

Determination of rheobase. The smallest strength of current in milliamperes which produces a visible muscle twitch is measured. In axonotmesis it is increased or infinite.

Determination of chronaxy. The smallest duration of impulse of current (in milliseconds) that will produce a visible muscle twitch at a constant strength of current (double the rheobase value) is measured. In axonotmesis it is prolonged or infinite.

Electromyography (EMG). Muscle action potentials are picked up by a needle electrode on voluntary contraction of the facial musculature. The EMG is of relatively little value in the acute phase of facial paralysis since denervation potentials only appear 12 days after the beginning of the paralysis.

Electroneuronography (ENoG). The sums of the action potentials of the facial musculature induced by contraction in response to maximal percutaneous faradic stimulation are measured. The proportion of degenerated fibers can be assessed approximately by comparison of the summation potential between the sound and the paralyzed side.

Nerve excitability test. The strength of current in milliamperes which suffices to induce a muscle twitch at a constant duration of impulse of 0.3 ms is determined. The threshold for the two facial nerves varies insignificantly (0.4 mA) in the same person. A difference in threshold between the two sides greater than or equal to 3.5 mA is abnormal. An increase in the threshold indicates progressive degeneration of the nerve fibers or progressive axonotmesis.

The results of determination of rheobase or chronaxy and those for ENoG provide important information in the acute phase of a paralysis about the extent of the degenerative processes in the nerve and their progress and are decisive in determining the choice of treatment.

Clinical Aspects of Diseases of the External Ear

Nonspecific Inflammation of the External Ear

Symptoms. In the *acute exudative inflammatory* phase the external auditory meatus is swollen and usually filled with fetid debris which can form a nidus of infection for gram-negative bacteria and anaerobes. The cartilaginous part of the meatus is painful; the tympanic membrane is intact but may be difficult to assess because of increased desquamation of the epidermis and accumulation of debris. Normal results of tuning fork and hearing tests with an open meatus indicate that the middle ear is not involved. However, regional retroauricular lymph nodes may be so enlarged and tender to pressure in serious cases that a picture of *pseudomastoiditis* is produced.

In the *chronic inflammatory phase* the meatus is wide, the epithelial lining is atrophic, and dry scales of epidermis accumulate. There is intense itching which causes the patient to scratch his external ear. This often causes damage and favors the development of a *superinfection* with acute dermatitis, with or without perichondritis (see also erysipelas, Color Plate **3b**).

Pathogenesis. Exogenous and endogenous factors such as maceration of the meatal skin by fluid, mechanical and chemical damage, allergy, and diabetes lead to a reduction of the elasticity of the meatal skin and to atrophy of the ceruminous and sebaceous glands. This causes loss of the protective film of secretion. The result is drying of the meatal skin, disturbance of its chemical balance, and increased susceptibility to infection by bacteria and fungi. The pH of the meatal skin is a very important factor in the growth of bacteria, in addition to the temperature, moisture content, and aeration of the external auditory meatus; alteration of aeration can lead to the growth of anaerobic bacteria. A rise of pH above 6.0 is a prerequisite for the development of infection.

Factors that encourage the elimination of pathogens in the meatal skin include:

- Low pH values
- Fatty acids in the secretions of the sebaceous glands
- Normal lysozyme content of the secretions of the ceruminous glands
- A normal self-cleaning mechanism by external migration of the meatal epithelium

Damage to these protective factors by displacement of the pH to alkaline values in allergy, reduction of the protective film, and changes in the composition of the secretions by mechanical stimulation or recurrent inflammation eventually cause a chronic otitis externa. This can lead to intermittent episodes of acute bacterial exudative inflammation.

Diagnosis and Differential Diagnosis

- The inflammation is localized to the auricle, external auditory meatus, and the regional lymph nodes.
- Extension to the outer and middle layers of the tympanic membrane (myringitis) only occurs exceptionally.
- The middle ear and mastoid are not affected by the disease.
- Conductive deafness due to obstruction of the external auditory meatus is unusual and mild in nature.
- It is important to exclude an acute otitis media, mastoiditis, and the acute phase of a chronic middle ear inflammation with cholesteatoma.
- Pain on pressure on the tragus strongly suggests otitis externa.

Investigations include otoscopy, a specimen of pus for bacteriology, possibly irrigation of the ear, hearing and tuning fork tests, audiogram, and radiology using Schueller's view to exclude mastoiditis.

Treatment. The external auditory meatus is cleaned manually under vision or by irrigation with water at 37 °C. The external auditory meatus is dried, and eardrops consisting of locally active broad-spectrum antibiotics and a corticosteroid are instilled several times a day during the moist phase. In severe cases systemic antibiotics are given. Once the acute inflammatory phase subsides, local applications of ointments based on a combination of an antibiotic and a steroid are used. However, certain antibiotics, notably neomycin, can themselves cause an allergic skin reaction. In these cases the local use of 70% to 80% pure alcohol is indicated, and in the *acute inflammatory phase* a fine gauze wick should be introduced into the ear. This is moistened repeatedly with alcohol which opens the external auditory meatus and reduces the swelling of the meatal skin by absorption of moisture.

Prophylaxis, course, and prognosis. The patient should be forbidden to clean his external auditory meatus with unsuitable instruments such as cotton Q-tips and matchsticks (see Color Plate **6a**). The otologist should clear the external auditory meatus regularly of debris as this is a culture medium for bacteria. Ointment should be applied locally to suppress the pruritis and to lubricate the skin. A very severe chronic recurrent form can occur which requires regular care by the otologist.

Specific Forms

Bacterial and Viral Diffuse Otitis Externa

A characteristic *erysipelas* occurs in streptcoccal infection. In *swimmer's otitis* due to maceration of the skin by halogen-containing swimming pool water and deep penetration of virulent organisms, there is usually a deep-seated *phlegmonous inflammation* with *perichondritis*. In addition to *swimmer's otitis externa* confined to the external ear, a tubal *swimmer's otitis media* may also occur.

Symptoms. These include fever, generalized illness, regional lymphadenitis, and pain on pulling on the auricle or pressure on the tragus. A phlegmonous form can extend to surrounding tissues and organs, such as the parotid gland, mastoid, and skull base, and in exceptional cases can cause osteomyelitis of the temporal bone and septicemia (*malignant otitis externa*, see p. 74). In severe cases of otitis externa, especially in infants and young children, there is complete obstruction of the external auditory meatus with an accompanying retroauricular lymphadenitis. The ear is displaced laterally, and the patient may appear to have mastoiditis.

Treatment. Systemic antibiotics; *local* reduction of the swelling of the skin of the external auditory meatus with 70% to 95% alcohol, chloramine in a 1 : 1,000 irrigation, or local application of topically active antibiotics.

Furuncle of the Ear

The patient is in good general condition but has local pain in the ear. Characteristic is a circumscribed, exquisitely painful swelling in the cartilaginous part of the external auditory meatus (hair follicles), a modest regional lymphadenitis, and pain on pressure on the tragus or pulling on the auricle.

Treatment. Alcohol-soaked (70% to 95%) gauze wicks are used until the furuncle points and bursts spontaneously. Incision and systemic antibiotics are only exceptionally indicated in patients with severe pain, a protracted course, or marked swelling.

Note: The glucose content of the urine and blood should be checked in patients with recurrent furunculosis of the external meatus.

Herpes Zoster Oticus (Color Plate **3c**)

This disease is characterized by multiple herpetic vesicles arranged in groups on the auricle, the external auditory meatus, and occasionally the tympanic membrane. In severe cases disorders of hearing and balance and facial paralysis may occur (see pp. 138 and 163).

Bullous Myringitis

This disease usually occurs in association with an influenzal infection. It is occasionally combined with otitis media in which case the patient has a conductive deafness. Initially there is a moist bluish-livid bullous inflammation which can extend to the tympanic membrane. After a few days the hemorrhagic vesicles dry out and heal without complications. The patient usually complains of extremely severe pain (Color Plate **7d**).

> *Note:* If the middle ear is invaded, systemic antibiotics must be administered immediately because of the danger of superinfection.

In most cases treatment is limited to simple toilet of the external meatus and otoscopic control. Antibiotics are only given to protect against secondary infection.

Malignant Otitis Externa

A severe necrotizing inflammation can develop from a commonplace otitis externa especially in diabetics, whether latent or manifest. The infection is generally caused by optionally anaerobic gram-negative organisms, usually *Pseudomonas aeruginosa*. The infection extends through the tissue clefts of the cartilaginous meatus and extends into the depths of the retromandibular fossa, along the base of the skull as far as the jugular foramen, and leads to an insidious osteomyelitis of the temporal bone.

Treatment. In addition to treatment for diabetes, and intensive antibiotic therapy, treatment rarely includes generous drainage of the retromandibular space, the infratemporal fossa, the pterygopalatine fossa, and the parotid space and generous debridement of the necrotic tissue from the external meatus, the temporal bone, and the parotid. Ligation or resection of the internal jugular vein may also be indicated if it is invaded.

The **prognosis** is poor despite massive antibiotics and extensive surgery because of septicemia and sinus thrombosis.

Otomycosis and Eczema

Otomycosis

Symptoms. The infection is caused by a fungus and is limited to the external auditory meatus. It produces a fine easily removable coating which is loose and fluffy, varying in color from whitish-yellow to greenish-black. The patient complains of itching, but seldom of pain.

Diagnosis. Culture and sensitivity tests demonstrate fungal mycelium.

Treatment. The mainstay of treatment is manual cleaning, but irrigation should be avoided if possible to prevent the formation of a "moist chamber" which encourages the growth of the fungus.

Antimycotic agents my be applied *locally* unless contraindicated by a perforation of the tympanic membrane. Antibiotics should not be used. Daily painting of the meatus with Merthiolate may help, and in severe cases systemic antimycotics may be used.

Course. The course is chronic and recurrent.

Eczema of the Ear

Symptoms. The disease follows an episodic course with intermittent acute exacerbations. The entry of fluid such as sweat or water during washing, or the presence of a moist exudate, favor colonization by pathogenic bacteria or fungi in the relatively enclosed external meatus.

In the acute stage there is deep-red inflammatory swelling with moist vesicles and pustules. Later, crusts accumulate. Rhagades form around the meatal introitus and fetid debris collects. The usual picture is a nonspecific acute otitis externa, but occasionally the appearances may progress to chronic myringitis with superficial granulations.

In the chronic stage the skin is atrophic, dry, scaly, and may in part be lichenified. The patient complains of chronic irritation. Occasionally stenosis may occur.

Diagnosis and Differential Diagnosis

Contact eczema may be due to cosmetic solutions, hair sprays, glasses frames made of metal or plastic, cement and flour dust, and drugs, e.g., antibiotics. Skin tests must be carried out to determine the antigen.

Microbial eczema is mainly due to infection with staphylococci or to oral mycosis. A swab should be taken for culture and sensitivity tests.

Seborrheic eczema is the most common form. It is often combined with acne.

Endogenous eczema is a localized manifestation of a generalized eczema.

Treatment includes elimination of the allergen and local treatment as detailed above.

Specific Chronic Inflammation

Tuberculosis and syphilis (stage 2) are rare nowadays. They cause local circumscribed lesions of the external ear and auditory meatus.

Trauma

Every injury to the auricle and cartilaginous part of the external auditory meatus may damage the perichondrium causing cartilaginous necrosis.

Furthermore, bacterial infection can cause perichondritis with partial or complete destruction of the cartilaginous framework leading to a cauliflower ear or atresia of the meatus. (See Color Plate **3a**.) Patients with partial or complete *amputation of the auricle* should be admitted immediately to the hospital along with the severed part of the auricle. Even large, completely severed parts of the auricle may be resutured by appropriate reconstructive techniques, provided the interval between the *injury* and the *operation* does not exceed 1 h.

Sharp and blunt trauma requires extensive debridement, primary suture, and antibiotic cover.

Hematoma of the auricle. This arises from closed blunt injury with dissection of the skin and perichondrial layer from the cartilage, and the formation of a subperichondrial hematoma (see Color Plate **2c**).

Treatment. A wide incision is made along the anterior edge of the helix, and necrotic tissue is removed by curettage. If necessary, a window is made in the cartilage to allow the two perichondrial surfaces to adhere and to prevent further accumulation of blood and serum between the cartilage and the perichondrium. An oiled silk compression dressing is used for 1 week, and antibiotic cover is given.

Note: Repeated aspiration may cause a seroma or superinfection leading to perichondritis.

If a hematoma is not treated, connective tissue organization, secondary calcification, and deformity of the auricle occur leading to a cauliflower ear (see Color Plate **2d**).

Frostbite

Grade 1 – cyanosis of the skin due to vascular spasm
Grade 2 – ischemia with formation of vesicles
Grade 3 – deep necrosis of tissue

Treatment. Sterile dressings, antibiotics, intravenous vasodilators, and possibly stellate ganglion block are employed depending on the severity of the injury. The part must be kept dry.

Burns require the same treatment as burns of the skin; particular attention must be paid to the close relationship between the skin and the cartilage.

Late complications include necrosis of the auricle and atresia or stenosis of the external auditory meatus.

Wax and Foreign Bodies

Note: Collections of wax and cell debris are unusual provided that the self-cleaning mechanism of the external auditory meatus is undisturbed. The present widespread habit of daily cleaning of the external ear using ready-made cotton Q-tips is an abuse which can sooner or later lead to the development of chronic otitis externa.

Wax is a yellowish-brown mass consisting of the secretion of the sebaceous and ceruminous glands, desquamated epithelium, hair, and particles of dirt. The normal symptom is deafness when the external auditory meatus is completely closed, but occasional complaints include a roaring noise in the head and a feeling of dizziness.

Differential diagnosis. This includes a plug of epidermis, a foreign body, dried blood, or purulent exudate.

Treatment. The ear is irrigated with water at 37 °C, provided that a perforation of the tympanic membrane is not hidden behind the plug of wax. This should be excluded by a careful history. If the patient does have such a perforation, the wax should be removed manually by a specialist. Hard wax should be first softened for 15 to 20 min by 3% hydrogen peroxide or one of the proprietary preparations. The moist external auditory meatus should be mopped out with cotton applicators. Local steroid or antibiotic creams or eardrops should be prescribed for patients with inflammation of the meatus. *The hearing should be tested after this procedure.*

A *plug of epidermis* is a compact white mass consisting of desquamated epithelial crusts which usually adhere firmly to the skin of the meatus.

Differential diagnosis. This includes a cholesteatoma of the meatus or of the middle ear. **Treatment.** Instrumental removal is performed by a specialist.

Foreign bodies are diagnosed by careful otoscopy. In children, a careful history should be taken to establish the nature of the foreign body.

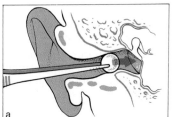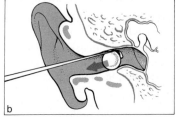

Fig. 1.**54a** and **b**   Attempts to remove a foreign body with simple forceps **(a)** displace the foreign body more deeply, and it may perforate the tympanic membrane causing dislocation of the ossicles and injury to the facial canal. The foreign body can be removed easily without danger to the patient by a hook under otoscopic control **(b)**.

Note: Foreign bodies that cannot be removed by syringing should be removed manually, using general anesthesia in small children.

If the patient is known or suspected to have a perforation of the tympanic membrane, the ear should not be syringed.

Blind attempts at extraction without otoscopic control, or attempts at extraction under vision with unsuitable instruments and unsatisfactory anesthesia, are negligent methods of treatment.

Removal of foreign bodies from the meatus should therefore only be carried out by a specialist, apart from the most simple cases.

Figure 1.**54a** and **b** shows the right and wrong methods of extraction of a foreign body from the meatus.

Tumors

Benign Tumors

These include retroauricular atheroma, cicatricial keloid, hemangioma and lymphangioma, dermoid tumors, fibroma, papilloma, keratoma, lipoma, and nevi.

Treatment. The tumor is surgically removed.

Meatal tumors include hyperostosis caused by periosteal stimulation which causes appositional bone growth with progressive narrowing of the lumen of the meatus and *exostosis,* a true bony tumor arising from the ossification centers in the anulus tympanicus. This tumor should only be removed if it causes stenosis (see Color Plate **5d**). *Condrodermatitis nodularis circumscripta helicis* causes painful nodes on the ear which should be distinguished from a premalignant lesion by the marked pain on pressure.

Treatment is excision.

Precancerous and Malignant Tumors

Classification, symptoms, diagnosis, and differential diagnosis are shown in Table 1.**10**.

Treatment. Premalignant lesions often progress to true carcinoma. Therefore, premalignant lesions should always be treated by radical surgery like a true tumor. Biopsy excision is not advisable, and every tumor of the external ear suspected of being malignant should be excised with a wide margin. The mainstay of treatment is surgery; radiotherapy or cryosurgery are second-best options (see p. 81).

Precancerous lesions such as senile keratosis or Bowen's disease are excised with a healthy margin. Periodic follow-up is necessary.

Table 1.10 Precancerous and Malignant Tumors of the External Ear

	Form	Color	Skin Surface	Cartilage Invasion	Regional Lymph Node Metastases	Differential Diagnosis
Cutaneous horn	A sharply limited warty growth of the epidmeris	Inconspicuous	Slightly nodular, intact	None	None	Senile papilloma: a smooth papillomatous tumor
Senile keratosis	Smooth mass with indistinct borders	Yellowish-brown	Rough, intact, occasionally covered by crusts	None	None	Basal cell carcinoma and eczema
Bowen's disease	Smooth round lump	Intensive brownish-red	Smooth but intact	None	None	Basal cell carcinoma
Basal cell carcinoma	Sharply demarcated smooth, slowly growing mass	Hyperemic, sometimes much more pigmented than the sorrounding skin (special form: pigmented basal cell carcinoma)	Often superficially ulcerated, crusted, raised edges with an atrophic center (or central ulcer)	Perichondrium sometimes infiltrated, Tumor relatively immobile on its base	Rarely	Squamous cell carcinoma, senile keratosis, Bowen's disease, eczema and chondro-dermatitis nodularis

Continued p. 80

Table 1.10 Continuation

Squamous cell carcinoma	Exophytic tumor of relatively rapid growth with indistinct margins	Often hyperemic	Ulcerated, raised edges, superficially nodular, firm	Always. The tumor is not movable; occasionally perichondritis.	20%	Basal cell carcinoma, senile keratosis
Malignant melanoma	A round mass sometimes verrucous, rapidly growing	Dark-brown to black, occasionally weakly pigmented, the amelonotic melanoma	Smooth to slightly nodular occasionally ulcerated or bleeds easily to touch	Perichondrium often infiltrated and the tumor is relatively immobile on its base	Frequent. Also early distant metastases, e.g., to the lung.	Pigmented cell nevus, a sharply demarcated flat mass, dark-brown in color, never ulcerated, and which does not grow or infiltrate as long as it remains benign. Seborrheic wart, a sharply demarcated verrucous tumor, dark-brown, nonulcerated, of slow, noninfiltrative exophytic growth.

Basal cell carcinoma (Color Plates **4a—d**):

A *nodular, secondarily ulcerated, basal cell carcinoma* can be treated by contact irradiation if it is confined to the auricle, as can a circumscribed, *atrophic, healing basal cell carcinoma.* However, the latter tumor is usually removed surgically. The *destructive, subcutaneously, infiltrating basal cell carcinoma* has a worse prognosis compared to the type mentioned above. It is treated by generous excision followed by reconstruction. Radiotherapy for basal cell carcinomas of the auricle greater than 1 cm in diameter carries the danger of damage to the perichondrium leading to perichondritis. Primary surgery is therefore the treatment of choice. Cryosurgery may be used for small basal cell carcinomas.

Keratinizing squamous cell carcinomas are infiltrating, often ulcerated, and in 20% of patients demonstrate early metastases to the regional lymph nodes (see Color Plate **5a** and **5b**). The treatment of choices is *radical surgery* paying no regard to the cosmetic result. Radiotherapy is only successful for tumors less than 1 cm in diameter that are not ulcerated, have not infiltrated the perichondrium, and have not metastasized to the regional lymph nodes. In all other cases, *partial or complete excision of the auricle* is the method of choice. Neck dissection is carried out for regional lymph node metastases.

Carcinoma of the external auditory meatus (see Color Plate **5b**) constitutes about 5% of all aural carcinomas. The prognosis is unfavorable compared to tumors of the auricle, because of late diagnosis, and because the tumor penetrates early into the parotid space or the middle ear. The *treatment of choice* is extensive resection of the tumor with radical neck dissection and parotidectomy if necessary. A *pigmented nevus* and a suspected malignant *melanoma* (see Color Plate **3d**) should be treated by *primary excision of the tumor* without a previous biopsy. Depending on the results of histology, it may be necessary to carry out a secondary surgical excision, dictated by the extent and depth of the tumor (see p. 519ff.), with a regional neck dissection or a radical neck dissection and, if necessary, parotidectomy. Postoperative radiotherapy, chemotherapy, or immunotherapy may also be necessary. Surgery should only be considered when distant metastases have been excluded. Mutilating operations for malignant tumors of the ear can be corrected by reconstruction of the auricle or by a prosthesis.

Congenital Anomalies

In addition to the large variation in site, size, and shape of the auricle, there are also numerous disfiguring anomalies. *Bat ear* is one of the most common of these, often caused by a hypertrophy or excess curvature of the conchal cartilage, or by a failure of folding of the auricle due to underdevelopment or absence of the anthelix.

Treatment. The deep conchal cavity is corrected, and an anthelixplasty performed. The angle between the auricle and the head is reduced to the ideal value of 30° and the conchalscaphoid angle to 90°. The operation should be carried out in the pre-school years.

Anotia (absence of the auricle) and *microtia* (a small, deformed auricle) are often combined with *stenosis* or *atresia* of the external auditory meatus and with an *anomaly of the middle ear* (see Color Plate **1b–d**).

Congenital aural fistulae and auricular appendages are usually situated in front of the auricle. They are due to incomplete closure of the first branchial groove or an incomplete fusion of the auricular hillocks. Three groups may be distinguished depending on the embryologic association and site (see Color Plates **1a** and **2a, b**).

1. Preauricular fistulae between the angle of the mouth and the tragus
2. Fistulae that begin in front of the ascending helix and lead toward the meatus, or open externally inferior to the angle of the jaw as a hyomandibular fistula
3. A small fistula or pitted depression affecting any part of the auricle

Treatment is excision, remembering the danger of damage to the parotid gland or facial nerve (see pp. 165, 554 ff.).

Reconstructive Operations on the Auricle

Reconstructive procedures on the auricle vary in difficulty. Whereas correction of an anomaly of the shape of the auricle (remodeling of the auricular cartilage) can be relatively simple, reconstruction of the entire auricle is one of the most difficult tasks of plastic surgery in this area. A thorough knowledge of transplantation of skin and cartilage are prerequisites for the success of this reconstruction. Provision of the skin required for the creation of the new auricle is not easy and requires the development of rotation and sliding flaps from the neck and from the region of the hairline. *Prostheses* should be considered as an *alternative* in difficult cases.

Reconstruction of the external auditory meatus and the sound-conducting apparatus are discussed in the section on anomalies of the middle ear (see p. 135).

Clinical Aspects of Diseases of the Middle and Internal Ear

Disorders of Ventilation and Drainage of the Middle Ear Spaces

Pathogenesis. The eustachian tube does not open regularly on swallowing due to one of the following factors:

- An inadequate tensor palati muscle

- Swelling of the tubal mucosa caused by chronic inflammation of neighboring structures such as the sinuses or tonsils or by allergy
- Obstruction of the ostium of the tube by hypertrophied adenoids in a child or adult
- Infiltration of the tube by a malignant tumor of the nasopharynx

The middle ear is thus no longer aerated, and the remaining air is resorbed, producing a decrease of pressure which acts as an irritant to the middle ear mucosa.

In *short-lasting tubal occlusion* or persistent reduced pressure in the middle ear, the following changes occur in the middle ear:

- Edema of the mucosa
- Exudate due to transudation of the constituent parts of the serum
- Stiffening of the ossicular chain with a retraction of the tympanic membrane.

Note: The cause of a disorder of ventilation and drainage of the middle ear is mainly a disordered opening mechanism of the tube, but mechanical obstruction of the tube by a lesion in the nasopharynx may also occur.

In *long-standing tubal occlusion* and reduced pressure the following occur:

- Metaplasia of the middle ear mucosa from the flat epithelial cells of the mucoperiosteum to columnar, ciliated, mucus-producing goblet cells
- Increase of the secretory activity of the goblet cells and mixing of the mucus with the transudate already present in the middle ear to cause a *seromucinous exudate*
- Formation of cholesterin-containing mucosal cysts (a cholesterol granuloma)

The seromucinous exudate and the change in the mucosa contribute considerably to reduction of the aeration of the middle ear, thus causing a vicious circle.

The metaplasia of the middle ear mucosa also affects the submucosa, causing first a proliferation of the connective tissue and second maturation of a local immunologically active cellular defense mechanism. The active secreting goblet cells produce the mucous blanket which serves to transport the newly formed immunoglobulins to the mucosal surface. The previously inactive mucoperiosteum of the middle ear is thus converted into a secreting hyperplastic respiratory mucosa characterized by its newly acquired property of responding to every new stimulus (mechanical, chemical, bacterial, enzymatic, allergic, or autoimmunologic) by a *completely mature defense mechanism*. This consists of the following:

- Mucociliary elements which form the *transport medium* for the superficially active *mucus blanket*
- Enzymatic elements which consist especially of bacteriocidal lysozymes and protease inhibitors
- Locally produced immunoglobulins

The result of the increased activity of the local and mucosal immune system is that each bacterial stimulus causes hyperplasia or metaplasia of the superficial epithelium and induces mucosal edema with a relatively cellular infiltrate. The resulting increase of volume of the middle ear mucosa thus sets up a *vicious circle of deteriorating ventilation and drainage*.

This hyperactivity of the middle ear mucosa continues after cessation of the external stimulus and finally leads to *tympanosclerosis*.

Enzymes and the pathologic concentration of metabolic products and mediators of inflammation (lipoids, mucopolysaccharides) cause a progressive metaplasia of the middle ear mucosa resulting in fibrosis and sclerosis of the middle ear and formation of cholesterol granulomas. These changes lead to an irreversible lesion called *tympanosclerosis*.

Basically, two main forms of disorders of ventilation and drainage can be distinguished: the first occurs acutely and is reversible, while the second follows a chronic course which is only partially reversible.

Acute Tubal Occlusion (Serotympanum)

Symptoms. A feeling of pressure in the ear occurs during a head cold (rhinopharyngitis), often accompanied by stabbing pain, deafness, and a crackling noise on swallowing.

Diagnosis. Otoscopy shows a retracted tympanic membrane (see Color Plate **7a**) and injection of the handle of the malleus and of the vessels of the tympanic membrane. If a transudate occurs, there is an amber discoloration of the pars tensa and, on occasion, a fluid level and air bubbles in the middle ear. The patient also has a mild to moderate conductive deafness.

Differential diagnosis. Otitis media must be ruled out.

Treatment. This is directed in the first place to the underlying disease: rhinopharyngitis is treated with decongestant nose drops, vasoconstrictors, and antihistamines to reduce hyperemia and edema in the tube. Antibiotics are given if there is danger of progression to otitis media. Hypertrophied adenoids are removed later if necessary, and sinusitis is treated.

Note: Oral analgesics rather than analgesic ear drops should be used for pain in the ear. Ear drops obliterate the otoscopic appearance of the tympanic membrane by macerating the superficial epithelium and can make recognition of otitis media difficult.

Course and prognosis. The symptoms usually resolve rapidly, but occasionally the disease progresses to a chronic seromucinous otitis media.

Note: The Valsalva maneuver or insufflation of air should not be carried out in the presence of inflammation in the nasopharynx because of the danger of transmission of organisms to the middle ear causing a tubal otitis media.

Chronic Seromucinous Otitis Media

Symptoms. There is a feeling of pressure and fullness in the ear often accompanying an infection of the upper airway and a considerable decrease in hearing on one or both sides. Noises are heard in the ear on yawning, swallowing, and sneezing. Pain is absent.

Pathogenesis. Tubal incompetence and the resulting reduced tympanic pressure are preeminent. Obstructive processes of the nasopharynx, disorders of tubal kinetics, especially incompetence of the muscles opening the tube in cleft palate, and virus infections are the most common underlying mechanisms.

Diagnosis. Otoscopy shows a markedly retracted tympanic membrane with localized protrusion, an exudate in the middle ear, and a dark discoloration behind the tympanic membrane (the so-called "blue drum") with a blackish fluid level or air bubbles. There is a conductive deafness for the entire frequency range of 40 to 50 dB. A typical impedance curve is found. Radiographs in Schueller's view often show opacity of the cell system as a result of the reduction of the air content and exudate. A search for the primary cause shows chronic inflammation of the adenoids, sinusitis, allergy, or tumor (see Color Plate **8b**).

Differential diagnosis includes hemotympanum (the dark-brown exudate behind the tympanic membrane on occasion lends this a bluish tinge) and chronic otitis media evidenced by a perforation, cholesteatoma flakes, and purulent exudate. Adhesions may occur after recurrent otitis shown by a markedly retracted tympanic membrane with thick scars, chalk deposits, and abnormal tubal function.

Treatment. If necessary, surgical restoration of tubal patency by adenoidectomy or re-adenoidectomy under direct vision and elimination of infection of the sinuses.

Paracentesis (Fig. 1.**55**) *and drainage of the middle ear.* The tympanic membrane is incised in the anteroinferior quadrant, under general anesthesia in children and under local anesthesia in adults. The middle ear effusion is aspirated out and long-term drainage is provided for at least 6 months by introduction of a drainage tube (or "grommet") (see Color Plate **7b**).

Steroid injections may be given under antibiotic cover. Mucolytic aerosols are used locally (tubotympanic application of sulfur-containing aerosols by inhalation). Alpha-chymotrypsin is given by tubotympanic, transtym-

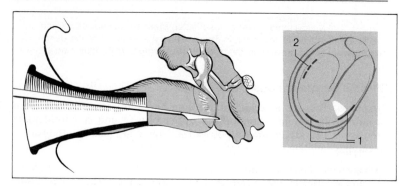

Fig. 1.**55**   Principle of paracentesis: on the left is shown the position of the myringo-tomy knife in relation to the speculum, the external meatus, and the tympanic membrane. On the right is shown the incision in the anterior and posterior lower quadrants of the pars tensa for acute otitis media posteroinferiorly and for drainage of the middle ear cavity, anteroinferiorly. 1, Correct; 2, paracentesis must *never* be done at this site.

panic, or systemic administration. Hyaluronidase and corticosteroids may be given by intratympanic application. Antiallergic treatment includes desensitization on positive evidence of allergies. It is now realized that radiotherapy or local radium to eliminate hypertrophic lymphatic tissue is contraindicated because the therapeutic effect is controversial and there is a danger of induction of cancer at a later period in life.

Course and prognosis. Long-term healing is only achieved in a proportion of patients. In the others there is a progressive chronic course leading to *adhesive processes* as a result of connective tissue organization of the seromucinous exudate and development of cholesterol granuloma and *tympanosclerosis* (see Color Plate **8d**). Hyaline degeneration of the muco-periosteum may also occur with the formation of sclerotic submucosal plaques as a result of local metabolic disturbances (see Color Plate **8b** and **d**).

Syndrome of the Patulous Eustachian Tube

Symptoms. These include *autophony* which is rumbling reverberation of the patient's own voice, and a noise in the ears synchronous with breathing as a result of movements of the tympanic membrane and resonance in the nasopharynx.

Pathogenesis. The symptoms represent a masking effect of the lower and middle tones evoked by resonance and respiratory noise. The primary cause is insufficiency of the closing mechanism of the tube (see p. 5). The secondary cause is disappearance of the fat bolster around the opening of the tube, a gaping ostium caused by hormonal disturbances, and possibly also by use of the contraceptive pill.

Diagnosis. The diagnosis is made by impedance audiometry and tubal function tests.

Treatment. If possible the basic cause is dealt with. The patient also requires an explanation of the cause of his symptoms.

Nonspecific Inflammation of the Middle Ear and the Mastoid

Note: The inflammatory diseases of the middle ear are important because of their frequency and their life-threatening complications due to the close relationship between the middle ear and the cranial cavity.

Acute Otitis Media

Symptoms. In the *first phase of exudative inflammation* which lasts for 1 to 2 days, there is an increase of temperature to 39° to 40°C, and in severe cases, rigors, and occasionally meningismus in children. The patient has a severe pulsating pain worse by night than by day. There is a muffled noise in the ear synchronous with the pulse, deafness, and sensitivity of the mastoid process to pressure. There is often no fever in older patients.

The *second phase of resistance and demarcation* lasts 3 to 8 days. The pus and middle ear exudate usually discharges spontaneously whereupon the pain and fever subside. This phase can be considerably shortened by early application of an appropriate antibiotic, which also prevents spontaneous perforation of the tympanic membrane.

In the *third healing phase* lasting 2 to 4 weeks, the aural discharge dries up and the hearing returns to normal.

Note: An acute middle ear inflammation may follow a serious course even if the tympanic membrane does not perforate.

Pathogenesis

Note: In healthy subjects the middle ear is sterile if the tympanic membrane is intact.

Routes of infection. The tubal route is the most common. *Hematogenous* infection is unusual and occurs in measles, scarlet fever, typhus, and septicemia. *Exogenous* infection requires rupture of the tympanic membrane or preceding perforation allowing penetration of bath water or dirt during irrigation of the ear. Incorrect methods for the removal of a foreign body from the external meatus are also another a cause.

Type of organism. In 90% of patients the infection is monomicrobial. The infecting organisms in decreasing order of frequency are: streptococci in adults, pneumococci in children, *Hemophilus influenzae,* staphylococci, and coliforms. A viral infection may prepare the way for secondary bacterial infection. The inflammation usually affects not only the mucosa of the middle ear, but also that of the entire pneumatic system.

Note: Every attack of acute otitis media is accompanied by mastoiditis.

Diagnosis. In the *first phase, otoscopy* shows hyperemia, then moist infiltration and opacity of the surface of the tympanic membrane. The contours of the handle of the malleus and its short process disappear (see Color Plates **7c**).

In influenzal otitis (see Color Plate **7d**), hemorrhagic bullae form on the external auditory meatus and the tympanic membrane. The patient has a conductive deafness. At the height of the exudative phase, the tympanic membrane bulges, especially its posterosuperior quadrant. Pulsation is also seen. The inflammation may extend to the external meatus obliterating the boundary between the meatus and the tympanic membrane. The mastoid process is tender to pressure as a result of the accompanying mastoiditis.

In the *second phase* of acute otitis media, immediately before spontaneous rupture, a pinhole-size fistula forms, usually in the posterosuperior quadrant. This discharges a pulsating, thin, fluid, odorless pus. *Radiographs* in Schueller's view show clouding of the cell system *without osteolysis,* i.e., the bony septa appear sharp.

In the *third phase* of acute otitis media, the inflammation and thickening of the tympanic membrane resolve, the pulsations disappear, and the discharge becomes mucoid and finally ceases. The perforation closes spontaneously leaving a fine scar. The hearing returns to normal. *Radiography* shows gradual clearing of the cell system.

Differential diagnosis. One must consider *otitis externa.* In the latter disease, there is pain on pressure on the tragus, the exudate is not pulsating, is usually fetid, and is never mucoid. There is little or no deafness, and the cell system appears normal on radiographs.

Treatment

1. Systemic antibiotics in high dosages are given, not only until the symptoms abate but for a further 10 days. Amoxycillin and other broad-spectrum penicillins are indicated.

2. Culture and sensitivity tests are performed and appropriate antibiotics given if the tympanic membrane perforates.
3. Nasal drops are given to decongest the mucosa of the nasopharynx around the opening of the tube.

Paracentesis (see Fig. 1.**55**) in the following circumstances:

- Marked bulging of the tympanic membrane
- Persisting high fever and severe pain
- Unsatisfactory spontaneous perforation with incomplete differentiation of the tympanic membrane
- As a diagnostic measure for the symptoms of early mastoiditis with discrete facial palsy, acute meningitis, or labyrinthitis when the appearances of the tympanic membrane are inconclusive

---

Note: Drops containing cortisone and antibiotic solution should not be used locally for aural discharge. They are useless, and also carry the danger of development of resistance to antibiotics. However, regular meatal toilet should be carried out for acute otitis media after the tympanic membrane perforates. The meatus may be irrigated at body temperature. The external meatus is then dried. The meatus is dusted with antibacterial and antimycotic powder. Closure of the meatus by cotton wool or gauze strips provides the ideal moist environment for inoculation with gram-negative bacteria or fungi. The meatus must therefore be kept open.

Aftercare. If the eustachian tube remains closed, it should be opened by politzerization or catheterization of the tube by an otologist. The paranasal sinuses and the nasopharynx should be checked, and adenoidectomy may be required later.

Course and prognosis. In the *first acute phase*, there is a danger of *early otogenic complications* depending on the virulence and resistance of the organism until the patient's own resistance develops and the bacterial infection is controlled by antibiotics.

In the *second phase*, complications occur very rarely. On the other hand, during this period, a *latent otitis media* and a consequent *occult mastoiditis* may develop due to an inadequate dose of antibiotics, increased resistance of the organism, or unsatisfactory resistance on the part of the patient. The general findings of otoscopy then do not correlate with the severity of the pathologic changes taking place in the middle ear and mastoid process. The *paucity of symptoms* leads to a false assumption that the otitis media has healed rapidly and completely. After an apparent *symptom-free interval, late otogenic complications* can occur in the *third phase* (see pp. 93, 108). This course resembles that of the previously dreaded pneumococcal-type III mastoiditis.

In the *third phase*, most cases of acute otitis media and its concurrent mastoiditis heal completely. However, if a *latent otitis media* and *mastoiditis* become established in the second phase, *late otogenic complications* may declare themselves within this third period, i.e., 2 to 3 weeks after the beginning of the otitis. The symptoms include:

- Reappearance of fever
- Recurrence of aural pain and discharge
- Headaches
- Worsening of the general condition
- Elevated erythrocyte sedimentation rate (ESR)

Specific Types

Acute Otitis Media in Infants and Children

Most patients heal without complications, but in a few patients there is a *severe form* characterized by:

- Severe general symptoms with high fever, meningeal and cerebral irritation, vomiting, refusal to eat, and disturbance of sleep
- Immediate improvement of the child's condition after spontaneous perforation or paracentesis
- A protracted course with numerous recurrences or exacerbations with combined otitis media and bronchopneumonia, digestive and feeding upsets, and pyelonephritis

> *Note:* The younger the child, the more severe the generalized symptoms are and the more discrete the local signs are. On occasion the gastrointestinal symptoms are the most pressing.

Infants and young children have a predisposition to tubal middle ear infection because of the short, straight, wide tube, the uniform character of the mucosa of the middle ear and the upper respiratory tract, increased frequency of infections of the respiratory tract, hyperplasia of the lymphoid tissue of Waldeyer's ring, poor aeration of the middle ear cavity which is still partially filled with myxomatous tissue or hyperplastic mucosa, and a difference in the reaction of the general and mucosal immune system determined in part by the genotype and in part by the phenotype.

Local symptoms. These include pressure in the ear, tugging on the diseased ear, and painful reactions to pressure and traction. The tympanic membrane is greyish-red in color and bulges only slightly. Spontaneous perforation is not common; its site of predilection is the anteroinferior quadrant. Discharge is uncommon because pus drains through the short, wide, straight eustachian tube. If a discharge occurs, then it is stringy and pulsating. Mucosal polyps may form in the middle ear; regional retroauricular lymphadenitis causes a swelling behind the ear. If the petrosquamosal fissure is open, the pus may penetrate directly from the middle ear beneath the periosteum causing marked swelling behind the ear.

Treatment. Treatment consists of parenteral antibiotics, nose drops, and analgesics. The ear is irrigated with physiologic saline solution at body temperature.

Paracentesis (see Fig. 1.55) should be carried out early if the tympanic membrane does not perforate spontaneously.

An *antrotomy* should be carried out early, even if the radiographs are normal, if it is indicated on clinical grounds.

Antrotomy is carried out under general anesthesia in infants and young children whose mastoid process is incompletely pneumatized or not pneumatized at all. The infected part of the mastoid process is cleared via a retroauricular access with wide opening and drainage of the *mastoid antrum* (see Fig. 1.56).

The **course** is usually protracted with intermittent exacerbations. There is often quick improvement and healing after surgical treatment of the diseased ear. The prognosis is good with correct treatment, but there is otherwise a danger of the development of a periantral osteomyelitis *(occult infant's antritis)* with vomiting and generalized toxic symptoms. In this case immediate antrotomy is indicated.

Influenzal Otitis

This is a hemorrhagic bullous acute middle ear inflammation (see Color Plate **7d**). Hemorrhagic vesicles form on the tympanic membrane and the skin of the meatus as a result of toxic *capillary damage* and extravasation into the tissues. The most common causative organism is *Hemophilus influenzae*. Primary infection with influenza A virus combined with a secondary bacterial infection *(Streptococcus pneumoniae)* can take a fulminating course and lead within a short time to complications such as facial paralysis, labyrinthine irritation, and meningitis.

Measles Otitis

This condition is a hematogenous viral otitis media with subsequent tubal secondary infection, often leading to a purulent mastoiditis. Because of the prominent general symptoms, it is often overlooked and is only recognized when complications occur.

Scarlatinal Otitis

This is an acute necrotizing inflammation during or following scarlet fever, with the formation of a subtotal perforation of the tympanic membrane, necrosis of the ossicular chain, and osteomyelitis of the temporal bone. It can be prevented by early treatment with antibiotics.

Mastoiditis

The most frequent complication of middle ear inflammation is *mastoiditis,* an extension of the infection from the middle ear cavity to the pneumatic system of the temporal bone. In contrast to the mucosal inflammation which always accompanies otitis media (see p. 87), the infection extends to and causes dissolution of bone. An unusually well-pneumatized bone infection may extend to the petrous pyramid *(petrositis)* and more rarely to the diploe of the *temporal bone* causing *osteomyelitis* of that bone.

Symptoms. Mastoiditis manifests itself by a change in the progress of resolution of acute otitis media.

General. Worsening of the general condition, rise of temperature, leukocytosis with a shift to the left, and markedly increased ESR.

Local. Increasing pain in the ear synchronous with the pulse radiating to the temporal bone and the occiput; reappearance or increase of the aural discharge which is creamy, odorless, and purulent. The patient also has a hearing loss.

Pathogenesis. Acute otitis media and its concomitant mastoiditis usually resolve without complications. Appearance of a complication depends on:

- The anatomic relations of the pneumatic system and the middle ear space. Because of the narrow connection between the antrum and the mastoid cells, there is poor aeration from the eustachian tube.
- The virulence and resistance of the organism.
- The local immune resistance of the mucosa.
- The general immune resistance of the patient.
- The general condition of the patient. Generalized diseases such as diabetes, allergy, and disorders of the liver and kidneys are important.

Diagnosis

- Aural discharge
- Tenderness to pressure over the mastoid
- Retroauricular swelling with a protruding ear

This *classical triad of symptoms* is now seldom seen because otitis media is treated with antibiotics. This is especially true of the critical period which used to occur in the 3rd week, during the preantibiotic era. The symptoms of mastoiditis are more discrete and its course more insidious than in former years so that this complication is easily overlooked. For this reason, the following *otoscopic findings* that are also present under antibiotic treatment must be treated with respect:

- A pale but still thickened tympanic membrane
- Circumscribed inflammation and thickening of the tympanic membrane in the posterosuperior quadrant
- Thickened opaque tympanic membrane
- Formation of a nipple on the tympanic membrane with a fine pinpoint fistulous opening
- Prolapse of the posterior meatal wall which occurs relatively often in small children (see p. 4)

Local Findings Over the Mastoid Process and the Surrounding Area

1. Soggy swelling of the skin is caused by edema due to extension of the infection.
2. Reddening and a taut, elastic, fluctuating swelling of the skin over the mastoid process due to a subperiosteal abscess occur (see Color Plate **8a**).

3. There is swelling of the zygomatic process with extension to the cheek and eyelids in an extensively pneumatized bone. This is relatively common in children.
4. Visible and palpable tender swelling of the lateral triangle of the neck with torticollis occurs. This is due to an abscess tracking from the mastoid apex in the fascial spaces of the digastric, sternocleidomastoid, splenius, and longissimus capitis muscles *(Bezold's mastoiditis).*
5. *Radiographs in Schueller's view* show a decrease in radiolucency due to reduction of the air content in the pneumatic system, *haziness and opacity of the mastoid cells,* haziness of the fine bony structures as a result of decalcification and liquefaction of the bony septa between the cells, and *bone destruction with foci of liquefaction.*

Differential diagnosis from pseudomastoiditis in otitis externa (see p. 73).
Furuncle. This causes a swelling restricted to the cartilaginous meatus and never causes prolapse of the posterosuperior meatal wall close to the tympanic membrane. Furthermore, the patient always has pain on pressure on the tragus. *Parotitis* should be differentiated from inflammation of the cells in the zygomatic process, as should a *cervical lymphadenitis.*

Treatment

Note: A mastoiditis in which the inflammation is no longer confined to the mucosa but has extended to the bone should be treated by surgery.

It is incorrect to assume that inflammation of the pneumatic system of the temporal bone can be healed by antibiotics if it has invaded the bony structures. The poor vascularization of the mucosa and bone prevents maintenance of a satisfactory concentration of antibiotic in the tissues. The poorly aerated cells filled with hyperplastic mucosa and granulations are an ideal culture medium for bacteria, especially of the anaerobic variety.

Indications for mastoidectomy. This operation is indicated at any stage of otitis media for the following:

- Symptoms of otogenic intracranial complications
- Signs of a subperiosteal collection
- A focus of liquefaction on mastoid radiographs in Schueller's view
- A facial paralysis

In the healing phase, i.e., in the critical 3rd week of otitis media, the operation is also indicated for:

- Recurrence of aural discharge, pain, and subfebrile temperature
- Worsening of the general condition and an increase of the ESR
- Aural discharge persisting for 4 to 5 weeks and resisting treatment, in the presence of good pneumatization of the temporal bone, with reduced air content on radiographs, and without serious generalized symptoms

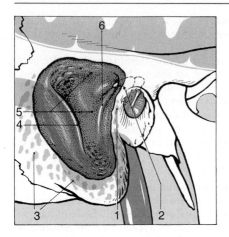

Fig. 1.**56** Principle of cortical mastoidectomy: posterior meatal wall (1) and attic wall (2) remain intact whereas the cell system of the mastoid process (3) is cleared via a retroauricular approach. The anatomy of the external auditory meatus is not changed by this operation. Sigmoid sinus (4), mastoid cavity (5) and facial nerve (mastoid segment) (6).

Principle of mastoidectomy. The diseased tissue in the cell system of the mastoid process is excised via a retroauricular skin incision under general anesthesia. A wide connection is created between the mastoid antrum and the mastoid cavity, and thus from the latter to the middle ear cavity (Fig. 1.**56**).

Antrotomy. See p. 91.

Course and prognosis. Two forms of true mastoiditis with bone destruction can develop from the *mastoiditis accompanying* otitis media, even under antibiotic treatment:

Acute mastoiditis. This is marked by purulent liquefaction of the bony septa of the pneumatic system with external rupture to form a subperiosteal or retroauricular abscess. The course is rapid and the symptoms marked. Paresis of the facial nerve is possible.

Chronic mastoiditis. This is partly a productive inflammation with obliteration of the spaces of the pneumatic system by inflammatory granulation tissue and partly a continuous inflammatory breakdown of bone. The course is therefore insidious, and the symptoms are initially mild.

Prognosis is good with correct treatment, but otherwise there is a danger of late otogenic complications.

Chronic Otitis Media

Chronic Mucosal Inflammation

Symptoms. *There is a chronic discharge of mucoid, purulent, odorless exudate.* The otitis demonstrates periods of complete freedom from symptoms, alternating with acute exacerbation. The exudate may be creamy and purulent in the acute phase and then becomes mucoid and stringy as the infection resolves. It is, however, always odorless.

Hearing. The patient has a conductive deafness.

Pain is absent, and the *general condition* is good.

Pathogenesis. This is not a disease with a unique cause, but it is the end result of several different primary disease processes. The inflammation remains confined to the mucosa but can in certain patients lead in time to a rarifying osteitis, i.e., a chronic inflammatory destruction of the ossicles, e.g., the long process of the incus. In contrast to cholesteatoma, this destructive process of bone is unusual and less likely to extend and progress. Vascular obliteration can occur due to heavy scar tissue deposits in the vascular subepithelial connective tissue layer, leading secondarily to nutritional disturbances of the neighboring bony tissue (aseptic bone necrosis).

Pathogenetic factors:

- Constitutional reduced mucosal (immunological) competence (see pp. 8–10)
- Type, pathogenicity, virulence, and resistance of the bacterial organisms
- Anatomic conditions of the middle ear such as pneumatization, and the connections between the attic, antrum, middle ear cavity, and eustachian tube
- Disordered function of the eustachian tube, i.e., in patients with cleft palate
- Generalized diseases such as allergy, immune defects, cachexia, and diabetes

Diagnosis

The history shows a chronic recurrent aural discharge with reduced hearing. *The otoscopic findings* include a central defect of the tympanic membrane (see Color Plate **8c**), scarring of the pars tensa, and occasionally aural polyps due to mucosal hyperplasia in acute exacerbations.

Radiographs. Schueller's view shows either reduced pneumatization or opacity of the cell system, if it is well pneumatized, and occasionally signs of bony destruction and formation of new bone (sclerosis). These are regarded as the signs of *chronic mastoiditis.*

The *audiogram* shows a conductive deafness.

Differential Diagnosis

Cholesteatoma is associated with a marginal defect of the tympanic membrane and a fetid discharge.

Aural tuberculosis shows several central perforations of the tympanic membrane with marked deafness.

Middle ear carcinoma causes a marginal defect with exuberant tissue extending into the meatus and bone destruction of the attic and the meatal wall.

Treatment

Conservative measures to dry up the middle ear. The external meatus is cleaned periodically. It may be irrigated with physiologic saline at body temperature. In the acute phase pus is taken for culture and sensitivity tests, and the appropriate systemic and local antibiotics are given, taking care not to use ototoxic drugs. In the chronic phase of slight otorrhea with mucosal hyperplasia, 3 % resorcinol-alcohol solution or 1 : 1,000 potassium permanganate solution may be used.

Note: This form of treatment by irrigation with these medications is not practiced in the United States.

Aural polyps are removed with a wire snare. Chronic infection of the nasopharynx and paranasal sinuses must be looked for.

Surgery. Mastoidectomy may be carried out to eliminate the foci of infection in the temporal bone and the middle ear cavity. A *tympanoplasty* may be carried out to reconstruct the sound-conducting apparatus, i.e., the tympanic membrane and the ossicular chain.

Course and prognosis. The course is episodic with exacerbations caused by exogenous infection from bath water, etc., and tubal infection. Complications are very rare. Progression to cholesteatoma is exceptional and deafness is usually progressive. The prognosis as regards life is good but as regards function is poor. Therefore, *an early tympanoplasty should be undertaken after intensive preparation* (see Fig. 1.**62a–l**).

Every patient with chronic mucosal inflammation should be treated as early as possible by *tympanoplasty* since the destruction of the sound-conducting apparatus increases with every inflammatory episode. If a hearing aid is necessary, a tympanoplasty is also indicated since chronic otorrhea renders the wearing of an earpiece impossible.

Note: Chronic mucosal inflammation is a form of chronic otitis media in which the inflammation is mainly confined to the mucosa. It usually does not cause progressive bone destruction and therefore is free of complication, but runs a protracted course.

Acquired Cholesteatoma of the Middle Ear

Symptoms

- Fetid otorrhea which is sometimes minimal or completely absent, when present always purulent, and never mucoid
- Progressive deafness, possibly dizziness

- Otalgia and fever in acute exacerbations
- Dull headaches or a feeling of pressure in the head

Pathogenesis

Note: An acquired middle ear cholesteatoma is not a tumor but a chronic inflammation which, unlike chronic mucosal inflammation, causes progressive destruction of the cells and bony structures.

Promoting Factors

- Disordered ventilation and drainage of the middle ear (chronic reduction of pressure) with hypopneumatization
- Displaced squamous epithelium as a result of increased capacity for growth of the meatal skin in the upper part of the anulus tympanicus (the papillary ingrowths form the later *matrix* either as a result of invagination of the pars flaccida or by formation of a retention pocket in the pars tensa)
- An increased proliferative tendency of the stratum germinativum (see Fig. 1.6) caused by the stimulus of inflammation
- Incompletely resolved embryonal hyperplastic mesenchymal remnants in the submucosa of the middle ear which later form the *perimatrix*

Histopathogenesis

A *cholesteatoma* may form a compact sac of desquamated lamellae arranged like the layers of an onion and connected with a fairly thick pedicle to its site of origin from the tympanic membrane (the pars flaccida or tensa). Alternatively, it consists of a widely fanned-out cholesteatoma matrix lining the antrum and mastoid cavity and sending off shoots into the furthest bony niches of the bony process. The latter type of cholesteatoma therefore shows a reticular or dendritic branched structure. The latter occurs more commonly in a tensa cholesteatoma than in a flaccida cholesteatoma. The *bone destruction* is caused first by *enzymes* (e.g., collagenase) formed in the perimatrix and second by *osteoclastic destruction* of bony tissue, i.e., a chronic osteomyelitis.

Note: A prerequisite for the development of a cholesteatoma is direct contact of the keratinizing squamous epithelium in the external meatus with mucoperiosteum of the middle ear which has been damaged by inflammation.

This can happen as a result of:

- A *marginal perforation* with a destruction of the protective barrier of the anulus fibrosus
- *Papillary ingrowths,* e.g., in the region of the pars flaccida or of the destroyed anulus fibrosus
- Formation of a *retraction pocket* of the pars tensa

- *Traumatic displacement of keratinizing squamous epithelium* after longitudinal pyramidal fractures or ruptures of the tympanic membrane with the development of a posttraumatic otitis media

The same pathogenetic factors (see p. 95) also apply to the genesis of cholesteatoma as to that of chronic mucosal inflammation.

Diagnosis. An inflammatory middle ear cholesteatoma may be classified from several different points of view (primary, secondary, or topographical anatomy). The method depending on the *site of origin* appears to be the most sensible from the diagnostic point of view and clearer than the above-named classifications. Cholesteatoma can thus be classified as follows:

- *Tensa cholesteatoma* (synonym: secondary middle ear cholesteatoma)
- *Flaccida cholesteatoma* (synonym: primary or genuine attic or epitympanic cholesteatoma)
- *Occult cholesteatoma* (synonym: cholesteatoma behind an intact tympanic membrane or a congenital cholesteatoma)

The *tensa cholesteatoma* (Fig. 1.**57**) develops from a *retraction pocket* caused by chronic inflammation usually in the posterosuperior quadrant of the pars tensa. It is characterized by a posterosuperior *marginal perforation.* Inflammatory *granulations,* fetid exudate with *flakes of cholesteatoma,* and circumscribed destruction of the surrounding *posterosuperior meatal wall* are often found in the region of the edge of the perforation. A conductive deafness is also present due to destruction of the ossicular chain. The site of predeliction is the incudostapedial joint.

The *flaccida cholesteatoma* (Figs. 1.**58a—c**, 1.**59a** and **b**; see Color Plate **9a** and **b**) arises from papillary ingrowth of the keratinizing squamous epithelium in the region of Shrapnell's membrane in the presence of simultaneous chronic epitympanitis. The stimulus of inflammation induces increased proliferation of the squamous epithelium. The characteristic of this type of cholesteatoma is therefore a circumscribed *perforation of the pars flaccida* often covered by a *crust* and usually also accompanied by *destruction of the lateral attic wall.* Medial to this lies *inflammatory granulation tissue* and fetid exudate with *flakes of cholesteatoma.* The patient has a conductive deafness and also involvement of the inner ear in the advanced stages.

Occult cholesteatoma develops gradually and remains for a long time without causing symptoms *behind an intact tympanic membrane* with no demonstrable perforation. In most cases, it is a *flaccida cholesteatoma* which develops *without a perforation* by papillary ingrowth into the epitympanum, extending from there to the neighboring middle ear space (Fig. 1.**60**). The pneumatization and the mucosal folds determine the pathways of spread of the cholesteatoma. In rare cases it may be a *congenital cholesteatoma.*

Fig. 1.**57**   Development of a tensa cholesteatoma. Chronic impairment of middle ear ventilation causes a reversible retraction of the pars
tensa in the posterosuperior quadrant. Intermittent middle ear infections lead to an atrophy
of the tympanic membrane (due to loss of its
supporting collagenous framework) and finally
to the development of a reversible, deep retraction pocket *(potential cholesteatoma)*. Repeated middle ear infections will then cause
adhesion to the promontory, to the long crus of
the incus, or to the facial nerve canal, trans-
forming the invaginated, atrophic tympanic
membrane into an irreversible, fixed retraction
pocket *(prospective cholesteatoma)*. Deprived
of its natural self-cleansing mechanism, the

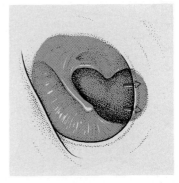

pocket tends to retain cellular debris, which forms a culture medium for gram-negative
proteolytic organisms. Bacterial endotoxins incite a papillary growth of the squamous
epithelium covering the inner surface of the retraction pocket, which eventually forms the
matrix for an *active tensa cholesteatoma* (see Color Plates **8b** and **9b**).

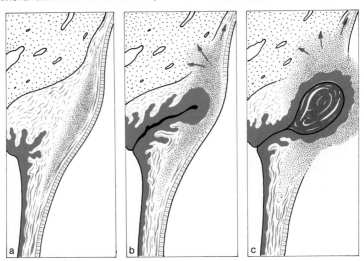

Fig. 1.**58a–c** Histologic pathogenesis of an attic cholesteatoma: **a.** Papillary down-
growth of the stratum corneum, the future matrix, of the pars flaccida toward the attic.
The connective tissue is loose, and the submucosa, the future perimatrix is hyperplastic and chronically inflamed. **b.** Invagination of the pars flaccida into the attic as the
result of hypoventilation and reduced pressure in the epitympanum. The future matrix
contacts the perimatrix and there is early bone destruction. **c.** Activation of the basal
cell layer of the matrix by chronic inflammation. Proliferation of keratinizing squamous
epithelium, destruction and undermining of the mucosa in the middle ear, replacement
by the "foreign" squamous epithelium from the invaginated pars flaccida, and formation
of a cholesteatoma sac.

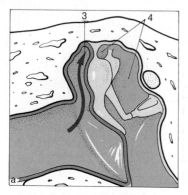
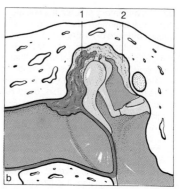

Fig. 1.**59a** and **b**   Development of an attic cholesteatoma. **a.** Retraction and invagination of the pars flaccida into the epitympanum occurs as a result of persistent reduced pressure in the middle ear. The keratinized squamous epithelium is thus displaced into the middle ear. **b.** Chronic inflammation causes hyperplasia of the mucosa of the attic and thus prevents satisfactory aeration of this region. 1, Cholesteatoma sac; 2, hyperplastic mucosa and "mesenchymal cushion" of the attic; 3, invaginated pars flaccida; 4, attic.

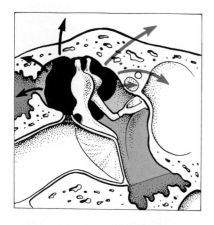

Fig. 1.**60**   Pathways of extension of a cholesteatoma: posteriorly toward the sigmoid sinus and the middle and posterior cranial fossa, or anteriorly toward the facial canal, the internal meatus, or the labyrinth. (See also Fig. 1.**4**.)

Common Diagnostic Characteristics

Radiography: Schueller's and *Stenvers' views* show limited pneumatization. *Axial and coronal high-resolution CT* of the temporal bone is now recognized as the most useful and versatile procedure for demonstrating bone destruction in the petrous pyramid, soft-tissue abnormalities in the middle ear, and extension of the cholesteatoma into the cranial cavity.

Audiometry. The *audiogram* shows a conductive deafness possibly combined with sensorineural deafness. Extension into the labyrinth causes progressive sensorineural deafness and facial paralysis.

Vestibular tests. Provided the labyrinthine capsule is intact, spontaneous and provoked vestibular nystagmus do not occur. Erosion of the lateral semicircular canal causes a positive fistula sign (see p. 69).

Facial nerve. Erosion of the bony canal of the facial nerve and its mastoid or tympanic segment, or extension into the internal meatus, first causes neurapraxia and later progressive axonotmesis.

Differential Diagnosis

- *Inactive chronic mucosal inflammation* with adhesions between the promontory and an atrophic pars tensa
- *Carcinoma of the middle ear or external meatus*
- *Tuberculosis of the middle ear*

Treatment

Conservative treatment with antibiotics, irrigation of the ear (also with a drainage tube), and antibiotic and corticosteroid-containing ear drops are ineffective because antibiotics (systemic or local) cannot control the local inflammation or the displacement of squamous epithelium into the middle ear space.

> *Note:* There are two goals of *surgery* for cholesteatoma: first, the *radical elimination of inflammation* by removal of the matrix, perimatrix, and invaded bone and second, *the maintenance and reconstruction of the sound-conducting apparatus.*

Before the discovery of chemotherapy and antibiotics, the *surgical treatment* of cholesteatoma was limited to the *radical* removal of the inflammatory process without regard to the maintenance or improvement of hearing since the elimination of a potential intracranial infection had first priority.

Radical operation (Fig. 1.**61**). The attic, middle ear cavity, antrum, and infected pneumatic spaces of the mastoid process are exposed by a retroauricular, or by endaural, access. Unlike a cortical mastoidectomy, the bony posterior meatal wall and the lateral attic wall are removed and the middle ear cavity thus brought into continuity with the external meatus. The cholesteatoma-matrix and perimatrix are removed radically under the microscope. The radical cavity heals in a matter of weeks by acquiring an epidermal layer. The disadvantage of this operation is that the sound-conducting chain is not reconstructed so that the functional result is generally poor. Furthermore, there is an open connection between the middle ear, the mastoid cavity, and the external auditory meatus so that chronic otorrhea is common due to tubal or exogenous infection.

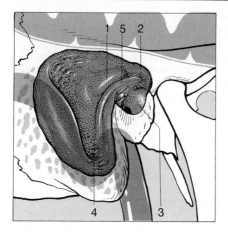

Fig. 1.**61**   Principle of radical mastoidectomy. The mastoid is eburnized and the antrum (1), the attic (2), the middle ear cavity (3), and the small mastoid cavity (4) are opened widely. Dissection of the bony facial canal up to the second knee (tympanic segment, (5). These structures are united in a common cavity opening into the external meatus. If a *tympanoplasty* is to be carried out, then a *modified radical operation* is performed, i. e., the middle ear cavity is closed off from the mastoid cavity and the sound-conducting apparatus is reconstructed.

Tympanoplasty (Fig. 1.**62a–l**)

Purpose of the operation:

1. Radical removal of the cholesteatoma with its matrix and perimatrix
2. Reconstruction of *sound pressure protection of the round window and of the sound pressure transformation between the tympanic membrane and the oval window* by means of:

● Closure of the perforation of the tympanic membrane with fascia or perichondrium
● Reconstruction of the direct connection between the tympanic membrane and stapes footplate if the ossicular chain is defective, i.e., construction of a columella to bridge the defect using a bone, cartilage, or synthetic prosthesis
● Separation of the middle ear cavity from the external meatus by reconstruction of the posterior meatal and lateral attic walls by bony or cartilaginous graft or preservation of the intact bony meatal wall

Radical elimination of the infection and reconstruction of the sound-conducting apparatus are now usually carried out in a one-stage procedure, but a *radical mastoidectomy* is still carried out occasionally in preference to a *tympanoplasty* for the following indications:

1. Cholesteatoma with intracranial complications
2. Cholesteatoma with facial nerve paralysis
3. Extensive reticular-dendritic cholesteatoma in a well-pneumatized temporal bone (see p. 97)

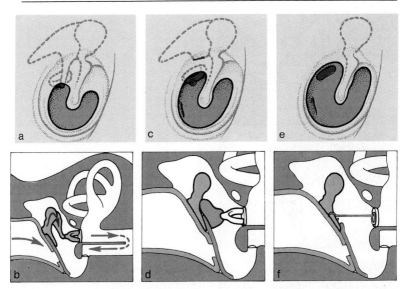

Fig. 1.**62** Principles of tympanoplasty (**a** through **f**). **a.** Simple perforation of the tympanic membrane; the ossicular chain is intact. **b.** Underlay graft of the defect in the pars tensa and reconstruction of the sound pressure protection and transformation mechanism. **c.** Tympanic membrane perforation with a defect of the long process of the incus. **d.** Closure of the perforation. Reconstruction of the sound-conductive apparatus by interposition of bone or cartilage between the malleus and the stapes, the columella effect. **e.** Defect of the incus and stapes with retention of the long process of the malleus and the footplate of the stapes in a subtotal perforation of the tympanic membrane. **f.** Bridging of the defect of the ossicular chain by interposition of a metal, synthetic, or ceramic prosthesis.

A *tympanoplasty* is then carried out at a second sitting after the infection has healed.

Course and prognosis (see Fig. 1.**60**). Untreated cholesteatoma is the most dangerous form of chronic middle ear inflammation. A patient who appears to be in perfectly good health and who has had no warning symptoms may at any time develop the following life-threatening intracranical complications:

- Labyrinthitis and meningitis
- Sinus thrombosis and septicemia
- Epi- or subdural abscess with meningitis
- Temporal lobe or cerebellar abscess

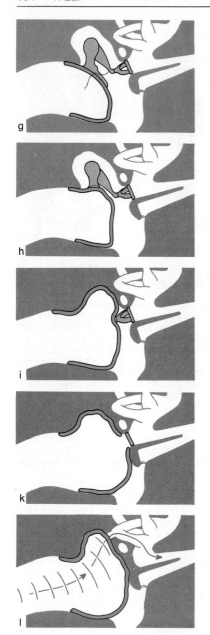

Fig. 1.**62.** The five classical types of tympanoplasty defined by Wullstein (**g** through **l**). Type I, simple myringoplasty. The perforation of the tympanic membrane is closed by fascia or perichondrium. **h.** Type II, reconstruction of the defective ossicular chain by bridging the defect with autologous bone or cartilage grafts, eventually with homograft ossicle substitution. **i.** Type III. Direct transmission of the sound waves from the tympanic membrane to the stapes by the columella effect. A shallow tympanum is created. **k.** Type IV. The ossicular chain is absent. The sound is transmitted directly to the oval window, and sound protection is provided for the round window. A small tympanum is formed. **l.** Type V. Here the oval window is completely closed by bony fixation of the footplate. A window is made into the horizontal semicircular canal so that sound is transmitted directly to this fenestration as in the similar operation for otosclerosis. Both type IV and V have now been abandoned in favor of the interposition of an artificial columnella (type IV) or instead of a type V by removing the footplate and interposing a bony, cartilaginous, or synthetic prosthesis as in stapedectomy for otosclerosis (see Fig. 1.**65**).

> *Note:* Conservative treatment almost never achieves healing of a cholesteatoma. Surgery is therefore always indicated (apart from occasional contraindications on general grounds) because of the danger of intracranial complications.

Congenital Cholesteatoma of the Temporal Bone

This is a rare cholesteatoma with no obvious connection with the external meatus or tympanic membrane. Usually, it is an occult cholesteatoma behind an intact tympanic membrane and only exceptionally does it develop from an embryonal ectodermal remnant within the temporal bone. It is also known as true or primary cholesteatoma.

Course of Specific Forms of Cholesteatoma

A cholesteatoma is rare in *infants and young children* but it increases in frequency after the age of 6 years.

Cholesteatoma is relatively rare in *old age*. It is then usually due to reactivation of an old inflammatory process which proceeds insidiously and can first manifest itself by the appearance of complications such as dizziness, rapidly progressive deafness, facial paralysis, or meningitis. The disease may be serious in *diabetics* because of reduction of general resistance and local tissue metabolic disorders, with progressive bone destruction, formation of sequestra, and invasion of the labyrinth, the facial canal, and the cranial cavity. A *petrositis* with an epi- or subdural abscess may develop insidiously, and the prognosis is then extremely poor. The postoperative healing process is often prolonged in diabetics with cholesteatoma.

A *meatal cholesteatoma* can arise either due to the pathologic proliferative tendency of the meatal epidermal lining in the bony part, or it may be the result of a rupture of a middle ear cholesteatoma from the antrum into the part of the meatus immediately lateral to the tympanic membrane.

A *posttraumatic cholesteatoma* arises as a result of a longitudinal pyramidal fracture extending into the external meatus. This allows meatal epidermis or a part of the tympanic membrane to be displaced into the middle ear space. This displaced keratinizing squamous epithelium first forms an innocent epidermal cyst; a bone-destroying cholesteatoma with a matrix and perimatrix arises later after the cyst becomes infected.

Adhesive Otitis (Middle Ear Fibrosis) (see Color Plate **8b**)

Symptoms. The tympanic membrane is retracted, scarred, and thickened but intact. The patient has a severe conductive deafness (see Color Plate **8b**).

Pathogenesis. The origin lies in recurrent otitis with cicatricial fibrosis of the poorly aerated middle ear, formation of cholesterol granuloma (see p. 83), and fixation of the ossicular chain.

Otogenic Infective Complications (Figs. 1.63 and 1.64)

Labyrinthitis

Symptoms. Dizziness, nausea, vomiting, whistling noises in the ears, and deafness develop within a brief period. The patient has no fever and no pain.

Pathogenesis. Toxins diffuse through the labyrinthine windows in *acute otitis media*, and the infection extends along the vessels (see p. 108).

In *chronic otitis media*, with cholesteatoma a fistula forms into the laby-

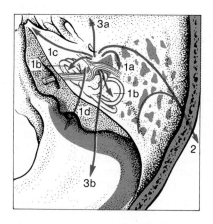

Fig. 1.**63** Pathogenesis and pathways of spread of otogenic complications. Intratemporal complications:
1a, Otogenic facial paralysis; 1b, labyrinthitis; 1c, petrositis; 1d, sinus thrombosis. Extratemporal complications: 2, external rupture of mastoiditis to form a subperiosteal abscess. Intracranial complications: 3a, extension into the middle cranial fossa to cause meningitis or temporal lobe abscess; 3b, extension to the posterior cranial fossa to cause meningitis or cerebellar abscess.

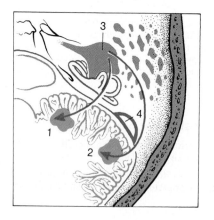

Fig. 1.**64** Extension of otitis media into the posterior cranial fossa and development of a cerebellar abscess: 1, presinus abscess; 2, postsinus abscess, 3, middle ear cavity; 4, sigmoid sinus.

rinth, and the infection extends directly into the perilymphatic space. After *a transverse fracture of the temporal bone or operative trauma*, there is direct damage to the membranous labyrinth with secondary infection.

Diagnosis. The patient has the cochlear and vestibular symptoms of a rapidly progressive inner ear failure.

Differential diagnosis. Ménière's disease, sudden deafness, and acute vestibulopathy.

Treatment. Intravenous antibiotics are administered in high doses by continuous infusion. The middle ear should be drained, and a mastoidectomy may need to be carried out. A radical mastoidectomy is carried out for cholesteatoma. Surgery is only undertaken after fractures if there is a simultaneous CSF otorrhea, facial nerve paralysis, or meningitis. Labyrinthectomy must be carried out for purulent labyrinthitis with meningitis.

Course and prognosis. Because of the varying pathologic anatomy, several different clinical forms of labyrinthitis are possible: serous in posttraumatic or viral cases, purulent due to bacterial invasion of the perilymphatic space, circumscribed due to a labyrinthine fistula in cholesteatoma, and generalized with involvement of the entire labyrinth due to extension of infection or generalized infection. In the latter form the course is fulminant with irreversible total loss of function. Possible extension of the infection to the meninges.

Epidural Empyema

Symptoms. Dull pulsating pain in the head, otorrhea, and subfebrile temperature occur. There is no completely characteristic pattern of symptoms.

Pathogenesis. Acute or chronic infection extends from the mastoid process into the epidural space due to destruction of the inner table by infection. The infection may also spread by preformed pathways along the perforating vessels in the bone which remains intact.

Diagnosis. This disease is characterized by a paucity of symptoms. It is usually an incidental finding at mastoidectomy, but may be demonstrated by neuroradiologic techniques including angiography and computed tomography.

Treatment. Immediate mastoidectomy with wide exposure of the dura, drainage, and antibiotics are indicated.

Course and prognosis. The prognosis is good if the disease is recognized early. Otherwise there is the danger of development of pachymeningitis with extension to the leptomeninges.

Subdural empyemata are rare and only occur during the course of a diffuse meningitis.

Otogenic Meningitis

Symptoms. These include headaches, stiffness of the neck, scaphoid abdomen, increasing loss of consciousness, photophobia, restlessness, tonic-clonic convulsions, and facial paralysis. Otorrhea, otalgia, and even deafness may be absent or occult. Typically there is bounding pulse, irregular breathing, and a fever of 39° to 40°C. The patient may have an oculomotor or abducens paralysis and abnormal optic fundi.

Pathogenesis. The cause is spread of an acute or chronic bacterial infection, usually due to pneumococci, into the subarachnoid space:

- By *direct continuity* due to inflammatory destruction of the bony walls
- *Along preformed pathways* via the perforating vessels and nerves in the bone, e.g., via the caroticotympanic nerves
- By a thrombophlebitis extending along the diploic veins
- *Via the labyrinth* and as a result of spread into the internal auditory meatus (this is rare)

Diagnosis. In addition to the typical clinical symptoms of acute meningitis, including abnormalities of the cerebrospinal fluid (CSF), there are signs of an acute, subacute, or chronic middle ear inflammation of varying degrees of severity. If the hearing is more or less normal, and the otoscopic findings are equivocal, the signs of the inflammation of the pneumatic system on radiographs of the temporal bone (in Schueller's view, Stenver's view, or tomography) can be decisive in making the diagnosis and the decision to operate.

The *CSF* shows pleocytosis, a marked increase of protein, and a reduced sugar and chloride content. The pressure is greater than 200 mm Hg. In the acute phase, bacteria, usually pneumococci, can be found in the fluid.

Differential diagnosis includes viral or epidemic meningococcal meningitis and tuberculous meningitis (low sugar level).

Treatment. Antibiotics are given intravenously in high dosages determined by sensitivity tests, e.g., penicillin 40 to 60 million U in 24 h for a pneumococcal infection. Repeated lumbar or suboccipital punctures are done.

The *blood-brain barrier* for antibiotics varies greatly depending on the severity of the meningitis. Some of the antibiotic is inactivated by binding to the CSF protein. Cephalosporins of third generation like ceftazidime (antipseudomonal cephalosporin and therefore useful for otogenic meningitis due to chronic otitis media), cefotaxime, and ceftriaxone penetrate the blood barrier very well. In contrast, the aminoglycosides including gentamicin, the broad-spectrum penicillins, and chloramphenicol do not penetrate well even in the presence of meningeal inflammation, and when they are used (rarely), they are given intrathecally. Intrathecal antibiotics are only used in exceptional cases. Immediate drainage of the middle ear cavity by mastoidectomy or radical mastoidectomy is required, with wide exposure of the dura.

Course and prognosis. The disease ends fatally if it is untreated or not treated correctly. The prospects of recovery are about 90% provided that the otitis media is recognized early as the cause of the meningitis and provided that energetic treatment is begun.

> *Note:* Any unexplained attack of meningitis must be suspected as having a nasal or aural cause.

In doubtful cases with obscure otoscopic and radiographic findings, the risk of an exploratory operation is less than that of an expectant policy if the middle ear space is infected. Intensive treatment by antibiotics does not cause resolution so long as the primary focus of infection has not been eliminated by surgery.

Otogenic Sinus Thrombosis

Symptoms. A perisinus abscess, periphlebitis, and incipient sinus thrombosis cause the same diagnostic difficulties as an epidural empyema. The release of emboli of infective thrombi alone causes the characteristic signs of *septicemia*. These include:

- Chills
- A spiking temperature chart, with several peaks on the same day
- Increased pulse rate
- Headaches
- Vomiting
- Somnolence
- Neck stiffness (accompanying meningitis)
- Dyspnea due to septic lung metastases or pneumonia
- Jaundice due to septic metastases in the liver or to nonspecific reactive hepatitis

Pathogenesis. Infection due to mastoiditis or cholesteatoma destroys bone in continuity so that it can rupture into the perisinus space. A perisinus abscess forms with periphlebitis of the sigmoid sinus followed by sinus phlebitis. The thrombus is initially mural but later it occludes the lumen and extends superiorly to involve the transverse and sagittal sinuses and the mastoid emissary vein and inferiorly toward the internal jugular vein.

The thrombus undergoes thrombolysis due to bacterial infiltration, and septic metastases are set up by blood-borne infected emboli.

Diagnosis. The following symptoms during acute otitis media or chronic otitis media with cholesteatoma suggest sinus thrombosis:

- High fever above 40 °C
- Spiking temperature with chills
- Swelling and sensitivity to pressure over the mastoid emissary foramen at the posterior border of the mastoid process *(Griesinger's sign)*
- Induration and tenderness of the internal jugular vein and of the anterior border of the sternocleidomastoid muscle
- Petechiae in septic coagulopathy
- Splenomegaly

Laboratory investigations. Blood culture is strongly positive. Urine testing shows hematuria due to septic interstitial focal nephritis, albuminuria, and cylinduria.

Radiography. Schueller's view shows osteolytic foci in the mastoid. CT shows bone destruction in the area of the sinus. Angiography shows narrowing or occlusion of the sigmoid sinus in the venous phase of carotid angiography.

Differential diagnosis includes miliary tuberculosis, typhus, malaria, brucellosis, viral pneumonia, and cystopyelitis.

Treatment. Immediate surgical excision of the primary inflammatory focus in the mastoid and sigmoid sinus by *cortical* (see p. 94) or *radical mastoidectomy* for cholesteatoma is performed (see p. 102). The sigmoid sinus must be exposed widely, the sinus wall is slit, and *thrombectomy* is carried out. The *internal jugular vein* is ligated and divided with a margin of healthy tissue. Parenteral *antiobiotics* are given in high dosages for a long period, if possible determined by the results of culture and sensitivity tests.

Course and prognosis. The disease is fatal if it is not treated correctly, or if the basic cause and its secondary consequences are not recognized promptly. Eighty percent of patients are cured with adequate treatment begun early.

Note: Every unexplained septicemia requires investigation not only of the tonsils but also of the ear since the otitis media which is primarily responsible may be unrecognized and only manifests itself by septicemia.

Otitic Hydrocephalus

This disease is caused by an increased intracranial pressure due to obstruction to drainage of CSF caused by a sterile otogenic sinus thrombosis.

Symptoms

- Failing vision
- Vomiting
- Double vision
- Jacksonian epilepsy
- Pareses and disorders of sensation

Pathogenesis. A relatively symptomless chronic mastoiditis follows an acute otitis media, leading to sterile erosion of perisinous bone and sigmoid sinus phlebitis with formation of a mural thrombus which extends to the confluence of the sinuses and the superior sagittal sinus. This causes occlusion of Pacchioni's granulations which interferes with resorption of CSF, leading to increased CSF pressure.

Diagnosis

- Abducens paralysis without Gradenigo's syndrome (see p. 113)
- Increased CSF pressure without pleocytosis
- Free CSF circulation without obstruction to the CSF
- Congested optic fundi with failing vision
- Normal air encephalogram since the ventricular system is not expanded
- Opacity and osteolytic perisinous lesions on mastoid radiograms
- A history of acute otitis media 3 to 5 weeks previously

Differential Diagnosis

- *Petrositis* (see p. 113) *with arachnoiditis in the cerebellopontine angle*
- Carotid aneurysm at the petrous apex

Treatment. Treatment includes a mastoidectomy, exposure of the sinus, thrombectomy, and neurosurgical decompression to allow drainage of the CSF.

Course and prognosis. These are good if the disease is recognized and treated early. Otherwise, the disease progresses to blindness and the development of Jacksonian epilepsy.

Otogenic Brain Abscess

Today this is a relatively unusual disease, but it was formerly one of the most serious late complications of chronic inflammatory middle ear cholesteatoma.

Symptoms. See Table 1.**11**.

Pathogenesis. The disease may spread as follows:

By *direct continuity* by one of the following pathways: (1) through the tegmen tympani to form a temporal lobe abscess; (2) through the sigmoid sinus to the posterior cranial fossa to form a cerebellar abscess; (3) from the labyrinth to the saccus endolymphaticus to form a cerebellar abscess.

Along preformed pathways via vessels (the diploic veins, advancing septic thromboangiitis of the cerebral veins) or via the internal auditory meatus in labyrinthitis.

Symptoms of temporal lobe abscess

- Speech disturbances revealed by a history of aphasia, and difficulty in understanding words. (This disorder of speech is exclusively sensory and is never motor.)
- Central hearing disorders which are mostly discrete
- Acoustic hallucinations
- Disorders of smell which are usually discrete
- Visual disturbances such as quadrantic hemianopsia and gaze paresis
- Cranial neuropathies of the IIIrd to VIIth cranial nerves
- Crossed lesions of the pyramidal tracts

Differential diagnosis. One must consider intracerebral tumor.

Symptoms of a cerebellar abscess. These include disorders of the oculomotor and postural system, a coarse spontaneous nystagmus to the side of the lesion, vestibular provocation nystagmus with irregular positional nystagmus, gaze-directional nystagmus due to secondary damage to the pons, and gaze-paretic nystagmus to the side of the lesion.

Further symptoms include ataxia, intention tremor, dysmetria, adiadochokinesia, hypotonia, and symptoms due to spread to neighboring organs such as paralysis of the IIIrd, Vth, VIth, VIIth, IXth, and Xth cranial nerves.

Differential diagnosis. Labyrinthitis, acute vestibulopathy, multiple sclerosis, cerebellar tumor, and cerebellopontine angle syndrome must be considered.

Table 1.11 Symptoms of Otogenic Brain Abscess		
1. Initial stage	Meningismus, nausea, headache, psychological changes, fever	The CSF shows pleocytosis and increase of pressure and protein
2. Latent stage	Epileptiform attacks, neurologic signs	Abnormal colloid curve
3. Manifest stage	Papilledema, psychological changes, focal signs of aphasia, alexia, agraphia, hemiplegia, epileptic attacks, and ataxia in cerebellar abscess. Symptoms due to spread to neighboring organs include cranial nerve paralyses, visual field defects, disorders of the oculomotor system and of posture.	Vomiting and bradycardia
4. Terminal stage	Stupor, coma, conjugated deviation to the side of the lesion, bradycardia, and Cheyne-Stokes respiration	

Investigations, in addition to otologic examination, include

- Neurootologic investigation: ERA, ENG, and electrodiagnostic methods for the facial nerve
- Neuroophthalmologic investigation of the optic fundi, visual field, and the ocular motor nerves
- Neurologic and neuroradiologic investigation including computerized axial tomography (CT) scan, MRI, EEG, brain scan, and possibly angiography, echoencephalography, and investigations of the CSF

Treatment

1. The primary focus is removed by mastoidectomy or radical mastoidectomy by an otologist *before a neurosurgical procedure to remove the abscess.*
2. *Primary removal of the brain abscess* is performed by a neurosurgeon. Treatment by aspiration has now been abandoned apart from a few exceptional circumstances because it is more logical to eliminate the focus of infection radically by surgery along the pathway of infection.
3. Appropriate, intense antibiotic therapy is administered.

Course and prognosis. Despite intensive surgical treatment, the mortality is still 20% to 30%. The defect often heals, but there may be neurologic deficits after neurosurgical excision of the abscess.

Petrositis

Previously, this was the most important site of origin of an otogenic intra-cranial complication. Nowadays, it is usually controlled by antibiotics and has therefore become rare.

Pathogenesis. Good pneumatization of the entire petrous pyramid is a prerequisite for the development of petrositis. As a result of extension of inflammation from the middle ear to the paralabyrinthine cells, purulent liquefaction is set up in the cells of the petrous apex often accompanied by osteomyelitis. The classic *Gradenigo's triad* is due to the close relationship of the pyramidal apex to the trigeminal nerve and the abducens nerve. The symptoms of this triad include otorrhea, ipsilateral irritation of the trigeminal nerve, and abducens paralysis. The facial, vagus, and glossopharyngeal nerves are also often paralyzed. Furthermore, the patient may have signs of labyrinthitis due to extension of the inflammatory process. With the advent of antibiotics, the symptoms of the primary otitis media may be hidden due to antibiotic treatment. Predisposing factors include advanced age and diabetes.

Diagnosis. The main symptoms are

- Trigeminal neuralgia
- Abducens paralysis with double vision
- Dizziness and deafness
- Deep throbbing headache
- Abnormal radiographs in Schueller's and Stenver's view and CT

Differential diagnosis. This includes brain abscess and sinus phlebitis.

Treatment. Massive and prolonged parenteral antibiotics are administered and mastoidectomy, and translabyrinthine clearance and drainage of the apical cells, with preservation of the facial nerve, are performed.

Prognosis. If the disease is recognized early and treated effectively, the prognosis is relatively good. However, the prognosis is poor in patients of advanced age and with diabetes (development of a circumscript meningitis at the base of the brain, with consecutive multifocal microinfarctions of the pons).

Specific Inflammatory Disease of the Middle Ear and the Mastoid Process

Tuberculosis

Tuberculosis of the middle ear may be due either to a miliary process or to tubal extension of a localized infection from the nasopharynx. It has practically disappeared nowadays and therefore only needs to be mentioned in passing.

Syphilis

Syphilis of the middle ear is exceedingly rare compared to syphilis of the internal ear and the auditory nerve.

Syphilis of the inner ear and the auditory nerve occur considerably more often than tuberculosis and is now increasing in frequency again. Syphilis manifests itself in the secondary and tertiary stages and also as metaluetic or congenital disease.

Symptoms. These include dizziness, tinnitus, rapidly progressive nonfluctuant hearing loss, and headaches due to chronic syphilitic meningitis.

Pathogenesis. The disease is due to a specific labyrinthitis and neuritis of the auditory nerve, the latter arising during the course of a meningovascular syphilitic meningitis. In the tertiary stage, and also in congenital and metaluetic disease, the nervous apparatus degenerates and atrophies due to a meningovascular or parenchymatous syphilis with progressive demyelinization of the auditory nerve.

Diagnosis. An apparently otherwise healthy young patient complains of progressive disorders of hearing and balance.

Main symptoms. Neurologic syphilis presents with bilateral high-tone sensorineural deafness, spontaneous and provoked nystagmus, disorders of vision, Argyll-Robertson phenomenon (fixed pupil, miosis, and anisochoria), and Hennebert's fistula sign in congenital syphilis in which adhesions form between the stapes footplate and the membranous labyrinth (see p.69).

Differential Diagnosis

- Ménière's disease that runs a fluctuating course
- A cerebellopontine angle tumor which has typical neuroradiologic findings
- Vertebrobasilar insufficiency which occurs in the older age group with discrete neurologic findings

Treatment. Long-term penicillin is given in high doses.

Course and prognosis. If the diagnosis is made early and correct treatment is given, both are good as regards life, but the outlook for restoration of function is poor.

Noninflammatory Diseases of the Labyrinthine Capsule

Otosclerosis

Otosclerosis is a localized disease of the bony labyrinthine capsule, the cause of which has still not been explained. The exact diagnosis is made by histology, but only 10% of patients with *histologic* evidence of the disease have *clinical otosclerosis:* 8% to 10% of whites, 1% of Japanese, and less than 1% of blacks have histologic diseases.

Symptoms. Depending on the site of the otosclerotic focus, the symptoms include:

- Conductive deafness of the middle ear type in about 80% of patients
- Mixed conductive and sensorineural deafness in about 15% of patients
- Pure sensorineural deafness in about 5% of patients

The disease declares itself *subjectively* by:

- A slowly progressive hearing loss which initially usually affects one ear, but later affects both ears in most patients
- Constant, progressive tinnitus

The disease never causes otalgia, otorrhea, dizziness, or disorders of balance.

Pathogenesis. This disease appears to have a multifactorial cause, with the following being the most important:

Heredity and Constitution

There is a familial disposition in 50% to 60% of patients with a dominant inheritance, which may be due to a hereditary enzyme defect. Because clinical otosclerosis only occurs in 10% of patients with histologic disease, a recessive pattern of inheritance is simulated. The chance of inheriting the disease from a parent with clinically manifest disease is about 20%, and from a parent with histologic disease is about 10%.

Disorders of Hormone and Bone Metabolism

Pregnancy coincides with a period of progression of clinically manifest otosclerosis in half of all female patients with the disease. Abnormal formation of lysosomes and increased enzyme activity of the histiocytes and osteocytes in the labyrinthine capsule, and enzymatic collagenolysis, and bony remodeling have been demonstrated. The newly reformed bone fixes the stapes footplate in the oval window (Fig. 1.**65**).

Note: Otosclerosis is due to an extremely localized disorder of mineral or bone metabolism with an abnormal increase of enzyme activity of the mesenchymal cells of the labyrinthine capsule determined mainly by genetics but also by hormonal disturbances.

Diagnosis. There is often a positive *family history. Otoscopy* occasionally shows hyperemia of the promontory shining through the tympanic membrane (Schwartze's sign). *Functional* symptoms include middle ear deafness, occasionally with an inner ear component. *Gellé's test* is abnormal (see p. 42). A pure-tone audiogram usually shows a pure middle ear deafness, occasionally a mixed deafness, and exceptionally a pure sensorineural deafness with positive recruitment. There is often a characteristic notch of the bone conduction curve at 2,000 Hz (the Carhart notch). *Impedance audiometry* usually shows a normal curve at normal pressures. However, the stapedius reflex is often suppressed due to otosclerotic fixation of the footplate.

Radiography usually shows very good pneumatization of the temporal bone.

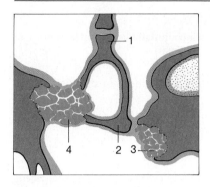

Fig. 1.**65** Histopathology of otosclerosis: 1, head of the stapes; 2, stapes footplate; 3, a facial nerve focus of otosclerosis; 4, a focus on the promontory.

Differential Diagnosis

- Congenital anomalies of the middle ear
- Posttraumatic dislocation or fracture of the ossicles
- Adhesive processes
- Tympanosclerosis

Treatment. *Stapedectomy* is performed (Fig. 1.**66**).

The *principle* of this operation is to open the middle ear and expose the stapes footplate in the oval window niche. Access is gained by incising the skin at the external canal lateral to the tympanic membrane. Canal skin and membrane are then turned forward. The fixed stapes is removed. The oval window is then closed by connective tissue and the stapes is replaced by a synthetic or wire prosthesis or by an autologous cartilage graft. The tympanic membrane and canal skin flap are then replaced. Alternatively, a hearing aid may be prescribed. Contraindications include advanced age, severe generalized disease, and severe inner ear deafness.

Course and Prognosis

Note: The earlier in life otosclerosis manifests itself the more rapid and unfavorable is its course.

If operation is not carried out for the pure middle ear type, the deafness progresses and eventually the patient has a high-grade hearing loss bordering on total deafness.

Results of stapedectomy. If inner ear function is normal, almost normal hearing for speech is restored in more than 80% of patients, and less than 1% of patients suffer complete deafness. If at all possible, the disease should be treated by surgery provided that the inner ear function is satisfactory. The use of a hearing aid is inferior to a stapedectomy since amplification has frequency limits.

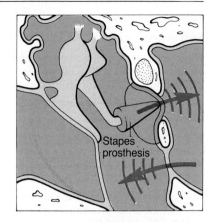

Fig. 1.**66** Principle of the stapedectomy by reconstruction of the sound-
pressure transformation mechanism.

Otologic Manifestations of Generalized Skeletal Disorders

The temporal bone, particularly the labyrinthine capsule, takes part in other
generalized skeletal disorders including osteogenesis imperfecta, Paget's disease,
localized osteitis fibrosa, and osteogenesis imperfecta tarda with blue sclera (Type
Lobstein). The development of osteosclerotic foci in the labyrinthine capsule can be
observed in all these diseases. It causes a typical progressive middle ear deafness,
and in some cases a secondary inner ear deafness.

Trauma of the Middle and Inner Ear

A thorough knowledge of injuries to the ear, and of their consequences, is
essential for every practicing doctor. These lesions are usually caused by
accidents, and such patients are therefore first seen by doctors working in
accident and emergency departments or by general practitioners.

Frequency. Although injuries to the ear constitute only 2% to 3% of all
injuries, 45% of fractures of the base of the skull extend to the temporal
bone affecting the middle and inner ear.

Note: The ear and nasal sinuses should be examined as early as possible
after every head injury. It ist the duty of the doctor who first sees the patient to
investigate the following:

- Fresh bleeding or CSF leak from the ear or the nose
- Evidence of blood or brain tissue in the external auditory meatus or the nose
- Facial paralysis
- Hemotympanum, rupture of the tympanic membrane, or a break in the out-
  line of the anulus tympanicus; see Color Plate **6b, c, d**
- Hearing loss
- Dizziness, disorders of balance, and nystagmus
- Bleeding from the nasopharynx

Temporal Bone Fracture

Pathogenesis

Direct fractures are caused by the effect of external violence concentrated on a small surface, e. g., by gunshot wounds. The result is a penetrating perforating fracture with brain damage.

Indirect fractures are due to diffused external violence. The course of the fracture may run either:

- Along the pyramidal axis (i. e., *a longitudinal fracture*) extending into the middle ear
- Across the pyramidal axis (i. e., *transverse fracture*) extending into the bony labyrinth and the internal auditory meatus

In both cases (Fig. 1.**67**) the dura may be torn, producing an open connection between the pneumatic system of the temporal bone and the subarachnoid space of the cranial fossae. The patient is then in danger of a latent infection ascending via the eustachian tube to the meninges.

Symptoms of longitudinal pyramidal fractures (mainly affecting the middle ear):

- Hemotympanum
- Tearing of the tympanic membrane (Color Plate **6c**)
- Bleeding from the external auditory meatus
- A break in the contour of the anulus tympanicus
- Step formation in the external auditory meatus, which should be differentiated from posterior displaced fracture of the mandibular condyle
- Middle ear deafness
- Facial paralysis in about 20% of patients, usually a neurapraxia or partial axonotmesis
- Occasionally CSF otorrhea

> ***Warning:*** Syringing or manipulations within the external auditory meatus must not be carried out.

Diagnosis. This rests on otoscopic findings, radiographs including Schueller's view, tomograms, and possibly CT in patients with facial paralysis or CSF otorrhea.

Symptoms of transverse pyramidal fractures (mainly affecting the inner ear):

- Intact external auditory meatus
- Intact tympanic membrane, possibly with a hemotympanum (see Color Plate **6d**)
- Hearing loss
- Vertigo

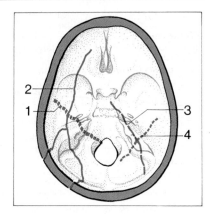

Fig. 1.**67** Temporal bone fractures: 1 and 4, transverse fractures; 2 and 3, longitudinal fractures; 2, combined frontobasal and longitudinal pyramidal fracture.

- Spontaneous nystagmus beating to the healthy ear
- Facial paralysis in about 50% of patients, usually showing an axonotmesis or neurotmesis
- Cerebrospinal fluid leak via the eustachian tube to the nasopharynx

Diagnosis. This is based on otoscopic and functional findings, radiographs in Stenvers' view, and tomograms. Additional investigations include EMG and neuronography, and Schirmer's test and gustometry for facial nerve paralysis (see p. 69).

Treatment of longitudinal and transverse pyramidal fractures. The treatment is dictated by the ever-present *danger of otogenic meningitis*. Therefore, *prophylactic antibiotics* are given consisting of high-dose, long-term parenteral broad-spectrum agents.

The temporal bone must be explored for early or late complications, as summarized in Table 1.12.

Emergency surgery must certainly be carried out, as soon as the general condition of the patient permits, for the indications detailed above. Since the patient has usually suffered multiple injuries, it is necessary to lay down priorities among the various disciplines as follows:

1. Traumatology
2. Neurosurgery
3. Otology
4. Maxillofacial surgery
5. Ophthalmology

Course and prognosis. The following complications are possible, especially as a result of unsatisfactory treatment or missed diagnosis:

Table 1.12 Pyramidal Fracture
Indications for early otologic intervention
• Early meningitis, treated by mastoidectomy
• Bleeding from the sinus, treated by opening of the mastoid and packing or ligature of the sinus
• Persistent CSF otorrhea, treated by repair of the dura
• Facial paralysis with signs of progressive axonotmesis, treated by decompression if there is more than 90% denervation shown by neuronography
• depressed fracture of the external auditory meatus, treated by reconstruction of the meatus because of the danger of secondary atresia
• Gunshot wounds of the temporal bone, treated by debridement of the fragmented area
Indications for late otologic intervention
• Antibiotic-resistant traumatic otitis media
• Chronic mastoiditis, treated by mastoidectomy
• Late facial nerve paralysis with symptoms of denervation, treated by facial nerve decompression (see p. 164)
• Posttraumatic deafness, treated by tympanoplasty
• Posttraumatic cholesteatoma, treated by radical mastoidectomy and tympanoplasty

Early complications:

• Acute otitis media with mastoiditis
• Extension of the above infection to the subarachnoid space causing *early meningitis* or an infected labyrinthitis extending to the meninges

Late complications:

• Chronic otitis media with mastoiditis
• *Late otogenic meningitis*
• Epidural abscess
• Otogenic brain abscess
• Posttraumatic cholesteatoma

Labyrinthine Concussion

Posttraumatic disorders of the inner ear function (deafness and dizziness) in the presence of normal otoscopic and radiographic findings are included under the term *labyrinthine concussion.*

Symptoms. These include tinnitus, unilateral or bilateral sensorineural deafness with positive recruitment and high-tone loss or a notch at 4,000 Hz, dizziness especially on change of position or rapid movements of the head, and disorders of balance.

Pathogenesis. This disease is usually due to organic mechanical damage to the membranous labyrinth similar to *acute acoustic trauma* (see p. 125). Microfractures of the labyrinthine capsule accompanied by bleeding into the peri- and endolymphatic space and mechanical disturbances of the microcirculation causing degeneration of the cochleovestibular sensory cells may also occur.

Diagnosis

- Normal otoscopic findings
- Normal radiographs (Schueller's and Stenvers' views; CT scan)
- A pure-tone audiogram showing a sensorineural deafness with a notch at 4,000 Hz (Fig. 1.**68**) or high-tone loss with recruitment
- Vestibular provocation nystagmus in the presence of vertigo, and more rarely spontaneous nystagmus, possibly reduced sensitivity to caloric stimulation

Differential Diagnosis

- Acute acoustic trauma in which vestibular symptoms are absent
- Posttraumatic psychogenic hearing loss in which the findings are inconsistent and vestibular symptoms absent

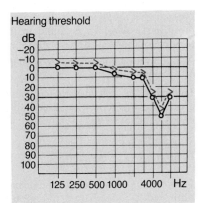

Fig. 1.**68** Posttraumatic dip at 4,000 Hz in a pure-tone audiogram.

Treatment. This includes intravenous low-molecular-weight dextran infusion, provided that there is no general contraindication, e.g., hypertension or allergy. Antivertiginous drugs are given for dizziness.

Course and prognosis. The disease usually settles rapidly in young patients and those with normal circulation. Otherwise, the symptoms, especially those of loss of cochlear function, only resolve incompletely. Irreversible vestibular defects are compensated centrally (see p.32). Cochleovestibular symptoms, especially dizziness, often progress in elderly patients.

Direct Injuries to the Middle and Internal Ear

Symptoms. *Injury of the tympanic membrane* is accompanied by momentary pain, slight bleeding from the ear, and modest deafness.

In *middle ear injuries,* there is profuse bleeding, pain and deafness, a pulsating sound in the ear, and occasionally facial paralysis.

In *inner ear injuries,* there is immediate tinnitus, deafness, dizziness, nausea, and vomiting.

Pathogenesis. Damage to the tympanic membrane and the middle and internal ear may be caused by introduction of pointed objects such as matchsticks, toothpicks, knitting needles, hairpins, and twigs into the ear, by careless removal of foreign bodies, by occupational injuries (hot cinders, welding sparks), by acid burns, or by gunshot wounds.

Diagnosis. *Otoscopic findings* include a tympanic membrane perforation with jagged, frayed, blood-streaked, and occasionally inrolled edges (see Color Plate 5c). Blood is found in the external auditory meatus mixed with perilymph in injuries to the inner ear. *Conductive deafness* is found in middle ear injuries, *sensorineural deafness,* or mixed deafness if the inner ear is involved, and in severe lesions there is *complete deafness and spontaneous nystagmus* to the sound side. An immediate total *peripheral facial nerve paralysis* is found in fractures involving the bony tympanic segment of the facial nerve canal (see Figs. 1.**20** and 1.**21**).

A bullet may be localized by *radiographs* in Schueller's or Stenvers' view or by tomograms.

Treatment. In *simple tympanic membrane rupture,* the fragments of the membrane are repositioned and splinted aseptically under the operating microscope. Systemic prophylactic antibiotics are given.

Warning: Unsterile instruments should not be used in the ear, and the ear should not be syringed.

Combined injuries of the tympanic membrane, middle ear, and inner ear are subjected to immediate exploration of the middle ear cavity and labyrinthine capsule under the operating microscope (tympanoplasty). A peri-lymph leak, e. g., from the round window, is stopped by closing the laby-rinthine fistula. Prophylactic antibiotics are given. A simultaneous facial nerve paralysis is treated by decompression of the facial nerve (see p. 164 and Fig. 1.77).

Course and prognosis. Simple injuries of the tympanic membrane and mid-dle ear usually heal smoothly and without functional deficit if they are treated in the correct manner by an otologist. Involvement of the labyrinth is usually followed by irreversible cochleovestibular failure. The prognosis for the facial paralysis is very good if continuity of the nerve has been pre-served, but after neurotmesis there is an irreversible paralysis if surgery is not undertaken.

Barotrauma

Symptoms. These include acute pain, pulsating noise in the ear, deafness, and occasionally vertigo and disturbance of balance.

Pathogenesis. Sudden changes in air pressure, producing an absolute or relative reduction of pressure in the middle ear, cause bleeding into the middle ear mucosa and into the tympanic membrane, and on occasion even rupture of the tympanic membrane and of the round window membrane. This may occur after rapid decom-pression or recompression from a low- or high-pressure chamber, a rapid dive from a great height in a nonpressurized aircraft, or after surfacing too quickly from deep-sea diving.

The disease is caused by a sudden closure of the tube which is compressed by the rapid rise of atmospheric pressure or by the associated increase of tissue pressure. After about 2 h of closure of the tube, the Valsalva maneuver and politzerization are ineffective since mucosal edema and serous-hemorrhagic exudate of the middle ear cavity have occurred due to the reduced pressure in the middle ear. This disorder is called aero- or barotitis.

Diagnosis. This is made from the history, from the otoscopic findings which show retraction of the tympanic membrane, occasionally subep-ithelial hemorrhage in the pars tensa, transudate behind the tympanic membrane, or a hemotympanum, and from the finding of conductive deafness.

Treatment. This includes decongestant nose drops, catheterization of the tube, possibly paracentesis, analgesics, and oral anti-inflammatory agents. *Prophylaxis* is important by avoiding flying and diving during inflamma-tion of the nasopharynx, nose, and paranasal sinuses. Anatomic deformi-ties in the nose and nasopahrynx obstructing nasal respiration and favor-ing the development of inflammatory diseases of the eustachian tube should be dealt with. These diseases include septal deformity, hypertrophy of the turbinates, and adenoidal hypertrophy. *Immediate tympanotomy* should be carried out for barotrauma with severe sensorineural deafness to allow the round window to be assessed so that a possible rupture of the round window membrane can be repaired.

Caisson Disease and Diving Accidents

These accidents occur in men working in water under several atmospheres of pressure. They can also occur in amateur sporting divers surfacing too quickly from too great a depth.

Symptoms

- Dizziness, vomiting, headache
- Noise in the ears and rapidly progressive hearing loss
- The above symptoms have a latent period of minutes to hours
- In severe cases disorders of vision, ataxia, and clouding of consciousness

Pathogenesis. When working under several atmospheres of pressure, either in a caisson or when diving to greater than 10 m, a considerable quantity of air, including relatively insoluble nitrogen, is taken into solution. Gaseous nitrogen is released into the blood if the patient decompresses too quickly from the caisson or surfaces too rapidly from depths greater than 10 m. This can lead to the formation of small gas emboli within the cerebral end arteries. These cause deficits in the area of supply of the cerebral vessels, including that of the inner ear. This explains the symptoms detailed above.

Diagnosis. There is a previous history of an accident, sensorineural deafness, spontaneous and provocation vestibular nystagmus, and in serious cases ataxia and neurologic deficits.

Treatment. Hyperbaric oxygen is given.

Course and prognosis. This depends on the degree of severity of the gas emboli and on the time taken to institute treatment. In serious cases, the patient may be blind or deaf, suffer from balance disorders, may be paralyzed, or may even die.

Acute Acoustic Trauma

Note: There is an important basic difference between explosion and gunfire injuries. The physical-acoustic properties of an explosion are qualitatively identical to those of gunfire but are completely different quantitatively. In an explosion there is a high-pressure wave but the shock wave lasts more than 1.5 ms, whereas with gunfire the peak of the pressure wave lasts less than 1.5 ms.

Symptoms. In *blast trauma* there is marked persistent earache, occasionally bleeding from the affected ear, deafness, and tinnitus.

In *gunshot trauma* there is a short stabbing pain in the ear, a marked continuous tinnitus, and deafness.

Pathogenesis. In both explosion and gunshot trauma, the cause is partly a direct and mechanical one due to bleeding and partly an indirect metabolic effect on the microcirculation causing partially reversible damage to the sensory cells of the organ of Corti. The severity and site of the lesion in the cochlea directly depend on the SPL of the acoustic energy and its maximum frequency. In explosion trauma, ruptures of the tympanic membrane and other middle ear lesions often occur.

Diagnosis. Only *explosion injury* causes abnormal otoscopic findings: also the audiogram shows a sensorineural or mixed deafness. In *gunshot trauma,* there is a notch at 4,000 Hz, or a high-tone loss, and positive recruitment (see Fig. 1.**68**).

Treatment. Low-molecular-weight dextran is infused intravenously within 24 h of the trauma if possible. Stellate ganglion block may help. A tympanoplasty must be carried out for middle ear injuries.

Course and prognosis. Traumatic *middle ear lesions* usually heal without complications or can be reversed by operation. The prognosis is good.

Inner ear lesions are partially reversible, but in certain patients there is continuing degeneration of sensory cells and secondary increased degeneration of the peripheral neurons.

Acoustic catastrophe. A pancochlear deafness arises after relatively mild acoustic stress. It is therefore better known as acoustically induced hearing loss to prevent confusion with acoustic trauma. The causes are not clear.

Chronic Noise Trauma to the Inner Ear

In contrast to acute acoustic trauma, this disease is the result of damage to the inner ear by weaker but more prolonged noise. Therefore, the severity of the lesion depends not only on the sound pressure peaks of the noise, but also on the exposure time and on the individual patient's sensitivity to the effect of noise. Emotional factors also play a considerable part and produce autonomic symptoms which have deleterious effects on the entire body.

Symptoms. *Subjectively,* there is a feeling of pressure in the ears and in the head, a feeling of deafness, generalized tiredness and lack of concentration, and often tinnitus. The subjective symptoms are often reversible since the patient becomes used to the noise. Few patients are aware of the developing deafness in the early phases. *Objectively,* a pure-tone audiogram initially shows a notch at 4,000 Hz, typically in both ears in chronic noise trauma. Later the threshold for the lower frequencies rises, and finally the deafness spreads to the speech frequencies. Further loss of hearing follows as a result of the physiologic aging process. In the early phases of its development, chronic noise deafness shows a certain tendency to recover when the patient is no longer exposed, but with increasing exposure this ability decreases.

Pathogenesis. The ear may react to sounds depending on the intensity and duration of exposure, in one of the following ways:

1. A physiologic *adaptation of threshold* may develop.

2. After more prolonged exposure, the ear may react by *fatigue* or by the appearance of a temporary threshold shift (TTS), which can be related directly to acoustic damage which is proportional to the exposure time and which has a linear relationship with the sound intensity. The "physiologic" TTS usually recovers within minutes and at the most 2 h after the end of exposure to the noise.

3. A *permanent threshold shift* (PTS) may develop which is an expression of pathologic fatigue and irreversible damage to the hearing organ. It is caused by a metabolic decompensation of the sensory cells due to a disturbed balance between supply and demand of energy metabolism. This is determined by increased oxygen consumption or by decreased supply during permanent intensive acoustic irradiation. The outer hair cells degenerate first, and the inner cells last.

Diagnosis. The deafness is of long standing, and a social history reveals occupational or lifelong social habits which are responsible. A pure-tone speech audiogram is important (Fig. 1.**69**).

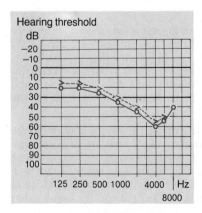

Fig. 1.**69** Pure-tone audiogram of chronic noise deafness.

Differential Diagnosis

- Endogenous heredodegenerative sensorineural deafness in which there is a positive family history
- Infective-toxic damage to the inner ear and auditory nerve, particularly by ototoxic antibiotics
- Progressive sensorineural deafness in severe generalized diseases such as diabetes, chronic nephritis, and hypertension

Note: The limits of noise causing damage to the ear are as follows:

- Equivalent continuous sound pressure (Leq) in the range 85 to 90 ($\pm$ 2.5) dB and higher must be regarded as damaging to the ear.
- Single sound impulses exceeding a peak of 135 dB also damage the ear.

Treatment. Active methods of treatment to deal with the cause are not available. If hearing in social situations becomes inadequate, a hearing aid should be prescribed. Prophylaxis including the provision of hearing protectors is very important.

Protection of Hearing

- Elimination or reduction of noise by technical improvements to machinery
- Protection of personnel against noise by ear protectors
- Limitation of the time of exposure to noise and frequent rest periods
- Medical prophylaxis against damage to the hearing prescribed by occupational medical health personnel

Note: A cotton wool plug does not protect against noise trauma to the ear.

Course and prognosis. The disease progresses to advanced deafness if protective measures are ignored.

Tumors of the Middle and Internal Ear, the Vestibulocochlear Nerve, and the Facial Nerve

Nonchromaffin Paraganglioma (Glomus Tumor)

This is the most frequent true tumor of the middle ear. It develops from neuroectoderm. The structure of the tumor is similar to that of the chemoreceptor tissue of the carotid body. It is characterized by extensive vascularity. Because of its structural and functional relationship to the carotid body, this tumor is also considered in the section on the *chemodectomas* (see p. 506).

Symptoms. These are very variable depending on the site of origin and extent of the tumor and include:

- Unilateral tinnitus synchronous with the pulse
- Unilateral hearing loss and feeling of pressure in the ear
- Disorders of balance
- Lesions of the lower cranial nerves causing facial paralyses, paralysis of the soft palate, hoarseness, disorders of swallowing, and paralysis of the tongue in the late stage

Pathogenesis. The tumor develops from nests of epithelial cells surrounded by a high vascular stroma. The sites of predilection are the bulb of the internal jugular vein, the tympanic plexus, and the lesser superficial petrosal nerve. They can be classified by site and extent as follows:

1. Glomus tympanicum tumors limited to the middle ear cavity
2. Glomus jugulare tumors limited to the middle ear cavity and the bulb of the jugular vein without destruction of bone
3. Glomus jugulare tumors destroying bone and invading the whole of the mastoid as far as the petrous apex
4. Glomus jugulare tumors with intracranial extension

Diagnosis. Otoscopy shows the tumor shining through the tympanic membrane (see Color Plate **9d**). The tumor is often red. If the tumor breaks through into the external meatus, a polyp which bleeds easily can be seen.

The deafness is conductive in the early stage, but is later sensorineural in type, and finally the patient may be stone-deaf if the tumor erodes into the labyrinth.

The hypoglossal, glossopharyngeal, or vagus nerves may be paralyzed in tumors arising primarily from the bulb of the jugular vein (the jugular foramen syndrome).

Intracranial extension is accompanied by pontine and cerebellar syndromes in addition to facial paralysis, trigeminal hypoesthesia, deafness, and vestibular symptoms.

Supplementary investigations include tomograms to allow comparison of both temporal bones in the anteroposterior and lateral projections, Mifka's views for the assessment of the jugular foramen, subtraction angiography (allows embolization of the main feeding vessels in selected patients at the same sitting), and finally computed tomography to demonstrate the foramen and the bulb of the internal jugular vein.

Treatment. Surgery is performed.

Tumors of groups 1 and 2 can be removed easily and radically by otologic surgery. Tumors of group 3 require a combined cervicotemporal access, and those of group 4 a two-phase neurootologic procedure designed to remove the tumor completely but to preserve the facial nerve. Embolization of the larger vessels and use of the cryoprobe reduce bleeding during the operation.

The results of radiotherapy are controversial so that surgery is the treatment of choice.

Course and prognosis. The tumor grows slowly. In advanced stages with extensive intracranial invasion, the patient may die due to compression of the brainstem or thrombosis of the carotid artery.

Bony Tumors

These rare tumors include:

- Osteoma
- Giant cell tumor
- Eosinophilic granuloma, a localized form of reticuloendotheliosis (see p. 134)
- Solitary plasmacytoma

Middle Ear Carcinoma

In most patients this is a keratinizing *squamous cell carcinoma* arising at the junction between the external auditory meatus and the tympanic membrane which has broken through into the middle ear.

Adenocarcinoma or adenoidcystic carcinoma arising primarily from the middle ear mucosa are very rare, as are *sarcomas*.

Symptoms

- Neuralgic pains around the ear
- Blood-stained otorrhea which is very fetid
- Progressive hearing loss
- Occasionally dizziness, disorders of balance, facial nerve paralysis, and intense headache if the tumor infiltrates the dura

Diagnosis

- Otoscopy showing a readily bleeding aural polyp
- Destruction of the tympanic membrane by hemorrhagic granulations
- Destruction of the posterior meatal wall
- A peripheral facial paralysis, enlargement of the regional lymph nodes, conductive deafness, combined conductive and sensorineural deafness, or even total deafness, spontaneous vestibular nystagmus to the healthy side depending on the extent of the tumor
- Radiographs, including tomograms which are essential, show extensive bone destruction of the temporal bone arising from the middle ear cavity and the external auditory meatus.

Treatment. Surgery and/or irradiation are implemented.

Depending on the extent and histologic type of the tumor, an extended mastoidectomy with radical neck dissection or a subtotal petrosectomy and parotidectomy if possible with preservation of the facial nerve may be undertaken. Postoperative radiotherapy may be used for extensive invasion of the temporal bone.

Course and prognosis. Despite combined surgery and radiotherapy, this tumor usually recurs locally and in the neck, with the exception of small localized early tumors. The prognosis is therefore poor since surgery is limited by the proximity of the base of the skull.

Acoustic Neuroma or Schwannoma

Symptoms. See Table 1.**13**.

Pathogenesis. This is a histologically benign tumor arising from the Schwann cells of the neurilemma. It usually arises in the transitional zone between the neuroglia and the neurilemma of the pars superior of the vestibular nerve.

Depending on their *site of origin,* these tumors may be divided into: *lateral acoustic neuromas* which lie in the internal auditory meatus and cause exclusively localized symptoms; *mediolateral acoustic neuromas* in the region of the porus, lying partly in the internal meatus and partly in the cerebellopontine angle and causing both localized symptoms and symptoms due to impairment of neighboring organs; and finally *medial acoustic neuromas* arising in the cerebellopontine angle and causing

---

Table 1.13   Subjective Symptoms of Acoustic Neuroma

Focal symptoms
- Tinnitus (incidence 70%)
- Unilateral progressive deafness (45%)
- Sudden hearing loss (40%)
- Fluctuating deafness (10%)
- Dizziness (30%)

Associated symptoms
- Unilateral facial nerve spasm or paralysis
- Double vision
- Ataxia
- Clumsiness on moving the arms
- Unilateral disturbances of sensation of the face

Symptoms of increased cranial pressure
- Occipital headache
- Projectile vomiting
- Decrease in vision and papilledema
- Personality changes

slight symptoms in the VIIIth cranial nerve but marked symptoms of involvement of adjacent cranial nerves, brain stem, and cerebellum, and finally the symptoms of increased intracranial pressure.

Three stages may be distinguished depending on the *size of the tumor* (Fig. 1.**70**):

1. Small intrameatal tumors of a diameter of 1 to 8 mm which cause focal symptoms
2. Medium tumors of a diameter of up to 2.5 cm with intrameatal and intracranial extent which cause focal symptoms and slight symptoms of involvement of neighboring neural structures
3. Large tumors greater than 2.5 cm in diameter causing focal symptoms, symptoms due to involvement of neighboring neural structures, and the symptoms of increased intracranial pressure, depending on their size

Diagnosis. See Table 1.**14**.

Diagnostic investigations include:

- Pure-tone and speech audiometry, stapedius reflex
- Electric response audiometry
- Vestibular tests with nystagmography
- CT with intravenous contrast enhancement
- MRI with gadolinium DPTA enhancement (for demonstrating intrameatal tumors smaller than 20 mm in diameter)

The standard Stenvers' and Towne's views often give false-negative findings in small or medial tumors. In small tumors the CSF often does not show the otherwise characteristic increase of *protein greater than 100 mg/100 ml without pleocytosis*.

Differential Diagnosis

- Ménière's disease (see p. 139)
- Sudden deafness (see p. 145)
- Primary congenital cholesteatoma of the cerebellopontine angle

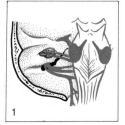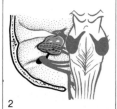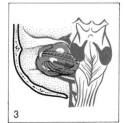

Fig. 1.**70**   The three stages of an acoustic neuroma: 1, intrameatal tumor; 2, intra- and extrameatal tumor; 3, a mainly extrameatal, medial tumor compressing the brain stem and the cerebellum.

Table 1.14   Objective Symptoms of Acoustic Neuroma

Focal symptoms
- *Retrocochlear sensorineural deafness,* with negative recruitment, abnormal SISI and threshold tests (see p. 48 ff.), abnormal decay on Békésy audiogram, and discrepancy between pure-tone and speech audiogram. Stapedius reflex is lost. Pathologic ABR and cochleography.
- *Vestibular symptoms* include spontaneous nystagmus to the healthy ear and loss of caloric and galvanic labyrinthine responses.

Associated symptoms
- Peripheral, usually slight, facial paralysis, neurodiagnostic axonotmesis and positive Hitselberger's sign
- Abducens paralysis
- Loss of the corneal reflex
- Hypoesthesia of the trigeminal nerve
- Occasionally palatal paralysis

Symptoms due to brain stem compression
include oculomotor disorders. In stage III tumors, pontine compression causes the following:
- Gaze-evoked nystagmus to the side of the tumor
- Direction-changing irregular positional nystagmus
- Abnormal or absent optokinetic nystagmus
- Pathologic ABR

Cerebellar symptoms
in stage III often include dysdiadochokinesia and ataxia.

Symptoms of increased intracranial pressure:
papilledema and projectile vomiting

- Secondary acquired occult middle ear cholesteatoma with paralabyrinthine extension and rupture into the internal auditory meatus (see p. 98)
- Meningioma and facial nerve neuroma
- Congenital syphilis causing vascular cochleovestibular symptoms (see p. 114)

Treatment. Neurosurgery or otologic surgery, or the two combined, is performed. (Fig. 1.71)

Intrameatal tumors (stage 1) may be removed by an extradural transtemporal or retrosigmoid approach, with no mortality, preservation of hearing in 20% of patients, and retention of facial nerve function in 95% of patients.

Medium-sized tumors (stage 2) are removed by a translabyrinthine or retrosigmoidal route. The mortality is nil, but 85% of patients become totally deaf. Facial nerve function, however, can be preserved in 85% of patients.

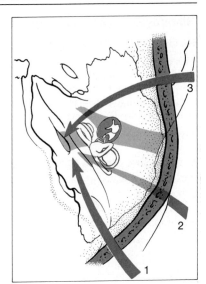

Fig. 1.**71** Neurosurgical and otologic routes of access to the internal meatus. 1, retrosigmoid and suboccipital; 2, translabyrinthine; 3, transtemporal through the middle cranial fossa.

Large tumors (stage 3) are dealt with by a retrosigmoid or suboccipital neurosurgical approach and a simultaneous transmeatal otosurgical approach. Mortality is less than 1%, and facial nerve function can be preserved in about 50% of patients.

Course and prognosis. The tumor grows slowly and in the early stages the symptoms are thus slight so that the diagnosis tends to be made late. The prognosis is good for small and medium-sized tumors.

Note: In every case of unilateral progressive sensorineural deafness or unilateral recurrent loss of hearing, the possibility of an acoustic neuroma must always be suspected, and a thorough neurootologic examination and neuroradiologic examination (including CT, ERA) carried out.

Note: Patients with von Recklinghausen's neurofibromatosis should be suspected as having one or more neuromas of the auditory or facial nerve.

Facial Nerve Neuroma

Symptoms. The tumor causes a slowly progressive facial paralysis or hemifacial spasm. Depending on its site, the tumor may cause symptoms similar to that of an acoustic neuroma.

Histiocytosis (Reticuloendotheliosis)

Hand-Schueller-Christian Disease of Children and Adolescents

This disease causes several bone defects due to granulomatous foci of infection in the skull. The *pathologic anatomy* is the formation of granulomatous reticulohistiocytes localized to the middle ear and mastoid.

Treatment includes chemotherapy, corticosteroids, and radiotherapy of the localized deposits in close cooperation with a medical oncologist.

Prognosis is poor.

Letterer-Siwe Disease (Disseminated Histiocytosis)

This disease follows a rapid course ending fatally with numerous disseminated deposits.

Eosinophilic Granuloma

This is a localized chronic form of reticular endotheliosis. The sites of predilection are the temporal bone and the ribs, the pelvis, and the long bones. *Aural symptoms* are caused by deposits in the temporal bone. The symptoms may simulate an otitis media with mastoiditis and formation of polypi in the external meatus.

Treatment includes chemotherapy, corticosteroids, surgery, and irradiation of localized deposits.

Prognosis is relatively good depending on the site. Conversion to a disseminated histiocytosis is possible, which ends fatally.

True Congenital Cholesteatoma (see p. 105)

Congenital Anomalies of the Middle and Internal Ear

Simultaneous congenital anomalies of the middle and internal ear are rare, but those affecting the middle and external ear together are common, occurring in 1 in 10,000 normal births.

Combined Anomalies of the External and Middle Ear

Symptoms

- Dysplasia
- Microtia
- Meatal atresia
- Facial deformities
- Deafness

The combination of microtia, meatal atresia, microgenia, and coloboma of the eyelids is known as mandibulofacial dysostosis or Treacher-Collins-Franceschetti syndrome.

Pathogenesis. The following may be responsible for the genesis of these anomalies:

- Genetic factors, chromosomal abnormalities, or mutation of genes
- Exogenous factors including hypoxia, radiation, ultrasound, and thalidomide
- Combined exogenous and genetic factors causing polygenic multifactorial anomalies

The development process (described on p. 1) is restricted or disturbed by these factors.

Diagnosis

- Inspection
- Radiographs including tomographs which are essential
- Audiometry with ERA
- Vestibular tests

Treatment. Surgery is performed or a hearing aid is prescribed.

Purpose of Treatment

1. Construction of an aesthetically satisfactory auricle and creation of an external meatus.
2. Improvement of hearing, either by reconstruction of the sound conducting apparatus by a tympanoplasty (see Fig. 1.**62a** and **b**) or by prescription of a hearing aid.

Timing of the Operation

A patient with bilateral meatal atresia with a conductive deafness of 50 dB should have an operation on one ear in the 3rd to 4th year of life.

However, it is preferable to reconstruct the external auditory meatus and to carry out a tympanoplasty *after completion of pneumatization and when the auricle has reached its final size,* i. e., after the 8th year of life. Otoplasty is carried out while the child is of school age.

Table 1.**15** Congenital Anomalies of the Internal Ear

- Mondini syndrome: isolated dysplasia of the cochlea
- Congenital CSF otorrhea: due to a fistula of the oval window with a patent cochlear aqueduct (Gusher Syndrome)
- Thalidomide embryopathy: a labyrinthine dysplasia with aplasia of the petrous pyramid
- Rubella embryopathy: labyrinthine anomalies with dysplasia of the middle ear

A bone conduction hearing aid is prescribed for patients with a bilateral atresia as early as possible, i. e., in the second half of the 1st year of life to allow the speech to develop normally.

Congenital Anomalies of the Internal Ear

These are rare and are summarized in Table 1.**15**.

Clinical Aspects of Cochleovestibular Disorders

Toxic Damage to the Hearing and Balance Apparatus

Exogenous ototoxins include drugs such as aminoglycosides and diuretics, industrial products, tobacco, and alcohol.

Endogenous ototoxins include bacterial toxins and the toxic metabolites of metabolic disorders such as diabetes and renal disease.

Symptoms

- Tinnitus is usually the first symptom.
- Hearing loss is found consisting of a progressive pure sensorineural deafness. Initially the loss is for the high tones, but later there is narrowing of the auditory field progressing from the high to the middle and lower frequencies. The deafness is always bilateral.
- Vertigo is present which is positional and is associated with nausea.
- There are disorders of balance with persistent vertigo and unsteadiness of gait.
- Oscillopsia, i. e., a weakness of fixation is present, due to a disorder of the vestibuloocular reflex.

Aminoglycoside Antibiotics

Pathogenesis. Because of their long half-life, aminoglycoside antibiotics are retained for a longer period and in a higher concentration in the inner ear fluids than in the other body tissues and fluids. This effect may be intensified by reduced renal excretion so that toxic concentrations may accumulate in the inner ear, leading to irreversible damage to the cochlear and vestibular end organs. The outer hair cells degenerate first, and then the inner hair cells at higher concentrations. Later the stria vascularis, the inner ear vessels, and the ganglion cells are damaged. It is not yet clear which structure is damaged primarily. These ototoxic aminoglycosides destroy both cochlear and vestibular sensory cells, and different agents have a different site of predilection: streptomycin is mainly vestibulotoxic, whereas dihydrostreptomycin is ototoxic. Neomycin and kanamycin are strongly ototoxic, and gentamicin is both oto- and vestibulotoxic.

Note: The development of inner ear damage depends on:

1. The dose of the ototoxic antibiotic and its half-life
2. Renal function
3. The condition of the stria vascularis and the resorptive cells in the inner ear

Diagnosis depends on:

- An audiogram which shows a progressive high-tone sensorineural deafness
- Vestibular tests which show a spontaneous nystagmus, depression of the thermal labyrinthine reaction, and abnormal vestibulospinal reflexes
- Abnormal renal function

Treatment. This includes immediate cessation of the aminoglycosides, intravenous infusion of low-molecular-weight dextran solutions to improve the peri- and endolymphatic metabolism in the inner ear, and possibly cortisone.

Course. The disease usually progresses for up to 6 months after the antibiotics are stopped; the prognosis must therefore be guarded because the inner ear damage is largely irreversible.

Note: Any patient being treated with aminoglycosides must have the following investigations:

1. Renal function tests
2. An audiogram once or twice a week during the course of treatment

Other ototoxic antibiotics include quinine and salicylates. Overdose causes metabolic damage to the hair cells of the inner ear which is reversible if it is recognized early. Prolonged use causes degeneration of the ganglion cells and the associated neurons.

Diuretics including furosemide and ethacrynic acid can also damage the inner ear. The extent of the lesion varies and affects mainly the outer hair cells, due to disturbance of the regulation of ion concentration caused by a lesion of the stria vascularis. These lesions are reversible in about 90% of patients.

Ototoxic Occupational Toxins:

- Arsenic compounds
- Mercury salts
- Lead salts
- Organic phosphate compounds
- Sulfur and tetrachlorocarbon compounds

- Carbon monoxide
- Benzol, nitrobenzol, and aniline

Carbon monoxide causes a peripheral cochlear and a central vestibular failure. The other substances cause degeneration of sensory cells and peripheral neurons, the central nuclei, and the neural pathways.

Inflammatory Lesions of the Hearing and Balance Apparatus

Herpes Zoster Otitis (Ramsay Hunt Syndrome)

The most common site of zoster infection in the head and neck, after herpes zoster ophthalmicus, is that affecting the ear.

Symptoms. Herpes zoster otitis may occur at any age, but it mainly does so between 40 and 60 years.

- The patient is generally unwell with a fever or subfebrile temperature.
- Erythema and vesicles are to be seen on the auricle and the external meatus (see Color Plate **3c**)
- Regional lymphadenitis is present (discrete).
- Severe neuralgic pain is found.
- Peripheral facial paralysis is found in 60%−90% of patients.
- Severe retrocochlear deafness is present in 40% of patients.
- Vertigo and disorders of balance are present in 40% of patients with release nystagmus to the healthy side.

Pathogenesis. The disorder is due to a viral infection. The portal of entry is unknown. The virus may spread by the bloodstream to the CSF and the meninges causing encephalomyelomeningitis with neuritis of the spiral or vestibular ganglion.

Diagnosis. Inspection and otoscopy show vesicles in the meatus or on the tympanic membrane. An audiogram shows retrocochlear deafness, and vestibular tests show spontaneous nystagmus and suppression of the thermal labyrinthine response. Electrodiagnosis of facial nerve function and Schirmer's test are also carried out. The glossopharyngeal and vagus nerves are relatively often affected presenting as paresis or an eruption in the pharynx.

Additional investigations include viral serology and examination of the CSF. The latter shows a slight increase in the number of cells and protein content, due to a *serous meningitis*. The disease often extends to the labyrinth causing a neurolabyrinthitis.

Differential diagnosis. Myringitis bullosa and idiopathic facial paralysis.

Treatment. Early cases are treated with acyclovir, an antiviral agent that inhibits the DNA synthesis of type I and II HSV as well as varicella-zoster virus. Cases at later stages are mainly treated symptomatically with analgesics, B complex vitamins, and electrotherapy of the paralyzed facial nerve to prevent disuse atrophy of the mimic musculature.

Course and prognosis. These are good for life, but poor for function. The facial nerve paralysis recovers slowly and often only partially. The cochleovestibular loss is usually irreversible.

Other Viral Infections

Influenza, measles, adenovirus, chicken pox, Coxsackie, and mumps viruses often cause a "neuritis statoacoustica" with corresponding symptoms.

The virus of *epidemic parotitis* has a particular affinity for the cochlea, usually causing a unilateral serous labyrinthitis, destruction of the hair cells, or degeneration of the organ of Corti. Neurolabyrinthitis with destruction of the spiral ganglion may occur. The vestibular part of the labyrinth is almost never attacked by the mumps virus.

Note: Infection with mumps virus is the most frequent cause of unilateral complete deafness in young children.

Course is usually mild or abortive with respect to the primary disease.

Prognosis is poor, with irreversible damage.

Serous Labyrinthitis

This condition is a toxic or virally determined abacterial serous inflammation of the peri- and endolymphatic spaces with partial or total destruction of cochlear and vestibular sensory cells. Loss of cochlear and vestibular function is usually irreversible (see p. 106).

Trauma

(See pp. 117–127).

Ménière's Disease*

Symptoms. The classic triad originally described by Ménière in 1861 consists of attacks of:

- Tinnitus
- Deafness
- Vertigo

---

* According to an inscription on the family grave in the Montparnasse graveyard, the name Ménière is spelled with é and è for the first and second *E*'s, respectively.

The *typical attack* begins acutely and consists of the three symptoms named above, followed by nausea, vomiting, and other autonomic symptoms. Characteristically there is no predisposing factor apart from psychological stress.

Symptoms are usually unilateral. In the disease-free intervals, the hearing often returns to normal and the tinnitus disappears, at least in the early phases of the disease. In the later stages there is *a fluctuating deafness in the low tones*. In the *end stage* the deafness is unilateral, severe, and pancochlear (Figs. 1.73 and 1.74). The patient also complains of persistent tinnitus. Initially the cochlear symptoms predominate.

Pathogenesis. The disease is caused by a disturbance of the *quantitative* relation between the volume of the peri- and endolymph. Furthermore, a disorder of the *qualitative electrolyte composition* of the two fluids causes *abnormal osmotic pressure regulation* within the membranous labyrinth. This causes an *endolymphatic hydrops* which has been demonstrated by histologic preparations of the temporal bone (Fig. 1.72).

The primary cause of this increase of pressure within the endolymphatic space is a disorder of resorption of the potassium-rich endolymph. This leads to an increase

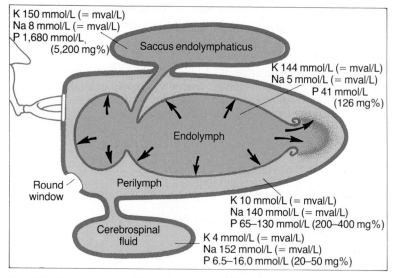

K 150 mmol/L (= mval/L)
Na 8 mmol/L (= mval/L)
P 1,680 mmol/L,
(5,200 mg%)

Saccus endolymphaticus

K 144 mmol/L (= mval/L)
Na 5 mmol/L (= mval/L)
P 41 mmol/L
(126 mg%)

Endolymph

Round window

Perilymph

Cerebrospinal fluid

K 10 mmol/L (= mval/L)
Na 140 mmol/L (= mval/L)
P 65–130 mmol/L (200–400 mg%)

K 4 mmol/L (= mval/L)
Na 152 mmol/L (= mval/L)
P 6.5–16.0 mmol/L (20–50 mg%)

Fig. 1.72   Pathogenesis of Ménière's disease (according to Schuknecht). The disturbance of the quantitative relationship between the volume of the perilymph and endolymph causes hydrops. Rupture of the membranous labyrinth initiates a pathologic displacement of the potassium and sodium ion concentrations in the inner ear fluids.

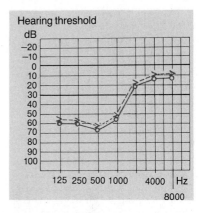

Fig. 1.**73** Typical low-tone deafness in early Ménière's disease.

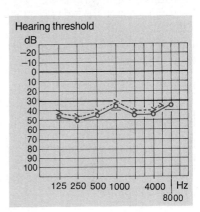

Fig. 1.**74** Typical   flat   pancochlear hearing loss in late stage of Ménière's disease.

of osmotic pressure. When this exceeds a certain level Reissner's membrane lying between the endo- and perilymphatic spaces ruptures, allowing the endo- and perilymph to mix. Histology has shown that the sites of predilection of the rupture are the helicotrema, the basal turn of the cochlea and the utricle, and part of the saccule lying opposite the ampulla of the semicircular canals. This explains the genesis of the cochleovestibular symptoms of the classic Ménière's attack.

The rupture of the hydropic labyrinth and the resulting mixing of the potassium-rich endolymph with perilymph which is normally low in potassium leads to a considerable rise of the potassium content in the intercellular spaces of the perilymphatic network in which the afferent neurons of the acoustic and vestibular nerves run. These are paralyzed by depolarization due to the increase of potassium, thus causing the symptoms of

Table 1.16 Synopsis of the Most Important Disorders of Balance and Hearing

Diagnosis	Subjective Symptoms	Audiogram	Vestibular Symptoms	Associated Neurologic Symptoms	Other Clinical Symptoms
Acute unilateral vestibular paralysis	Acute rotatory dizziness and prolonged dizziness, possibly positional. Nausea, vomiting, no loss of consciousness, normal hearing and no tinnitus.	Normal	Spontaneous nystagmus to the sound side, possibly positional nystagmus, no response to caloric stimulation, ataxia. Galvanic tests are usually abnormal, with an increased threshold.	None	Often diabetes, acute infection by viruses or toxoplasmosis, or hyper- or hypotension, immune disorder
Ménière's disease	Episodic vertigo, unilateral tinnitus, unilateral deafness, and fluctuating hearing loss	Unilateral fluctuating sensorineural hearing loss with positive recruitment, and often a flat or low tone curve	Spontaneous nystagmus to the healthy side after the attack, reduced caloric response, normal galvanic test	None	None
Acoustic neuroma	Progressive unilateral hearing loss, progressive disorder of balance, occipital headache, occasionally also recurrent hearing loss with partial remission, tinnitus	Unilateral retrocochlear sensorineural deafness, at first for the high tones. Stapedius reflex lost. Absent recruitment and marked loss of discrimination for speech and with a discrepancy between the pure-tone and speech audiograms, and an abnormal ERA level.	Spontaneous nystagmus to the healthy side, possibly gaze-evoked nystagmus to the diseased side, positional nystagmus, abnormal caloric and galvanic responses, possibly abnormal opto-kinetic responses in the presence of compression of the brain stem and cerebellum.	Associated symptoms, absent corneal reflex, abnormal glabellar tap, facial weakness, and positive Hitselberger sign, papilledema, and abducens paralysis in large tumors	None

Table 1.17 Subjective Symptoms of a Peripheral Vestibular Disorder
• Rotatory dizziness • Lateropulsion • Unsteadiness Provided that these symptoms • Occur in attacks • Are accompanied by deafness • Are induced by change of position, or • Are combined by otorrhea and facial paralysis

cochleovestibular failure. This process may last a few minutes to several hours and is reversible in the early phases of the disease, which explains the clinical recovery, especially of the fluctuating hearing loss (Figs. 1.73 and 1.74).

Psychological factors such as stress can act as a trigger mechanism for an attack, but are not primarily responsible for the development of the disease.

Diagnosis. See Tables 1.16 and 1.17.

Treatment during an attack. This consists of bed rest, intravenous infusion of fluid and electrolytes for prolonged vomiting, and intravenous antivertiginous and antiemetic drugs. Low-molecular-weight dextran infusions are given to improve the labyrinthine circulation and to increase the flow of peri- and endolymph. Psychotropic drugs should not be given during an attack because of the danger of central disinhibition of the vestibular system causing worsening of the symptoms.

In the symptom-free interval, the patient requires psychological support, possibly psychiatric investigation, and if necessary psychotropic drugs.

A protracted course with repeated attacks which disable the patient should be treated by *destroying* the vestibular end organ while retaining *social hearing.* The affected sensory cells of the vestibular endorgan, inducing the spells of dizziness, are selectively destroyed by *local application of gentamicin* to the round window. Patients resistant to treatment are managed by transtemporal approach to the internal meatus and selective vestibular neurectomy.

In cases with poor hearing and marked tinnitus, the treatment of choice is total elimination of the severely damaged inner ear by transtympanic *labyrinthectomy,* or in resistant cases by *translabyrinthine exposure of the internal meatus with resection of the intrameatal portion of the vestibulocochlear nerve.* This operation causes complete deafness. Surgical exposure of the ductus endolymphaticus and drainage of the endolymphatic sac is an operation based on a speculative hypothesis (decompression of the hydrops), and it must be regarded both from a pathophysiologic point of view as well as from clinical experience as of doubtful value and should therefore be rejected.

Course. One of the characteristics of Ménière's disease is that its course is unpredictable. At one end of the spectrum are *abortive forms* which heal after a few attacks without permanent deafness. At the other end of the spectrum the disease may progress episodically over several years with symptom-free intervals of varying duration. However, in the course of time the fluctuating deafness becomes irreversible. In addition, there is also an *acute form* in which a number of attacks lead rapidly to almost complete deafness and to great disability because of the disturbance of balance. In these cases, elimination of the diseased vestibular part of the inner ear by the transtympanic application of gentamicin or by one of the surgical routes described above is indicated. Bilateral disease is relatively uncommon, occurring in only 10% of patients.

Acute Vestibular Paralysis (Vestibular Neuronitis)

Symptoms. See Table 1.**18**.

Pathogenesis. So far this condition is largely unexplained. The disease may be caused by a *disturbance of the microcirculation* due to an infection, an autoimmune disease, or a metabolic disorder reducing the suspension stability of the blood causing *sludging*. This may happen, e. g., in diabetic angiopathy. Other cases may possibly represent direct inflammatory damage to the vestibular end organ, the peripheral vestibular neurons, or the higher primary centers in the medulla oblongata due to meningoence-

---

Table 1.**18** Symptoms of Acute Vestibular Paralysis (Vestibular Neuronitis)

A previously healthy patient suffers from

- Rotatory dizziness
- Nausea and vomiting
- Dizziness persisting for days or weeks
- Ataxia

Typically the following are absent:

- Tinnitus
- Deafness
- Loss of consciousness
- Double vision or visual field defects

phalitis caused by a neurotropic virus or other agents such as Rickettsiae, or protozoa such as Toxoplasma gondii. The generalizéd descriptive term of vestibular "neuronitis" is therefore wrong, as it only applies to some patients. This disorder shows some similarities to sudden deafness in its course, unilateral involvement, and acute onset.

Diagnosis. See Table 1.**16**.

Differential diagnosis. See Tables 1.**16** and 1.**18**.

Treatment. In the early acute phase, treatment is mainly symptomatic by antivertiginous drugs and sedatives, plus intravenous rheomacrodex. Antibiotics are given if there is objective evidence of bacterial infection, and corticosteroids are given if an autoimmune disease is suspected. Active physiotherapy, including exercises to train the balance, should begin as soon as possible. Psychotropic drugs should not be given in the acute phase!

Course and prognosis. These depend first upon *site* (end organ, peripheral neuron, primary centers of the brainstem), *cause* (diabetes or infection), and *age*. End organ lesions in young patients usually resolve rapidly and completely. In contrast, central vestibular deficits in elderly patients require weeks or months to compensate, and recovery is the exception.

Sudden Deafness

Note: This disease is a medical emergency.

Symptoms

- Initially a feeling of pressure in the ear followed by
- Tinnitus which is usually marked followed by
- Severe hearing loss beginning within minutes and occasionally leading immediately to complete deafness

The following symptoms are absent:

- Dizziness
- Balance disorders
- Neurologic and ophthalmalogic symptoms

Pathogenesis. As in vestibular neuronitis this is largely unexplained. The lesion is almost always localized to the inner ear and is rarely retrocochlear. It is probable that the cause is a *disorder of microcirculation,* but it may be an autoimmune disease.

Diagnosis. The symptoms are usually unilateral. An audiogram shows a sensorineural deafness restricted to the higher and middle frequencies with recruitment or complete deafness.

Differential Diagnosis

1. Acoustic neuroma

> *Note:* Neuromas of the VIIIth cranial nerve can often cause sudden hearing loss with partial hearing damage without obvious accompanying subjective symptoms. These initial symptoms must be respected and investigated by neurootology and radiology (see p. 130).

2. Acute tubal occlusion causing pain, conductive deafness, and typical otoscopic findings.

3. Impacted cerumen

4. Epidemic parotitis

5. Herpes zoster oticus

Treatment. Low-molecular-weight dextran is infused intravenously. If an autoimmune disease is suspected, prolonged corticosteroids are given, initially under antibiotic cover. Hyperbaric oxygen is technically demanding and the results dubious. Stellate ganglion block may also be used (see p. 489).

Course and prognosis. If treatment is instituted within 24 h, there is often partial or complete recovery within several days. Spontaneous remission also often occurs. The prognosis is poor in diabetics and elderly patients with already established irreversible vascular disease.

Symptomatic Cochleovestibular Disorders

Pathogenesis. This term covers a group of cochlear or vestibular symptoms of different origin, due partly to *circulatory disorders* (diabetes, hypertension, disorders of cerebral circulation, e.g., vertebrobasilar insufficiency), partly to *trauma* (posttraumatic cervical syndrome, commotio cerebri), and partly to *inflammatory-degenerative* lesions of the cervical spine (cervical syndrome).

Syndrome of benign paroxysmal positional nystagmus:

The characteristic symptoms are ascribed to a peripheral lesion (*cupulolithiasis*). Deposition of inorganic substances in the cupula of the posterior semicircular canal increases the sensitivity of the sensory end organ to linear as well as centrifugal acceleration. This results in physiologic stimuli inducing a positional nystagmus.

The *cervical syndrome* includes cervicobrachial neuralgia, and brief attacks of dizziness dictated by the position and changes in position of the head, occasionally associated with tinnitus and pains in the nape of the neck which may radiate to the occiput and the forehead area. Objective findings: CS-Torsion-nystagmus. The cause is a lesion of the joints of the cervical spine and of the muscles of the back of the neck (see p. 18).

The *posttraumatic cervical syndrome* is mostly due to a whiplash injury and causes almost the same symptoms after a symptom-free interval of several weeks but the objective vestibular signs, such as positional nystagmus, are more pronounced.

Vertebrobasilar insufficiency causes central vestibular symptoms (spontaneous nystagmus), irregular provoked nystagmus, disorders of coordination of the oculomotor system demonstrated by optokinetic tests (see p. 68), disturbances of vision, drop attacks, and brief loss of consciousness. The latter are important in distinguishing this syndrome from the cervical syndrome. The subclavian steal syndrome also belongs in this group: the blood flows in the wrong direction in the vertebral artery due to stenosis of the proximal part of the subclavial artery on the same side so that blood is "stolen" from the vertebrobasilar circulation to compensate for the peripheral shortage of blood. The result is transient, i. e., reversible ischemia in the brainstem with corresponding symptoms (see p. 482 ff.). Diabetes, hypertension, and vascular disorders predispose to vertebrobasilar insufficiency.

Presbycusis

Symptoms. These include hearing loss, usually on both sides, for the high tones initially and later for the middle frequencies. A "social deafness" is gradually established, i. e., the patient can no longer take part in conversation with several people at the same time. The hearing for speech is affected by loud noise, and loud sounds cause discomfort due to positive recruitment. The pure-tone hearing is often better than the hearing for speech, and the hearing for syllables often better than that for sentences *(schizacusis).* Other symptoms include noises in the ears and psychological disturbances which increasingly isolate the elderly deaf patient from his environment causing depression, mistrust, and delusions of persecution.

Pathogenesis

Physiologic presbycusis. This is a degenerative process in the inner ear and CNS without exogenous damage.

The *cause* of the degenerative process is a disorder of DNA synthesis, deposition of pigment (lipofuscine), extracellular deposition of cholesterin and lipids, conversion and breakdown of collagen substances, and loss of intercellular fluid.

The changes first appear in the fifth to sixth decades of life.

Pathologic presbycusis. Supplementary inner ear and CNS lesions are caused by exogenous factors such as environmental noise and by the life style such as diet, social toxins, physical and psychological stress, hypertension, and maturity-onset diabetes. In summary, this is a multifactorial disease within the peripheral and central auditory systems beginning earlier than the physiologic presbycusis.

Four types of presbycusis may be distinguished on the basis of morphologic degenerative lesions:

1. *Sensory presbycusis* due to hair cell degeneration. The audiogram shows high tone loss.
2. *Neural presbycusis*. A large part of the population of cochlear neurons is lost so that the predominant symptom is loss of discrimination for speech.
3. *Strial type of presbycusis* due to degeneration of the stria vascularis. This causes abnormalities in endolymph production and secretion with repercussions on the energy metabolism of the hair cells. An audiogram shows a flat curve of pancochlear hearing loss with retained discrimination for speech.
4. *Conductive cochlear presbycusis*. An age-determined degenerative process in the cochlear duct causes physicoanatomic lesions of the structure of the basilar membrane. This affects the stimulus transport in the cochlea (see p. 20) which is demonstrated on an audiogram by bilateral symmetrical sensorineural deafness causing a characteristic sloping curve, with a linear increase of hearing loss above 1,000 Hz.

Diagnosis. The patient has a bilateral (usually symmetrical) sensorineural deafness. The audiometric curve depends on the type (see Fig. 1.**75**).

Differential diagnosis. A marked unilateral sensorineural deafness must be distinguished from an acoustic neuroma or a cerebellopontine angle tumor. Marked unilateral or bilateral tinnitus, synchronous with the pulse, must be differentiated from an intracranial aneurysm of the posterior cranial fossa or a glomus tumor.

> *Note:* Elderly deaf patients require early rehabilitation of communication to the same extent as young deaf patients provided that their mental powers are not severely limited.

Treatment. A hearing aid, auditory training, and a lip reading course are prescribed. The family must be given an explanation about how to deal with the deaf patient. The patient should be returned to society.

Course and prognosis. See Table 1.**19**.

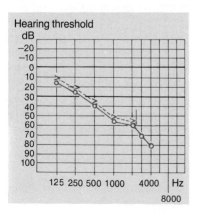

Fig. 1.**75** Audiometric findings in presbycusis. *Pure tone audiogram:* severe presbycusis with an average hearing loss of 55 dB in the major speech frequencies.

Table 1.19 Synopsis of Hearing Disorders and Their Treatment

Conductive deafness (middle ear)

Anatomic Substrate	Function	Type of Disorder	Effect on Hearing	Treatment	Prognosis for Auditory Rehabilitation
Middle ear	Conduction	Discontinuity due to infection of the ossicular chain, ventilation disorders of the middle ear, or stiffening of the ossicular chain and the tympanic membrane with increasing acoustic resistance i.e. increased impedance	*Quantitative* hearing loss due to mechanical loss of sound energy	Surgery or a hearing aid	Good

Table 1.19 Synopsis of Hearing Disorders and Their Treatment (Continuation)

Sensorineural deafness (inner ear)

Anatomic Substrate	Function	Type of Disorder	Effect on Hearing	Treatment	Prognosis for Auditory Rehabilitation
Inner ear	Mechanical frequency analysis, stimulus transformation of a mechanical into a bioelectrical stimulus, and possibly coding	Destruction of the sensory cells in the inner ear due to traumatic, vascular, metabolic, toxic, or inflammatory damage	*Quantitative* hearing loss combined with a *qualitative* worsening of speech intelligibility, due to loss of frequency analysis and stimulus transformation coding; distortion effect due to recruitment	Hearing aid, hearing training, and lip reading. Trial of medical treatment.	Relatively good. Depends on the degree of hearing loss.
Peripheral neuron	Coding, transmission of nerve impulses; lateral inhibition and interneural inhibition assure acoustic selectivity	Degeneration of the peripheral neuron due to inflammatory, vascular, traumatic, or metabolic injury	*Quantitative* and *qualitative* deterioration of hearing for speech due to abnormal coding, loss of neurons, unsatisfactory selectivity, and inability to discriminate	Hearing aid, hearing training, and lip reading	Doubtful

Table 1.19 Synopsis of Hearing Disorders and Their Treatment (Continuation)

Auditory perception (central)

Anatomic Substrate	Function	Type of Disorder	Effect on Hearing	Treatment	Prognosis for Auditory Rehabilitation
Central auditory pathways and centers	Integration, i.e., assembly of individual nervous impulses in a functional modulated activity; storage of auditory memory; decoding of acoustic information	Degeneration of the central pathways and the ganglion cells in the primary and secondary hearing centers due to inflammatory, vascular, traumatic or metabolic lesions	Mainly complete loss of the information content due to unsatisfactory integration and decoding of the acoustic signal. Partial loss of the auditory memory. The final phase is complete central deafness.	Hearing aid useless. In selected cases hearing training or lip reading.	Poor

Table 1.20 Genetic Forms of Deafness	
Sporadic-recessive deafness	Progressive morphologic lesion present at birth, usually with total degeneration of the cochlea and the peripheral cochlear neuron
Type • Michel • Mondini • Scheibe	Hypo- or aplasia of the labyrinth with almost complete loss of function of the cochlea and vestibule
Dominant hereditodegenerative deafness	Progressive disorder with an irregular course. First manifests itself at or after puberty. Often combined with other inherited symptoms to form a circumscribed syndrome such as those detailed below.
• Waardenburg's syndrome	Congenital anomalies of the facial skeleton, dystopia canthorum; blepharophimosis; disorders of pigmentation of the eyes, hair and skin (albinism); degenerative atrophy of the cochlea and the ganglion cells
• Usher's syndrome	Hereditary progressive sensorineural deafness with retinitis pigmentosa. Degeneration of the cochlea and the spiral ganglion.
• Refsum's syndrome	The same symptoms are found as in Usher's syndrome with the addition of polyneuropathy and ataxia. Often this condition first manifests itself between the ages of 10 and 20 years.
• Alport's syndrome	Progressive inner ear deafness, bilateral, but often asymmetrical beginning in the second decade of life associated with a nonspecific chronic glomerulo and interstitial nephritis. The frequency is 1 in 200000 births. The renal disorder is inherited, and the inner ear lesion may be a secondary nephrogenic effect.
• Pendred's syndrome	Perceptive deafness with labyrinthine dysplasia associated with thyroid gland disorders.
Chromosomal anomalies	Anomalies of the external and middle ear associated with numerous other organ anomalies and developmental disorders of the inner ear.
• Trisomy 13	Labyrinthine hypoplasia with aplasia of organ of Corti and the stria vascularis
• Trisomy 18	Similar changes with atresia of the auditory nerve
• Cri-du-chat syndrome	Similar malformations associated with laryngeal anomalies

Sensorineural Deafness Due to Other Causes

Deafness in Children (Pediaudiology).

See Tables 1.**20** through 1.**23**.

Clinical Aspects of Central Deafness

Acoustic Agnosia

Synonyms include sensory aphasia, psychogenic or word deafness, sensory deaf mutism, and central deafness.

Symptoms. The main symptom is the delayed development of speech which unfortunately is often recognized late since the child is often mistakenly diagnosed as suffering from delayed mental development or autism. Other symptoms include acoustic inattention due to the absence of acoustic ability to differentiate, disturbances of perception, slurred articulation, animated gestures, and miming. Directional hearing is lost and the patient suffers paramusia, amusia, and loss of musicality.

Pathogenesis. Causes may be cerebral and skull trauma, encephalitis, and pre-, peri-, and postnatal damage to the central nervous system.

Diagnosis. A clinical diagnosis of acoustic agnosia can only be made after observation over a period of time. Investigations include electroencephalography, computed tomography, ERA, and psychotechnical investigation which allow a defini-

Table 1.**21** Prenatal Acquired (Exogenous) Deafness	
Infections from the mother	
• Rubella embryopathy	Developmental disorders of the middle and inner ear, severe bilateral sensorineural deafness
• Congenital syphilis	Progressive degeneration of the inner ear and the peripheral neuron associated with interstitial keratitis and dental defects (Hutchinson's triad)
• Toxoplasmosis	Inflammatory damage to the inner ear
• Viral infections	Mumps, herpes zoster, poliomyelitis, influenza, cytomegalus
Toxic damage due to:	Quinine, aminoglycosides, and thalidomide which causes multiple anomalies
Further exogenous damage due to:	Diabetus mellitus of the mother, fetal hypoxia, irradiation

Table 1.22 Perinatal Acquired (Exogenous) Deafness	
Perinatal hypoxia	Injury of the cochlea and its centers in the brain stem
Premature birth	Hemorrhage into the cochlea
Kernicterus (perinatal hyperbilirubinemia)	Rh-incompatibility, massive deposits of bilirubin in the cochlear centers and occasionally in the cochlea itself with corresponding cochleoneural deafness

Table 1.23 Postnatal Acquired (Exogenous) Deafness	
Infective diseases	
• Meningitis and meningoencephalitis	Labyrinthitis and cochleovestibular neuritis with damage to the sensory cells and peripheral neurons; central lesions
• Mumps	Cochlear and neural lesions (see pp. 139, 540 ff.)
• Measles	Degeneration of the cochlea and its peripheral neurons due to infective damage, serous labyrinthitis
• Otitis media	Recurrent otitis, infective toxic damage to inner ear associated with sensorineural deafness

tive diagnosis to be made after consultation between an otologist, a pediatric neurologist, a pediatric psychiatrist, and a child psychologist.

Treatment. Long-term treatment includes acoustic differentiation exercises, articulation training, and prescription of a hearing aid for an objectively demonstrated sensorineural deafness. A hearing aid is useless for a true sensory agnosia. Rhythmic exercises, music therapy, and exploitation of visual observations build up the patient's conceptual store (lip reading).

Audimutism

This term is inaccurate since it does not adequately characterize delayed development of speech. The child is mute although he can hear. The term audimutism in its strictest sense should be confined to those children who after the 3rd year of life can only make themselves understood by gestures, are unable to speak any words, but are not mentally defective, and demonstrate normal hearing. There is a connection between audimutism and brain damage in early childhood. The term deaf *mutism* has therefore been abandoned and replaced by that of "absent or delayed development of speech."

Basis of Rehabilitation of Deafness in Children and Adults

Note: An assessment of deafness with respect to the potential for social rehabilitation should be based not only on the degree of severity and the site of the hearing loss, but equally on the age and the physical, mental, and speech development of the patient.

Classification of Deafness Depending on the Degree of Severity

Normal hearing. The hearing threshold of the pure-tone audiogram does not exceed 20 dB for any frequency.

Slight deafness. On the pure-tone audiogram, there is a hearing loss of > 20 dB, or at the most 40 dB within the entire frequency range. Deafness of this degree does not usually cause delay in development of speech in a child of normal intelligence.

Conductive deafness can usually be treated medically. Sensorineural deafness must be treated individually with a hearing aid, supplemented by language training from a hearing therapist. Individual schooling and hearing training are not indicated.

Moderate deafness. In this case the average hearing loss within the main speech frequencies of 250 to 4,000 Hz is between 40 and 60 dB. This causes considerable difficulty in understanding speech so that the development of speech is delayed. The prescription of a hearing aid is absolutely indicated, and children require early hearing and speech education. Initially, the child should attend a special school for the deaf but he can usually attend a normal school later, provided he has a hearing aid and normal intellectual development.

Severe deafness. The average hearing loss within the main speech frequencies is greater than 60 dB, and the tones above 1,000 Hz are most severely affected. Provided that the child has normal intellectual development, a hearing aid is certainly indicated since a high degree of communication by speech can be developed from even the smallest remnant of hearing using electroacoustic methods and early speech and hearing training. These children should attend special schools for the deaf. Severely deaf adults whose hearing and speech were previously normal should be treated by a hearing aid and intensive exercises to distinguish vowels, consonants, and loudness while using that hearing aid. They should have several years training in lipreading to encourage visual compensation for the loss of auditory function.

Bilateral *complete deafness* is fortunately very rare. Even patients with almost total deafness often have remnants of hearing which can be shown by electroacoustic methods, and these islands can be utilized by high-performance hearing aids. The child should be educated in separate schools for the deaf. In these schools sign language has been replaced currently by the use of real speech: articulated speech is practiced using the vibration sense and lip reading training partly directly and partly by a video recorder. In selected cases children as well as adults can be considered for a *chochlear implant,* which involves the implantation of a multi-channel cochlear prosthesis.

Multiple handicap. This is a special group of deaf children who in addition show intellectual retardation, behavioral disturbances, extensive organic brain damage, or delay in motor development causing failure to speak. An exacting therapeutic program must be set up for this group requiring the combination of an otologist, a phoniatrist, a neurologist, a child psychiatrist, psychologist, and a logopedist.

Voice and speech disorders due to deafness. Deafness mainly affects the ability to communicate in children, but it can also affect adults. Physio-

Table 1.24 Timetable of Speech Development (adapted from *Kussmaul*)	
Up to the 7th week	Crying
6 weeks–6 months	First babbling period, beginning of auditory feedback
6– 9 months	Second babbling period, hearing predominant
8– 9 months	Echolalia, imitation and first understanding of speech
9–12 months	Beginning of deliberate speech
13–15 months	Early precise use of significant words, symbolic function of speech
12–18 months	One-word sentences, developmental stammering
18–24 months	Two-word sentences; unformed sentences of several words, first age of questioning
End of 2nd year of life	Non-grammatical sentences, establishment of consciousness of symbols
from 3 years onward	Formed sentences of several words, adoption of first grammatical principles
from 4th year of life	Second questioning age, first establishment of logical and emotional relationships, maturation of the thinking-speaking process

logic *auditory verbal communication* requires both a normal voice and speech apparatus and also normal feedback through the ear.

The change of speech in those born without hearing, or those who become deaf or partially deaf in later life, is defined as *otogenic dyslalia*.

Table 1.**24** gives **a review of speech development** in childhood.

The Completely Deaf Child

In a *child with no hearing or only residual islands of hearing,* auditory feedback is absent, and the child develops a typical monotonous speech which distinguishes the totally deaf child from a child with normal hearing or a partial hearing loss.

The best rehabilitative results are achieved by:

- Early diagnosis and treatment
- Early prescription of a hearing aid
- Prolonged auditory training and early voice and speech training in special preschools and deaf schools to develop the missing sound components of speech and speech content,
- Cochlear implant in selected cases

The Cochlear Implant

The cochlear implant consists of a directional microphone, which picks up speech sounds and transmits them to a speech processor. This device encodes speech information, which is transmitted through the intact skin by radio waves to a receiver-stimulator implanted in the mastoid bone. A multi-electrode array implanted into the basal turn of the cochlea simulates normal sound encoding by electrical stimulation of the remaining auditory nerve fibers in the inner ear. This electronic device enables about 30% of patients to comprehend running speech in an open field without benefit of lip reading. In the rest it affords significant improvement of communication through the partial restoration of acoustic perception.

Hearing Aids

The prescription of a *hearing aid* is indicated if a deafness cannot be relieved or improved by other means such as surgery. This is *a functional prosthesis* and must be prescribed by the specialist after a thorough audiometric investigation.

A hearing aid comprises a microphone, an amplifier (consisting of transistors), and an electromagnetic headphone driven by a battery. Many hearing aids are provided with a directional microphone. The sensitivity of this microphone depends on the direction of the sound. The sound is con-

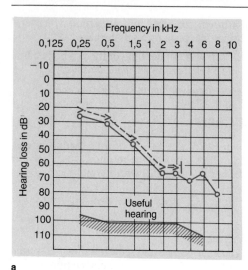

a

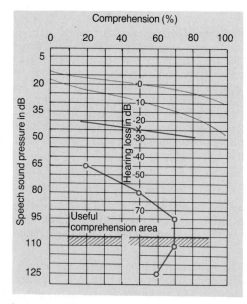

b

Fig. 1.**76a** and **b**   Comparison of the *useful hearing* of the pure-tone audiogram with the *useful intelligibility level* on the speech audiogram indicates the threshold of discomfort (Lehnhardt). The speech audiogram is mainly responsible for expressing the indications for prescription of a hearing aid. The problem is to find an apparatus that not only reflects the frequency characteristics of the pure-tone threshold, but also one with an automatic volume control which takes account of loudness in the suprathreshold area. The *threshold of discomfort* is decisive in determining the upper limit of amplification. The threshold is that level at which sounds are uncomfortable but not painful. The remaining *useful hearing range* lies between this and the hearing threshold. The *speech field* of the deaf patient which is to be amplified by a hearing aid is encompassed by this range.

ducted from the hearing aid into the patient's ear by a tube and an earpiece. A bone conduction aid can be supplied if an earpiece cannot be used because of chronic meatal or middle ear inflammation and discharge, congenital anomalies, or allergies to the earpiece, and so forth. The choice of hearing aid, e.g., between a behind-the-hear or in-the-ear device, one that is part of the spectacles, or a pocket apparatus is determined initially by *electroacoustic properties*. These include amplification, frequency characteristics, maximal output sound pressure peak, and automatic amplification regulation such as automatic gain control or peak clipping. These properties must correspond to the type of deafness and its site, middle or inner ear, taking particular account of recruitment, and furthermore to the hearing threshold within the frequency range to be amplified, the patient's hearing dynamics, and the shape of the discrimination curve (see pp. 43–57 and Table 1.3). This requires accurate audiometric investigation (Fig. 1.76a and b).

The *pure-tone audiogram* shows whether the deafness is conductive or sensorineural in type. Furthermore, it demonstrates the patient's hearing threshold in the frequency and hearing dynamic range whose upper limit is the threshold of discomfort (see pp. 26, 48).

A *speech audiogram* provides information about the hearing loss for numbers and the patient's word comprehension (see pp. 52 ff.) so that the deafness can be classified. Furthermore, it provides information about the patient's *minimal discrimination loss* and the *maximal comprehension* of the tested ear. If a monaural hearing aid is to be used, the ear with the least discrimination loss is chosen. The shape of the *discrimination curve* provides important information regarding the choice of an automatic volume control which is usually built into most hearing aids nowadays: the peak of *maximal comprehension* is crucial to the choice of the required amplification level. The *discomfort threshold for speech* is also an important parameter for the upper limit of amplification. It forms a limit that should not be exceeded during transmission of speech through the hearing aid; otherwise an undistorted loudness discomfort occurs which can be accompanied in sensorineural deafness by a further loss of discrimination and associated subjective distortion.

Speech discrimination or maximum understanding for speech (PB words) is more important in the assessment of a hearing aid than the hearing loss for understanding of test words of two syllables or greater.

Note: Deafness always affects the ability to communicate. Deafness should therefore be detected, diagnosed, and treated adequately as early as possible.

This involves both the medical profession and the supplementary professions. The foremost duty of the medical profession is not only to treat the afflicted but also to improve public awareness of the deaf patient and his problems.

Clinical Aspects of Central Balance Disorders

Symptoms. The following symptoms indicate a central cause for a balance disorder:

- Sudden attacks of dizziness of short duration (1 to 2 s)
- Fluctuating dizziness with *loss of consciousness*
- Dizziness with *"drop attacks"* which are short-lasting attacks of loss of muscle tone in which the patient sinks to the ground but does not become unconscious
- Dizziness with double vision and other *disturbances of vision* such as hemianopsia, scotoma, etc.
- Dizziness with *dysarthria and change of personality*

Pathogenesis. Central vestibular disorders are usually the result of *multifocal lesions* of the brain stem. Therefore, they are usually accompanied by symptoms of disorders of the visual oculomotor and somatosensory system (Tables 1.**25** and 1.**26**).

Table 1.25 Pathogenesis of Central Vestibular Disorders

Inflammation	• Meningitis
	• Meningoencephalitis
	• Cerebellar abscess
Trauma	• Cerebral concussion and contusion
Space-occupying processes	
	• Infratentorial tumors
	• Cerebellopontine angle tumors
	• Glomus tumors
	• Arachnoid cysts
Vascular processes	
	• Vertebrobasilar insufficiency
	• Basilar artery migraine
	• Arteriovenous anomalies
Intoxication	• Barbiturates
	• Alcohol
Degenerative diseases of the central nervous system	
	• Multiple sclerosis
	• Syringobulbia
	• Cerebellar degeneration

Table 1.26 Synopsis of Central Balance Disorders

	Neurootologic symptoms	Neurophthalmologic symptoms	Neurologic symptoms
Encephalitis	Spontaneous nystagmus, often disassociated; positional nystagmus (irregular); gaze-evoked nystagmus; pathologic optokinetic reflexes	Papilledema	Meningismus, somnolence, restlessness, cerebellar symptoms, focal neurologic symptoms, abnormal spinal fluid chemistry
Cerebral concussion	Positional (provocation) nystagmus, pathologic vestibulospinal reflexes	—	Headaches, memory defects, poor mental concentration
Infratentorial tumor with brain stem compression	Spontaneous nystagmus, positional nystagmus (irregular) gaze-evoked and gaze-paretic nystagmus, pathologic optokinetic nystagmus, pathologic vestibulospinal reflexes with ataxia, pathologic caloric responses	Eye muscle paresis, papilledema, horizontal and vertical gaze paresis	Focal neurologic symptoms of Vth, VIth, IXth and Xth, cranial nerves, dysphagia, pyramidal signs, extremity paresis, dissociated sensation, headache, vomiting
Vertebrobasilar insufficiency with involvement of pons and medulla	Vestibular spontaneous nystagmus, vestibular provoked nystagmus, pathologic vestibulospinal reflexes, pathologic optokinetic reflexes	Horner's syndrome	Cerebellar ataxia, motor hemiparesis, disturbed sensation, involvement of Vth, VIIth, IXth, and Xth cranial nerves

Table 1.26 Continuation

Multiple sclerosis	Vestibular spontaneous nystagmus, irregular positional nystagmus (irregular), gaze-evoked and gaze-paretic nystagmus, abnormal caloric responses, abnormal optokinetic reflexes, pathologic vestibulospinal reflexes, ataxia	Dissociated (disconjugated) nystagmus horizontal and vertical gaze paralysis, bilateral internuclear ophthalmoplegia, retrobulbar neuritis	Multiple attacks of multilocular demyelinating disorders of the central nervous system with spastic paralysis, urinary incontinence, intention tremor, dysdiadochokinesis, and para- and dysesthesia
Barbiturate intoxication	Vestibular spontaneous nystagmus, irregular positional nystagmus (irregular), gaze-evoked nystagmus Abnormal vestibular ocular and optokinetic reflexes	Oculomotor disorders	Cerebellar ataxia, dysarthria, somnolence

Clinical Aspects of Disorders of the Facial Nerve

The *symptoms* and *differential diagnosis* of a *central* and a *peripheral lesion of the facial nerve* have already been discussed (see pp. 18, 69). Therefore, only the consequences of a *peripheral lesion of a facial nerve* and its cause, characteristics, and treatment will be discussed here.

Inflammatory or Otogenic Facial Paralysis

A peripheral facial paralysis which is at least partly reversible may be caused by neurotropic viruses such as herpes zoster (see p. 138), Coxsackie, or poliomyelitis virus, by a neuroallergic polyradiculitis, Guillain-Barré disease, or by sarcoidosis. The latter is also known as Heerfordt-Mylius syndrome, with uveitis and parotitis in addition to facial paralysis (see p. 544). However, for the otologist the most important and commonest form is *otogenic facial paralysis*.

This may occur first as an immediate complication of an *acute otitis media or mastoiditis* which is *treated* by antibiotics and immediate mastoidectomy; the lesion is usually a neuropraxia. Second, paralysis may arise as a complication of a *middle ear cholesteatoma* invading the bony facial canal. Extension of the inflammation to the nerve sheath, the epi-, peri-, and endoneurium causes axonal degeneration and demyelinization of the mastoid, tympanic, and labyrinthine segments. The *treatment* is radical mastoidectomy and decompression of the nerve.

The *prognosis* for the first type is always good provided that the patient does not suffer from latent or manifest diabetes. The prognosis in the second type is occasionally poor, despite intensive antibiotics and decompression of the facial nerve since the nerve is usually only partially reinnervated and therefore cannot heal completely.

Idiopathic Facial Paralysis (Bell's Palsy)

The **cause,** as the name indicates, is unknown. It may be a disturbance of the microcirculation leading to a serous inflammation with the formation of edema. The bony canal is unyielding, and compression of the nerve leads to ischemia and venous congestion so that a vicious circle is set up. A virus infection may also be responsible.

Electrodiagnosis in about 80% of patients shows *a neurapraxia* with a good prognosis. In 20% of patients there is partial *axonotmesis*. In about 5% to 10% of patients with idiopathic facial paralysis, the axon degeneration progresses between the 4th and 10th days despite treatment with corticosteroids. If *neuronography* shows more than 90% of degenerated neurons, a *decompression is indicated*.

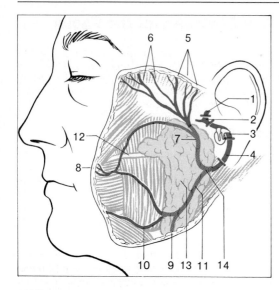

Fig. 1.77 Anatomy of the course of the facial nerve relative to exposure of the nerve.
1, Meatal segment;
2, labyrinthine segment;
3, tympanic segment;
4, mastoid segment;
5, temporal rami;
6, zygomatic rami;
7, temporofacial portion;
8, buccal rami; 9, cervical rami; 10, marginal mandibular ramus; 11, cervical facial portion;
12, parotid duct;
13, parotid gland;
14, extratemporal part of the facial nerve.
1–4 intratemporal section, 5–11 extratemporal section.

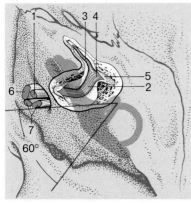

Fig. 1.78 Operative approach to the inner auditory canal and the intratemporal facial nerve segments. 1, Meatal segment; 2, labyrinthine segment; 3, greater superifical petrosal nerve; 4, geniculate ganglion; 5, beginning of the tympanic segment of the facial nerve; 6, cochlear nerve; 7, superior and inferior vestibular nerve.

Treatment. This includes injection of steroids, stellate ganglion block, and low-molecular-weight intravenous infusion of dextran.

Schedule for prednisone in the treatment of idiopathic facial paralysis: 60 mg for 4 days reducing by 5 mg daily to 5 mg on the 15th day, followed by intermittent dosage of 5 mg for 10 days.

Immediate *decompression* of the nerve should be undertaken for progressive denervation (Figs. 1.**77** and 1.**78**) after careful assessment of the indication (see pp. 69, 163).

The *principle of treatment* is to decompress the nerve fibers by exposure of the nerve and slitting of its sheath.

Electromyography in the first 2 weeks of the paralysis does not provide prognostically valid information. During this time, therefore, electrodiagnostic and neuronographic investigation should be carried out every 2 days to identify those patients requiring decompression.

An unusual form of idiopathic facial paralysis is the *Melkersson-Rosenthal syndrome.*

Symptoms

- Recurring facial paralysis
- Furrowed tongue and cheilitis
- Facial edema

The cause is unknown, treatment with steroids is unsatisfactory, and the prognosis is dubious.

Traumatic Facial Paralysis

Causes include fracture of the base of the skull, blast and gunshot injuries, iatrogenic lesions during middle ear operations and parotidectomy.

Frequency. A facial paralysis occurs in 10% to 20% of all longitudinal pyramidal fractures and in 50% of all transverse fractures. Seventy-five percent of all paralyses developing completely within 24 h of the trauma and 90% of late-onset paralyses resolve spontaneously.

Prognosis. The outcome of a paralysis in pyramidal fracture is determined by the type of the lesion, such as depression of the canal, damage to the nerve by a splinter of bone, shearing of the nerve without fracture of the bony canal, or a nerve sheath hematoma leading to edema. Electrodiagnosis is the only reliable method of determining those patients who will develop rapid degeneration of the axons and will therefore not recover fully without decompression (see Fig. 1.**78**).

Treatment. The same basic rules for decompression apply as for idiopathic facial palsy. Conservative treatment is limited to steroids in the first 6 days after the trauma provided that there is no contraindication.

Reconstructive Surgery After Facial Paralysis

Facial paralyses are due to various lesions of the facial nerve. Their severity depends on the extent to which the continuity of the nerve has been preserved and which segment of the nerve is affected (see Fig. 1.**77**).

In crushing and constricting injuries, depression of the bony canal, and direct injury of the nerve by bone splinters, exposure of the nerve within its intratemporal course, so far as the bone has been damaged, suffices to decompress the nerve. Occasionally slitting of the nerve sheath must also be performed to release a hematoma. Lesions of the facial nerve in the facial region due to skull fractures, knife and stab wounds, and operative trauma are relatively unusual. A lesion of *all* nerve branches is caused solely by damage to the main trunk of the nerve (see Figs. 1.**20** and 1.**77**); peripheral injuries usually only affect individual branches.

Principles of Treatment

The site of injury to the nerve should be looked for, if possible within 48 h: the nerve should be resutured by microsurgery, if necessary using a nerve graft from the great auricular or sural nerve. An *old* injury should be managed by an attempt at nerve reconstruction in the region of the lesion, and if this is not possible, by anastomosing the branches of the facial nerve to the opposite side by a "crossover" graft according to Scaramella.

A *loss of continuity* may be due either to a clean division of the nerve or to an extensive defect requiring one of the following procedures.

1. *End-to-end suture* is indicated after division of the nerve, if the proximal and distal stumps can be brought together without tension after resecting the epineurium (Fig. 1.**79**).
2. *Rerouting* consists of exposing the damaged nerve over a wide area and shortening its route by lifting the nerve out of the bony canal. This allows an end-to-end suture without tension, even for extensive defects (see Figs. 1.**79** and 1.**80**).
3. *Autogenous nerve grafts* using a free graft from the great auricular or sural nerve are used for large defects if the freshened nerve stumps cannot be apposed without tension (Fig. 1.**81**).

In most cases of irreversible facial nerve damage, satisfactory recovery of function can be achieved by one of these operative techniques. In extensive damage of the nerve and its immediate surroundings, and especially for defects in the cerebello-

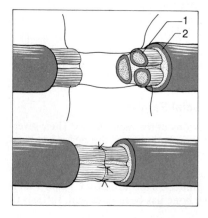

Fig. 1.**79** Fascicular nerve suture. Perineural reconstruction begins with the central fascicle. 1, Perineurium; 2, Epineurium.

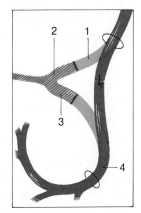

Fig. 1.**80** Facial nerve repair by rerouting of the damaged facial nerve in its intratemporal course. 1, Meatal segment; 2, labyrinthine segment; 3, tympanic segment; 4, mastoid segment. Defect in segments 2 and 3.

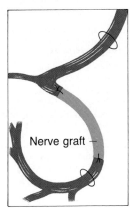

Fig. 1.**81**   Facial nerve repair by a nerve graft.

pontine angle, reneurotization of the mimic facial musculature is only achieved by *nerve replacement techniques*. There are basically two methods: first, the peripheral stump may be anastomosed with a cranial nerve such as the hypoglossal or accessory on the same side. Second, individual branches of the still-functioning healthy side may be anastomosed by free autologous nerve grafts with the facial nerve using a cross-face (or faciofacial) anastomosis. The best results are achieved by a *hypoglossal-facial anastomosis* which must include resection of the epineurium. The results of faciofacial anastomosis cannot yet be assessed fully. In cases of defects in the facial nerve in the area of the cerebellopontine angle after tumor resection, end-to-end anastomosis with fibrin adhesive or nerve transplantation is carried out (Dott's operation).

Long-standing paralyses lead to degeneration of motor end plates and disuse atrophy of the muscle fibers. The critical period for end plate degeneration is 1 year after denervation. A replacement graft is useless in these circumstances and a muscle fascia sling is therefore introduced.

Synopsis of Ear Symptoms

See Tables 1.27 and 1.28.

Table 1.27 Local Symptoms of Ear Disease	
Pressure feeling	*Uni- or bilateral, constant or intermittent:* cerumen, tubal problem, Ménière's disease, glomus tumor
Pain (otalgia)	*Dull, penetrating sensation:* beginning otitis media or parotitis *Pulsating:* caused by acute otitis media or furuncle in the external canal *Stabbing or intermittent:* otalgia secondary to radiation therapy; bad teeth; temporomandibular joint syndrome; parotitis; tumor of the base of the tongue, tonsil, hypopharynx, or larynx
Aural discharge (otorrhea)	*Smell:* fetid in otitis externa and cholesteatoma *Color:* yellow with cerumen and pus; hemorrhage in influenzal otitis *Consistency:* watery in cerebrospinal otorrhea, mucoid in chronic secretory otitis, greasy in external otitis and cholesteatomas *Pulsating:* otitis media with perforation *Nonpulsating:* external otitis

Table 1.**28** Functional Ear Symptoms

Tinnitus	*Type:* whistling, buzzing, ringing, hissing; crackling are often due to tubal problems *Occurrence:* constant, intermittent, may occur in attacks as in Ménière's disease *Character:* synchronous with pulse in hypertonia, cranial aneurysm, or glomus tumor
Deafness	High-tone loss caused by acoustic trauma or presbycusis Low-tone loss caused by Ménières disease, otitis media, otosclerosis Decreased speech intelligibility, due to a loss of discrimination (inner ear or VIIIth cranial nerve lesion) Fluctuating, episodic as in Ménière's disease and sudden hearing loss Improvement in noisy environment, said to be typical of conductive deafness Unilateral in Ménière's disease, VIIIth cranial nerve tumors Bilateral in age- and noise-induced losses
Vertigo	Turning vertigo in Ménière's disease and acute vestibular paralysis (vestibular neuronitis) Elevator and swing vertigo due to inner ear affections Blackout spells due to extravestibular or orthostatic cause Episodic in Ménière's disease Continuous vertigo occurs in vestibular paralysis Spontaneous and episodic in Ménière's disease Provoked by head movement and position change of the body, caused by the inner ear, the cervical syndrome, vertebrobasilar insufficiency Unsteadiness in gait and standing is caused by central vestibular disturbance and multiple sclerosis *Combined with vertigo:* • Nausea, vomiting – occurs in acute vestibular paralysis and Ménière's disease • Double vision-indicates a brain stem lesion • Loss of consciousness – is due to a brain stem or a space-occupying intracranial.lesion.

2. Nose, Nasal Sinuses, and Face

Applied Anatomy and Physiology

Basic Anatomy

External Nose

The supporting structure of the nose consists of bone, cartilage, and connective tissue. Figure 2.1 shows the most important elements. The *bony*, superior, part of the nasal pyramid is often broken in typical fractures of the nasal bones, but it may also be fractured in injuries of the central part of the face. The *cartilaginous*, inferior portion is only slightly at risk, at least in mild blunt trauma because of its elastic structure, but it is at risk in stab wounds, lacerations, and gunshot injuries. The shape, position, and properties of the bone and cartilage of the nose influence considerably the *form* and aesthetic *harmony* of the face (see p. 282) and the *function* of the nasal cavity.

The following *blood vessels* of the external nose are of practical importance:

- Facial artery and its branches
- Dorsal nasal artery arising from the ophthalmic artery

Profuse hemorrhage may arise from these vessels in injury to the central part of the face.

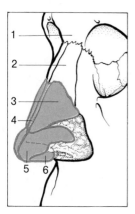

Fig. 2.1 Nasal skeleton: 1, glabella; 2, nasal bone; 3, lateral nasal cartilage; 4, upper edge of the cartilaginous nasal septum; 5, greater alar cartilage; 6, medial crus of (5).

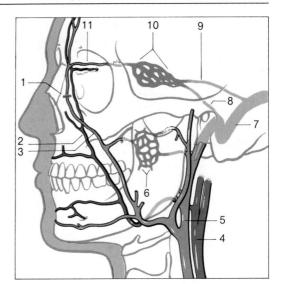

Fig. 2.**2**   Important vascular relationships of the face. 1, Site for ligation of the angular vein; 2, facial artery; 3, facial vein; 4, common carotid artery; 5, internal jugular vein; 6, pterygoid plexus; 7, sigmoid sinus; 8, inferior petrosal sinus; 9, superior petrosal sinus; 10, cavernous sinus; 11, superior ophthalmic artery and vein.

The angular vein is also clinically important: a thrombophlebitis arising from a furuncle of the upper lip or the nose can spread via the ophthalmic vein to the cavernous sinus to cause a cavernous sinus thrombosis (see p. 250 and Fig. 2.**2**).

The external nose derives its sensory *nerve supply* from the first and second branches of the trigeminal nerve (see Fig. 2.**13a** und **b**). The muscles derive their motor *nerve supply* from the facial nerve.

Nasal Cavity

The interior of the nose is divided by the nasal septum into two cavities, which are usually unequal in size. Each side may be divided into the *nasal vestibule* and the *nasal cavity* proper (Fig. 2.**3a** and **b**). The nasal vestibule is covered by epidermis containing hairs (vibrissae) and sebaceous glands. The latter are the site of origin of a nasal furuncle which can thus only develop in the nasal cavity in the vestibule.

The medial wall of the nasal vestibule encloses the supporting structure of the anterior part of the cartilaginous septum and the connective tissue septum, i. e., the *columella*. The roof of the vestibule is formed by the horseshoe-shaped lower lateral or alar cartilage whose medial crus extends into the columella and whose lateral crus supports the external wall of the vestibule (see Figs. 2.**1** and 2.**3a** and **b**). The alar

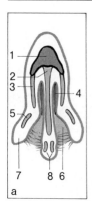

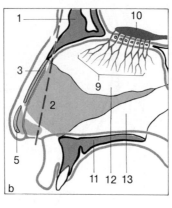

Fig. 2.**3a** and **b**   **a.** Section through the anterior nose showing the vestibule and the limen nasi. The limen nasi lies at the junction of the pink and red areas. **b.** Medial nasal wall. 1, Bony nasal bridge; 2, nasal septum; 3, lateral nasal cartilage; 4, nasal cavity; 5, alar cartilage; 6, nasal vestibule; 7, nasal ala; 8, nasal columella with medial crus of the cartilaginous ala; 9, filaments of the olfactory nerve; 10, olfactory bulb; 11, palatine bone; 12, perpendicular plate of the ethmoid; 13, vomer. The dashed line shows the plane of section of (a).

cartilage thus determines the shape of the nasal tip and the nasal apertures. Correction of this area is thus often an important part of rhinoplasty.

A very important structure from the physiologic point of view is the *internal nasal valve* or limen nasi. This lies at the junction of the vestibule and the nasal cavity. It is formed by a prominence of the anterior edge of the upper lateral or triangular cartilage on the lateral wall of the nose (see Fig. 2.**3a**). The internal nasal valve or limen nasi is normally the most narrow point of the entire cross section of the nasal cavity, and thus has an important influence on nasal respiration (see p. 182).

The *nasal cavity* extends from the internal nasal valve to the choana. The structure of the floor and roof of the nose, of the medial wall, and of the *nasal septum* can be seen in Figure 2.**3a** and **b**.

The outline of the *lateral wall of the nasal cavity* is more complex than that of the medial wall. It contains several structures that are important in the function of the nose and nasal cavity (Fig. 2.**4**):

- Three nasal turbinates
- Ostia of the nasal sinuses, with the exception of that for the sphenoid sinus
- Opening of the nasolacrimal duct

The superior, middle, and inferior meatus lie inferior to the three turbinates (Fig. 2.**4**), and the nasal sinuses and the nasolacrimal duct open into them. Thus, they are of diagnostic and therapeutic significance.

a. The *inferior meatus,* lying between the floor of the nose and the insertion of the lower turbinate, does not contain a sinus ostium, but does

Fig. 2.4 Lateral nasal wall. I, Superior meatus; II, middle meatus; III, inferior meatus. 1, Nasal vestibule; 2, opening of the nasolacrimal duct; 3, origin of the inferior turbinate; 4, maxillary ostium; 5, insertion of the middle turbinate; 6, sphenoid sinus; 7, insertion of the superior turbinate; 8, frontal sinus; a, drainage of the antral cavity; b, drainage of the frontal sinus through the nasofrontal duct; c, drainage of the anterior ethmoid cells;

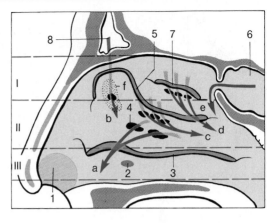

d, drainage of the posterior ethmoid cells; e drainage of the sphenoid sinus; f, area of infundibulum (black dotted area).

have the opening of the nasolacrimal duct lying about 3 cm posterior to the external nasal opening (see Fig. 2.**4**).

b. The *middle meatus,* between the inferior and middle turbinate, is of clinical importance because the nasofrontal duct, the anterior ethmoid cells, and the maxillary antrum open into it (see Fig. 2.**4**).

c. The *superior meatus,* between the middle and superior turbinate, contains the opening for the posterior ethmoid cells (see Fig. 2.**4**). The sphenoid ostium lies on the anterior wall of the sphenoid sinus at the level of the superior meatus (see Fig. 2.**4**).

The nasal cavity is lined by two different types of epithelium: *respiratory and olfactory* (Fig. 2.**5a–d**).

The *respiratory epithelium* lines the entire airway and its projections and offshoots, (e.g., the nasal sinuses and the middle ear) from the nasal introitus to the bronchi. It shows morphologic variation in different parts of the respiratory tract. Figure 2.**5b** shows the structure of the respiratory epithelium of the nasal cavity. The epithelium is columnar-ciliated with goblet cells and a layer of mixed glands, a fairly well-marked lymphoid cell zone, and fairly well-developed venous cavernous spaces in the turbinates and around the ostia (see Fig. 2.**5a**).

The *olfactory mucosa,* innervated by fibers of the olfactory nerve, covers the area of the olfactory cleft, the cribriform plate, part of the superior turbinate, and the part of the septum lying opposite it. The structure is shown in Figure 2.**5d**, and its topographic extent in Figure 2.**5c**. Bowman's glands occur specifically in this area. They produce a lipolipid secretion which covers the olfactory region and aids olfactory perception, along with the enzymes it contains. It is entirely dissimilar to the secretion of the glands of the respiratory epithelium.

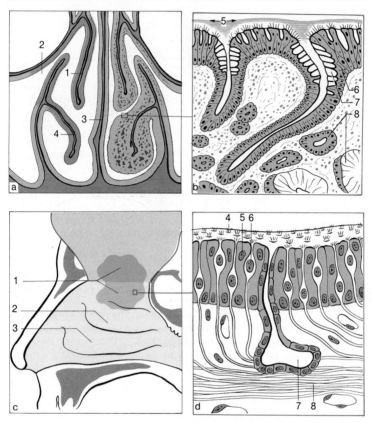

Fig. 2.**5a—d**   **a.** Frontal section through the nasal cavity. On the left the nasal mucosa is constricted, and on the right the nasal mucosa is normal. **b.** Respiratory mucosa. 1, Middle turbinate; 2, antrum with ostium; 3, nasal septum; 4, inferior turbinate; 5, layer of mucus; 6, respiratory epithelium with cilia; 7, goblet cells; 8, mucosal glands. **c.** Sagittal section through the nose with the septum turned upward. **d.** Olfactory mucosa. 1, Olfactory region; 2, middle turbinate; 3, inferior turbinate; 4, olfactory zone with cilia; 5, supporting cell; 6, olfactory cell; 7, Bowman's gland; 8, olfactory fibers.

Nasal Sinuses

The nasal sinuses are prolongations of the nasal cavity into the neighboring bone of the skull (Fig. 2.**6**).

The *maxillary sinus* is the largest sinus, with an average size of 15 ml. The paired sinuses are often developed asymmetrically, and the resulting dif-

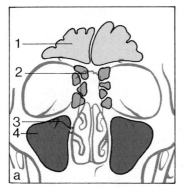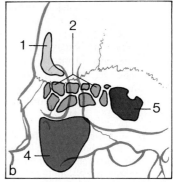

Fig. 2.**6a** and **b**   Nasal sinuses. a. Frontal section. b. Sagittal section. 1, Frontal sinus; 2, ethmoid sinus; 3, maxillary ostium; 4, antral cavity; 5, sphenoid cavity.

ferent thickness of bony wall may give rise to incorrect radiologic diagnoses. The sinus usually consists of one chamber only, but it may have niches, and indeed may even contain separate loculi. These may cause difficulties in diagnosis and treatment. The ostium of the maxillary sinus lies in the superior part of the medial wall of the sinus and opens into the nose in the middle meatus (see Fig. 2.**6a**). This position of the opening does not favor spontaneous emptying of the cavity since it does not lie at the deepest point of the cavity in the upright position, but indeed lies almost at the top of the cavity.

The *superior or orbital wall* of the maxillary sinus also forms the floor of the orbit. The infraorbital nerve runs within it.

The *medial wall* is also the lateral wall of the nasal cavity. It contains the maxillary ostium and the accessory ostia.

The *anterior wall* contains the infraorbital foramen.

The *posterior wall* forms the dividing wall between the sinus and the pterygopalatine fossa. The maxillary artery, the pterygopalatine ganglion, and branches of the trigeminal nerve and autonomic nervous system lie within the pterygomaxillary fossa (see Fig. 2.**10**).

The *floor* of the maxillary sinus is related to the tooth roots in the alveolus, particularly those of the second premolar and the first molar. This is the site of origin of an odontogenic sinusitis (see Fig. 3.**16a** and **b**).

Before the second dentition appears, i.e., until about the 7th year of life, the maxillary sinuses are usually very small since the maxilla contains the tooth buds of the second dentition. The maxillary sinus only develops its final form and size after the second dentition appears.

The *frontal sinus* varies in form and extent more than the maxillary sinus. The average frontal sinus has a capacity of 4 to 7 ml. The difference in size between the right and left cavities is often considerable in the same person. The frontal sinuses may be completely absent on one or both sides in 3 % to 5 % of subjects, but they may also be very extensive and demonstrate loculi. The latter favor the development of inflammatory complications. The bony nasofrontal duct runs a curved course to open in the nose under the head of the middle turbinate in the infundibulum of the hiatus semilunaris (see Fig. 2.**4**).

The frontal sinuses develop after birth and are only completely formed in the 2nd decade of life. A bony septum lies between the two sinuses. The floor of the frontal sinus forms part of the roof of the orbit and is one pathway for the spread of inflammatory orbital complications. The canal of the supraorbital nerve runs in the floor of the frontal sinus.

The posterior wall of the frontal sinus forms part of the bony anterior cranial fossa, and is thus a typical pathway of spread for rhinogenic intracranial complications due either to frontonasal injury or as a complication of sinusitis (see p. 248).

The *ethmoid labyrinth* consists of six to ten air-containing cells of a total volume of 2 to 3 ml. Clinically, *anterior and posterior* ethmoid cell groups may be distinguished, derived from an embryologic paired anlage which coalesce in the 1st year of life to *one* ethmoid cell. There are communications between *all* the ethmoid cells of one side, and often also common ostiums for the anterior ethmoid complex in the middle meatus and for the posterior ethmoid complex in the superior meatus (see Fig. 2.**4**).

Unlike all the other nasal sinuses, the ethmoid labyrinth is fully formed at birth.

Superiorly, it is related to the anterior part of the base of the skull and is a pathway of spread for rhinogenic intracranial infections.

Laterally, the lamina papyracea separates the ethmoid cells from the orbital cavity and is a pathway of spread for orbital complications.

Posteriorly, the ethmoid labyrinth is related to the sphenoid sinus. The optic nerve often runs very close to the posterior ethmoid cells or even within them. This may explain some cases of retrobulbar neuritis (see Figs. 2.**36** and 2.**53**).

Medially, the ethmoid labyrinth is related to the middle and superior turbinates.

The *sphenoid* is the most posterior of the sinuses. It lies in the skull base, at the junction of the anterior and middle cranial fossae in the body of the sphenoid bone. There are marked individual variations in shape and size, the capacity of the sinus being 0.5 to 3 ml. The sphenoid sinus may be entirely absent in 3 % to 5 % of subjects. The ostium of the sphenoid sinus lies on the anterior wall of the body of the sphenoid bone in the sphenoethmoidal recess behind and somewhat above the superior turbinate (see Fig. 2.**4**).

The sphenoid sinus does not begin to develop until 6 years of age.

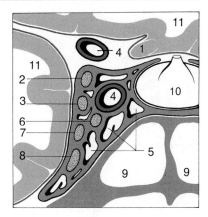

Fig. 2.**7** Frontal section through the sphenoid sinus. 1, Optic nerve; 2, oculomotor nerve; 3, trochlear nerve; 4, internal carotid artery; 5, cavernous sinus; 6, abducens nerve; 7, ophthalmic nerve; 8, maxillary nerve; 9, sphenoid sinus; 10, pituitary gland; 11, brain.

The *superior* wall of the sphenoid sinus is related to the anterior and middle cranial fossae and is the pathway of spread of rhinogenic intracranial complications. The optic chiasma and the optic foramen are close relations. Furthermore, the sella turcica and the pituitary gland lie on the roof of the sphenoid sinus, which can thus be used for access in operations on the pituitary through the sphenoid sinus.

On the *lateral wall* of the sphenoid sinus lie the cavernous sinus, the internal carotid artery, and the IInd, IIIrd, IVth, Vth, and VIth cranial nerves. The optic canal may lie free in the lateral wall of the sphenoid sinus, as may the internal carotid artery and the IIIrd and VIth cranial nerves (Fig. 2.**7**).

The *floor* of the sphenoid sinus is related to the roof of the nasopharynx and the choana.

Behind the very thick *posterior wall* lies the posterior cranial fossa and the pons. Its relations are shown in Figures 2.**7**, 2.**34a** and **b**, 2.**36a–c**, and 2.**53** (pp. 242, 245, 275).

The *mucosa* lining the paranasal sinuses is simpler than that of the nasal cavity. Cavernous erectile tissue may be found within the mucosa around the ostia, and this can influence the patency of the ostia (see p. 185). This variability of the opening of the ostia is supplemented by simultaneous variations in volume of the neighboring turbinates (see Fig. 2.**5**; Fig. 2.**8**). In a functional sense they thus form the *ostiomeatal unit*.

The *blood supply* of the nasal cavity and the nasal sinuses is provided by both the internal and external carotid artery and their accompanying veins. Figure 2.**9** shows the blood supply of the *medial* nasal wall, and Figure 2.**42a** shows the supply of the *lateral* nasal wall.

The *external* carotid artery supplies the nose internally via the internal maxillary and externally via the facial artery. The sphenopalatine artery is an important branch of the internal maxillary artery.

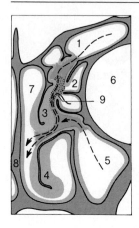

Fig. 2.**8**   Ostiomeatal unit. 1, Frontal sinus; 2, ethmoid sinus; 3, middle turbinate; 4, inferior turbinate; 5, antral cavity; 6, orbit; 7, nasal cavity; 8, nasal centrum; 9, infundibulum under the anterior end of the middle turbinate (black dotted area).

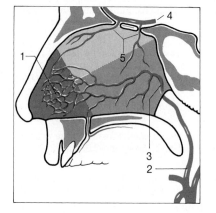

Fig. 2.**9**   Vasculature of the nasal cavity: 1, Kiesselbach's area; 2, internal maxillary artery; 3, sphenopalatine artery; 4, ophthalmic artery; 5, anterior and posterior ethmoid arteries.

■ Kiesselbach's area

■ Area supplied by external carotid artery

░ Area supplied by internal carotid artery (schematic)

The branches from the *internal* carotid artery run via the ophthalmic artery and from there via the anterior and posterior ethmoidal arteries.

A particularly rich and relatively superficial plexus of small vessels *(Kiesselbach's plexus)* lies on the anterior part of the nasal septum (see Fig. 2.**9;** Color Plate **11c** and **d**). It is supplied ultimately by both the internal and external carotid artery.

Venous drainage is provided by the ophthalmic and facial veins, and the pterygoid and pharyngeal plexus. It is thus partly intracranial to the cavernous, coronary, and transverse sinuses, and is also partially extracranial (see Fig. 2.**2**).

The *cavernous spaces* within the mucosa of the nasal turbinates are very important clinically, as are those on the nasal septum and around the ostia of the nasal sinuses. The filling of these spaces with venous blood varies greatly and is under autonomic control. It regulates the thickness of the mucosa and therefore the cross-sectional area of the nasal cavity and of the ostia of the nasal sinuses. It thus controls respiration, ventilation, and drainage (see Figs. 2.**5a** and 2.**8**).

The *lymphatic drainage* consists of two parts: first, an *anterior system* which collects the lymph from the nasal pyramid and which drains to the submandibular superficial cervical lymph nodes, and second, the *posterior system* that drains the posterior part of the nasal cavity and the nasopharynx to the retropharyngeal lymph nodes and the jugular nodes (see Fig. 6.**11**).

Nerve supply. The nasal cavity and nasal sinuses have a sensory and autonomic (secretory and vasomotor) nerve supply. In addition, they have the special sensory function of the olfactory nerve.

The *sensory nerve supply* is provided by the first and second branches of the trigeminal nerve. The complex *autonomic* innervation for secretion and vasomotor supply is shown in Figure 2.**10**.

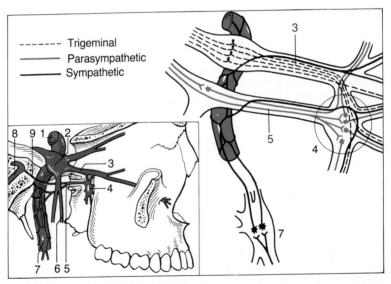

Fig. 2.**10**   Nerve supply of the nasal mucosa. 1, Internal carotid artery with sympathetic plexus; 2, Gasserian ganglion; 3, maxillary nerve; 4, pterygopalatine ganglion; 5, nerve of the pterygoid canal; 6, mandibular nerve; 7, superior cervical ganglion; 8, facial nerve with nervus intermedius; 9, greater petrosal nerve. Inset shows the course of fibers in the pterygopalatine ganglion: black line equals sympathetic fibers; solid red line equals parasympathetic fibers; dotted black line equals trigeminal nerve.

Autonomic innervation. The *sympathetic* fibers for vasoconstriction arise from the first to the fifth thoracic segments of the spinal cord, and synapse in the superior cervical ganglion. The postganglionic fibers run with the blood vessels to the mucosa of the nose and nasal sinuses. Some fibers run without synapsing through the pterygopalatine ganglion.

The pathway for the *parasympathetic* fibers for vasodilatation is from the nucleus lacrimomuconasalis along the nervus intermedius to the geniculate ganglion and then along the facial nerve, the greater superficial petrosal nerve, and the nerve of the pterygoid canal to the pterygopalatine ganglion.

The preganglionic parasympathetic fibers synapse in the pterygopalatine ganglion. From here they supply the mucosa of the nose and nasal sinuses with secretory and vasodilator fibers.

The *pterygopalatine or sphenopalatine ganglion* has a key role in the function of the nose and nasal sinuses. It is the main site of its autonomic innervation and possesses three roots:

1. Parasympathetic fibers which supplement secretory and vasodilator functions
2. Sympathetic fibers for vasoconstriction and inhibition of secretion
3. Sensory fibers from the trigeminal nerve arising in the trigeminal ganglion and running in the maxillary nerve

The nose and the maxillary sinus are closely related both anatomically and functionally to the *maxilla.* This bone forms the upper half of the masticatory system and also forms the main part of the middle third of the facial skeleton. The upper jaw is important in diseases of the nose because of its immediate relationship to the nose and nasal sinuses, because it is frequently damaged in injuries of the face and sinuses, and because tumors arising in the nose often extend into it. Figure 2.**47** shows its anatomy (see also Fig. 2.**69a** and **b**).

Basic Physiology and Pathophysiology

The nose is both a *sense organ* and a *respiratory organ*. In addition, the nose performs an important *function* for the entire body by providing *both physical and immunologic protection from the environment*. Finally, it is also important in the formation of speech sounds.

The Nose as an Olfactory Organ

The human sense of smell is poorly developed compared to most mammals and insects. Despite that, it is still very sensitive in the human and is almost indispensable for the individual. For example, taste is only partially a function of the taste buds since these can only recognize the qualities of sweet, sour, salty, and bitter. All other sensory impressions caused by food such as aroma and bouquet are mediated by olfaction. This *gustatory olfaction* is due to the fact that the olfactory substances of food or drink pass through the olfactory cleft during expiration while eating or drinking. The sense of smell can *stimulate appetite* but can also *depress it*. It also provides *warning* of rotten or poisonous foods and also of toxic substances, e. g., gas. The sense of smell is particularly important in the field of psychology: Marked affects may be induced or inhibited by smells. It should also be remembered that a good sense of smell is essential for those in certain occupations, e. g., cooks, confectioners, wine, coffee, and tea merchants, perfumers, tobacco blenders, and chemists. Finally, the physician needs a "clinical nose" for making his diagnosis.

The *olfactory area* of the nose is relatively small (see Fig. 2.5c). It contains the olfactory cells, i. e., the *bipolar nerve cells,* which are to be regarded as the sensory cells and first-order neurons. They are collected into about 20 fibers in the olfactory nerves which run to the *primary olfactory center of the olfactory bulb* (see Figs. 2.3b and 2.11).

From here the neurons of the bulb run via the *olfactory tract* to the *secondary olfactory center.* The *tertiary cortical olfactory field* lies in the dentate and semilunate gyri.

The mode of action of the scent molecules on the olfactory cells is not known with certainty. There are numerous current theories of the mechanism of action, including: emission of scent corpuscles, selective absorption, specific receptors on the sensory cells, enzymatic control, molecular vibrations, electrobiologic processes such as changes in cell membrane potential, etc.

It is certain that only *volatile* substances can be smelled by humans. These substances must be soluble in water and lipids. Only a few molecules suffice to stimulate the sense of smell. 10^{-15} molecules per ml of air are sufficient stimulation on average to exceed the threshold.

It is said that there are about 30,000 different olfactory substances in the atmosphere; of these, humans can perceive about 10,000 and are able to distinguish among 200.

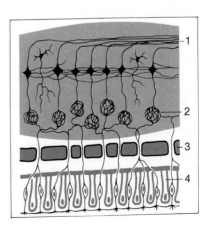

Fig. 2.11 Olfactory organ. 1, Olfactory fibers in the olfactory bulb; 2, olfactory glomeruli; 3, cribriform plate; 4, olfactory epithelium.

The sense of smell, like other senses, demonstrates the phenomenon of *adaptation*. The sensitivity of the olfactory organ depends also on hunger: several olfactory factors can be smelled better if the subject is very hungry than shortly after eating, a very useful physiologic regulation.

Anosmia and hyposmia may be caused by obliteration of the olfactory cleft (polyps, etc.), causing *respiratory anosmia*. Inability of the olfactory substances in food and drink to pass from the mouth and throat to the olfactory epithelium of the nose because of obstruction of the nasal cavity or the choana is described as *gustatory anosmia*. *Central anosmia* is caused by a disorder of the central nervous parts of the olfactory system in the presence of a patent airway. Causes include: traumatic rupture of the olfactory nerve, cerebral contusion, and cerebral diseases. *Essential anosmia* is due to local damage to the olfactory epithelium, e.g., due to influenza, with an open olfactory cleft.

The Nose as a Respiratory Organ

In the human the only physiologic respiratory pathway is via the nose. Mouth breathing is unphysiologic and is only brought into play in an emergency to supplement nasal respiration. The physiology of the airstream through the normal nose in inspiration and expiration may be summarized as follows:

The average ventilation through a normal nose in physiologic breathing is 6 l/min, and 50 to 70 l/min in maximal ventilation.

The internal nasal valve or limen nasi is the most narrow point in the normal nose. It thus acts like a nozzle, and the speed of the airstream is very high at this point.

The nasal cavity between the valve and the head of the turbinates acts as a *diffusor,* i.e., it slows the air current and increases turbulence. The central part of the nasal cavity with its turbinates and meatus is the most important part for nasal respiration. The column of air consists of a laminar and a turbulent stream. The proportion between laminar and turbulent flow considerably influences the function and condition of the nasal mucosa.

The airstream passes in the reverse direction through the nasal cavities on *expiration*. The expiratory airstream demonstrates considerably less turbulence in the central part of the nose, and thus offers less opportunity for heat and metabolic exchange between the airstream and the nasal wall than on inspiration. The nasal mucosa can thus recover during the expiratory phase. Inspiration through the nose followed by expiration through the mouth leads rapidly to drying of the nasal mucosa.

The nasal resistance, i.e., the difference of pressure between the nasal introitus and the nasopharynx, is normally between 8 and 20 mm H_2O. If the values exceed 20 mm H_2O, the internal nasal valves expand during breathing. Supplemental mouth breathing begins at values greater than 40 mm H_2O.

Complete exclusion of the nose from breathing leads in the long term to deep-seated mucosal changes. Mechanical obstruction within the nose, e.g., due to septal deviation, hypertrophy of the turbinates, cicatricial stenoses, etc., can lead to mouth breathing and its damaging consequences (see p. 321) and can also cause mucosal diseases of the nose and nasal sinuses.

The *nasal patency* can be influenced by many different factors, including temperature and humidity of the surrounding air, the position of the body, bodily activity, changes of body temperature, the influence of cold on different parts of the body, e. g., the feet, hyperventilation, and psychological stimuli. The state of the pulmonary function, of the heart, and of the circulation, endocrinologic disorders such as pregnancy, hyper- or hypofunction of the thyroid gland, and some local, oral, or parenteral drugs, e. g., rauwolfia and ephedrine, may have considerable influence on the patency of the nose (see p. 217). Methods for measuring this are described on p. 193.

During normal nasal respiration, the inspired air is *warmed, moistened, and purified* during its passage through the nose.

The *warming* of the inspired air through the nose is very effective, and the constancy of the temperature in the lower airways is remarkably stable. The nasal mucosa humidifies and warms the air. The temperature in the nasopharynx during normal (exclusively nasal) respiration is constant at 31° to 34 °C independent of the external temperature. The heat output of the nose increases as the external temperature falls so that the lower airways and the lungs can function at the correct physiologic temperature.

The *optimal relative humidity* of room air for subjective well-being and function of the nasal mucosa lies between 50% and 60%. The water vapor saturation of the inspired air in the nasopharynx lies between 80% and 85%, and in the lower airway is fairly constant between 95% and 100%, independent of the relative humidity of the environmental air. The water vapor secreted by the entire respiratory tract per 1,000 liters of air can reach 30 g. Most of this is supplied by the nose. On the other hand, the mucosal blanket renders the nasal mucosa watertight and prevents release of too much water into the air, which would cause drying of the mucosa.

The *cleaning function* of the nose includes: first, cleaning of the inspired air from foreign bodies, bacteria, dust, etc., and second, cleaning of the nose itself (see below). About 85% of particles larger than 4.5 μm are filtered out by the nose, but only about 5% of particles less than 1 μm in size are removed.

Foreign bodies entering the nose come into contact with the moist mucosal surface and the mucosal blanket, which continually carries away the foreign bodies. The details are described below.

Note: The nose warms, moistens, and cleans the atmospheric air.

The Nasal Mucosa as a Protective Organ

In addition to warming, humidifying, and cleaning the inspired air, the nose also has a *protective function* consisting of a highly differentiated, efficient, and polyvalent resistance potential against environmental influences on the body. A basic element of this defensive system is the *mucociliary apparatus,* i.e., the functional combination of the secretory film and the cilia of the respiratory epithelium by which the colloidal secretory film is transported continuously from the nasal introitus toward the choana. A foreign body is carried from the head of the inferior turbinate to the choana in about 10 to 20 min. The efficiency of this cleansing system depends on several factors such as pH, temperature, condition of the colloids, humidity, width of the nose, toxic gases, etc. Disturbances in the composition or in the physical characteristics of the mucosal blanket or of the ciliary activity can have marked influences on the physiology of the nasal cavity.

The nasal mucosa protects the entire body by making contact with and providing resistance against animate and inanimate foreign material in the environment. *Two defense zones* can be distinguished in the nasal mucosa: first, the mucosal blanket and the epithelium, and second, the vascular connective tissue of the lamina propria.

Resistance factors of the second defensive zone include: (1) nonspecific protective factors and structures such as the ground substance and fibrils, micro- and macrophages, mast cells, vessels, the autonomic nervous system, hormones, interferon, protease inhibitors, complement, etc.; and (2) specific defensive factors such as sensitized B- and T-lymphocytes, eosinophil granulocytes, immunoglobulin IgG, IgM, IgE and lymphokines.

The Nose as a Reflex Organ

Specific nasal reflex mechanisms may arise:

- Within the nose and affect the nose itself
- From other parts of the body or organs and affect the nose
- In the nose and affect other parts of the body

A reflex system which is obviously confined to the nose but whose purpose is unknown is the nasal *cycle.*

One cycle lasts between 2 and 6 h. Provided that both halves of the nasal cavity are of normal patency, the lumen widens and narrows alternately, lowering or increasing the respiratory resistance in each half of the nose. However, the resistance of the entire nose remains constant in the ideal case. This reflex phenomenon is controlled by the action of the autonomic nervous system on the cavernous spaces of the vascular system of the nasal mucosa.

Nasopetal reflexes arise, e.g., from cooling of the extremities, which changes the respiratory resistance. They may also arise from the lungs and bronchi and from other autonomic control points.

Important *nasofugal* communications exist between the nose and the lung, the heart and circulation, the metabolic organs, and the genitals.

In addition, there are sneezing, lacrimal, and cough reflexes, and under certain emergency situations, reflex respiratory arrest.

Influence of the Nose on Speech

The nose influences the sound of speech. During the formation of the resonants "m," "n," and "ng," e.g., the air streams through the open nose, whereas during the formation of the vowels the nose and the nasopharynx are more or less closed off by the soft palate from the resonating cavity of the mouth.

Function of the Nasal Sinuses

The biologic purpose of the nasal sinuses is largely speculative. It is obvious that the pneumatized cavities of the bone of the skull reduce the weight, at the same time increasing the superficial extent of the bones of the skull.

The existence of the *ostia* causes particular pathophysiologic problems affecting *ventilation and drainage*.

Ostial obstruction interrupts the self-cleaning mechanism of the affected sinus; therefore, the secretions stagnate and change in composition. The retained secretions form an ideal medium for saprophytic bacteria which are often present in normal sinuses.

Ostial obstruction often also causes a vicious circle, illustrated in Figure 2.**12**.

The causes of closure of the ostium include:

1. Environmental factors such as relative dryness of the nose, toxic gases, or agents in the air.
2. Local congenital or acquired anomalies, including: deviation of the septum, scars, lesions of the turbinates, infections of the nose or nasal cavities, dental diseases, allergic diseases of the nose or nasal sinuses (particularly in children), vasomotor dysfunctions with a neurogenic or hormonal basis, metabolic diseases such as avitaminoses, diabetes, disordered electrolytes, mechanical obstruction due to crusts, polypi, foreign bodies, prolonged use of a nasogastric tube or prolonged nasal tracheal intubation, and benign and malignant tumors.

The vicious circle of ostial occlusion can only be broken in the long term by dealing with the causal factors by appropriate medical or surgical measures.

The nasal sinuses are only minimally involved in the respiratory phases of the nasal cavity.

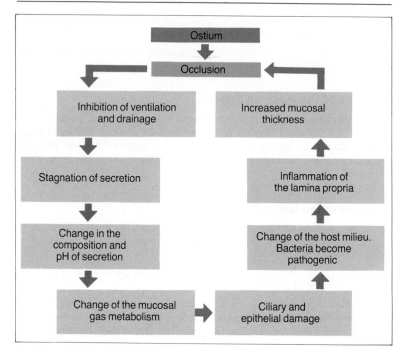

Fig. 2.**12**   Results of occlusion of a sinus ostium.

The change in pressure which can be recorded in the sinuses during respiration is relatively slight. When the ostium is occluded, a relatively small fall of pressure in the sinuses from −20 to −50 mm H_2O occurs that is enough to cause the symptoms of the incorrectly termed *vacuum sinusitis*. These include fairly marked headaches that disappear when ventilation of the sinus is restored.

Methods of Investigation of the Nose, Paranasal Sinuses, and Face

External Inspection and Palpation

Attention is paid to the following points:

- The properties of the overlying skin, e.g., hardness, firmness, discolorations, inflammatory swellings, and tenderness to pressure

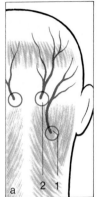
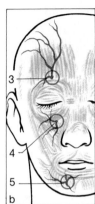

Fig. 2.**13a** and **b** Clinically important sites of exit of nerves. **a.** At the occiput. 1, Lesser occipital nerve; 2, greater occipital nerve. **b.** On the face. 3, Supraorbital nerve; 4, infraorbital nerve; 5, mental nerve.

- Externally visible changes in shape of the cartilaginous or bony structure due to congenital or acquired deformities, e.g., saddle nose, hump nose, broad nose, or scoliotic nose; the early or late results of trauma; painful swelling due to inflammation; nonpainful swelling due to tumor
- Palpable masses of neighboring structures, e.g., the forehead, the cheeks, the upper lip, or the eyelids; proptosis, displacement of the bulb or limitation of its movement
- The nasal alae during respiration, inspection for indrawing or flaring of the ala
- The nasal vestibule, the anterior border of the nasal septum, the roof of the vestibule, and the internal part of the nasal cavity, inspection by lifting the tip of the nose
- Crepitation and mobility of the nasal bony framework
- The sites of exit of the various nerves (Fig. 2.**13a** and **b**)
- Sensitivity to pressure of the forehead, the cranial vault, or the cheek

Anterior Rhinoscopy

Anterior rhinoscopy using a nasal speculum, a strong light source, and a head mirror or a head lamp is only carried out *after* inspection *without* instruments (Fig. 2.**14a–c**). The method of using the nasal speculum is shown in Figure 2.**15a** and **b**. Usually, the left hand holds the speculum when inspecting *both* nasal cavities.

Technique. The speculum is *introduced* into the nasal vestibule with its *blades together*. The point of the speculum is directed somewhat laterally in the nasal vestibule.

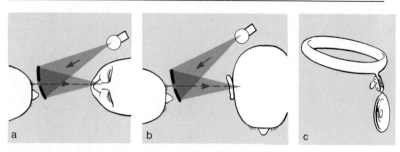

Fig. 2.**14a–c**   **(a)** Direction of beam of light on anterior rhinoscopy using a head mirror; **(b)** direction of beam of light for examination of the ear with the head mirror; **(c)** head mirror with central aperture.

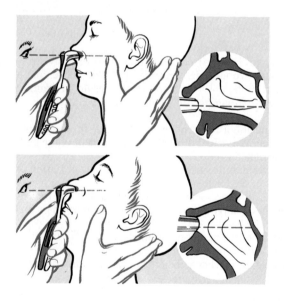

Fig. 2.**15a** and **b** Anterior rhinoscopy. **(a)** Position I, **(b)** position II.

The speculum is now opened out in the nasal vestibule and fixed to the nasal alae with the index finger. The instrument is held *slightly* open while *removing* it to prevent pain due to avulsion of vibrissae. The right hand is used to adjust the position of the face and head. As shown in Figure 2.**15a**, the patient's head is initially in the vertical position, allowing the examiner's gaze to be parallel to the floor of the nose and along the inferior turbinate and the inferior meatus *(position I)*. If the nasal cavity is wide, the choana and the posterior wall of the nasopharynx can be seen in this position. The patient's head is tilted slightly backward to allow the upper part of the nasal cavity to be examined. The middle meatus, which is of great clinical importance, and the middle turbinate are thus brought into view *(position II)* (Fig. 2.**15b**). If the head is tilted strongly backward, the olfactory cleft may also be visible *(position III)*.

In small children and infants, it is advisable to use an ear speculum rather than a nasal speculum for anterior rhinoscopy.

When the position of the head has been adjusted satisfactorily, the hand holding the speculum may be used simultaneously to fix the head. The right hand is then free for manipulating instruments, performing aspirations, etc., within the nasal cavity.

Note: The nasal mucosa is often so turgescent that the view of the nasal cavity is minimal. In such cases a decongestant spray is introduced into the nose and allowed to act for 10 min. A good view then usually can be obtained.

The following are noted during anterior rhinoscopy:

- The nasal secretions, their color, quantity, and properties; mucus, pus, and formation of crusts
- Localization of abnormal secretion
- Swelling of the turbinates, narrowing or widening of the nasal meatus
- Properties of the mucosal surface (including its color), e. g., whether it is moist, dry, smooth, cornified, or uneven
- Position of the nasal septum and septal deformities
- Sites of major blood vessels, e. g., Kiesselbach's plexus
- Abnormal pigmentation or color of mucosa
- Presence of abnormal tissue
- Ulcerations or perforations
- Foreign bodies

The clinically important region of the middle meatus can be anatomically narrow and difficult to examine. It can be visualized by a long Killian's nasal speculum [Fig. 2.**16** (2)] provided that local anesthesia of the nasal mucosa has been induced (e. g., by local application of Xylocaine or 1 % pantocaine with 1:1,000 adrenaline, one drop to one ml of anesthetic solution).

Rigid or flexible endoscopes are nowadays often used to assess inaccessible areas such as the ostia, the infundibulum, and the posterior part of the nasal cavity (see Fig. 2.**23**).

The important nasal instruments in common use are shown in Figure 2.**16**.

Posterior Rhinoscopy

Indirect Examination

Figure 2.**17a** and **b** shows the method of examining the nasopharynx with a mirror, with a composite view of the region obtained. Posterior rhinoscopy is used to examine the posterior part of the nasal cavity: the choana,

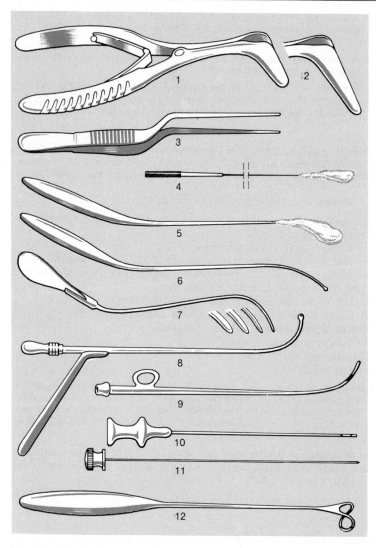

Fig. 2.**16**   Nasal instruments. 1, Normal nasal speculum; 2, long nasal speculum (Killian); 3, bayonet forceps; 4, cotton applicator; 5, curved applicator; 6, nasal probe; 7, Ritter's bougies in different sizes; 8, cannula for postoperative irrigation of sinuses; 9, cannula for irrigation the maxillary antrum via the middle meatus; 10, Liechtwitz cannula for antral lavage via the inferior meatus; 11, trocar for use in 10; 12, palatal retractor.

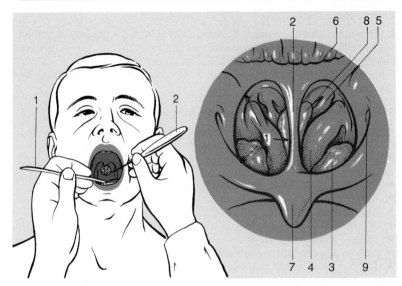

Fig. 2.**17a** and **b**   Posterior rhinoscopy. Method of holding the tongue depressor (1) and mirror (2). The inset shows a composite picture of the nasopharynx composed of individual views: 1 choana, 2 posterior edge of septum, 3 inferior turbinate, 4 middle turbinate, 5 superior turbinate, 6 adenoid, 7 uvula, 8 septum padding 9 tubal ostium.

the posterior ends of the turbinates, the posterior margin of the septum, and the nasopharynx together with its roof and the ostia of the eustachian tube.

Technique. Posterior rhinoscopy requires much practice on the part of the examiner and cooperation by the patient. A tongue depressor is placed on the center of the base of the tongue with one hand, and the base of the tongue is pressed slowly downward. The distance between the surface of the tongue and the soft palate and the posterior pharyngeal wall thus is increased. A small mirror is warmed on the glass side, and then is tested on the hand to make sure that it is not too hot. The other hand is used to introduce the mirror into the space between the soft palate and the posterior pharyngeal wall. The mirror must not touch the mucosa, otherwise it elicits the gag reflex. If the soft palate remains tense, the patient is asked to breathe gently through the nose, to sniff, or to say "ha." The palate thus relaxes and provides a free view into the nasopharynx. A view of the different parts of the nasopharynx is obtained by moving and tilting the mirror (see Fig. 2.**17b**). The vertical posterior edge of the septum is used for orientation to locate the normal structures. If a satisfactory view is not obtained because of the gag reflex, a successful examination may often be achieved by inducing local anesthesia of the oropharynx, particularly of the soft palate and the posterior wall of the pharynx, by a 1 % Xylocaine spray.

Endoscopic Examination

If it is not possible to examine the nasopharynx with the method described above, either *endoscopy* (see p. 202) or *palatal retraction* (or both combined) may be carried out. Figure 2.**18** shows the principle of palatal retraction, although this technique has been rendered largely obsolete by the use of endoscopy.

The following points are to be noted during *posterior rhinoscopy:*

- The opening and width of the choanae
- The shape of the posterior end of the inferior and middle turbinates
- Evidence of scars or deformities in the nasopharynx, e.g., due to trauma
- The shape of the posterior part of the nasal septum
- Nasal polypi
- The shape of both tubal ostia and Rosenmüller's fossa
- Obstruction of the nasopharynx by enlarged adenoids in children
- Tumors of the nasopharynx
- Abnormal secretions in the choanae
- The properties of the mucosa of the posterior part of the nose and the nasopharynx, e.g., for moisture, dryness, thickening, and color

Computed tomography is used to evaluate the spread of paranasal sinus lesions to adjacent structures, particularly the skull base, cranial cavity, retromaxillary space, and orbits. Also used in trauma patients, CT is indispensable for the differentiated evaluation of bony structures. It is supplemented by MRI for soft-tissue investigations.

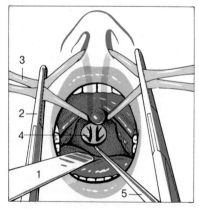

Fig. 2.**18**   Palatal retraction. 1, Tongue depressor; 2, forceps; 3, rubber catheters; 4, view in the posterior nasopharyngeal mirror; 5, mirror handle. Local anesthesia of both nasal cavities, and the nasopharynx and oropharynx is induced by a spray or topical application. A thin rubber catheter or suction tube is passed through the nasal cavity on each side. The ends lying in the nasopharynx are grasped through the mouth with the forceps and are pulled forward, putting the soft palate under tension. The two ends of the tube are clamped and fixed in this position. The nasopharynx may now be examined either by a warmed mirror or by an endoscope.

A *palatal retractor* [see Fig. 2.**16** (12)] may occasionally be used rather than introduction of a catheter.

Assessment of Nasal Patency

This is achieved by *rhinomanometry*. In practice, the following directly measurable parameters of the respiratory flow (see p. 182) are available:

- The nasal differential pressure (ΔP), i.e., the difference between the pressure at the nasal introitus and the nasopharynx
- The volume flow ($\dot{V}$), which is the volume of air passing through the nose in unit time
- The nasal resistance (W)

$$W = \frac{\Delta P}{\dot{V}}$$

Usually, measurements are carried out during spontaneous respiration (Fig. 2.**19a**). The volume of air passing through the nose during active nasal respiration is recorded at the same time as the pressure differential across the nose. The results may be recorded either by a pair of curves (Fig. 2.**19b**) or as an *xy* function (Fig. 2.**19c**) and provide information about unilateral or bilateral nasal patency (see p. 182).

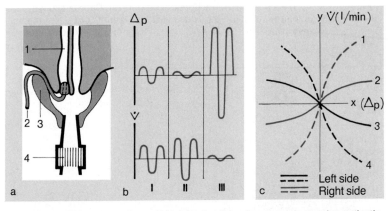

Fig. 2.**19a–c** Rhinomanometry. a. Principle of unilateral measurement, using patient's own air flow measurement. 1, Right nasal cavity; 2, pressure tubing with olive; 3, face mask; 4, flow resistance (Fleisch). b. Recording of two simultaneous curves. I, normal; II, above-average nasal patency; III, reduced nasal patency. c. xy plot: inspiration is shown on the right of the y axis and expiration is on the left. Inspiration is recorded right and above, and expiration left and below. 1, Respiratory resistance curve, right side, with good nasal breathing; 2, respiratory resistance curve, right side, with poor nasal breathing; 3, respiratory resistance with poor nasal respiration on the left; 4, respiratory resistance curve with good nasal respiration on the left.

A rough *qualitative* test of nasal patency can be achieved by holding a polished metal plate in front of the nose during inspiration and expiration. The surface area of the resulting fogging gives an approximation of the patency of the two sides of the nose.

In *infants* the nasal patency is tested by holding a wisp of cotton wool or a feather in front of the nose.

Olfactometry

The following tests of olfaction are available: first, a rough *qualitative* test; second, a semiobjective *quantitative* test in which olfactory substances are presented; third, a quantitative *and* objective assessment by simultaneous computer recording and evaluation of the induced cerebral responses. The latter ist known as ERO (evoked response olfactometry) analogous to evoked response audiometry. Qualitative testing is particularly useful in

Table 2.1 Some Known Olfactory Substances			
	Stimulation of		
Substance	The Olfactory Nerve	The Sensory Part of the Trigeminal Nerve	The Chorda tympani (VIIth cranial nerve) and the Glossopharyngeal Nerve (IXth cranial nerve)
Coffee	+		
Wax	+		
Vanilla	+		
Lavender oil	+		
Turpentine oil	+		
Birch tar	+		
Cinnamon	+		
Benzaldehyde	+	+	
Menthol	+	+	
Turpentine	+	+	
Petroleum	+	+	
Peppermint	+	+	
Camphor	+	+	
Alcohol	+	+	
Formaldehyde	+	+	
Acetic acid	+	+	
Ammonia		+	
Chloroform	+		+
Pyridine	+		+

Table 2.**2** Causes of Olfactory Disorders

Intranasal

Mechanical obstruction of the airway
    Septal deviation
    Posttraumatic obstruction of nasal respiration
    Rhinitis (infective, vasomotor, or allergic)
    Sinusitis
    Nasal polypi
    Tumors of the nose or nasopharynx
    Choanal atresia
    Laryngectomy

Lesions of the olfactory receptors
    Atrophic rhinitis and ozena
    Vitamin A deficiency
    Chronic inhalation of industrial toxins, smoking
        Toxic damage by cadmium, chromic acid, varnish and solutes, osmium
        tetroxide, sulfur dioxide, sulfuric acid, heavy metals, e.g., lead and zinc.
        One-time contact with butylene glycol, benzolic acid, putrid gases,
        poison gas, or selenic acid can cause permanent damage.
Side effects of drugs such as amphetamine, coumarin, kanamycin, cocaine,
meprobamate, morphine, neomycin, phenothiazine, penicillamine, procaine,
streptomycin, etc.

Intracranial

Trauma
    Damage to the olfactory bulb, tract or nerve
    Bleeding around the frontal part of the base of the brain
    Fracture of the cribriform plate

Infection
    Virus diseases
    Frontal lobe abscess
    Syphilis of the CNS

Tumor
    Frontal lobe tumor
    Esthesioneuroblastoma
    Vascular tumors of the anterior cranial fossa
    Meningioma in the course of the olfactory nerve
    Pituitary or parasellar tumors

Vascular
    Arteriosclerosis of the anterior cerebral arteries

Systemic diseases
    Diabetes mellitus
    Vitamin B deficiency anemia (pernicious)

Congenital olfactory disorders, e.g., aplasia of the olfactory bulb in Kallmann's
    syndrome (olfactogenital dysplasia)

Hormonal olfactory disorders

Psychotic olfactory disorders

practice. A small battery of glass tubes with ground glass stoppers is kept available containing the different test substances. The patient is asked to sniff the opened tubes, with a rest between tubes. Substances that stimulate the olfactory nerve exclusively (smell) must be differentiated from substances that also stimulate the trigeminal nerve (sensation), and also from those that stimulate the sense of taste subserved by the glossopharyngeal nerve (taste) (Table 2.1).

The ability to identify different substances may be of importance in neurologic differential diagnosis.

Two different parameters can be tested: (1) the *threshold* at which the substance is *perceived* and (2) the *threshold* at which it is *recognized*. The first threshold is of lesser magnitude than the second.

All the methods named so far depend on the subject's cooperation, and the results are therefore largely subjective. Objective results can only be obtained by *computer olfactometry* (ERO).

Tests for simulation are possible with computer olfactometry or with the cinnamon test. The taste of cinnamon is mediated by the olfactory nerve. Cinnamon cannot be recognized in the absence of the ability to smell.

Anosmia is complete loss of the ability to smell, *hyposmia* indicates reduced ability to smell, and *parosmia* indicates the state in which the subjective impression does not correspond to the substance offered. In *cacosmia* all smells appear to be offensive. Cacosmia is often an indication of a central nervous system lesion.

The causes of olfactory disorders are summarized in Table 2.2.

Note: The sense of smell should always be tested thoroughly before any operation on the nose or sinuses, for medicolegal reasons.

Radiology of the Nose and Sinuses

Diagnosis of diseases of the nasal sinuses is hardly possible without the use of radiology.

Radiographs of the nose in the lateral projection are necessary to demonstrate a fracture of the nasal bone. They may also be used if an intranasal foreign body is suspected.

The radiologic demonstration of the different *sinus cavities* is complicated by their position in the bony skull, their close relationship to the base of the skull, and the resulting inevitable overlapping of the contours in the roentgenogram. There is no single projection that allows *all* sinuses to be assessed; therefore, *several* views are necessary. The most important routine projections, the main sinuses which they demonstrate, and the indica-

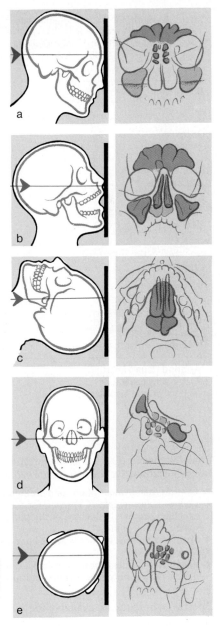

Fig. 2.**20a–e** The most important radiographic projections for the nasal sinuses: (a) occipitofrontal; (b) occipitomental; (c) axial; (d) bitemporal; (e) Rhese's lateral oblique.

Table 2.3 Important X-Ray Projections for the Diagnosis of Sinus Disease

X-Ray Direction	Frontal Sinus	Maxillary Sinus	Ethmoid Sinus	Sphenoid Sinus	Structures Best Visualized
Posteroanterior	+	(+)	+	–	Frontal bone, mandible, zygoma, orbit
Occipital mental	+	+	(+)	(+)	Zygoma, orbit, midface nasal cavities,
Caudal-cranial submental vertical	–	–	+	+	skull base, nasal cavities, nasopharynx, zygomatic arch
Modified axial (after Welin)	+	–	–	–	Deep extension of the frontal sinus
Lateral bitemporal	+	(+)	(+)	+	Sella turcica, epipharynx, nasal root, midface position,
Rhese oblique lateral	–	–	+	–	Orbit, optic foramen

+   good visualization.
(+) fair visualization.
–   poor or non-visualization.

tions for their use are summarized in Figure 2.**20a–e** and Table 2.**3**. The following adjunctive procedures are required less often:

- *Contrast examinations* of one or more sinuses
- *Computed tomography (CT) scans,* for extension of sinus disease to surrounding structures, especially the base of the skull, the cranial cavity, the retromaxillary space, and the orbit
- *Scans* to assess metabolically active bone diseases and tumors
- *Stereoscopic views*
- *Angiography* of the internal or external carotid artery to demonstrate intracranial rhinogenic complications, tumors, and space-occupying lesions
- *Xeroradiography*

Special techniques are available for the maxilla, the mandible, the temporomandibular joint, the zygoma, the zygomatic arch, and the alveolar process. Orthopantomograms are also used to demonstrate the jaws and teeth.

Magnetic resonance imaging (MRI) is still in the clinical testing stage. It provides a new method of morphologic assessment of the head and neck without exposing the patient to ionizing radiation.

Ultrasound can also be used to investigate the nasal sinuses. Its advantage is that the patient is spared exposure to radiation. Its disadvantage is that the findings are less detailed and technical faults are more likely.

Lavage of the Sinuses

The maxillary sinus, the frontal sinus, and the sphenoid sinus may be irrigated, but not the ethmoid sinuses. There are two purposes for irrigating the sinuses. First, on *diagnostic grounds* to allow aspiration and lavage of abnormal secretions, bacteriologic and cytologic examination of the secretions, and possibly the introduction of a contrast medium for radiography. Second, the sinuses may be irrigated for *therapeutic purposes* to allow drainage of abnormal secretions and introduction of locally active substances into the sinuses.

Lavage of the maxillary antrum. Two different methods are in routine use: (1) access via the *inferior meatus* (sharp puncture) and (2) access via the *middle meatus* (blunt puncture) (Fig. 2.**21a** and **b**).

Principle of lavage through the inferior meatus. Local anesthesia of the *inferior* meatus is induced. A Liechtwitz trocar is placed against the lateral nasal wall beneath the origin of the inferior turbinate (see Fig. 2.**21a**). After pushing the cannula

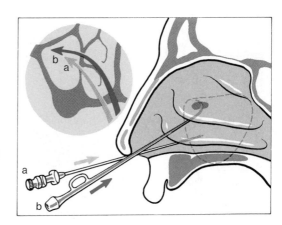

Fig. 2.**21a** and **b** Antral lavage. **a.** Sharp puncture via the inferior meatus. **b.** Blunt irrigation via the ostium of the middle meatus.

through this usually thin part of the lateral nasal wall, aspiration, lavage, or the introduction of drugs may be carried out through the cannula.

Principle of lavage via the middle meatus. Local anesthesia of the *middle* meatus is induced. The ostium of the maxillary antrum is sought, and a blunt curved cannula, such as that described by Siebenmann (Fig. 2.**21b**), is introduced through it. Aspiration, lavage, and introduction of medicines then can be carried out through the cannula.

A *long-term drain* may be introduced for conservative treatment, especially in children (see p. 243).

Complications during blunt puncture are very unlikely if it is carried out expertly. The point of the cannula may be pushed into the soft tissues of the cheek, into the pterygopalatine fossa, or into the orbit by incorrect technique during sharp puncture.

> *Note:* Air must never be used to blow out the irrigated sinus since it can cause an air embolus. The symptoms are collapse, loss of consciousness, cyanosis, possibly hemiplegia, amaurosis, and sudden death.

Lavage of the frontal sinus. Because of marked variation in the convoluted course of the frontonasal duct, probing and lavage of the frontal sinus via the duct are difficult. It is estimated that the mucosa is damaged in 50% of

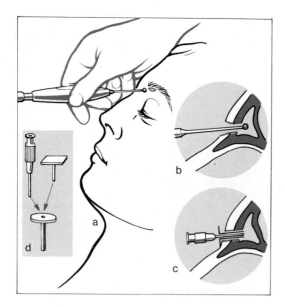

Fig. 2.**22a–d**   Kuemmel-Beck's frontal sinus trephine. (a) Access and position of the drill; (b) bore hole in the anterior wall of the frontal sinus; (c) guide tube and lavage cannula installed; (d) guide tube with lavage cannula and occlusion plate.

patients by the instrument. This difficulty is overcome by external access via the anterior wall of the sinus.

Puncture (as described by Kuemmel and Beck) (see also p. 240) can be carried out using a fine drill under local anesthesia. It allows *irrigation* for both *diagnostic and therapeutic* reasons and also *prolonged drainage* of the frontal sinus for 1 or 2 weeks, thus allowing daily administration of drugs. The principle of puncture is shown in Figure 2.**22a–d**.

Technique. Anteroposterior and lateral radiographs of the sinuses must be carried out first. If the frontal sinus has not developed or is very shallow, there is a danger that the frontal lobe may be punctured.

Irrigation of the sphenoid sinus can be carried out with special cannulas by the specialist.

The *ethmoid labyrinth* does not possess a defined ostium, and therefore cannot be irrigated. However, pathologic secretions can be evacuated by means of suction.

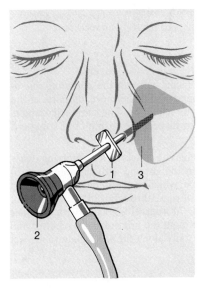

Fig. 2.**23** Sinoscopy. **a.** The optic is introduced either through the medial central wall (as shown) or through the oral vestibule. (1) By means of a trocar passed through a tube into the antral cavity; (2) rigid telescope in the antral cavity; (3) antral cavity.

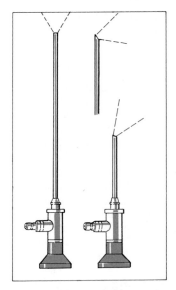

Fig. 2.**24** Various endorhinoscopes.

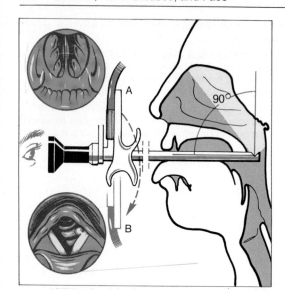

Fig. 2.**25** Stuckrad's loupe endoscopy. Position A: inspection of the nasopharynx; position B: inspection of the hypopharynx and larynx. The illustration (B) shows a polyp on the left vocal cord.

Nasal Endoscopy

Most parts of the *nasal cavity* can be inspected with the *operating microscope* after the mucosa has been decongested. Furthermore, all parts of the cavity may be inspected with a fiberoptic telescope. The same telescope is used for *antroscopy* and can be used to inspect the frontal and sphenoid sinuses also (Figs. 2.**23** and 2.**24**).

The *nasopharynx* may be inspected using von Stuckrad's magnifying *endoscope* under optimal illumination with cold light and with variable magnification. Figure 2.**25** shows this endoscope, which may also be used to inspect the hypopharynx and larynx if it is turned through 180° (see p. 397). Other useful instruments are the 30° or 70° (nasal) telescope with a caliber of 2.7 mm, which can be introduced through the inferior nasal meatus, and the 120° scope, which is inserted transorally along the soft palate to inspect the nasopharynx.

Specific Diagnostic Methods

1. *Biochemical and immunologic investigation of the secretions.* Biochemical and immunologic analyses of nasal secretions are being used increasingly for routine diagnosis in everyday practice.
2. *Cytology.* Smears of the secretions or smears taken from the mucosa can be assessed by cytology. This is useful in the differential diagnosis between catarrh, bacterial infection, allergic rhinitis, and mucosal mycoses.

3. *Allergic investigation.* Investigations carried out on patients include skin tests (scratch, prick, intracutaneous, or friction) and provocation tests (conjunctival and intranasal). *Laboratory investigations* include the total IgE in the serum (PRIST) and specific IgE in the serum [radioallergosorbent test (RAST)]. Eosinophil counts in the blood and in the nasal secretion are less informative.

4. *Biopsy.*

> *Note:* In all cases where the diagnosis *is not clear,* particularly if a tumor is suspected, a *biopsy* provides the diagnosis. If the results of biopsy are negative, but the clinical suspicion of malignancy persists, the biopsy must be repeated on several occasions with the specimens taken from different sites.

Clinical Aspects of Diseases of the Nose, Sinuses and Face

The *chief symptoms* of disease of the nose and sinuses are:

- Increased nasal secretion (Table 2.**4**) is found.
- Nasal obstruction (Table 2.**5**) occurs.
- Bleeding or hemorrhagic secretion (Tables 2.**8** and 2.**9**) is present.
- Fetor (Table 2.**6**) is present.
- Altered or absent sense of smell (see Table 2.**2**) is noted.
- Pains in the head or face (Table 2.**7**) occur.
- Disease of neighboring organs such as the teeth, the lacrimal apparatus, the eyes, the mouth, and the throat is present. Important symptoms of eye disease include abnormalities of refraction, limitation of the visual field, acute loss of vision, and displacement of the orbit. Diseases of the mouth and throat may be symptomatic, or a change in quality of the voice and speech.

Inflammatory Diseases of the Nose and Paranasal Sinuses

Inflammations Confined Mainly to the External Nose

The skin of the nose and the face may be affected by the common typical skin diseases which affect the rest of the skin, such as *impetigo, acne, trichophyton, rosacea,* and *lupus erythematosus.* These diseases are treated by the appropriate dermatologic methods.

There are other skin diseases that are particularly important in the nasal area. These are described below.

Nasal Eczema

Symptoms. The disease is moist in the early phases with vesicles and pustules. Later, crusts form, and then painful rhagades. In the chronic stage, there is itching, burning, and desquamation. The disease is localized to the external nose and the skin of the nasal vestibule and never affects the nasal mucosa.

Pathogenesis. The disease often is caused by abnormal nasal secretions, but may also be due to a contact allergy (sensitivity testing!). Promoting factors include diabetes mellitus, generalized eczema, and dietary sensitivity in children.

Treatment. The crusts should be softened with mild greasy ointment followed by a corticosteroid. Rhagades are treated with 5% to 10% silver nitrate solution. The cause should be looked for and treated or eliminated.

Folliculitis of the Nasal Vestibule (Sycosis) and Nasal Furuncle (see Color Plate **10c**).

Symptoms. Increasing pain, marked sensitivity to pressure, and feeling of tension in the tip of the nose is followed by reddening and swelling of the tip of the nose, of the nasal ala, and of the upper lip. The area becomes edematous, and the patient may have a fever. The swelling may begin to resolve before suppuration occurs. Otherwise, a typical furuncle forms, containing pus and a central necrotic cove.

Pathogenesis. A pyodermia, usually due to staphylococcal infection, arises from the hair follicles of the nasal vestibule or the upper lip, often close to the nasal tip. The disease is always limited to the skin and never affects the mucosa.

Treatment. Antibiotic creams are applied to the nasal vestibule as long as the disease remains a circumscribed folliculitis. Manipulation in the nose is forbidden. If it is suspected that a furuncle is forming, high-dose oral or parenteral antibiotics are given, possibly combined with local antibiotics. They must be continued for several days after the symptoms have subsided (Do not discontinue too early or use too low a dosage)! It may be necessary to prescribe a fluid diet and voice rest to immobilize the tip of the nose and the upper lip. Soaks of alcohol or ice water are used on the external nose. It may be necessary to admit the patient to the hospital in severe cases.

> *Note:* A furuncle on the nose or upper lip must never be squeezed because of the danger of spreading of the infection and of complications such as thrombophlebitis and cavernous sinus thrombosis (see p. 250). The veins of the nose and upper lip drain to the venous system of the neck via the facial vein, but also drain via the angular and ophthalmic veins through the orbit to the cavernous sinus. Figure 2.**2** shows the appropriate anatomy, and the point at which the angular vein may be divided on suspicion of an early thrombophlebitis.

Frostbite and Burns

The nose is particularly at risk of frostbite and sunburn under extremes of weather and temperature. The damage is divided into three grades of severity, the most severe being dry or moist tissue necrosis.

Treatment is as for thermal damage to other parts of the body.

Erysipelas

Symptoms. There is an incubation period of several hours to 2 days. The disease begins with a high fever and possibly chills. There is marked pain and closely demarcated reddening of the edematous skin. Often there is extension on both sides of the nasal pyramid in a butterfly shape. The disease often resolves within 1 week with proper treatment.

Pathogenesis. The organism is usually a streptococcus. The portal of entry is often a small abrasion of the skin.

Differential diagnosis. Angioneurotic edema, acute dermatitis, and herpes zoster must be considered.

Treatment. Antibiotics are continued for 8 days after the exanthem subsides, and local moist dressings are applied.

Prognosis is good.

Rhinophyma
(See Color Plate **10b**).

Symptoms. The disease begins with coarsening of the skin over the cartilaginous part of the nose. A lumpy bluish-red pseudotumor forms and slowly progresses to a markedly protuberant lobular swelling of the anterior part of the nose which may even obstruct breathing and eating. This disease usually occurs in older men.

Pathogenesis. It is said that this disease may be associated with rosacea, but it may also be due to massive hypertrophy of the sebaceous glands of the nasal skin.

Treatment. The disease is treated surgically. The tissue is removed in layers with a scalpel or CO_2 laser and is sliced off down to the level of the normal nasal contour. The area then is allowed to heal spontaneously or is covered with a split skin graft.

Lupus Vulgaris of the Nose

Symptoms. Fine red nodules are found on the nasal vestibule, the head of the inferior turbinate, and the septum lying opposite to it. The nodular stage is followed by central necrosis, with ulceration and formation of granulomas, and finally scarring with deformity of the underlying cartilage. The nasal introitus becomes stenosed, and the cartilaginous framework of the nose collapses.

Pathogenesis. The disease is due to tuberculous infection in the presence of relatively robust immunologic resistance (the proliferative form). The organism responsible is the mycobacterium tuberculosis, either of the human or bovine type.

Diagnosis. The diagnosis is reached by demonstration of the infectious agent and by biopsy. Diagnosis of the disease is notifiable.

Differential diagnosis. Eczema of the nasal introitus, anterior rhinitis sicca, perforating ulcer of the septum, syphilis, mycosis, lupus erythematosus, sarcoid, and malignancy. Tuberculosis usually attacks the cartilaginous part of the nose, and syphilis the bony part.

Treatment. Long-term triple combinations of tuberculostatic drugs (see p.331) and vitamin D_2 are given.

Sarcoid of Besnier-Boeck-Schaumann

Symptoms. Sarcoid may occur as an isolated lesion in the nose. It begins with bluish-red to brownish nodules and infiltration of the facial skin. Regional lymph nodes are firm and enlarged.

Diagnosis. See p. 498.

Differential diagnosis. This includes rhinophyma, lupus, gumma, and malignancy.

Treatment. Steroids are administered under the supervision of an internist. Surgery should only be considered for solitary nodules and pressing symptoms.

Syphilis

Symptoms. Stage 1 is similiar to a primary chancre of the skin and is rare. Stage 3 shows gummatous infiltration with painful swelling of the *bony* part of the nose, foul-smelling secretions, formation of sequestrae, sharply demarcated ulceration, and usually a regional lymphadenopathy. Finally, the typical saddle nose is produced affecting the *bony* part of the nose, and firm, radiating scars form within the nose.

Pathogenesis. This illness is due to an infection with *Treponema pallidum*. Intrauterine infection may cause an early congenital syphilis within the first months of life, or late congenital syphilis beginning between the age of 3 and puberty but accompanied by the triad of interstitial keratitis, Hutchinson's teeth, and inner ear deafness. The infection may also be acquired (extrauterine) after birth.

Diagnosis. This is based on history, serology (which is not always positive in stage 3), Nelson's test (TPI), and biopsy.

Differential diagnosis. Tuberculosis and malignancy must be considered.

Treatment. Antibiotics are administered, usually under the supervision of a venereologist. Local treatment may be required in stage 3. Once the lesion has healed, reconstruction of the defect may be required.

Rhinoscleroma

Epidemiology. This disease occurs in Eastern Europe, North Africa, Central and South America, and Asia.

Symptoms. The disease begins with an atypical rhinitis with purulent secretion and crusts. A flat, nodular infiltrate then appears in the nasal mucosa. There is increasing coarsening of the external nose (tapir nose). The lesion heals with extensive scars.

Pathogenesis. The infectious organism is *Klebsiella rhinoscleromatis.*

Diagnosis. This depends on the history, with particular attention to foreign travel, and on the results of biopsy and microbiologic examination.

Differential diagnosis. This consists of tuberculosis, syphilis, sarcoid, mycoses, and Hodgkin's disease.

Treatment. Antibiotics are given, dictated by culture and sensitivity tests.

Prognosis. The outcome is dubious and recurrence is possible.

Leprosy

Epidemiology. This disease occurs in tropical and subtropical areas.

Symptoms. A bulbous thickening in the nasal vestibule, obstruction of the nasal cavity, extensive crusting, fetid secretion, ulceration and liquefaction of the nasal framework, and leonine facies occur.

Pathogenesis. The disease is due to an infection with *Mycobacterium leprae* (Hansen).

Diagnosis. This is based on history of contact, symptoms of infection of other parts of the body, and neurologic lesions which are exclusively sensory. Culture and the lepromin reaction also form part of the investigations.

Treatment. Long-term diaminodiphenylsulfone and also tuberculostatic drugs are given. The organism may become resistant to the latter.

Inflammations Localized Mainly in the Nasal Cavity

In the following section, diseases arising primarily within the nasal cavity are dealt with separately from those arising in the nasal sinuses, although disease of the nose may originate in the sinuses and vice versa.

Acute Forms

Acute Rhinitis

Symptoms. Since the common cold may be due to different organisms, the symptoms are not uniform. In the *common* form, there is a *dry prodromal stage* with generalized symptoms including chills and a feeling of cold alternating with a feeling of heat, headache, fatigue, loss of appetite, possibly subfebrile temperature, but often a high temperature in children, as well as itching, burning, a feeling of dryness in the nose and throat, and nasal irritation. The nasal mucosa is usually pale and dry. The *catarrhal stage* usually begins a few hours later with watery secretions, nasal obstruction, temporary loss of smell, lacrimation, rhinolalia clausa, and worsening of the constitutional symptoms. The nasal mucosa is deep red in color, swollen, and secretes profusely. After several days, the disease changes to a *mucous phase.* The generalized symptoms begin to improve, the secretions thicken, the sense of smell improves, and the local symptoms gradually regress. Resolution should be achieved within a week.

Secondary bacterial infection may occur. The secretions are then greenish-yellow, and the disease resolves more slowly.

Initial catarrh occurs in influenza and infection with other types of viruses such as parainfluenza, adenovirus, rheovirus, coronavirus, enterovirus, myxovirus, and respiratory syncytial virus. The symptoms are as described above, but are complicated by other manifestations such as involvement of the entire respiratory tract, the gastrointestinal tract (causing diarrhea), the meninges, the pericardium, the kidneys, and the muscles.

Pathogenesis. The infection is caused by a rhinovirus. More than 100 types have been isolated, belonging to the Picorna group. The disease may also be caused by numerous other viruses. The incubation period of the rhinovirus is from 1 to 3 days. The disease is spread by droplet infection and is potentiated by cooling of the body.

Diagnosis. Initially, it is often not clear whether catarrh is the initial symptom or an accompanying symptom of a severe virus infection.

Differential diagnosis. This often can be made only after a few days. It includes the initial phase of an acute exanthem, allergic or vasomotor rhinitis, congenital syphilis, or nasal diphtheria (usually in children).

Treatment. There is no treatment for the basic cause. *Symptomatic treatment* includes decongestant nose drops or oral decongestants. Antibiotics should only be given for secondary bacterial infection, and culture and sensitivity tests should be taken first. Steam inhalations, treatment with infrared lamps, and analgesics and bed rest should be prescribed if necessary.

Prophylaxis. While there is no scientific evidence that prophylaxis is possible, measures to improve general health may be helpful. These include building up the patient's general resistance by sauna baths, therapeutic regimens at health resorts, hydrotherapy, participation in sports, administration of vitamin C, and careful hygiene, especially when in contact with young children. Adenoidectomy may be necessary in children (see p. 321). Immunization against the coryza virus is not yet possible, but there are vaccines against influenza.

Allergic Rhinitis

The most common form is hay fever, but other allergens may be responsible.

Symptoms. These include itching in the nose, nasal obstruction, sneezing attacks, and a clear, watery nasal discharge. The patient may also have a feeling of fullness and irritation of the entire head, possibly conjunctivitis, a feeling of being unwell, temporary fever, loss of appetite, autonomic symptoms, possibly inability to work, and temporary hypo- or anosmia. Secondary infection is possible.

Pathogenesis. An inhalation allergy is the cause. The shock organ is usually the nasal mucosa, but it may also be the conjunctiva or other mucous membranes. The disease is often hereditary.

Seasonal allergic rhinitis is caused by pollen.

Perennial allergic rhinitis is due to an inhaled allergen independent of the season. The allergens include fungi, animal hair, house dust, mites, houseplants such as primulas and roses, and also foods such as fish, strawberries, nuts, eggs, milk, and flour. There are occupational allergies, e. g., to flour for bakers, to hair and epithelial scales for hairdressers, etc., and other allergies to bacteria and parasites.

Infection and allergy. Bacteria and viruses can act as allergens, but the practical significance of this is still controversial. Three pathogenetic mechanisms are possible:

1. There is an allergic reaction to bacteria or viruses without clinical infection, e. g., to nasal saprophytes.
2. There is an allergic reaction to bacterial or viral infection, e. g., chronic bacterial rhinitis or sinusitis with resultant sensitivity to the causal organism.
3. Secondary infection in a tissue already altered by allergic reaction is present. In this case, the infective agent is not the same as the antigen.

Form 2 corresponds to the term "infection allergy". Its time course puts it in the class of *late allergic reaction* (Coombs/Gell type IV).

If an infective allergy is supected, then tests should be carried out for the antigen (i. e., the positive cutaneous late reaction to a bacterial extract), and antibiotics are given depending on the sensitivity tests. The long-term value of hyposensitization has not yet been confirmed in clinical practice.

Diagnosis. This is made from the typical history, cytology of the nasal secretions, intracutaneous tests, prick tests, and patch tests, intranasal challenge with rhinomanometry, estimation of serum and secretion IgE, and the RAST.

Local findings. The nasal mucosa is livid and pale. In acute stages the mucosa may also be deep red. The turbinates are swollen, and there are large amounts of clear secretion.

Differential diagnosis. Vasomotor rhinitis and coryza must be considered (see Table 2.**4**).

Treatment. *Causal.* Specific desensitization, based on allergen tests, should be carried out (for pollen allergies before the pollen season, in autumn), and continued for several years thereafter. Allergen avoidance may mean a change of climate, or a change of occupation may be necessary. Local or systemic sodium chromoglycate inhibits the liberation of H substances (histamine, serotonin, etc.) from mast cells.

Symptomatic treatment includes antihistamines, steroids (special preparations for local use in the nose, e. g., beclomethasone diproprionate spray), and decongestant nasal drops (see p. 224). The patient should be watched for possible signs of steroid side effects. Polyps or persistent edematous swellings should be removed (see p. 217 ff.).

Prognosis. This is in general good. The disease gradually regresses as the patients get older, but progression to bronchial asthma (or vice versa) is possible.

Complications. Involvement of the nasal sinuses and the lower respiratory tract, and polyps of the nose and sinuses are possible.

Vasomotor Rhinitis

Symptoms. These are the same as for perennial allergic rhinitis. The course is usually paroxsysmal.

Local findings include a livid, pale nasal mucosa. During an attack there is profuse watery secretion and swelling of the nasal turbinates.

Pathogenesis. This is a neurovascular disorder of the blood vessels of the nasal mucosa, affecting the parasympathetic system particularly. Allergens to specific antibodies cannot be demonstrated. It is a nonspecific reflex hypersensitivity of the nasal mucosa. An attack may be caused by various influences, e. g., change of temperature or humidity, alcohol, dust, smoke, mechanical irritation, stress, anxiety neurosis, endocrine disorders, drugs (e. g., antihypertensive agents such as reserpine or beta-blockers, oral contraceptives), and drug abuse (imidazoline and catechol derivatives, clomethiazole, etc.). See also Rhinitis of Pregnancy (p. 217).

Diagnosis. The typical history and exclusion of allergic rhinitis by negative allergen tests and no elevated IgE in the secretion provide the diagnosis.

Differential diagnosis. This includes allergic rhinitis, a foreign body in the nose (particularly in children), and the early phases of a cold (see Table 2.**4**).

Conservative treatment. This includes elimination of all recognizable irritant factors (although this is seldom possible); administration of antihistamines, decongestant nose drops or oral decongestant drugs, steroids (e.g., beclomethasone) in very small doses for a limited period; treatment of the metabolic and endocrine systems where necessary; and sedatives, but imidazoline preparations should be avoided for long term application because of the potential for habituation.

Surgery may succeed if conservative treatment fails. There are several possibilities in increasing order of extent: (1) puncture of the inferior or middle turbinate with electrocautery, cryosurgery, and laser treatment (see p. 215 ff. and Fig. 2.**26a**); (2) removal of any possible mechanical points of irritation such as septal spurs or deviations (see p. 260); (3) reduction of the inferior and, at times, the middle turbinate, and removal of the posterior end of a hypertrophic turbinate by conchotomy (see p. 216; Fig. 2.**26c**); (4) division of the parasympathetic nasal fibers, either the nerve of the pterygoid canal, vidian nerve, or the greater petrosal nerve in the middle cranial fossa. Both methods of nerve interruption are still in a highly experimental stage and therefore not yet commonly recommendable. This latter procedure is, of course, highly experimental and should not be used in the US in the present litigious climate.

Prognosis is uncertain. The disease often improves suddenly but occasionally is resistant to treatment.

Foreign Bodies in the Nose (see Color Plate **12a**)

These are usually found in children and may be retained for a very long time. They include coins, metal fragments, peas, etc.

Symptoms. These include unilateral nasal obstruction, a worsening chronic purulent rhinitis or sinusitis, unilateral fetid secretions, and formation of a rhinolith due to deposition of calcium around the foreign body.

Diagnosis. This is based on anterior rhinoscopy and radiology. A foreign body is often an incidental finding. The nose is inspected and probed, using an endoscope if necessary, after decongestion and induction of local anesthesia.

Treatment. The foreign body is removed instrumentally, at times under a short general anesthetic since long-standing foreign bodies are often firmly fixed and provoke brisk bleeding when they are mobilized.

> *Note:* Unilateral chronic purulent rhinorrhea in a small child should suggest the diagnosis of a foreign body, and the child should be examined by a specialist.

Chronic Forms

Rhinitis Sicca Anterior

Symptoms. These include a feeling of dryness, irritation, and formation of crusts in the nose and also mild occasional nasal bleeding.

Pathogenesis. Several factors are responsible such as injury of the exposed parts of the anterior nasal mucosa, dust, nose picking, extremes of temperature, etc.

Diagnosis. The nasal mucosa on the anterior part of the nasal septum immediately posterior to the mucocutaneous junction is dry. The mucosal surface is raw, roughened, and granular. Crusts form, followed by ulceration and at times a later septal perforation.

Differential diagnosis. Included here are chemical injury in chromium workers, iatrogenic septal perforation after operations or incorrect cautery, trauma, lupus, leprosy, and syphilis.

Treatment. Nasal ointments containing oil are applied. Septal perforation is dealt with on p. 262.

Table 2.4 Causes of Acute Nasal Discharge

	Etiology	Occurrence and Age of Predilection	Subjective Symptoms	Nasal Secretion	Condition of the Nasal Mucosa	Course	Complications	Diagnosis
Acute rhinitis coryza, common cold	Viral infection with possible secondary bacterial infection	Any age	Sneezing secretion, nasal obstruction, pressure feeling in head	Serous, becoming mucopurulent after several days	Mucosal swelling and redness	3–8 days	Acute sinusitis, pharyngitis, otitis media, laryngotracheitis, bronchitis	Evidence of infection, history
Vasomotor rhinitis	Neurovascular reaction to several mechanical and chemical stimuli, also to stress and psychological factors	Episodic after exposure to the stimulus or after psychological stimulation, often beginning in middle age	Attacks of sneezing, massive watery secretion, obstructed nasal respiration, pressure feeling in head	Profuse clear thin fluid secretion, poor in protein	Pronounced mucosal swelling with little reddening. In symptom-free intervals the mucosa is pallid. There is rapid swelling of the turbinates and profuse secretion on exposure.	Usually minutes to hours, often relapsing	Reflex asthma, erythema of the external nose, swelling of the face	History, determination of the inciting stimulus. Allergy tests are negative.

| Allergic rhinitis | Antigen-antibody reaction in the nasal mucosa to specific stimuli, e.g., (1) * pollen (grass or trees); (2) house dust, animal hair, feather beds, mould, fungus; (3) food-stuffs and occupational antigens | Usually occurs for the first time in young patients. (1) Seasonal (spring, summer, early autumn) (2) and (3) perennial | Irritation in the nose and eyes, nasal obstruction, attacks of sneezing, conjunctivitis, watering of the eyes, and pressure feeling in head | A very rich watery or thin mucous, which later may be mucopurulent | In the acute phase there is mucosal swelling and redness. Between attacks the mucosa is livid and pallid | (1) Pollinosis lasts 1 to 2 months every year at the same time. (2) and (3) last weeks to months but may be chronic, depending on the degree of sensitivity of the antigen and exposure. | Bronchial asthma, chronic sinusitis, otitis media (seldom purulent), nasal polypi | History: evidence of allergens shown by testing intracutaneous, intranasal; possibly eosinophilia in the nasal secretions; increase of specific immunoglobulins in the nasal secretions |

* Numbers in parentheses refer to categories enumerated in "Etiology" column.

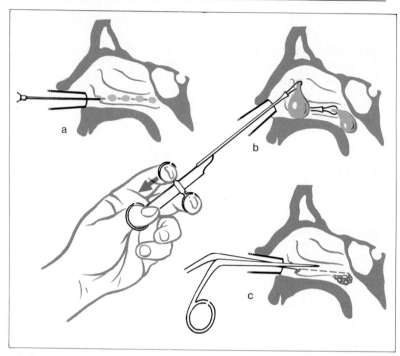

Fig. 2.**26a–c** Endonasal operations. **(a)** Electrocautery of the inferior turbinate; **(b)** snaring of polypi with the wire loop; **(c)** inferior turbinectomy with removal of the posterior end of the turbinate.

Chronic Rhinitis

This is a collective term for chronic irritation or inflammation of the nasal mucosa with hypertrophy of the nasal mucosa, especially around the nasal turbinates. It is characterized by either hyperemia and edema, or true tissue hypertrophy.

Symptoms. The main symptom is nasal obstruction that fluctuates markedly in the early stages and also alternates from side to side. Later, it is continuous and severe and usually affects both sides. The secretions are tough, stringy, colorless, and only rarely purulent. Postnasal catarrh is particularly prominent with sniffles and compulsive clearing of throat. Other symptoms include rhinolalia clausa, epiphora, secondary dacryocystitis, and secondary pharyngitis. In severe cases, fatigue, sleeplessness, an unsteady or woozy feeling in the head, and, occasionally, headache and a feeling of pressure in the head may occur. There is a general loss of psychological and physical well-being.

Pathogenesis. Many causal factors are possible such as recurrent acute inflammation with gradual irreversible damage to the mucosa; infection in the sinuses, obstruction of nasal drainage due to enlarged adenoids or a nasopharyngeal tumor; vasomotor diseases of the mucosa, chronic inflammation due to tobacco smoke and dust, chemicals, acquired toxins, persistent extremes of temperature, excessive and abnormal humidity, pregnancy, menstruation, menopause, endocrine disturbances (e. g., of the thyroid and adrenal glands, diabetes), diseases of the heart and circulation, side effects of drugs (see below), and infective allergy (late-type allergy, see p. 209).

Diagnosis. The disease is long-standing, and the history often shows one or more of the toxins named above. Examination shows a dark red and partially bluish-violet swelling, affecting the inferior turbinate especially. The nasal lumen is narrowed or obstructed. The thickened mucosa responds to decongestant nose drops in simple chronic rhinitis, but true tissue hypertrophy in chronic hyperplastic rhinitis does not.

In the *later stages,* the mucosa over the turbinates assumes a slightly granular surface, which gradually becomes nodular and demonstrates micropolyps. These edematous processes can develop into single or multiple *nasal polypi* (see Color Plates **11a, 12c** and **26a**), especially around the inferior turbinate. Often this true *tissue hypertrophy* begins at the posterior ends of the turbinates, usually the inferior (see Color Plate **25a**). The choanae are then blocked by mulberry-like masses which can be demonstrated only by *endoscopic examination of the nasopharynx* or by indirect examination with the mirror.

Differential diagnosis. This includes sinusitis, foreign bodies, specific infections of the nasal mucosa (see p. 220), adenoidal hypertrophy, allergy, Wegener's granuloma, and tumors. Biopsy should be carried out if necessary (see Table 2.**5**).

Treatment. *Conservative.* Any known or suspected etiologic agents should be dealt with. Some medicines may need to be curtailed, drug overuse controlled, and the patient may need endocrinologic investigation by an internist. Attention to the environment and occupation may prove valuable. Symptomatic medical treatment by decongestant nose drops, etc., is only of short-term benefit (see p. 223). In the long term, uncritical symptomatic treatment not only is valueless but is even damaging.

Surgical in increasing order of extent:

1. *Reduction of the inferior turbinate* by sclerosing agents, the cryoprobe, or the laser. *Electrocoagulation* is carried out with a differential needle electrode pushed into the mucosa at several sites in the lower turbinate (and occasionally the middle turbinate) under local anesthesia (see Fig. 2.**26a**). This produces multiple, localized scars in the nasal mucosa.

Table 2.5 Causes of Nasal Obstruction

Nostrils, nasal cavity, nasal sinuses

Short history
  A furuncle and eczema of the nostrils
  Acute infective vasomotor or allergic rhinitis or sinusitis
  Trauma, edema, submucosal hematoma, and fracture
  Foreign body

Long history
  Collapsing nasal alae
  Stenosis of the nostrils
  Anterior rhinitis sicca with crust formation
  Septal deviation and septal spurs
  Chronic rhinitis and sinusitis, which may be allergic
  Hypertrophy of the turbinates, including hypertrophy of the posterior ends
  Nasal polypi
  Bullous concha
  Synechiae or incorrectly managed trauma; occasionally septum perforation
  Rhinitis medicamentosa
  Bleeding polyp of the septum
  Foreign body and rhinolith
  Atrophic rhinitis and ozena
  Tumors
  Congenital anomalies

Nasopharynx

Short history
  Pharyngitis
  Retropharyngeal abscess

Long history
  Adenoid hypertrophy
  Choanal polyp
  Choanal atresia
  Nasopharyngeal angiofibroma
  Adhesions between the soft palate and the posterior pharyngeal nerve
  Tumors, especially malignant

Cryosurgery using a fine probe filled with liquid nitrogen produces partial obliteration of the mucosa of the turbinates.

The CO_2 or argon laser also produces mucosal scars by evaporation or coagulation of tissue.

2. Turbinectomy or mucotomy. A strip of tissue is removed from the lower edge of the inferior turbinate, occasionally from the middle turbinate, and from the enlarged posterior ends of the turbinate using scissors or a wire loop. The purpose is to reduce the volume of the turbinate, but atrophic rhinitis can occur if too much tissue is removed (see p. 218).

Pregnancy Rhinitis

Increasing swelling and obstruction of the nose may occur, especially in the second half of pregnancy. The symptoms resolve after delivery.

Rhinitis Medicamentosa

There is reversible or irreversible damage to the mucosa caused by topically or systemically applied drugs.

Mucosal swelling leading possibly to hyperplastic rhinitis may be caused by acetylsalicyclic acid, oral contraceptives, guanethidine, hydantoin, estrogens, paraaminosalicylic acid, phenothiazine, rauwolfia preparations, beta-blocking drugs, and tetraethyl ammonium.

Dryness of the nasal mucosa is caused by atropine, belladonna preparations, corticosteroids, imidazoline, or catecholamine derivatives.

Toxic rhinopathy is caused by abuse of decongestant nose drops (see p. 224).

Nasal Polypi
(See Color Plates **11a** and **12c**).

Nasal polypi are benign pedicled or sessile masses of nasal or sinus mucosa caused by inflammation.

Symptoms. These include mechanical obstruction to nasal breathing, mechanical anosmia, epiphora, colorless stringy or purulent secretion, postnasal catarrh, headache, snoring, and rhinolalia clausa. Abnormal growth of the facial skeleton in children leads to a broad, bony nose, the so-called frog face. Chronic sinusitis may be caused by obstruction of the sinus ostia. Polypi can also arise in one or all sinuses even if the nasal cavity is free.

The *choanal polyp* is a polyp on a long pedicle usually arising in the antrum. It may block the choana or the nasopharynx completely.

Pathogenesis. Nasal polypi are often due to mucosal allergy (the late type); allergy tests are positive in 25 % of all patients. They may also be due to the common chronic rhinitis or sinusitis, particularly of the ethmoids. The triad of nasal polypi, aspirin sensitivity, and asthma is quite common.

Diagnosis. The typical findings on anterior rhinoscopy are solitary or multiple glazed, transparent, smooth-walled, whitish-yellow masses, mobile to pressure with a probe, usually the middle meatus or the choana. They are often bilateral.

Note: Polypoid sinusitis often develops in addition to nasal polypi. The sinuses therefore should always be investigated by radiography and possibly by endoscopy in patients with nasal polypi (see p. 227).

Differential diagnosis. This includes encephalomeningocele (excluded by radiography and probing), a bleeding polyp of the septum (see p. 254), malignant nasal tumors, or a pituitary tumor, e. g., an adenoma.

Treatment. Although nasal polypi shrink or disappear completely under steroids, this treatment is not appropriate because the polyps recur once the steroids are stopped. If an allergen can be demonstrated, it should be eliminated. Polyps cause irreversible damage to the nasal cavity, to the external part of the nose in young patients, and indeed to the entire body; polypectomy therefore is needed.

Polypectomy: Polypi (see Fig. 2.**26b**) are removed under local or general anesthesia, often combined with ethmoidectomy or antrostomy (see p. 238).

Prognosis. Polyps have a marked tendency to recur, particularly if they are due to allergy.

Atrophic Rhinitis and Ozena

Atrophic rhinitis may or may not be accompanied by a foul smell from the nose. In the former case the disease is described as ozena.

Symptoms. This disease occurs mainly in women, often beginning at puberty. The face is typically flattened and broad.

The nasal cavity usually is filled completely by greenish-yellow or brownish-black crusts. Once the crusts are removed, it can be seen that the nasal cavity is very wide. The mucosa is atrophic and dry due to fibrosis of the subepithelial layer, and the inferior turbinate is atrophic. In ozena there are a fetid secretion and crusts. The repulsive smell considerably hinders social contact. The patient herself has anosmia so that she is unaware of the unpleasant smell that she produces. She does, however, have a sensation of nasal obstruction. There are often severe mucosal changes including dryness and dry, thick crusts involving the entire pharynx, larynx, and trachea.

Pathogenesis. This is not known with certainty, but is probably multifactorial. The disease is more common in orientals than in whites, and more common in the latter than in blacks. There is a geographic concentration, e. g., in Eastern Europe and in India. The nasal cavity is abnormally wide due to atrophy of the mucosa and of the bony nasal skeleton. The mucosal glands and the sensory nerve fibers degenerate, the respiratory epithelium undergoes squamous metaplasia, and the mucociliary cleaning system is destroyed. The thick, gluey secretions are decomposed by bacterial proteolysis.

Secondary atrophic rhinitis is due to trauma to the nose or too extensive surgery to the nose and sinuses and to occupational exposure to glass, wood, asbestos, etc.

Table 2.6 Causes of Nasal Fetor
Atrophic rhinitis with fetor (ozena).   Both sides of the nose are full of foul-smelling crusts.
Tumors of the nose and sinuses.   There is a putrid smell due to breaking down of the tumor.

Purulent rhinitis and sinusitis.
   Unilateral or bilateral purulent secretion.
   There is *considerable* fetor especially in sinusitis of dental origin.

Rhinolith and foreign body   cause unilateral nasal obstruction and foul-smelling secretion.
Gumma due to stage III syphilis   causes a marked fetid purulent secretion due to breaking-down of the gumma.
Nasal diphtheria and nasal tuberculosis   cause a sweetish smell.
Glanders   causes foul-smelling, purulent nasal secretion.

Diagnosis. The nose contains gluey, dry, greenish-yellow secretions and crusts, occasionally lining the entire nasal cavity. Once the nasal cavity has been cleaned, it is seen to be very wide, and the turbinates to be very small. The crusts give off a smell in ozena.

Differential diagnosis. See Table 2.6.

Treatment. *Conservative.* The nose is cleaned by douching several times a day with dilute salt water and by the introduction of large, cotton wool tampons impregnated with greasy ointments. Local applications include *oily* nasal drops, emulsions, or ointments, and possibly vitamin A supplements. Steam inhalations with saline solution are given, and osmotic powders, e.g., dextrose, are sniffed up the nose.

Operative treatment may be used to prevent drying out of the nose by narrowing of the nasal cavity. Two main procedures are available.

1. Bolstering of the nasal mucosa (Fig. 2.**27a**) with autologous or homologous tissue (cartilage or bone chips)
2. Median displacement of the lateral nasal wall (see Fig. 2.**27b**) by internal rotation of the mobilized lateral nasal wall, which is fixed in its new position to produce narrowing of the nasal cavity

Nasal Diphtheria

This usually occurs in children older than 6 months. The secretions may be hemorrhagic and purulent or exclusively purulent with crusts and rhagades around the

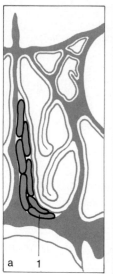
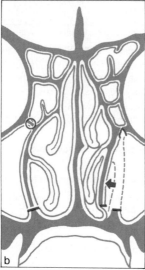

Fig. 2.**27a** and **b** Operations for atrophic rhinitis. **(a)** Submucosal supplementation with cartilage chips (1); **(b)** mobilization and medial displacement (right of illustration) of the lateral nasal wall as described by Lautenschlaeger. The red circle shows the point of rotation of the lateral nasal wall.

nostrils. The disease is rare in adults. Nasal diphtheria can occur isolated or in combination with pharyngeal diphtheria (see p. 346).

Diagnosis is made by culture. *This is a notifiable disease.*

Treatment is by antitoxic serum (see p. 347).

Tuberculosis of the Nasal Cavity

Two forms may be distinguished: (1) lupus (see p. 205) and (2) exudative ulcerative mucosal tuberculosis. This is usually the result of hematogenous or intraluminal dissemination in pulmonary tuberculosis. The mucous membrane shows moth eaten ulcerations.

Diagnosis. This is determined by bacteriology and biopsy.

Syphilis of the Nasal Cavity

Stage I (infection from instruments!) and stage II are very rare; stage III is more common (see p. 206). The **diagnosis** is made by serology and biopsy and possibly identification of the organism.

Sarcoidosis, see pp. 206 and 498.

Scleroma of the Nasal Cavity, see p. 206.

Leprosy of the Nasal Cavity, see p. 207.

Glanders

Epidemiology. This disease occurs mainly in Eastern Europe and North America. The causative organism is *Malleomyces mallei*. It is transmitted by ungulates.

Symptoms. Purulent, foul-smelling nasal secretions, granulations, and ulcers are found on the nasal mucosa. The disease may extend to the external nose and surrounding areas.

Diagnosis. This is made by culture, an agglutination test, and biopsy. *The disease is notifiable on suspicion.*

Treatment. Antibiotics are administered.

Blastomycosis

Epidemiology. This disease occurs in North, Central, and South America and is caused by several types of blastomyces (yeasts).

Symptoms. Crusts and mucosal ulcers are found which may extend to the external nose. The regional lymph nodes are usually enlarged.

Diagnosis. Culture and biopsy provide the diagnosis.

Treatment. Amphotericin B is given, and may be followed by excision of the diseased skin or mucosa.

Rhinosporidiosis

Epidemiology. The disease occurs in India, Ceylon, Africa, and North and South America and is caused by *Rhinosporidium seeberi.*

Symptoms. These include polypoid, reddish nodular granulations of the anterior part of the nasal cavity which bleed easily. The disease may extend to the nasal sinuses and pharynx.

Diagnosis. This is made by culture and biopsy.

Treatment. The polypi are removed and the base is cauterized, but there is a danger of bleeding.

Other mycoses that can occasionally cause nasal symptoms include moniliasis, aspergillosis, mucormycosis, and coccidioidosis.

Wegener's Granulomatosis

Symptoms. This nasal disease presents with increasing nasal obstruction, epistaxis, nasal discharge, combination of crusts, mucosal granulations, and later septal perforations and saddling of the *cartilaginous* skeleton. There is progressive loss of tissue. In addition, the patient has pulmonary symptoms (chronic bronchitis) and generalized symptoms such as malaise, tiredness, night sweats, and intermittent limb pain.

Pathogenesis. The cause of this disease is not clear. It may be an autoimmune disease with granulomatous arteritis, perivasculitis, and necrotizing vasculitis. Generalized manifestations affect other parts of the body such as the lungs, kidneys, liver, middle ear, larynx, and trachea.

Diagnosis. The diagnosis rests on the clinical picture, the local findings, the course of the disease, and on biopsy. The erythrocyte sedimentation rate (ESR) is usually markedly elevated. Electrophoresis shows reduced albumin and increased globulin. The most specific test at present is the determination of nuclear antigens (ANPA = anti-nuclear cytoplasmatic antibody) in the cytoplasm of white blood cells. The lungs should be investigated carefully by radiography. Renal investigations should also be done.

Differential diagnosis. This includes midline granuloma, leukemia, malignant lymphoma, and sarcoid.

Treatment. Steroids in high doses begun as early as possible, combined with immunosuppressive agents. Chemotherapy or radiotherapy may also be used.

Prognosis is poor. Death is often due to renal failure.

Lethal Midline Granuloma

This is a monolocular disease. The nasal prodroma are similar to that of Wegener's granuloma. Progressive ulceration of the central part of the face extends also to the maxilla.

Pathogenesis. The cause is unknown. The disease may be due to an immune deficiency, but may also be related to malignancy of the reticulohistiocytic system.

Diagnosis. Typically, the disease is localized to the central part of the face. The ESR is elevated, and there is a hypochromic anemia.

Differential diagnosis. The includes Wegener's granuloma, glanders, scleroma gumma, noma, blastomycosis, and histoplasmosis.

Treatment. A combination of radiotherapy, steroids, chemotherapy, immunosuppressive agents, and antibiotics is applied. Occasionally extensive excision is required.

Prognosis. With early diagnosis and energetic treatment the outlook is not necessarily unfavorable.

Basics of Local Conservative Treatment of the Upper Respiratory and Digestive Tract

The following factors facilitate treatment of diseases of the upper respiratory and digestive tract:

- Easy accessibility for local medical treatment
- Local and systemic medical treatment may be combined
- Easy accessibility for physical methods of treatment such as inhalation, irradiation, health cures, ionizing radiation for malignancy, etc.

Physical Treatment

Inhalation. Two main methods are possible:

1. *Steam inhalation.* Steam is used for its therapeutic affect or to carry active agents. A steam kettle or tent may be used. The droplet size is greater than or equal to $30\,\mu$m so the vapor is unstable and rapidly precipitates. Steam is often supplemented by the addition of salts, ether oils, active agents, detergents, and wetting agents, or agents active on mucopolysaccharide secretions. Precipitation occurs mainly in the nose, mouth, pharynx, and larynx.

2. *Aerosol inhalation.* A true aerosol is used with a droplet size less than $30\,\mu$m in a quasistable suspension of fluid in air. The smaller the particles the further they penetrate into the airway. The optimal droplet size for the nose and pharynx is 10 to $15\,\mu$m (up to $50\,\mu$m), for the trachea 5 to $10\,\mu$m, and for the bronchi and alveoli less than $5\,\mu$m. Jet nebulization is better for the upper and middle airways than *ultrasound* or a *gas-driven apparatus.* Drugs to be used in the aerosol include vasoactive substances to decongest the mucosa, secretolytic agents, antiallergic substances, steroids, antibiotics, chemotherapy, antiasthmatic drugs, and vitamin preparations.

Rules for inhalation therapy:

● The droplet size of the aerosol should be chosen to correspond to that of the principal diseased part of the respiratory tract.
● Medications used should have a pH around 7.0, should be water soluble, approximately isotonic, nontoxic and nonirritant, well retained, and capable of being atomized.
● Inhalation treatment should last 10 to 15 min.

Local thermal treatment. At the present, warm methods are preferred using microwaves, with a wavelength of less than 1 m, for the sinuses, larynx, etc. Infrared rays with a wavelength of less than 760 nm are used for superficial soft tissue inflammation, and originate as an electric light with carbon filament lamps which have rich infrared emission, and are particularly effective in chronic catarrhal rhinosinusitis. Light in the visible spectrum, especially red light with a wavelength between 760 and 400 nm, is used for superficial soft tissue inflammation as are moist warm dressings, mud, and heating pads.

Warmth produces hyperemia both by direct and reflex action on the deep tissues, and this accelerates and intensifies the anti-inflammatory processes in the tissues. Application of cold, on the other hand, retards the circulation and thus inhibits the inflammatory process.

Spa treatment. This form of treatment is popular in Europe. In chronic mucosal diseases of the upper respiratory tract, the following are indicated: exposure to the sun or bathing in sulfur springs; exposure to the dry stimulating climate of the high mountains for chronic catarrh with increased secretions; exposure to a moist stimulating climate in patients with dry chronic catarrh. Treatment in spas or health resorts should last for at least 4 to 6 weeks, and even several months in children.

Medical Treatment

Principles of Topical Drug Administration

● Drugs that are active only on the mucosal *surface* (e.g., drugs soluble in oil) should be distinguished from those that are absorbed and act *within the mucosa* (e. g., water-soluble drugs).

- Occasionally water-soluble solutions may be absorbed through the mucosal surface as fast as intravenous injection.
- The drug must not damage the cilary activity, the mucosa, or the superficial film of secretions.
- The pH of the drug should lie around 7.0 and its osmotic pressure should be between 0.5 and twice isotonic.
- Locally applied drugs should not have systemic effects and should be neither antigenic nor carcinogenic.

Groups of Medicines

Vasoactive substances, e. g., adrenalin or imidazoline derivatives such as Privine, Nasivine, and Otrivine shrink the mucosa by vasoconstriction. Uncritical persistent use carries the danger of habituation, leading to a rhinitis medicamentosa and resistant mucosal swelling, failure of the autonomic vascular regulation, and organic mucosal damage. Local or systemic decongestant agents of any type should therefore be used for a brief period only, i. e., for 1 to 2 weeks at the most at a time.

> *Note:* In infants and small children, there is a danger of acute intoxication due to the use of nose drops. Special preparations should therefore be used for children.

Antibiotics. Topical antibiotics should in rare cases be used if oral or parenteral administration is not sufficiently active, and it should then be dictated by culture and sensitivity tests. Large-molecule antibiotics should be chosen for their action on the mucosal surface, e. g., neomycin, bacitracin, and gramicydin, because they are absorbed poorly or not at all. Their effect and side effects should be weighed carefully before they are prescribed, taking into account the development of resistance, allergic sensitivity, change of the local flora leading to secondary mycosis, and side effects on other organs.

Corticosteroids. These should *not* be used for viral infections. Only topical preparations that are not absorbed and do not produce side effects, e. g., beclomethazone diproprionate, should be used. Oral or parenteral steroids should be restricted to disease that has resisted other forms of treatment and to emergency situations, e. g., life-threatening edema. Contraindications include diabetes, tuberculosis, peptic ulcer, adrenal insufficiency, etc.

Antiallergic treatment should be directed toward the *cause* if possible, i. e., desensitization after appropriate tests for allergens or withdrawal from the allergen. If this is not possible, symptomatic antihistamines may be given orally or sodium chromoglycate, and possibly ipratropium (Atrovent), locally or steroids if possible also given locally.

Inflammation of the Sinuses

General Principles

Etiology, pathophysiology, pathology, and clinical findings in inflammation of the different nasal sinuses are often identical or very similar. They are therefore

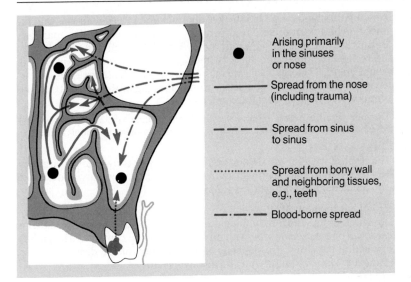

Arising primarily
in the sinuses
or nose

Spread from the nose
(including trauma)

Spread from sinus
to sinus

Spread from bony wall
and neighboring tissues,
e.g., teeth

Blood-borne spread

Fig. 2.**28** Sites of origin of sinusitis.

described together. Nonspecific infection is much the most common: specific infections occur by extension from the nasal cavity but are very rare.

Sinusitis is a very common disease: it is estimated that 5 % of the population of Central Europe suffer from chronic sinusitis. The maxillary antrum is the most commonly affected in adults, followed in decreasing order of frequency by the ethmoids, frontal, and sphenoid sinuses. In children the ethmoid sinuses are most frequently affected. Infection of several sinuses is described as *polysinusitis,* and of all the sinuses as *pansinusitis,* unilateral or bilateral.

Pathophysiologic mechanisms of the ventilation and drainage of the sinuses are illustrated on p. 186. Figure 2.**28** shows the sites of origin and pathways of spread. The most frequent cause of sinusitis is extension of infection from the nasal cavity into one or several sinuses. Even a common cold causes mucosal inflammation of the sinuses, but this very often does not produce symptoms.

Pathogenesis. The organisms include viruses, pneumococci, hemophilus influenzae, hemolytic streptococci, staphylococci, *Escherichia coli,* and rarely anaerobes. Mixed infection often occurs, and infection with fungi may also occur. The course of the infection is also influenced by immunologic factors such as allergy and anergy and interaction between the organisms and resistance, e. g., in infective allergy, superinfected allergy, and the sinobronchial syndrome. Ten percent of infections of the maxillary antrum are due to diseased tooth roots. A dental granuloma, especially of the second premolar and the first molar, causes a maxillary sinusitis of dental origin. The organisms are mainly anaerobes, the secretion is characteristically fetid, and the course is chronic. Healing of this form of sinusitis is impossible without dental treatment.

An acute sinusitis occurs in *swimmers and divers*. Organisms are forced into the nose and sinuses during diving. Irritation by chlorine in swimming pools is also possible.

The respiratory tract can demonstrate hereditary or congenital deformities. The nasal sinuses are then inevitably involved, e. g., in mucoviscidosis and in Kartagener's syndrome (see p. 244).

Pathologic anatomy. Depending on the organism, its virulence, pathophysiologic factors, and immunologic resistance, sinusitis may take either a *catarrhal* or a *purulent* form, with mixed forms being common. The pathology within the sinus also depends on the duration of the disease process. *Acute and chronic sinusitis* may be distinguished.

Symptoms. These include *pains in the face and the head*. Characteristically, these become worse on bending, lifting, coughing, etc., which increase the pressure in the sinuses.

The pains are usually worse in acute sinusitis than in chronic sinusitis, in which pain may be entirely absent. The characteristics of sinus pain are a feeling of pressure in the skull, or a lancinating, boring, pulsating pain especially in the anterior part of the skull (Table 2.7 and Fig. 2.**29**). Sensitivity to pressure or tapping over the affected sinus is common, i. e., over the cheek in maxillary sinusitis, over the forehead in frontal sinusitis, and in the medial canthus in ethmoiditis. The first and second divisions of the trigeminal nerve may be affected by direct stimulation of the nerves running in the walls of the sinus. Sphenoiditis causes a typical pain in the occiput, but also in the temporal region, and in the center of the skull (see Fig. 2.**29**).

Symptoms of sinusitis in children are described on p. 243.

Secretion. Unilateral nasal discharge, especially in adults, is always suspicious of sinusitis. The secretion may be colorless and of variable viscosity but is usually colored, being yellow, green, or mixed with blood (see Color Plate **12b**). The pus is inspissated and sometimes friable. The secretion is often odorless and is only fetid if the sinusitis is of dental origin. The secretion drains both from the front of the nose and into the nasopharynx, particularly in infection of the posterior sinuses. Typical streams of pus occur from the ostia of the sinuses (see Fig. 2.**4**) and on the posterior wall of the pharynx.

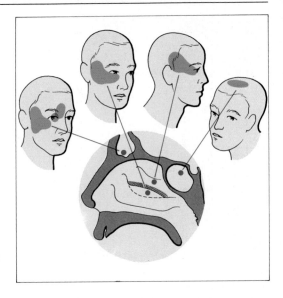

Fig. 2.**29**   Referred pain from several intranasal trigger points.

Nasal obstruction. This may be intermittent or permanent. Unilateral nasal obstruction should always lead to a suspicion of sinusitis.

Abnormalities of smell. Hyposmia or anosmia is common; cacosmia may occur in dental empyema and in chronic sinusitis.

Eczema of the nostrils and conjunctivitis. These are especially common in children.

Extension to the lower airway causes coughing, hoarseness, or bronchitis (see p. 243).

Generalized symptoms. These include lethargy, disinclination to work, and mental symptoms including depression. Fever only occurs as a result of a generalized infection or is a sign of early complications.

Diagnosis

- Anterior and posterior rhinoscopy (see pp. 187, 189)
- Nasoendoscopy (see p. 202)
- Radiography, possibly including a contrast medium (see p. 196)
- Tomography (p. 198) and computerized axial tomography (CT) scan
- Ultrasound (see p. 199)
- Puncture and irrigation (see p. 199)
- Sinoscopy by Beck's trephination (see p. 201)
- Bacteriologic examination of the secretions
- Exploration of the sinuses and biopsy

Table 2.7 Common Causes of Pain in the Head and Face

Etiologic Group and Subgroup	Site of Predilection of Pain	Typical Symptoms
Headache of nasal and sinus origin		
Furuncle of the nose and lip	Initially localized to the nose, lip, and cheek and then becomes diffuse	Stabbing, burning pain on contact
Nasal obstruction Septal deviation Hypertrophy of the turbinates Foreign bodies Synechias Tumors	Diffuse, intermittent, localized in the central part of the forehead and between the eyes	Mainly a feeling of fullness and pressure
Vasomotor and allergic rhinitis	Diffuse in the central forehead area and between the eyes	Feeling of fullness with prickling and itching in the nose, and attacks of sneezing in the early phases
Frontal sinusitis	Forehead, usually unilateral, anterior wall of the frontal sinus, floor of the frontal sinus sensitive to pressure	Begins with catarrh gradually increasing; remission at certain times of day is possible; the pain worsens on bending, straining, and lifting, is mainly a dull ache.
Maxillary sinusitis	Cheek, upper jaw, often the forehead on one or both sides	
Ethmoidal sinusitis	Root of the nose, medial canthus	
Sphenoidal sinusitis	Skull, center of the skull, occiput	
Atrophic rhinitis and ozena	Diffuse	Dull headache and feeling of dryness

High or low pressure in the sinuses	over the affected sinus	Prolonged pain
Tumors in the nose, sinuses, and nasopharynx	Depends on the site of tumor, is often felt deeply within the skull	Prolonged headache which becomes intolerable when the dura is invaded
Vasomotor headache		
Vasomotor cephalgia	Often maximal over the forehead, the temple, and the vertex; usually bilateral	Diffuse, dull, often pulsating, often induced by a change of weather, lack of sleep, or alcohol abuse. Pain may last for hours or days
Migraine	Usually restricted to one half of the head but may change in side; characterized by periodic attacks, increasing and decreasing. The temporal vessels may be tortuous and prominent.	Periodic, hammering, pounding, boring and deep-seated; occasionally preceded by visual symptoms (scotoma); often combined with nausea and vomiting. Pain lasts many hours. The beginning and end of migraine attack are clearly demarcated.
Erythroprosopalgia (Horton's syndrome, cluster headache, histamine cephalgia)	Strictly unilateral, affects the temporal region and the eye, pain radiates over the entire half of the head, and scalp is supersensitive	Periodic, intensive, stabbing cirumscribed pain and reddening of the eye, epiphora and nasal discharge, nasal obstruction; mainly affects men, often at night. Lasts 1–2 hours. Can be relieved by nitroglycerine or histamine.

Table 2.7 Continuation

Etiologic Group and Subgroup	Site of Predilection of Pain	Typical Symptoms
Neuralgias		
Trigeminal neuralgia	Unilateral, usually lancinating, extremely intensive attacks, always localized to the same area, mainly the area of distribution of the second division of the maxillary nerve. The trigger zones include the infraorbital foramen, the upper jaw, and the cheek. The ethmoidal nerve may be affected: its trigger zone is the junction of the nasal bone and nasal cartilage. Palpebral and parietal points also occur. The third division of the trigeminal, the mandibular nerve, may be affected. The pressure points include the mental foramen, the lower jaw, and the tongue. The first division of the trigeminal nerve, the ophthalmic nerve, is only rarely affected. The pressure point is then the supraorbital foramen, the forehead, the eye, or the bridge of the nose.	Sudden shooting attacks, tic douloureux, particularly on contact, eating, or speaking, with free intervals. It begins without recognizable cause, and the pain is intensified by external stimuli. There are typical trigger zones. Idiopathic and symptomatic forms should be distinguished. The latter may be due to trauma. The pain lasts less than 1 minute.
Glossopharyngeal neuralgia	Unilateral, localized to the base of the tongue, the tonsil, the hypopharynx, the palate, and the ear. The trigger zone is the hypopharynx.	Lancinating intensive attacks of pain radiating to the ear, caused by eating or speaking. The head is held to the sound side.

Vagus neuralgia	Unilateral pain of the neck, from the ear to the larynx or the sternum. The trigger zone is the thyrohyoid membrane or the greater hyoid cornu.	Drawing pain (see also superior laryngeal nerve).
Auriculotemporal neuralgia	Pre- and periauricular, temporal, deep in the ear.	Burning pain with reddening of the skin, profuse sweating, hyperesthesia, often induced by chewing and eating warm or hot food. Occasionally it is due to parotid disease, and may also be caused by occlusal defects.
Nasociliary neuralgia; pterygopalatine ganglion neuralgia (Charlin's syndrome)	Medial canthus, nasal bridge. The trigger zone is the inner canthus. The eye symptoms are prominent.	Periodic, usually not persistent pain, reddening of the forehead, swelling of the nasal mucosa, epiphora, conjunctivitis, unilateral sniffling. Abolished by anesthesia of the ciliary nerve.
Sluder's neuralgia (lower half headache; pterygopalatine ganglion neuralgia)	Nasal roof, or orbital cavity, root of the nose, upper jaw, and possibly teeth, radiating to the temporal area and the mastoid. The nasal symptoms are prominent.	Continuous or episodic severe pain especially at night, often combined with sneezing attacks and unilateral sniffles. Mainly occurs in women, can be relieved by anesthesia of the pterygopalatine ganglion.
Hunt's neuralgia Geniculate ganglion neuralgia	Preauricular and in the meatus and roof of the palate. Paroxysms deep in the ear.	Periodic, boring pain, abnormal sense of taste, occasionally facial paralysis, often combined with herpes zoster oticus
Facial Pain of Dental Origin		
Pulpitis	Localized to the affected tooth and the surrounding tissue, radiating to the ear	Boring, thumping pain, often becomes intolerable under stimulation, often nocturnal

Table 2.7 Continuation

Etiologic Group and Subgroup	Site of Predilection of Pain	Typical Symptoms
Unerupted teeth	Pain on pressure on the posterior molars	Intermittent pain, particularly on chewing, trismus
Periodontitis and parulis	Deep pain around the affected tooth, irradiating to the ear	Agonizing, intensive persistent pain induced by thermal stimuli and chewing
Inflammation of the jaw	Localized around the site of the dental infection	Very severe, persistent pain, soft tissue swelling, and possibly trismus
Mandibular facial pain		
Osteomyelitis	Diffuse irradiating to both sides of the head	Severe and boring pain
Arthritis and arthrosis in the mandible, tempo-romandibular joint syndrome, Costen's syndrome	Temporomandibular joint, irradiating to the ear, sensitivity to pressure over the temporomandibular joint	Stabbing or pressing pain on movement of the jaw; malocclusion
Pain in The Head and Face Due to Eye Disease		
Keratitis	Pain localized to the anterior part of the eye	Persistent pain as long as a corneal ulcer or foreign body is present. Can be interrupted by corneal anesthesia.
Disorders of accommodation and refraction	In or behind the eye, often irradiating to the temple	Drawing, pressing, dull pain. Headache on reading for long periods.
Muscular asthenopia	Orbit and periorbital tissues	Feeling of tension, pressure, may have a migrainous character

Iridocyclitis	Eye, radiating to the forehead and temple, often also to the occiput	Feeling of pressure; dull, boring pain within the eye; photophobia
Neuritis of the optic nerve	Deep in the orbit	Boring, tearing, or dull pain; increasing loss of vision; trigeminal nerve also occasionally involved
Acute glaucoma	Radiating from the eye to the forehead, the temple, the cheek, the upper jaw, the teeth, or the occiput. Projection of pain in or behind the eye.	Pain occurs suddenly, pressure; also tension. Hard tense bulb, ciliary injection.
Chronic glaucoma	In and over the eyes	Continuous by changing dull pain; also headache
Pharyngeal Headache		
Acute tonsillitis and peritonsillar abscess	Diffuse pain in the oropharynx	Pressure, dysphagia
Retropharyngeal abscess	The nape, radiating to the occiput	Oppressive pain, dysphagia
Styloid process syndrome	Nasopharynx radiating to the ear	Fluctuating, may be brought on by movements of the head; sensitivity to pressure on the tonsillar bed
Tumors of the oro- and hypopharynx	Depends on site of the tumor	Persistent pain
Headache of Vertebral Origin		
Cervical spondylosis, whiplash injury, myalgia, tension headache	Occipital, may be restricted to one half of the head, irradiates to the top of the skull, possibly pains in the arm also. The site may vary.	Occipital trigger zone (greater and lesser occipital nerve); often brought on after persistent unfavorable position of the head. Begins and ends gradually, affects the „helmet" area.
Cervical migraine	Episodic, restricted to half the head	Nausea, vertigo, and tinnitus

Table 2.7 Continuation

Etiological Group and Subgroup	Site of Predilection of Pain	Typical Symptoms
Otogenic Headache		
Otitis externa and meatal furuncle	Meatus, preauricular, temporomandibular joint, often radiating to the temple and occiput	Severe stabbing pains, pain on pressure on the tragus
Herpes zoster oticus	Meatus, preauricular, temporomandibular joint, often radiating to the temple and occiput	Severe stabbing pains, with vesicles in the meatus and on the auricle
Acute otitis media	Deep in the ear, irradiating to the temple	Stabbing, pounding pain, worse at night, pulsating tinnitus
Mastoiditis	Mainly retroauricular, mastoid process	Pounding pain, sensitivity to pressure on the mastoid process
Cholesteatoma	Lateral skull and occipital region	Dull pain, usually not very severe
Infection of the petrous pyramid	Apical headache, unilateral headache, projected within the head	Dull pain, Gradenigo's syndrome with abducens paralysis and trigeminal neuralgia
Tumors of the ear and temple bone	Depends on the site of the tumor	Persistent pain, becoming almost intolerable when the dura is involved
Otalgia		
Neuralgias of the facial and glossopharyngeal nerves, the vagus nerve and its auricular branch	Site depends on the nerve involved. Pain arises deep in the head or neck, irradiates to the ear.	Pain is usually sudden and stabbing.

Superior laryngeal nerve	Stabbing paroxysmal pains on the lateral part of the neck.	There is sensitivity to pressure on the thyrohyoid membrane, triggered by swallowing, coughing, and yawning.
Great auricular nerve, and trigeminal nerve	The pain radiates to the ear.	
Intracranial Causes		
Cerebral infarct and intracerebral bleeding	Unilateral headache	Sudden pain, possibly with vomiting, and focal symptoms
Subarachnoid hemorrhage	Diffuse, seldom unilateral	Sudden pain, possible disturbances of consciousness, vomiting, meningismus, focal symptoms
Inflammatory intracranial diseases, e.g. Meningitis, encephalitis	Diffuse	Meningismus and possibly focal symptoms
Cerebral tumor, subdural hematoma, brain abscess	Diffuse, seldom localized	Deep boring pain, signs of increased intra-cranial pressure, papilledema, focal symptoms, and possibly vomiting
Intermittent obstruction of CSF drainage	Diffuse, possibly unilateral	Sudden pains, possibly with change in position, accompanied by vomiting and confusion
CSF hypotension	Diffuse	Pain often occurs on sitting or standing, and disappears when lying down or on pressure on the internal jugular vein

Table 2.7 Continuation

Etiologic Group and Subgroup	Site of Predilection of Pain	Typical Symptoms
Other causes		
Hypertension	Diffuse	Maximum in the morning and on waking
Hypertensive crises	Diffuse	Episodic, possibly vomiting, confusion
Hypotension	Diffuse	Comes on after standing up quickly, with giddiness, vertigo
Temporal arteritis	The temple on one or often both sides	Temporal artery is painful to pressure. Usually occurs in old patients. Danger of involvement of the optic nerve
Toxins and drugs	Diffuse	Depends on the cause
Febrile infections	Diffuse	Depends on the type of infection
Preuremia	Diffuse	Disturbances of vision, loss of appetite, attacks of vomiting, itching of the skin, thirst
Psychogenic headache	Variable, usually irradiating, often bilateral	Mental stress

Differential diagnosis. The different causes of pain in the head and face are summarized in Table 2.7.

Basic Principles of Conservative Treatment of Sinusitis

1. *Acute sinusitis*
   Decongestant nose drops are given several times a day, particularly to decongest the sinus ostia. Cotton pledgets soaked in vasoconstricting agents may be introduced.

Local applications of heat or microwaves, etc. (see p. 223), are used. Cold applications may be tried if heat is not tolerated.

In the early phases of the disease hot packs, hot baths, etc., often abort the attack. Bed rest may be necessary if the patient feels unwell.

The choice of antibiotics should be dictated if possible by culture and sensitivity tests. The procedures described in the paragraph on "Subacute sinusitis" below should be used for a fulminating infection.

2. *Subacute sinusitis*
   If improvement does not occur within a week by the above measures, the sinus should be punctured and washed out (see p. 199). A topically active antibiotic may be instilled depending on the result of sensitivity tests. Systemic antibiotics may also be prescribed depending on the course of the infection. All the measures decribed in the paragraph on "acute sinusitis" above should also be applied.

3. *Chronic sinusitis*
   A course of sinus lavages should be tried, possibly using an indwelling catheter (see p. 199) especially in children. Antibiotic instillation may be used on occasion. Operation should be advised if the disease has not resolved after six to ten lavages. If there is an allergic component the measures described in paragraphs (1) to (3) above should be combined with antiallergic treatment, i. e., tests, hyposensitization, and local or general steroids. Spa treatment may also be prescribed.

Details of Disease of the Individual Sinuses

Maxillary Sinus

Symptoms of acute maxillary sinusitis. These include acute pain in the central part of the face and the face on the same side, hyperesthesia of the facial skin, but occasionally only a feeling of pressure or fullness. Sensitivity to tapping over the cheek, swelling of the turbinates on the same side, and a stream of pus in the middle meatus and on the floor of the nose are other features.

Symptoms of chronic maxillary sinusitis. Pain is often slight, and there is often only a feeling of pressure. Symptoms also include chronic nasal obstruction, mucoid or purulent secretion, and neuralgias in the distribution of the infraorbital nerve, disorders of smell including cacosmia, nasal

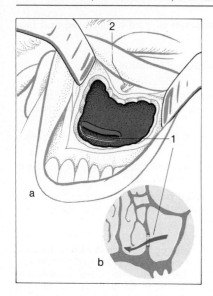

Fig. 2.**30a** and **b**   Radical antrostomy. **(a)** View of the open sinus with a window into the inferior meatus (1) and the infraorbital nerve (2). **(b)** Position of the window between the maxillary sinus and the inferior meatus.

fetor, chronic rhinitis, and hypertrophic turbinates, streams of secretion, and possibly, polyps.

Treatment

For *conservative* treatment, see p. 237. Lavage is described on p. 199.

Surgical treatment is by Caldwell-Luc radical antrostomy (Fig. 2.**30a** and **b**).

Principle. Local or general endotracheal anesthesia is used. Access is obtained via the oral cavity. The soft tissues of the cheek are elevated from the canine fossa, and a window is created in the anterior wall of the antrum. The diseased antral mucosa is removed, and a large window is created in the lateral nasal wall leading from the antrum into the inferior meatus.

An intranasal antrostomy may also be performed.

Principle. This is a palliative procedure for recurrent catarrhal maxillary sinusitis. Local or general anesthesia is used. A large window is created between the inferior meatus and the antral cavity, with the physician working from the nasal cavity.

Ethmoid Sinuses

Symptoms of acute ethmoiditis. These often include a feeling of pressure or fullness between the eyes, at the root of the nose, or in the temporal area. Marked pain is unusual. Symptoms also include disorders of smell, nasal

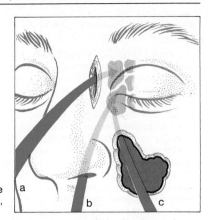

Fig. 2.**31a–c** Surgical access to the ethmoid. **(a)** External, **(b)** transnasal, **(c)** transmaxillary.

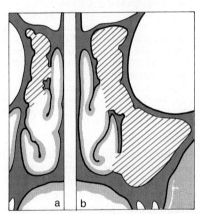

Fig. 2.**32a** and **b** Condition after ethmoidectomy. **(a)** Intranasal ethmoidectomy, **(b)** transmaxillary ethmoidectomy.

obstruction, increased secretion, hypertrophy of the turbinates, particularly the middle turbinate of the diseased side, and a stream of pus from the central or superior meatus.

Symptoms of chronic ethmoiditis. The diagnosis is often difficult since the symptoms are often atypical. They include chronic unilateral nasal discharge and fatigue. A globus sensation may also be caused. Symptoms also include postnasal drip, mucosal swelling in the middle meatus, nasal polyps, and hyposmia or anosmia. The *anterior* ethmoid sinuses especially are often a concealed focus of infection and require tomography and endoscopy for diagnosis.

Treatment. Conservative treatment is described on p. 237.

Surgical treatment. Three routes of access. All may be carried out under local or general anesthesia.

1. Intranasal (Figs. 2.**31b** and 2.**32a**). The middle turbinate is carefully displaced medially. A prior submucosal resection of the septum may be necessary to provide access. The ethmoid complex is entered lateral to the middle turbinate, and the ethmoid cells are cleared piecemeal with forceps. The advantages of this method are that there is no external scar and that the maxillary antrum remains intact. The disadvantage is the narrow operative field so that vision is often restricted, leading sometimes to complications such as injury to the anterior cranial fossa or to the orbital contents. The risk of complications is greater than with routes of access described in paragraphs (2) and (3) below.

2. Transmaxillary (see Figs. 2.**31c**, 2.**32b**). Access is gained to the maxillary antrum by a Caldwell-Luc approach (see p. 238). The ethmoid complex is opened via this incision, and the diseased mucosa is cleared completely. The advantage of this procedure is good access and a satisfactory view of the ethmoids. The disadvantage is that the antrum must be opened, but this is often necessary in any case for a simultaneous maxillary sinusitis.

3. External approach (see Fig. 2.**31a**). A curved incision is made in the medial canthus. A window is then made in the bony nasal pyramid through which the ethmoid cells are cleared. The advantage of this procedure is that it gives the best view of the ethmoid sinus, and it is possible to work tangential to the bony base of the skull which is well exposed. The disadvantage is an external scar on the lateral part of the nose.

4. Conservative endonasal microsurgery is also possible if it is likely that resolution can be obtained by dealing with minor mechanical obstructions such as mucosal prolapse.

Frontal Sinus

Symptoms of acute frontal sinusitis. These include severe pain in the forehead and head, sensitivity to pressure or tapping on the forehead and on the sites of exit of the supraorbital nerve, and a stream of secretions or pus on the anterior part of the middle meatus. The mucosa of the middle meatus is often glazed, swollen, and red.

Symptoms of chronic frontal sinusitis. Here a mild feeling of pressure in the forehead, sensitivity of the supraorbital nerve to pressure, and chronic unilateral nasal discharge are found. Hyposmia and cacosmia are also possible. Large frontal sinuses are more often chronically infected than small ones. Polypi form relatively often in a diseased frontal sinus, but rarely extend into the nasal cavity.

Treatment

Conservative treatment is described on p. 237.

Surgical treatment. All frontal sinus operations may be carried out under local or general endotracheal anesthesia.

The principle of *Beck's trephine* is shown in Figure 2.**22a–d** and described on p. 201. A burr hole is made in the anterior wall of the sinus in the supraorbital region. A short blunt cannula is introduced through which the cavity of the frontal sinus may be aspirated, irrigated, and filled with antibiotics. The cannula should not be retained for more than 8 days because of the foreign body reaction of the sinus mucosa.

Principle of the Various Frontal Sinus Operations

1. *Jansen-Ritter's method.* A curved incision is made near the medial canthus and is extended into the eyebrow. A window is created in the floor of the frontal sinus, and the mucosa is cleared completely from the sinus [Fig. 2.**33a** (II)]. Next, wide drainage is created into the nasal cavity. A permanent communication between the nose and the frontal sinus is secured by a Uffenorde's mucosal flap or a large synthetic stent for at least 8 days. The advantage of this procedure is a cosmetically acceptable external incision. The disadvantage is that the procedure can only be used for relatively small frontal sinuses. The procedure is not suitable for dealing with trauma to the anterior base of the skull.

2. *Killian's method.* Access is obtained as in method (1) above. In addition, a window is created in the anterior wall of the frontal sinus with retention of the bony orbital arch to preserve the profile [see Fig. 2.**33a** (III)]. The operation then proceeds as in paragraph (1) above. This procedure is indicated for very large frontal sinuses since it guarantees access to all the loculi of the sinuses, and thus allows removal of all parts of the mucosa. The contour of the forehead is preserved.

3. *Riedel's method* [see Fig. 2.**33a** (IV)]. Access is obtained by method (1) above. The floor and anterior wall of the frontal sinus are removed, and the operation continues as in paragraph (1) above. The advantage of this procedure is that it guarantees clearance of the sinus and postoperative obliteration of the frontal sinus area. The disadvantage is the cosmetic deformity of the face due to sinking in of the forehead. Later correction is then necessary using a synthetic implant.

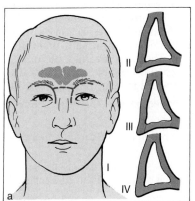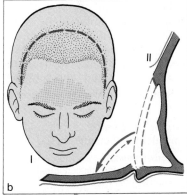

Fig. 2.**33a** and **b**   **a.** Incision (I): principle of a frontal sinus operation as described by Jansen-Ritter (II), by Killian (III), and by Riedel (IV). **b.** Osteoplastic frontal operation. Incision (I) and temporary osteoplastic flap (II).

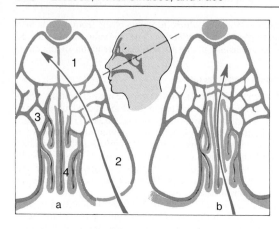

Fig. 2.**34a** and **b**   Sphenoid sinus operations. **(a)** Transmaxillary procedure, **(b)** transseptal procedure. 1 Sphenoid sinus, 2 maxillary sinus, 3 ethmoid sinus, 4 nasal cavity.

4. *Osteoplastic method* (see Fig. 2.**33b**). A curved incision is made within the hairline. The borders of the frontal sinus are cut on three sides, a bone flap is turned forward, and the diseased mucosa is removed. Trauma to the anterior base of the skull can also be dealt with by this approach. The bone flap and the scalp are replaced. The advantage of this method is an excellent view of the frontal sinus and the anterior base of the skull even in a very large sinus. The scar is invisible if the patient has hair. The disadvantage is that it is a relatively large access that is not suitable for small frontal sinuses.

Sphenoid Sinus

Symptoms. There are no characteristic symptoms. The patient may complain of a pain or a feeling of pressure within the skull irradiating to the occiput or the temple (see Fig. 2.**29**). Deep pain in the eyes is also possible. Nasal respiration is usually not obstructed. Secretions usually drain into the nasopharynx causing a postnasal drip. There is a stream of pus on the posterior wall of the pharynx or in the superior meatus. Suspicion of disease of the sphenoid sinus goes halfway toward making the diagnosis.

Treatment. *Conservative treatment* is described on p. 237. Lavage is possible.

Surgical treatment by a sphenoid sinus operation may be carried out under general intubation anesthesia.

1. *Transethmoidal access* (Fig. 2.**34a**). After ethmoid surgery as described on p. 240, the operation is extended into the sphenoid sinus lying immediately adjacent to the posterior ethmoid cells.
2. *Transseptal access* (Fig. 2.**34b**). An incision is made in the nasal septum. The posterior end of the nasal septum anchored in the anterior wall of the sphenoid (the rostrum) is sought. The bone of the septum and the anterior wall of the sphenoid sinus is removed. The sphenoid sinus is cleared and packed via the nasal cavity.

Both routes may also be used for transnasal access to the pituitary. The transethmoidal route is used more often.

Specific Types of Sinusitis

Pansinusitis

The symptoms are those of disease of the various sinuses combined, and may be bilateral. The diagnosis can often only be confirmed by radiography.

Treatment. This should be conservative in the acute phase. If this is not successful, if the disease has already had a prolonged course, or if there are severe symptoms, an appropriate combination of the operations described above should be carried out on the affected sinuses, if necessary on both sides.

Sinusitis in Children

The symptoms may be the same as in adults, but symptoms are often slight (occult or latent sinusitis), and the inflammation is chronic catarrhal in type. Hyperplasia of the adenoids is often responsible. Ethmoiditis may even occur shortly after birth. Maxillary sinusitis is very rare in infants but increases in frequency in children over the age of 4 years. Infection of the frontal and sphenoid sinuses does not usually begin until the 5th to 12th year of life. Occult chronic sinusitis in children is most common between the ages of 7 and 12 years and is often responsible for secondary diseases of the bronchi and lungs, developmental disorders, unexplained fever, and disorders of the stomach, intestine, and kidneys. Differentiation is required from cystic fibrosis (see p. 244).

Symptoms. These include dry cough, sniffles, chronic nasal catarrh, recurrent colds, loss of appetite, and failure to thrive. Radiography is required for diagnosis.

Treatment. Conservative treatment is described on p. 237.

Special treatment includes *adenoidectomy,* infrared, or microwave and possibly a retained irrigation catheter. A fine silicone tube is introduced into the lumen of the sinus via a thick cannula. After removal of the cannula, the silicone tube remains with its end in the sinus. The other end is fixed to the cheek and is then available for attachment to a syringe. Other forms of treatment include building up the resistance and antrostomy (see p. 238).

Extensive surgery should be avoided if at all possible.

Pathophysiologic Relationships Between the Sinuses and the Rest of the Body

1. *The nasal sinuses and the bronchial system (sinobronchial syndrome).* Common membership of the functional airway system requires that the nervous and

humoral control of all parts of the system work in harmony. Reactions at each site may have repercussions on other parts of the system. This may be descending (rhinobronchial) or ascending (bronchorhinologic).

2. *Mucoviscidosis, cystic fibrosis,* is the most frequent congenital disorder of children. The function of the exocrine glands is abnormal, causing a constant increase of chloride and sodium in the sweat and saliva, and an abnormal tough secretion. The main symptoms are pulmonary (progressive bronchial obstruction) and abdominal due to deficiency of pancreatic enzymes, rectal prolapse, and cirrhosis. Nasal manifestations include sinusitis and polypi of the nose and sinuses.

3. *Kartagener's triad* is a congenital disease consisting of bronchiectasis, situs inversus (dextrocardia), and nasal sinus disorders (sinusitis and polypi). Genetic defects of the cilia, immotile cilia syndrome, are also observed.

Mucoceles and Cyst

Mucoceles or pyoceles are caused by obstruction of the drainage of a sinus and by resulting retention of secretion in the sinus. The frontal, ethmoid, sphenoid, and maxillary sinuses are affected, in decreasing order of frequency. The cause may be inflammation, trauma, surgery, or tumor. In the absence of spontaneous drainage, the increasing internal pressure gradually converts the bony sinus wall into a fibrous capsule that extends in the direction of least resistance such as the floor of the frontal sinus or the lamina papyracea (see Color Plate **15a**).

Main symptoms include displacement of the orbit externally or inferiorly and limitation of movement of the bulb leading to disorders of vision and double vision. Optic atrophy and amaurosis can occur in extreme cases. Mucoceles of the posterior sinuses can cause an orbital apex syndrome (see p. 247) or simulate a hypophyseal or cerebral tumor. Lesions arising in the maxillary sinus cause increasing distension of the cheek, but eye symptoms are unusual.

Diagnosis. This is by radiography including tomography.

Differential diagnosis. Early inflammatory complications, malignancy, and meningocele must be considered.

Treatment. Clearance of the affected sinus and creation of a wide communication with the nasal cavity must be attained.

Cysts

These arise principally from the maxillary sinus and may be *dental* radicular (arising from a tooth root) or *follicular* (arising from a displaced tooth germ). They produce typical radiologic findings (Fig. 2.**35a** and **b**).

Treatment. This is either by removal of the cyst via the antral cavity or from the mouth by an oral surgeon for radicular cysts.

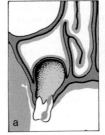
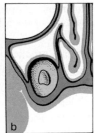

Fig. 2.**35a** and **b** Dental maxillary cysts. **(a)** Radicular, **(b)** follicular.

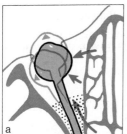
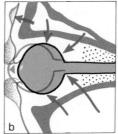
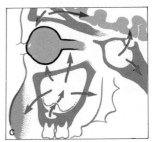

Fig. 2.**36a–c** Inflammatory complications of sinusitis. **a.** Horizontal section. Rupture from the ethmoid cells into the orbit with displacement of the bulb. **b.** Sagittal section. Rupture from the frontal cavity or the maxillary sinus into the orbit, to the lids, and to the forehead. **c.** Sagittal section showing directions of rupture from the maxillary sinus to the soft tissues of the cheek and to the orbit; extension from the teeth to the maxillary sinus; extension from the frontal sinus to the orbit and the frontal lobe; and extension from the sphenoid sinus into the cranial cavity and to the base of the skull. Dotted area shows region of the orbital apex.

Complications of Sinus Infections

Extension to the External Soft Tissues (see Color Plates **13b, 14c, 15b**)

This may be due to a frontal sinusitis which causes swelling of the soft tissues of the forehead or the upper eyelid, to an ethmoiditis which causes swelling of the eyelids, especially the lower, or to a maxillary sinusitis which causes swelling of the cheek and edema of the lower eyelid. The cause is usually an *acute* sinusitis or an *acute* exacerbation of a chronic sinusitis. The typical pathways of extension are shown in Figure 2.**36a–c**. The soft tissues over the point of rupture show a boggy swelling which is usually red and painful on pressure.

Diagnosis. This rests on the history, the clinical findings, and radiography.

Treatment. Appropriate antibiotic therapy and if indicated, operative drainage of the affected sinus must be carried out.

Orbital Complications (see Color Plates **13a, c, 14a**)

These are relatively common and very serious. The ethmoid and frontal sinuses are usually the site of origin, and the maxillary only rarely. The following degrees of severity may be distinguished (Fig. 2.**37**):

- A prodromal stage of orbital edema
- Orbital periostitis (see Fig. 2.**37a**)
- Subperiosteal abscess (see Fig. 2.**37b**)
- Orbital phlegmon (see Fig. 2.**37c**).

Orbital edema may occur as collateral concomitant lid swelling or as *inflammatory* edema and is more common in children than adults.

Symptoms. The eyelids are boggy, glazed, and swollen. Complete resolution is possible with conservative treatment of the sinuses (see p. 237), and antibiotics particularly in children.

Orbital Periostitis

This is the first destructive stage of an orbital complication due to rupture of the pus through the bony orbital wall (see Fig. 2.**37a**).

Symptoms. These include swelling of the lids and circumscribed pain on pressure on the bone around the site of rupture, which is usually mostly in the area of the medial canthus.

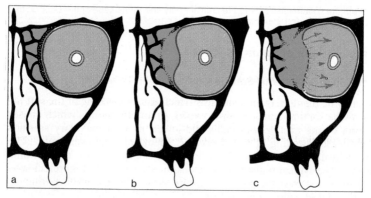

Fig. 2.**37a–c**   Orbital complications arising from the ethmoids. **(a)** Orbital periostitis; **(b)** subperiosteal abscess; **(c)** orbital phlegmon.

Treatment. Surgery to the sinus of origin is mandatory, otherwise a subperiosteal abscess will form.

Subperiosteal Abscess with Periorbital Edema (see Figs. 2.**36** and 2.**37b**)

Symptoms. Swelling of the lids, pain, displacement of the bulb laterally and inferiorly are noted. Rarely protrusion of the bulb may be present, and even more rarely enophthalmos depending on the point of rupture. Chemosis is also possible, and fever may occur in children. If the *abscess* spreads to the *eyelid* there is pain, redness, and a tight swelling of the eyelid. The typical sites of rupture are shown in Figure 2.**36a, b.**

Treatment. Immediate surgical drainage of the sinus of origin and drainage of the subperiosteal abscess are indicated.

Orbital Phlegmon (see Fig. 2.**37c**; Color Plates **13c** and **14a**)

An orbital phlegmon forms the most extreme and immediate danger for the eye.

Symptoms. These include marked edema and discoloration of the lids, chemosis, marked protrusion of the bulb, and rapid worsening of vision, severe pain which increases on pressure on the bulb or movement of the eye, and limitation of movement of the eye due to damage to the ocular muscles and their nerves. Later features include complete paralysis of the orbit, congestion of the retinal veins, papilledema, and possibly panophthalmitis. Secondary intracranial extension to the cavernous sinus is possible.

Treatment. Immediate wide exposure of the sinus of origin and *immediate* ophthalmologic consultation are necessary.

Differential diagnosis. This depends on radiography, computed tomography, and ophthalmologic findings. Malignancy of the orbit, mucoceles, benign tumors (e. g., osteoma), inflammation of the lacrimal drainage system, cavernous sinus thrombosis, noninflammatory orbital diseases, and erysipelas must be excluded.

The **orbital apex syndrome** (see Fig. 2.**36a–c**) is due to a lesion of the orbital apex affecting the nerves and vessels traversing the optic foramen and the superior orbital fissure. The main symptoms are loss of vision, ptosis, double vision, severe temporoparietal headache, and exophthalmos due to compression of the IInd, IIIrd, IVth, Vth, and VIth cranial nerves. *Causes* include trauma, neoplasms, and extension of an ethmoidal or sphenoidal sinusitis. *Treatment* is by immediate decompression because of the danger of amaurosis.

Rhinogenic retrobulbar optic neuritis (see Fig. 2.**36a–c**) is due to extension of inflammation of the sphenoid or posterior ethmoid sinuses to the retrobulbar space. It is rare. *Symptoms* are primarily ophthalmologic. *Treatment* is by operative drainage of the appropriate sinus if there is *absolute* evidence of the presence of infection of that sinus.

Malignant exophthalmos due to thyrotoxicosis may be dealt with by a nasal operation (see p. 525). Edema of the soft tissues of the orbit with resulting effects on the circulation and an actual increase in tissue leads to increased intraorbital pressure causing injury to the bulb and the optic nerve. Decompression may be achieved by removing the bony floor of the orbit, the ethmoid cells, and the lamina papyracea with preservation of the infraorbital nerve.

> *Note:* Any unilateral or bilateral loss of vision or oculomotor disorder causing double vision requires thorough rhinologic investigation.

Intracranial Complications

Figure 2.**38** shows the principal pathways of spread of rhinogenous (usually sinus) infections into the intracranial cavity. These may be explained anatomically as follows:

- Direct extension after destruction of the bone by circumscribed osteitis, and necrosis of the bony wall of the sinus, possibly due to trauma
- Extension via osteomyelitis (see p. 251)
- Extension via blood vessels, usually the veins in the bone, which communicate between the sinus and the intracranial cavity
- Extension via the general circulation (hematogenous metastases)

Epidural Abscess

Symptoms. There are no typical symptoms of this disease. Symptoms may include subfebrile temperature, headache and pressure in the head, and exhaustion. Usually there are no signs clearly indicating the local disease. The findings in the cerebrospinal fluid (CSF) are unremarkable. Epidural abscess is often only discovered coincidentally at an operation on the

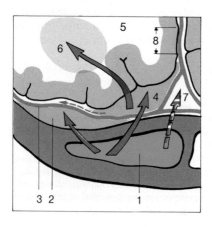

Fig. 2.**38** Genesis of intracranial complications of sinusitis. 1, Frontal sinus with empyema; 2, epidural abscess; 3, dura; 4, subdural abscess with marginal adhesion (8) or with extension as meningitis in the direction shown by the small dashed arrow; 5, brain; 6, abscess; 7, extension to the sagittal sinus.

sinus of origin which demonstrates osteitis or bony necrosis, e.g., of the posterior wall of the frontal sinus.

Supplementary diagnostic procedures. These include radiography of the sinuses, angiography, and CT scans.

Differential diagnosis. This is epidural hematoma.

Treatment. This consists of drainage of the sinus of origin with wide exposure of the inflamed dura until healthy tissue is exposed on all sides and drainage into the nasal cavity.

Subdural Abscess

Symptoms. Again there are no typical symptoms as is indeed the case in epidural abscess. The patient may occasionally complain of headache and increasing signs of meningeal irritation shown by a pleocytosis of the CSF. Gradually the symptoms of meningitis or brain abscess develop such as clouding of the sensorium, neurologic irritation, neurologic signs, convulsions, hemiparesis, etc. The CSF may be normal or show the changes of inflammation, and the CSF pressure may be raised. A meningitis of unfavorable prognosis may occur.

Diagnostic methods. These include radiography of the sinuses, CT scan, neurologic investigation, electroencephalography, and carotid angiography.

Differential diagnosis. This is subdural hematoma in which there is blood in the CSF.

Treatment. Drainage of the sinus of origin, and of the subdural abscess (via the pathway of spread) must be undertaken. High-dose antibiotics are given.

Rhinogenic Brain Abscess

This usually arises from the frontal sinus, and only rarely from the ethmoid sinus. Even rarer is a hematogenous *frontal lobe abscess.*

Symptoms. Frontal lobe abscesses cause relatively few localizing symptoms. Four stages of a rhinogenic frontal lobe abscess may be distinguished: initial, latent, manifest, and terminal. General symptoms, the symptoms of increased intracranial pressure and focal symptoms are usually pronounced. Confirmatory signs include deteriorating general condition, occasionally fever, increasing, boring headache, and sensitivity to pressure on the vault of the skull, nausea, vomiting, slowing of the pulse, papilledema, unilateral anosmia, disordered sensorium, increasing somnolence, decreasing interest in the environment, and loss of concentration, generalized mental slowing, and altered behavior such as inappropriate joking and excessive euphoria, restlessness, coma, and cranial nerve paralysis (particularly of the Ist, IIIrd, and VIth cranial nerves).

Supplementary diagnostic methods. These include radiography of the nasal sinuses, CT scan, carotid angiogram, electroencephalogram (EEG), echoencephalogram, and olfactometry.

Treatment. Therapy depends on the stage of the disease and the size and site of the abscess. The mainstay of treatment of abscesses arising from the nose or sinuses is combined neurosurgery and nasal surgery to excise the abscess accompanied or followed immediately by drainage of the appropriate sinus.

Sinus Thrombosis (see p. 109, analogous)

Cavernous Sinus Thrombosis

Symptoms. These include edema of the upper and lower lid, oculomotor disorders, proptosis, papilledema, increasing loss of vision possibly ending with blindness, chemosis (see Color Plate **14b**), a septic temperature chart with chills, a high continuous or remitting irregular fever, headache, variable pulse rate, and increasing clouding of consciousness. Examination of the CSF shows increased cell count and increased protein content. The generalized symptoms of sepsis, with splenomegaly and a typical blood picture, may also be found.

Pathogenesis. A propagated thrombophlebitis arising from an upper lip or nasal furuncle and spreading via the angular vein, a septal abscess, sphenoiditis with neighboring osteomyelitis, acute osteomyelitis of the frontal bone, orbital phlegmon, or petrositis with extension to the cavernous sinus may all be causes (see Figs. 2.**2** and 2.**36c**).

Differential diagnosis. This includes orbital phlegmon, dental or tonsillar phlegmons and septicemia, otogenic sinus thrombosis, and hematogenous spread (i.e., staphylococcal sepsis).

Treatment. Broad-spectrum antibiotics should be given in *high dosages for a prolonged period* at the earliest suspicion of a thrombophlebitis, if possible determined by culture and sensitivity tests. Treatment also includes bed rest and fluid diet and the use of anticoagulants (Liquemin). In a furuncle of the nose or upper lip, the angular vein should be divided by electrocautery or partially resected, depending on the local findings (see Fig. 2.**2**).

In advanced cases, an attempt may occasionally be made to drain the cavernous sinus surgically.

Prognosis is very bad.

Complications. These include meningitis and septic metastases in the pulmonary and general circulation.

Rhinogenic Meningitis

Symptoms of typical purulent meningitis. High fever, hyperesthesia, photophobia, variable pulse rate, neck stiffness, headache, vomiting, Jacksonian attacks, and symptoms of motor irritability (floccilation) are present. Kernig's, Lasègue's, and Brudzinsky's signs are positive, and later there is opisthotonus and scaphoid abdomen.

The cranial nerves, i.e., IIIrd and IVth, are affected. Examination of the CSF shows high-grade pleocytosis (the normal is up to 12/3 cells/ml), a markedly raised pressure (normal 7 to 12 cm H_2O), increased protein (normal 25 to 40 ml/100 ml), and decreased sugar (normal 40 to 90 mg/100 ml). The organism may also be isolated.

Supplementary diagnostic procedures. These include lumbar or suboccipital puncture, neurologic investigation, and bacteriologic examination of the CSF.

Differential diagnosis. Nonrhinogenic meningitis, e.g., epidemic meningitis, viral meningitis, subarachnoid hemorrhage, and other cerebrospinal diseases must be considered.

Treatment. This consists of immediate surgical drainage of the sinus of origin and exposure and closure of any defects found in the dura. High-dose antibiotics are given, and a lumbar puncture is repeated frequently until the cell count falls below 100 ml.

Bony Complications

Osteomyelitis of the Flat Bones of the Skull (see Color Plate **14c**)

This is a life-threatening disease which *may spread directly* from a frontal sinusitis due to inflammatory disease or trauma, but may also be due to *hematogenous* spread (Fig. 2.**39**).

The course is often fulminating because the diploic of the vault of the skull (spongiosa, medullary space, diploic veins) possesses no anatomic barriers. Thus, infection which has broken through into the diploic spreads like wildfire in all directions, and then breaks out of this layer into the intracranial cavity allowing the development of typical intracranial complications (see p. 248). External rupture to form a subperiosteal abscess is also possible.

Symptoms. Adolescence is the age of predilection. The course can be stormy but it may also be indolent.

Main symptoms. High fever, chills, poor general condition and exhaustion, severe headache, clouding of consciousness, tenderness of the frontal region and the vault of the skull, and a boggy soft tissue swelling over the diseased part of the bone occur. In addition, there may be clear symptoms

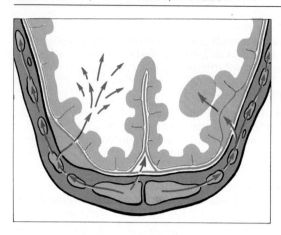

Fig. 2.**39** Genesis of osteomyelitis of the flat bones of the skull. Extension from a frontal sinus empyema to the diploe and marrow spaces of the vault followed by an epidural or subdural abscess, sinus thrombosis (sagittal sinus), diffuse or circumscribed encephalitis, and brain abscess.

of the development of an intracranial complication, over a long or shorter period (see p. 248).

Diagnosis. This rests on the demonstration of frontal sinusitis, radiographs that show typical radiolucency of the bones of the skull, which only appears after the 2nd week, a shift to the left in the blood count, and an increased ESR. Papilledema and abnormal findings in the CSF indicate an intracranial complication.

Differential diagnosis. This includes erysipelas and other septic diseases.

Treatment. High-dose antibiotics are urgently indicated, but are not sufficient alone, and the frontal sinus or the sinus of origin should be drained immediately. The bone of the vault of the skull should be exposed widely with a healthy margin with removal of the external table, decortication, and removal of the diploë, and occasionally the internal table of the vault of the skull. If necessary, surgical management of an already manifest intracranial complication must be carried out.

Osteomyelitis of the Upper Jaw

This condition is not common. Its cause is usually dental disease; more rarely it is due to hematogenous spread, or may originate from the sinuses, i.e., in trauma. It may also arise from bony necrosis after infectious fevers such as typhus, measles, and scarlet fever or from radionecrosis due to radiotherapy.

Symptoms include swelling of the cheek, pain in the face, abscesses pointing into the mouth, the antrum, or externally.

Treatment. Removal of the (dental) cause is indicated. Antibiotics are administered and the diseased bone removed.

Osteomyelitis of the Upper Jaw in Infants

This condition is accompanied by acute swelling of the cheek, signs of local infection, and an abscess pointing either into the mouth or externally.

Cause. Possibly infection of the antral cavity which is still very small in infants.

Treatment. This consists of high-dose antibiotics, and possibly careful drainage from the vestibule of the mouth, taking care not to damage the follicles of the teeth.

The causes of swelling of the face are shown in Table 2.**11**.

Epistaxis

Although the course of this disease is usually harmless, and the cause often banal and non-specific, epistaxis may be a life-threatening disease which is extremely difficult to treat, whose causes may not be remediable, and which may lead to death. Therefor epistaxis should not be regarded as a harmless event either from the diagnostic or therapeutic point of view. The most common *sources of bleeding* are shown in Fig. 2.**9**. Depending on the *cause,* it is possible to distinguish *epistaxis due to local causes* from *symptomatic nosebleeds* with a generalized cause. The most important causes are summarized in Table 2.**8**. Two important points that must be made are:

1. Much the most common source of bleeding (in about 90% of cases) is *Kiesselbach's plexus* (see Fig. 2.9 and Color Plate **11c** and **d**) on the anterior portion of the septum. The mucosa in this area is very fragile and is tightly adherent to the underlying cartilage, and thus offers little resistance to mechanical or functional stress.
2. *A bleeding polyp of the septum* is an alternative source of bleeding which may occasionally be found on the anterior third of the septum. This is a circumscribed dark-red benign angiomatous neoplasm thought to be caused by mechanical irritation.

Diagnosis. Table 2.9 shows the necessary diagnostic steps. Occasionally, it may be very difficult or even impossible to localize the source of bleeding with certainty. Bleeding from the posterior part of the nasal cavity and from the middle and superior meatus (see Fig. 2.9) is not harmless and requires immediate expert investigation and treatment. It may arise from the anterior or posterior ethmoidal artery or the sphenopalatine artery.

Differential diagnosis. This includes bleeding which does not arise in the nose but in which the blood escapes through the nose, e. g., due to tumors of the nasopharynx or the larynx, hemoptysis, bleeding esophageal varices, and bleeding due to injury to the vessels around the base of the skull (e. g., the internal carotid artery) escaping via the sphenoid sinus or the eustachian tube.

Table 2.8 Epistaxis

Local causes of epistaxis

Idiopathic principally this refers to mild recurrent nosebleeds in children and adolescents.

Vascular, microtrauma to Kiesselbach's plexus. This is usually mild, brief and a single occurrence.

Anterior rhinitis sicca. This involves chemical or thermal injury to the nasal mucosa; or septal perforation, frequently involving slight bleeding or blood-stained nasal discharge, often with a feeling of dryness or crusting in the nose.

Environmental influences such as living at high altitudes, reduced air pressure, or drying due to air conditioning may be implicated.

Trauma, e. g., fractures of the nasal bone or the nasal septum, injuries of the facial skeleton or the anterior base of the skull. There is usually severe profuse bleeding as an immediate result of the trauma. The internal carotid artery may be damaged and this may be an immediate life-threatening problem, or there may be an interval before the formation of aneurysm and attacks of bleeding.

Foreign body in the nose or rhinolith. This may cause unilateral mild bleeding and fetor and purulent secretion in the long term.

Bleeding polyp of the septum. This refers to histologically telangiectatic granuloma or hemangioma with a marked tendency to bleed when it is disturbed.

Tumors, particularly malignant tumors of the nose or sinuses. These often cause blood-stained secretion only.

Tumors of the nasopharynx, especially *nasopharyngeal angiofibroma,* may cause massive life-threatening attacks of bleeding.

Causes of Secondary Epistaxis

Infections, especially acute *infectious diseases* such as influenza, measles, typhus, and catarrh may be involved. The epistaxis usually involves slight, short lived bleeding, principally in children and adolescents.

Vascular and circulatory diseases such as arteriosclerosis and hypertension may be present. The bleeding is arterial, often pulsating and spurting. It affects the middle-aged and elderly and tends to recur.

Blood diseases and diseases of coagulation
   Thrombopathy, e. g., thrombocytopenic purpura, Werlhof's disease or idiopathic thrombocytopenic purpura, sickle cell anemia, leukemia, Glanzmann's disease or thromboasthenia and Willebrand-Juergen's constitutional thrombopathy.

Coagulopathy, e. g., hemophilia, Waldenström's disease, prothrombin deficiency or overdosage with anticoagulants, fibrinogen deficiency, and deficiency of vitamins K and C.
Vasopathy, e. g., as scurvy, Möller-Barlow disease or infantile scurvy, and Henoch-Schönlein purpura. The bleeding in this group is mainly a superficial trickle of relatively dark blood.

Uremia and liver cell failure

Endocrine causes, e. g., vicarious menstruation, epistaxis during pregnancy, and pheochromocytoma which causes hypertensive crises due to circulating catecholamine.

Hereditary hemorrhagic telangiectasia with typical mucosal lesions (Osler's disease). This causes recurrent mild to modest, obstinate, and often multifocal bleeding, principally in the anterior and posterior part of the septum.

Table 2.**9** Epistaxis (Diagnostic steps)

1. History

2. Localization of the source of bleeding and determination of its cause
   Anterior: Nose picking, idiopathic epistaxis, rhinitis anterior, infectious diseases
   Posterior or middle: Hypertension, arteriosclerosis, fractures, tumors
   Superficial: Hemorrhagic diatheses, coagulation disorders, Osler's disease

3. Measurement of the blood pressure and assessment of the circulation

4. Analysis of blood coagulation

Possibly:

5. Radiographs of the skull, the nose, and sinuses, and possibly tomograms

6. Examination by an internist to exclude generalized causes (see Table 2.**8**)

Treatment (Table 2.**10**)

General Symptomatic Treatment

- Preserve a calm atmosphere.
- The patient should sit with the upper part of the body tilted forward and the mouth open so that he can spit out the blood and not have to swallow it. The upper part of the body at least should be upright.
- Cold compresses are applied to the nape of the neck and also to the dorsum of the nose.
- Mild pressure is applied to both nasal alae for several minutes.

Table 2.**10**   Treatment of Epistaxis

General measures
  Calming of patient (if necessary with medication)
  The patient should sit up
  Application of cold to the nape of the neck
  Lowering of the blood pressure in hypertension
  Administration of fluid and plasma expanders
  Blood transfusion if the hemoglobin falls below 50%
  Discontinuation of anticoagulants

Local measures
Occlusion of the bleeding source by
  Local application of hemostatic agents such as Privine cotton packing or
  other hemostatic substances such as thrombin, gelatin tampons,
  oxycellulose, and fibrin
  Infiltration of the bleeding area with vasoconstricting agents
  Cautery, galvanocautery, or laser application to a small bleeding point
  Anterior packing or inflatable tampons
  Posterior packing (balloon catheter, Bellocq)

Vascular ligation
Depending on the source of the bleeding and providing that the bleeding
cannot be arrested by any other method the following blood vessels may be
divided:
  Internal maxillary artery
  Anterior and posterior ethmoidal arteries
  External carotid artery

Substitution in bleeding disorders
  Fresh blood transfusions, vitamin C, and systemic hemostatic agents in
  thrombopathies
  Fresh blood transfusion, Cohn fraction, vitamin K for coagulopathy
  ACTH, steroids, calcium, vitamin C, and estrogens for vasopathy

For Osler's disease
  Septal dermoplasty (Saunder's plasty)

Local Procedures

The following may be used for a bleeding point localized to Kiesselbach's plexus.

A. *Cautery*

Technique

1. Privine 1:1,000 is sprayed on the mucosa of the bleeding side of the nose to produce mucosal vasoconstriction.

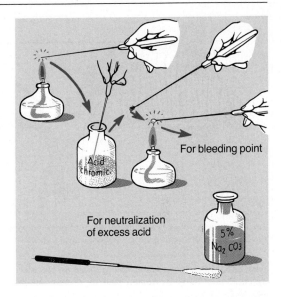

For bleeding point

For neutralization
of excess acid

Acid
Chromic

5%
Na₂ CO3

Fig. 2.**40**   Preparation
of a chromic acid bead.

2. After a 5-min wait, a cotton pledget soaked in pontocaine 1% to 2%, or Xylocaine 1% and Privine, is placed in the anterior nasal cavity and left in place for 5 to 10 min to produce local surface anesthesia and vasoconstriction. During this period the cauterizing material, e.g., a chromic acid bead (Fig. 2.**40**) or 40% to 70% trichloroacetic acid on a cotton applicator, is prepared.
3. After removing the cotton pledget, the bleeding point is touched with the chromic acid pearl until a yellow crust due to superficial necrosis forms. Excess material is neutralized immediately with 5% silver nitrate solution or sodium bicarbonate applied with several cotton pledgets which are changed frequently.

Instead of chromic or trichloroacetic acid, hemostasis may be secured with cold cautery, electrocautery, or laser. The anterior part of the nasal cavity should be packed when cautery does not stop the bleeding.

> *Note:* *Both* sides of the septum should never be cauterized at a similar point at the same sitting because of the danger of septal perforation. Very *fine* cotton tipped applicators should be used, the cauterizing surface should be small and applied to a small area only. A hemostatic wad of cotton saturated with ferrous chloride should never be introduced into the nose because of the danger of severe damage to the mucosa or of a septal perforation.

B. *Anterior Nasal Packing*

Technique. Topical anesthesia of the nasal mucosa is first induced [see section (A) above]. Two to four cm wide strips of ointment-saturated gauze are introduced in layers from above downward or from behind forward into the nasal cavity. The

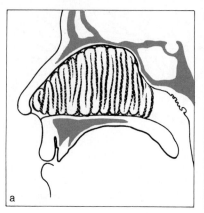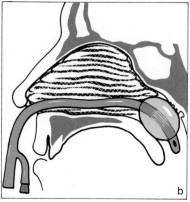

Fig. 2.**41a** and **b**   Nasal packing: **(a)** Anterior nasal packing in vertical layers; **(b)** anterior and posterior packing using horizontal layers and an inflatable balloon.

pack should produce satisfactory pressure on the bleeding source (Fig. 2.**41a** and **b**). As an alternative, *pneumatic* packing with an inflatable balloon may be used.

The following procedures may be required to achieve hemostasis if anterior packing is inadequate for profuse hemorrhage, e. g., after trauma, vascular rupture in hypertension, or if the source of bleeding is concealed and lies far posteriorly.

C. *Posterior Nasal Packing*

This procedure is very painful and requires, if possible, general anesthesia and intubation, or at least, a very good topical anesthesia.

Principle. A gauze or sponge pack with a stay suture is used to close off the choana and is fixed in the nasopharynx to prevent the escape of blood from the nose into the nasopharynx. Anterior packing is then performed. The original packing described by Bellocq placed a considerable burden on the patient, required skill on the part of the surgeon, as well as satisfactory anesthesia. The posterior part of the nasal cavity may be closed off from the nasopharynx more simply and more efficiently by a catheter with an inflatable cuff (see Fig. 2.**41b**).

Technique. A Foley catheter is passed into the nasopharynx down the side of the nose that is bleeding, under general anesthesia or, if necessary, with topical anesthesia. Its cuff is then filled with water until the nasopharynx is occluded securely and the flow of blood posteriorly has been stopped. The anterior part of the nose then is packed, and the end of the catheter coming out of the nose is fixed.

An inflatable catheter of this type should always be available in every clinic and ENT practice.

A severe septal deviation or prominent spur may necessitate surgical correction of the septum.

Note: A catheter left within the nose or a stay suture attached to a postnasal pack must not exert pressure on the nasal alae or the columella. Necrosis can occur rapidly, causing scars of the tip of the nose and the anterior part of the nasal cavity. A posterior nasal pack should not be left in for longer than necessary and never for more than 5 to 7 days. Antibiotic cover should be given while the packing is in place because of the danger of sinusitis or otitis media since the pharyngeal ostium of the eustachian tube is blocked if the packing is in the correct position.

D. *Vascular Ligation*

This procedure must be carried out for uncontrolled life-threatening epistaxis if the methods described above have not been effective. Depending on the source of the bleeding, it may be necessary to ligate the internal maxillary artery in the pterygopalatine fossa (Fig. 2.**42c**), the anterior and

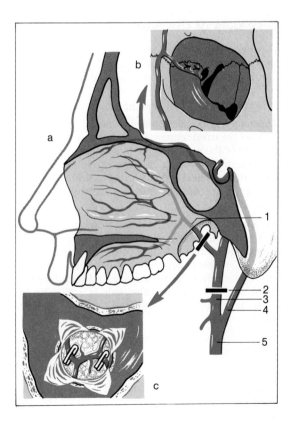

Fig. 2.**42a–c** Sites for ligation in severe epistaxis. **a.** Overview, 1, A. internal maxillaris; 2, ligation of the external carotid artery; 3, external carotid artery; 4, internal carotid artery; 5, common carotid artery. **b.** Ligation of the ethmoidal arteries. **c.** Ligation of the internal maxillary artery in the pterygopalatine fossa.

posterior ethmoidal arteries (see Fig. 2.**42b**), or the external carotid artery at the anterior border of the sternocleidomastoid muscle above the origin of the lingual artery (see Fig. 2.**42a**).

E. *General Therapeutic Measures for Severe Nosebleeds*

These measures are summarized in Table 2.**10**.

F. *Hereditary Telangiectasia* (Rendu-Osler's disease) (see Color Plate **16c** and **d**)

Local procedures to achieve hemostasis and blood replacement may be inadequate in the long term because of the multiple bleeding points and a chronic course in severe cases. The diseased nasal mucosa containing abnormal fragile blood vessels is then removed and replaced by split skin graft (Saunder's dermoplasty).

Diseases of the Septum

Few people have a perfectly straight and perpendicular nasal septum. The septum usually shows slight bends and spurs. Provided that these do not hinder nasal respiration, they are not to be regarded as abnormal.

Deviation of the Nasal Septum

This may first be *developmental* due to unequal growth of the cartilage and bone of the nasal septum; second, it may be *traumatic* due to facial fracture, fracture of the nose or septum, or possibly due to injury at birth. The parts of the septum are then either too large for the given skeletal space, or are dislocated and heal in an incorrect position. In these cases deviations, spurs, and crests are caused which reduce the patency of the nasal cavity (see Color Plate **11e**).

Symptoms. These include nasal obstruction, which is often unilateral and may be intermittent, hyposmia or anosmia, and headaches which can vary depending on the condition of the nasal cavity. A subluxation of the septum, i. e., displacement of the ventral edge of the septum and obstruction of the nasal introitus to one side and septal deviation with obstruction of the nasal cavity on the other side is especially likely after *trauma*. This combination of factors can lead to complete bilateral obstruction of the nasal cavity (Fig. 2.**43a**).

Tension septum. The septum is too large for the space available so that it is then under tension. This can cause nasal obstruction and headaches; it can also distort the profile of the nose (e.g. humped).

Diagnosis. The diagnosis is based on rhinoscopy and possibly rhinomanometry.

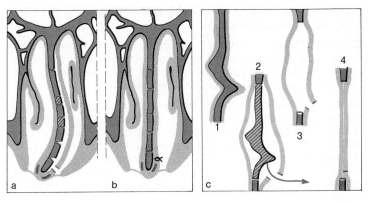

Fig. 2.**43a–c** Operations on the nasal septum. **a.** Septal deviation with incisions and segmental resection. **b.** Final condition. **c.** Submucosal septal resection by Killian's method: 1, septum with spurs; 2, submucosal dissection of the cartilaginous bony septum and partial removal; 3, mucosal pocket after septal resection; 4, final condition with mucosal layers replaced.

Treatment is by *surgery*.

1. *Septoplasty*. Figure 2.**43a** and **b** shows the principles. It is possible to remove all parts of the septum and to reimplant them if necessary after shifting and remodeling. However, the function of the nasal cavity can often only be restored satisfactorily by simultaneous correction of the external nasal pyramid (see section on *septorhinoplasty*, p. 282).

2. *Killian's submucous resection of the septum* (see Fig. 2.**43c**). After creating a mucosal tunnel, all deviated cartilaginous and bony parts of the nasal septum may be removed, straightened, and reimplanted if necessary.

Complications of (1) and (2) above include septal perforations (see below). If too much cartilage is resected, the cartilaginous part of the nose may fall in, causing an anterior or inferior saddle, or duckbill nose (see pp. 262, 283). In both cases reconstructive procedures are available and indicated.

Septal Hematoma and Septal Abscess (see Color Plate **11b**)

These are usually caused by trauma, and usually occur in children. Blunt nasal trauma with a sheering effect leads to elevation of the mucoperiosteum from its cartilaginous or bony attachment. A hematoma forms in the newly created perichondrial-periosteal space, and it may often be bilateral. Infection leads to a septal abscess.

Symptoms. Include increasing nasal obstruction, tenderness, and pain are symptomatic. If an abscess forms, local pain increases, and the patient complains of headaches, fever, pain on pressure, and reddening of the bridge of the nose. In the long term, the cartilaginous part of the nose undergoes necrosis and sinks in.

Diagnosis. The history reveals an incident of trauma. Examination shows that the hematoma is usually located to the most anterior part of the septum. It also shows a swelling of the septum which occludes the lumen of both nostrils and is cystic when palpated with a probe.

Treatment. Wide incision and drainage of the hematoma is carried out, followed by packing of the nostrils to encourage the mucoperichondrium and the mucoperiosteum to readhere. If infection is found, the incision must be held open by a drain to prevent cartilaginous necrosis leading to deformity of the external nose or septal thickening due to fibrosis. Antibiotic cover is given. If necrosis occurs, the nonviable fragments are removed, and it may be necessary to implant preserved cartilage to support the nose.

Complications. If an infection is not drained, it may extend to the meninges or the cavernous sinus.

Septal Perforation

This condition is usually the result of trauma, nasal operation, rhinitis sicca anterior, frequent nose picking, cocaine sniffing, infection (lupus, syphilis, etc.), or occupational injury.

Symptoms. These include crusting, fetor (possible but rare), slight recurrent nosebleeds, and a whistling noise on inspiration and expiration if the perforation is small. Large perforations lying posteriorly may cause no symptoms.

Treatment. *Surgical* treatment. The perforation is closed by mucosal transposition or bridge flaps or by free fascial grafts.

Conservative treatment. The local symptoms of crusting and epistaxis are alleviated by daily nasal douches and mild ointments. An attempt may be made to close the perforation with a collarstud obturator made from soft plastic. However, an obturator is a foreign body, and a plastic reconstruction is therefore preferred.

Saddlenose of the Cartilaginous Part of the Nose (Duckbill)

This condition results from trauma, an incorrectly executed nasal operation, or a septal abscess, but it may also be congenital. The septal cartilage is partially or completely absent.

Symptoms. The profile of the nose is typical (Fig. 2.**56b**), and the patient may also complain of nasal obstruction because of the absent support for the nasal introitus.

Treatment. Rhinoplasty is performed with implantation of a strut (Fig. 2.**59a** and **b**).

Trauma to the Nose, Paranasal Sinuses, and Facial Skeleton

Trauma to the Nose

Symptoms. These include a visible deformity, lateral dislocation or depression of the nasal pyramid, hematoma of the soft tissues, orbital hematoma, swelling of the overlying soft tissue, pain on pressure on the nasal pyramid, possibly headaches, epistaxis, nasal obstruction, and disorders of smell.

Pathogenesis. This is circumscribed trauma to the nose from in front (Fig. 2.**44a**) or from the side (Fig. 2.**44a** and **b**). The nasal injuries may also form part of a severe injury to the face and skull (see Fig. 2.**46** and 2.**47**).

Causes include traffic accidents, accidents at work, blows, brawls, falls, etc. The injuries may be divided into closed and open. In *closed* injuries due to blunt trauma, the injury is not penetrating and the nasal skeleton is covered completely with soft tissues with *no* external communication. In *open* injuries due to abrasions, cuts, or stab wounds, the cartilaginous or bony part of the nasal skeleton is exposed.

Diagnosis. This begins with the history and examination, which show deformity and abnormal mobility of the external nose, soft tissue injuries over the nose, and crepitation of the fragments on lateral pressure on the nose. Radiography of the nasal pyramid using lateral *soft tissue* views (with dental film) can be done as well as olfactometry. Involvement of the paranasal sinuses and the anterior base of the skull must be excluded (see p. 275).

Note: A greenstick fracture in young patients or apparently harmless soft tissue swelling may initially conceal a fracture and severe skeletal injury. If fracture of the nasal bone is suspected, *thorough* investigation should always be carried out for functional, cosmetic, and legal reasons.

Treatment. An open injury is first carefully cleaned. The wound edges and the nasal bones are checked, the displaced fragments are replaced, and the soft tissues are repaired with atraumatic sutures. Antibiotic cover is necessary.

Repositioning of a Simple Fracture of the Nasal Bone

This should be carried out *within the first 24 h,* within 48 h at most, because the fracture can be easily reduced. Delay can have considerable cosmetic and functional sequelae because the fragments heal in a displaced position.

Technique. Short-acting intravenous or intubation anesthesia is used. The deviated part of the skeleton is replaced, and the depressed part of the skeleton is elevated as

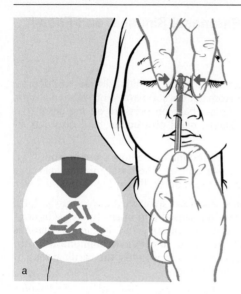

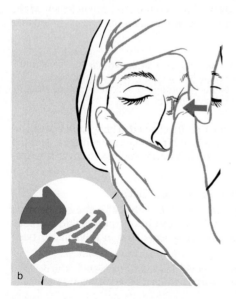

Fig. 2.**44a** and **b**   Fracture of the nasal bone: **(a)** by violence from in front, and its reposition; **(b)** by violence from the side, and its reposition.

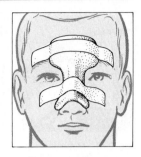

Fig. 2.**45**   Fixation of the replaced fracture by a splint.

shown in Fig. 2.**44a** and **b**.If the fragments are already fixed or wedged, they must be refractured in the direction opposite that of the original trauma or even repositioned by osteotomies. The septum should be checked and corrected if necessary. Anterior nasal packing is introduced, and an external splint (Fig. 2.**45**) is worn for 8 days to ensure fixation.

Management of a Compound Fracture of the Nasal Bone or Nasal Pyramid.

The affected part of the skeleton is examined and debrided carefully through the soft tissue wound which may need to be extended. The fragments are replaced and fixed, if necessary, using wires. The soft tissues are sutured, packing is introduced, and a splint applied (see Fig. 2.**45**). Antibiotic cover is given.

If the soft tissues have been extensively damaged with contamination, swelling, or necrosis, treatment of a compound fracture of the nasal bone may have to be delayed for 8 to 14 days until the acute tissue reaction has settled. The decision about timing of surgery for a fracture of the nasal bone must be made by the rhinologic surgeon.

Complications. These include septal deviation (see p. 260) and septal hematoma and abscess (see p. 261). Long-term cosmetic defects may be caused by poor initial management or secondary infection. Extensive and difficult plastic surgery is then needed, often in several stages (see p. 282).

Trauma of the Middle Third of the Face and the Sinuses

Fig. 2.**46** shows typical examples of the mechanism.

Maxillary Fracture

Sagittal, vertical fractures are unusual, and the most common is a transverse fracture involving both sides of the face and always the antral cavity. It may also involve the other nasal sinuses and the anterior base of the skull. Figure 2.**47** shows the three typical horizontal fractures of the middle third of the face. These are usually classified by the Le Fort system.

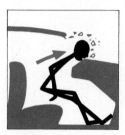
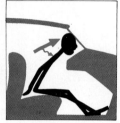
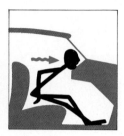

Fig. 2.**46** Mechanism of injury of the facial skeleton and the base of the skull in a traffic accident (see Fig. 4.**15a–c**).

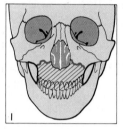
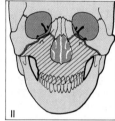
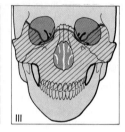

Fig. 2.**47** Types of central middle-third fracture (Le Fort classes I, II, III).

Symptoms

1. In *Le Fort class I,* low maxillary horizontal fractures, the upper alveolus is detached. The patient has abnormal occlusion and a hematoma or fracture of the wall of the antrum.
2. In *Le Fort class II,* pyramidal fractures, the upper jaw is detached and the fracture passes through the nasal bone, the frontal process of the maxilla, the medial orbital floor, and the zygomaticomaxillary suture. In this form of fracture, there often is considerable dislocation and depression of the central part of the face with involvement of the ethmoids, the orbital contents, and the lacrimal apparatus, and an increase of the interpupillary distance causing hypertelorism.
3. In *Le Fort class III* fractures, the facial skeleton is separated from the base of the skull. The fracture usually runs along the zygomaticofrontal, maxillofrontal, and nasofrontal sutures. The ethmoids, sphenoids, and often the frontal sinus and the orbit and its contents are involved, as are all the structures of the central part of the facial skeleton, often with massive depression of the middle third of the face and multiple frac-

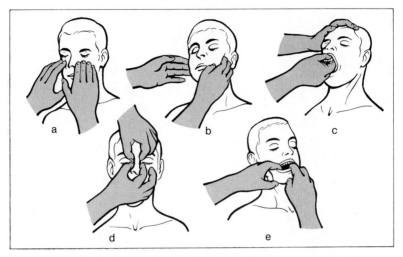

Fig. 2.**48a−e**   Palpation of central middle-third fractures. **(a)** Bony orbital rim; **(b)** zygomatic bone; **(c)** upper jaw; **(d)** nasal pyramid; **(e)** mandible.

tures of the bones of the face, the so-called dish face. This type of fracture usually extends also to the anterior part of the base of the skull (see p. 275).

The typical symptoms of shock, concussion, and cerebral contusion almost always occur immediately after the injury.

For facial swelling as a symptom, see Table 2.**11**.

Pathogenesis. Central middle-third fractures are typical high-speed injuries, mainly due to traffic accidents and more rarely to occupational injuries.

Diagnosis. A *history* is taken with respect to the type, direction, and force of the trauma. *Inspection* often shows massive skeletal fractures, dislocations, and depression with little soft tissue injury. The symmetry of the central middle third of the face and frontal area should be inspected (Fig. 2.**48a−e**). The inside *and* outside of the nose should be inspected. The orbit and its contents should be inspected also, looking for unilateral or bilateral hematoma, eye movement, and double vision. Vision is assessed. *Palpation* is directed to tenderness on pressure, abnormal movement of the upper jaw (see Fig. 2.**48c**), a break in the normal facial contour, steps and defects in the bony skeleton, especially of the orbital rim, trismus, and crepitation of the root of the nose. The movement of the mandible in all

Table 2.11 Facial Swelling

Site	Cause	Typical Symptoms
Forehead and upper lid	Frontal sinusitis and complications	Soft tissue edema, sensitivity to pressure, reddening
	Osteomyelitis of the frontal bone	Boggy, soft tissue swelling, sensitivity to pressure on the vault of the skull, rapidly progressive edema, chemosis, swelling of the lids, swinging temperature chart
	Mucocele of the frontal sinus or the ethmoid sinus	Resilient, nontender, noninflamed swelling, grows slowly
	Encephalocele	Noninflammatory pulsating swelling at the root of the nose
	Tumors	Noninflammatory, firm, usually immobile swelling; may be edema and pain on pressure
	Trauma	Edema, often hematoma of the upper lids, signs of fracture, pain on pressure
Upper jaw, cheek, and lower lid	Maxillary and ethmoidal sinusitis	Soft tissue edema of the cheek, the lower lid, medial canthus; pain on pressure, reddening
	Mucocele of the antrum or ethmoids	Resilient noninflammatory swelling of the cheek or the medial canthus, not tender and not inflamed
	Osteomyelitis of the upper jaw, due to sinusitis, dental causes, or radiotherapy	Painful inflammatory swelling and redness
	Zygomatic abscess, due to otitis media	Painful inflammatory swelling of the temple and zygoma with edema of the lid, and ear symptoms

Parotitis	Inflammatory swelling of the preauricular area and cheek, severe pain and tenderness
Sialadenosis of the parotid gland	Painless, occasionally fluctuating, marked preauricular swelling
Parotid tumors	Benign: slow-growing, no pain, no facial nerve paralysis Malignant: rapid growth, pain, and possibly facial paralysis
Inflammatory dental disease	Painful swelling of the cheek, edema of the lids, and possibly trismus
Odontogenic cysts	Painless swelling of the cheek and slow growth
Dacryocystitis	Very sensitive to pressure, inflammatory swelling, possibly fluctuation in the medial canthus, drainage of pus from the lacrimal punctum (see Color Plate 15c)
Tumors	Firm, usually poorly mobile swelling, usually not very tender
Trauma	Edema, often a hematoma of the lower lids, possibly the sign of a fracture and sensitivity to pressure
Angioneurotic edema	Allergic edema with a feeling of tension and pruritus, facial swelling particularly of the lip and the lid, coming on suddenly and recurrent

Table 2.11 Continuation		
Site	Cause	Typical Symptoms
Mandible	Osteomyelitis due to dental diseases or radiation	Inflammatory painful swelling, possibly with trismus
	Inflammatory dental disease	Painful swelling and possibly trismus
	Odontogenic cysts	Painless slow-growing swelling
	Masseteric hypertrophy	Painless, thickening of the masseter muscle on mastication
	Sialadenitis of the submandibular gland	Inflammatory swelling in the submandibular region
	Sialadenosis of a major salivary gland	Painless swelling, slow growth
	Tumors	Firm, usually poorly mobile swelling
	Trauma	Swelling, often a hematoma on the injured area und possibly the signs of a fracture

Diffuse facial swellings may also occur in nephroses, chronic nephritis, endocrine disorders such as myxedema, and Cushing's disease.

directions, the occlusion, and the state of the teeth are assessed, and *defects* of sensory or motor *innervation, a CSF rhinorrhea,* and *prolapse of the brain tissue* are looked for.

Radiography. Skull radiographs and special views are obtained. Impacted foreign bodies are searched for if they are radiopaque. Angiography, CT scan, and olfactometry may also be needed.

A maxillofacial surgeon, an ophthalmologist, a neurologist, or a neurosurgeon may need to be *consulted.* In multiple injuries, the advice of a general or orthopedic surgeon may be necessary before treatment begins. The priority of timing of the various procedures should be mutually agreed.

> *Note:* Skeletal asymmetry or deformity is often concealed in middle-third fractures by the rapid soft tissue swelling or bloody effusion. Furthermore, apparently harmless soft tissue injuries in the region of the base of the skull may conceal serious life-threatening skeletal injuries.

Treatment. At the site of injury, the traumatologic ABC should be observed:

A = Airway. The airway is secured and aspiration prevented.
B = Bleeding. This must be controlled.
C = Circulation. Shock must be treated.

> *Note:* Every patient with a fracture of the middle third of the face should be *hospitalized.* Admission to which department is decided by the extent and type of the injury to the skull, and the other injuries to the extremities, thorax, and abdomen. Since patients with head injuries very often require immediate treatment by special traumatologic teams consisting of a neurosurgeon, a rhinosurgeon, a maxillofacial surgeon, and an ophthalmic surgeon, immediate admission to a suitably equipped large traumatologic center is indicated.

The purpose of definitive surgery is the reconstitution of the normal anatomy and function by debridement, ventilation, and drainage. The specific functions of the *rhinologic surgeon* are, first, the treatment of the soft tissue injury and management of the nose and sinuses by debridement, drainage, and ventilation; second, assessment of the base of the skull (because of the frequent combination with a fracture of the anterior cranial fossa and the pterygopalatine fossa); and third, correction of the facial skeleton and the bony orbit (see pp. 272 and 273). The definitive surgery for middle-third fractures should be carried out as *quickly* as possible since the fracture may heal very rapidly in the wrong position due to the formation of callus. The management of simultaneous frontobasal injuries is described on p. 275.

Fractures of the Zygoma and the Bony Orbit

Combined fractures are frequent, involving the trifurcate zygoma with the zygomatic arch and also the orbital rim with the orbital floor (lateral mid-face fracture). Isolated blowout fractures of the orbital floor and isolated fracture of the zygomatic arch may also occur. Fractures of the zygoma and orbit may also form part of a more severe mid-face fracture or frontobasal fracture. The antrum is almost always involved (Fig. 2.**49b**). The mechanism of fracture is usually blunt violence to the lateral part of the face by a blow from a fist, a traffic accident, or a fall down stairs. The fracture is almost always depressed. Dislocation of the fragments may be minimal, but there may be extensive comminution with multiple fragments which can only be repositioned and fixed with great difficulty (Fig. 2.**49a** and **b**).

Symptoms. These include orbital hematoma, swelling of the eyelids, asymmetry of the middle third of the face with a sunken contour of the cheek on the side of the fracture, inferior displacement and possibly enophthalmos on the side of the fracture, a step in the bony wall of the orbit inferiorly or laterally, rarely of the upper rim, and possibly trismus. The soft tissues in the zygomatic area swell initially, but the underlying bony outline is flattened. The sensation of the infraorbital nerve be lost. In a blow-out fracture, there is partial limitation of the movements of the eye, with double vision due to trapping of the inferior rectus or inferior oblique muscles.

Diagnosis. This rests on the history of the type and direction of trauma, inspection, and bimanual palpation, which shows asymmetry of the facial skeleton, a step in the orbital wall, or limitation of movement of the lower jaw (see Fig. 2.**49**). *Radiography* includes standard views of the nasal sinuses, and special views for the zygomatic arch, and tomograms. Ophthalmologic examination should be carried out.

Note: Fractures of the zygoma are relatively frequent. They are often overlooked initially because of the soft tissue swelling of the cheek and of the lateral part of the face. They are thus recognized late, after bony consolidation in the incorrect position. Even after relatively mild trauma to the middle third of the face, from in front, or from the side, asymmetry of the facial skeleton or a step in the orbital wall or loss of sensation of the infraorbital nerve should always be looked for by bimanual palpation to allow comparison of the two sides.

Treatment. There are several operations available to accomplish the *repositioning and stabilization* of fractures of the zygoma (Fig. 2.**50a** and **b**):

1. Access from the vestibule of the mouth and from the maxillary antrum
2. Access from the temporal region
3. Access directly through the overlying soft tissues

Fig. 2.**49a** and **b**   Zygomatic fracture. **a.** Lateral.
1, Zygomatic arch;
2, mandible; 3, coronoid process; 4, temporomandibular joint.
b. From in front. 5, Body of the zygomatic bone;
6, Medial palpebral ligament. The inset shows involvement of the orbit, antral cavity and ethmoids.

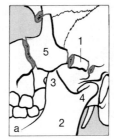
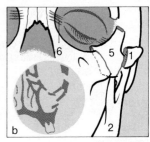

Fig. 2.**50a** and
b   Management of a typical zygomatic fracture. **a.** Soft tissue incision to allow repositioning of the fragments and fixation, and access for elevation; **b.** condition after repositioning and wiring.

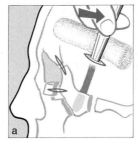
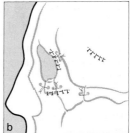

The use and combination of repositioning and methods of stabilization, such as single-pronged retractors, wiring, etc., depend on the type and severity of the fracture. External fixation is usually not necessary for zygomatic fractures. If there is loss of sensation of the infraorbital nerve, the nerve must be exposed and decompressed.

Isolated Blowout Fracture

This is caused by violence localized to the orbital contents by a blow from a fist, a tennis ball, a champagne bottle cork, etc. The thin bony floor of the orbit fractures and prolapses into the antral cavity (Fig. 2.**51a**). This can lead to trapping of the orbital contents (fat, ocular muscles such as the inferior rectus and inferior oblique muscles) by the fragments and to prolapse of the fractured floor of the orbit into the antral cavity.

Symptoms. These include enophthalmos, double vision, limitation of movement of the eye, which is most obvious when looking upward due to trapping of the lower ocular muscles, and disorders of sensation of the infraorbital nerve.

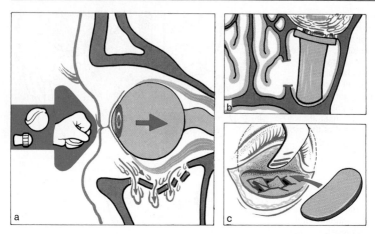

Fig. 2.**51a–c**   Blowout fracture. **(a)** Mechanism; **(b)** prop fixation of the orbital floor via the antral cavity; **(c)** fixation via the orbit with bridging of the defect.

Diagnosis. This depends on radiographs, tomograms, and ophthalmologic examination.

Treatment. The antral cavity must be explored as early as possible (see p. 238). The bony fragments are exposed and the prolapsed part is replaced, possibly combined with bridging or stabilization of the bony defect with lyophilized dura or cartilage or by the temporary introduction of a plastic prop into the antrum (see Fig. 2.**51b**). *Alternative or supplementary measures* include access via the orbit through an incision in the lid and introduction of lyophilized dura or a sheet of silicone or Teflon to support the orbital contents (see Fig. 2.**51c**). If the fracture heals in an incorrect position, the resulting enophthalmos can be corrected by supporting the orbital contents with an implant, preferably of autologous rather than synthetic material.

Barotrauma of the Sinuses

This is caused by the considerable difference between the air pressure in the sinus and the environment, if rapid equalization of pressure is not possible because of anatomic abnormalities. Flyers, divers, and parachute jumpers are most often affected.

Symptoms include sudden, severe, stabbing pain in the region of the nasal sinuses, usually the frontal and rarely the antrum, during and after a temporary marked pressure difference. The result may be a nosebleed or sinusitis due to severe mucosal damage of the affected cavity.

Treatment includes decongestion of the nasal mucosa, symptomatic measures, possibly antibiotics, and as a prophylactic measure surgery to the nose and sinuses, e.g., septal correction, conchotomy, etc.

Frontobasal Injury to the Anterior Cranial Fossa and the Neighboring Sinuses

Trauma to the frontal area and to the root of the nose usually is incurred in traffic accidents but occasionally also in occupational injuries. It causes a fracture which first affects the upper sinuses (the frontal, the ethmoid, and the sphenoid sinuses), and from there extends into the anterior cranial fossa. Alternatively, the fracture may primarily affect the upper part of the frontal bone together with the dura and the intracranial structures, and the fracture line may extend from here into the nasal sinuses. Frontobasal fractures occur in 70% of all fractures of the skull base. There are typical fracture lines in the anterior cranial fossa , the rhinobasis, similar to the fracture lines in laterobasal fractures (see p. 118, Figs. 2.**52a–d** and 2.**53**).

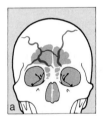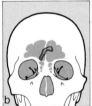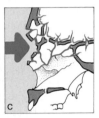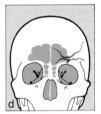

Fig. 2.**52a–d**   Frontobasal fracture. **a.** High fracture (Escher type I). **b.** Middle fracture (Escher type II). **c.** Deep fracture (Escher type III). **d.** Lateroorbital fracture (Escher type IV).

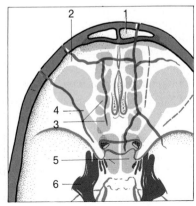

Fig. 2.**53**   Typical fracture lines of the anterior base of the skull. 1, Frontal sinus; 2, orbit; 3, ethmoid; 4, optic nerve; 5, sphenoid sinus; 6, Gasserian ganglion.

Dural tears and brain injuries, which may be open or closed, thus often arise in the anterior cranial fossa (see Color Plate **16b**). Infection ascending to the intracranial cavity is possible through the fracture line from the nose or the sinuses. This may occur immediately after the accident (early infection) or years later (late infection) as a *meningitis* or *brain abscess* (see Fig. 2.**38**).

Symptoms. *Cardinal symptoms* include CSF rhinorrhea, brain prolapsing from the nose or from the external wound of the nasofrontal area, extensive facial hematoma, possibly surgical emphysema, proptosis with or without loss of vision, and frontal pneumoencephalocele.

Symptoms also include cerebral concussion or contusion, unilateral or bilateral hematoma of the eyes, which is *not* conclusive evidence of fronto-basal injury (see Color Plate **16a**), and occasionally severe bleeding from the pharynx, mouth, and nose. Cerebrospinal fluid rhinorrhea is a *certain* sign of a dural tear, but dural tears are possible without a CSF leak. Anosmia occurs in 75% of patients, and the IInd cranial nerve, and, more rarely, the IIIrd, IVth, Vth, and VIth cranial nerves may be injured. External soft tissue injuries are slight or even absent in 20% of all patients. On occasion, signs of imminent increased intracranial pressure such as bleeding, pulse rate alteration, homolateral dilatation of the pupil, and fixed pupil are present.

Diagnosis. This rests on the history and type of accident, radiographs of the skull in two planes, radiographs of the sinuses in several different projections (occipitomental, occipitofrontal, axial; and overextended axial), tomograms, and computed tomograms.

Evidence of a CSF rhinorrhea is obtained from a positive glucose test and increased protein content in the fluid, compared to that in nasal secretions, isotope localization of the dural defect, and possibly the fluorescein test.

Treatment. As soon as the patient has been stabilized by treating shock, the anterior cranial fossa and the affected nasal sinus should be exposed to allow debridement and watertight closure of the intracranial cavity by dural repair. The procedure is performed through the nasal sinuses. Injuries of the nasal sinuses are repositioned.

Three groups of indications for operative intervention include:

1. *Vital indications,* operative intervention immediately
- Life-threatening increase of intracranial pressure due to intracranial bleeding
- Life-threatening bleeding into the sinuses, nasopharynx, or base of skull
2. *Absolute indications,* operative intervention as soon as possible
- Evidence of a dural tear such as CSF rhinorrhea, pneumoencephalocele
- Open brain injury
- Early or late intracranial complications such as meningitis, extradural abscess, subdural abscess, or cerebral abscess

- Impacted foreign body
- Orbital complications
- Osteomyelitis of the frontal bone
- Depressed fracture with a suspected dural tear
- Cranial nerve lesions which require decompression
- Impaling injuries

3. *Relative indications,* operative intervention within 1 to 2 weeks
- Fractures affecting the frontal, ethmoid, or sphenoid sinus in which the dura may be involved, but this has not been proved with certainty
- Depressed fractures, and fractures with obvious displacement of fragments, with or without the suspicion of a dural tear
- Injuries to the nasal sinuses with penetrating soft tissue injuries
- Infection of the nasal sinuses already present at the time of injury
- Posttraumatic sinusitis and mucopyocele

The purpose of the operation is wide exposure of the injured area together with the dura to allow removal of fragments and management of injury to the brain and the base of the skull. This is followed by closure of the dura with fascia or galea and provision of free drainage of the affected sinus by one of the typical rhinologic sinus operations (see pp. 238ff.).

The three typical routes of access are shown schematically in Figure 2.**54** (a) frontoorbital (extracranial), (b) transfrontal-extradural (rhinologic-rhinosurgical access), and (c) transfrontal-intradural (neurosurgical access).

The choice of procedure and the order of the operative steps depend on the individual patient and on joint treatment planning by the neurosurgeon, the rhinologist, and the maxillofacial surgeon, possibly with the ophthalmic surgeon, and the general surgeon or traumatologist in patients with multiple injuries.

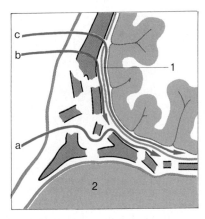

Fig. 2.**54** Routes of access for management of frontobasal fractures. (a) Frontoorbital extracranial, (b) transfrontal-extradural rhinosurgical, (c) transfrontal-intradural neurosurgical. 1. Dura; 2, nasal cavity.

Complications. These include CSF fistula, recurrent late meningitis, early or late brain abscess, osteomyelitis of the flat bones of the skull (see p. 251), and formation of muco- or pyoceles (see p. 244).

Other Possible Injuries of the Facial Skeleton

Injury to the facial nerve (see p. 165).

Injury to the lacrimal system (see Fig. 2.55) quite commonly is combined with injuries of the sinuses and the central middle part of the face. If possible, these should be repaired at the same time as the injuries to the sinuses and face. If this is not possible, or is not successful, stenosis or complete obstruction of the lacrimal sac or nasolacrimal duct occur (see Color Plate **15c**), requiring correction (dacryocistorhinostomy) (see Fig. 2.55) either by the ophthalmic or rhinologic surgeon.

Injuries of the mandible and of the temporomandibular joint are managed by the maxillofacial surgeon, who is also responsible for restitution of correct occlusion.

The main symptoms of mandibular fractures include swelling of the lower part of the face, abnormal movement or deformity of the mandible, anomalies of occlusion, pain on movement, compression or torsion of the mandible, and possible trismus.

Immediate first aid measures should be undertaken for comminuted fractures, particularly of the chin with extensive soft tissue injury. The patient should be intubated, or a tracheotomy should be carried out, because of the danger of respiratory obstruction. Profuse bleeding should be arrested, if necessary by a pressure dressing. Soft tissue defects or scars are dealt with in the usual way by plastic surgery reconstructive procedures.

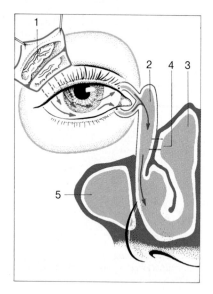

Fig. 2.**55** Eye and nose. 1, Lacrimal gland; 2, lacrimal sac with lacrimal ducts; 3, nasal cavity; 4, site for dacryocystorhinostomy; 5, antral cavity.

Congenital Anomalies and Deformities of the Nose

Congenital Anomalies of the Nose

The embryonal face is formed from nine processes. Development is complex so that congenital anomalies are relatively frequent, even if they are often only slight. Anomalies incompatible with life, e.g., *arhinia,* are extremely rare.

Cleft Face and Nose

Oblique facial clefts, even in a rudimentary form, are rare, as are *transverse* facial clefts in which the angle of the mouth lies near the tragus, causing macrostomia.

Median clefts are more common but are usually only rudimentary. They range in extent from *hypertelorism,* with or without true median facial cleft and with or without meningoencephalocele, to *dog nose, proboscis,* or even *doublenose.*

Treatment is by plastic surgery.

Cleft Lip, Jaw, and Palate

These anomalies are relatively common and affect $1\%_0$ of whites.

Treatment is by reconstructive surgery, occasionally in stages, and orthodontic and prosthetic procedures. In addition, speech therapy may me needed. The planning of treatment is described on p. 374.

Cleft lip and palate provide several tasks for the rhinologist: first, the anomalies of the external nose such as a flattened nasal ala and anomalies within the nose such as dislocation of the septum; second, speech disorders such as rhinolalia aperta of varied severity; and third, the almost constant abnormalities of tubal aeration causing seromucotympanum or chronic otitis media.

Nasal Fistulae, Nasal Cysts, Dermoid Cysts, and Gliomas

Median nasal fistulae, from which cloudy secretion may drain, usually end blindly at the level of the glabella or in the ethmoid-septum region. This is also true of *congenital nasal cysts* that lie in the same position, but also may arise in the nasal vestibule or nasal septum.

Dermoid cysts are more common. They often contain hair and accessory structures such as ectodermal inclusions which lie above, below, or within the frontal bone.

Gliomas are tumors of the frontal region or the root of the nose in the midline and consist of solid glial tissue.

All these anomalies must be removed surgically.

Meningoencephalocele

Dural and brain herniations (hernias and celes) may be found in the nose and be confused with nasal polyps. They may also lie extranasal and be related to the frontal bone, the ethmoid, or the nasal septum. The *causes* are incomplete closure of the neuropore during the 3rd embryonal week and trauma.

Diagnosis is made by tomography, arteriography, and brain scan.

Treatment is by operative removal, closure of the dura, and possibly osteoplastic correction of any existing hypertelorism.

Stenosis and Atresia of the Nostrils

These are usually congenital but may also be acquired, due to trauma or destructive infections.

Treatment is by plastic surgery.

Choanal Atresia (see Color Plate 26b)

This is a bony or membranous occlusion of the posterior nasal opening which may be bilateral. Girls are more affected than boys. Hereditary factors have been demonstrated. The disorder is usually congenital but may also be acquired due to trauma. Incomplete atresias (= stenoses) also occur.

Symptoms. These include chronic purulent nasal discharge, inability to breathe through the nose or to sneeze, and anosmia.

> *Note:* *Bilateral* atresia in the *newborn* is a *life-threatening situation.* The infant is unable to breathe through the mouth satisfactorily because of the relatively high position of the larynx and must also depend on nasal respiration during feeding. There is thus a danger, in bilateral atresia at least, of asphyxia, cyanosis, atelectasis of the lungs, or aspiration pneumonia. Spontaneous feeding is difficult or impossible.

Diagnosis. This is made by probing the nose, endoscopy of the nose and nasopharynx, and by radiography with a contrast medium to fill the nose in the supine position.

Differential diagnosis. This includes all those disorders that cause nasal obstruction, especially polypi, foreign bodies, encephalocele, and tumors.

Treatment. In *bilateral atresia* in the newborn: if the child is in danger of asphyxiating an intubation, or a tracheotomy is carried out, and a feeding tube is passed. Immediate palliative measures are given, such as penetration of the atresia (mechanically or by laser) on one side at least and introduction of a plastic tube through the opened choana. These procedures are continued for the first few weeks until the infant has learned to mouth breathe. Definitive surgery of the atresia is not advisable before the end of the 1st year of life. A *transpalatal* procedure is then carried out to expose the atretic plate, the area is excised extensively, and mucosal flaps are turned in to epithelialize the choanal opening. An intranasal procedure is also available. Operation may be deferred in *unilateral* atresia to a later date.

Disorders of Shape of the External Nose

Anomalies of shape of the external nose (see Fig. 2.**56a–e**) often require rhinoplasty both on aesthetic grounds and because of disordered function.

Anomalies of shape of the nose may be due to the cartilaginous or bony parts of the internal or external nose skeleton being too large or too small, or being improperly positioned in relation to each other or to surrounding structures. Certain parameters as illustrated in Figure 2.**57** are used for the analysis of the deformities on standardized photographs. Certain angles in the facial contour are also to be taken into account (see Fig. 2.**57**).

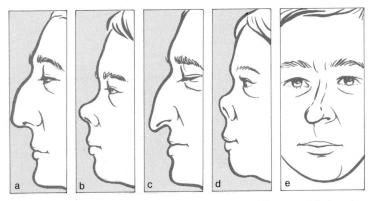

Fig. 2.**56a–e** Different nasal types. **(a)** Hump nose, **(b)** saddle nose, **(c)** drooping nasal tip, **(d)** short nose, **(e)** scoliotic nose.

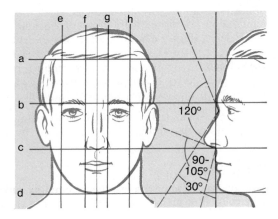

Fig. 2.**57** Relations of the normal face and important profile angles.

Basics of Rhinoplasty

There are two requirements of rhinoplasty. First, it should restore a normal form to the nose so that it harmonizes with the rest of the face. Second, the function of the nose and nasal sinuses with respect to respiration, olfaction, etc., should be maintained, improved, and returned to normal. This double goal often requires correction of both the outside and inside of the nose, i. e., a *septorhinoplasty*. These operations should be carried out by a suitably trained rhinologist.

Corrective and reconstructive operations should be distinguished. In *corrective* rhinoplasty, especially correction of the supportive framework of the nose, all operative steps are carried out from inside the nose without an external incision.

The principal steps of *rhinoplasty* are:

- An incision in the nasal vestibule
- Elevation of the soft tissue covering the nasal skeleton
- Isolation, mobilization, and correction of all skeletal elements
- Union of the mobilized and corrected skeletal parts to form a pleasing nasal framework and a functionally favorable nasal cavity
- Fixation of the mobilized, corrected skeletal elements in the required position

Anomalies of the *cartilaginous* part of the nose include *anomalies of shape of the base of the nose,* e. g., a *hanging nasal tip,* a tip too flat, too wide, too cleft, too long, or too short: *nasal alae* that are flaccid, too arched, or asymmetrical; a *nasal columella* that projects too much, is too retracted, too thick, too short, or too bent. The entire nose may also be too long or too short, etc.

Anomalies of the *bony part of the nose* include anomalies of shape of the *bridge of the nose,* e. g., hump nose, saddle nose, twisted nose, broad nose, or narrow nose; of the *root of the nose;* and of the *nasal septum.* Usually the *bony and cartilaginous* nose require correction *together.*

In *reconstructive* rhinoplasty, partial loss of the soft tissue, of the skeleton of the nose, or total loss of the nose are dealt with, and a complete nose is rebuilt. Local or distant flaps are used, depending on the type and extent of the defect (Figs. 2.**62a** and **b** and 2.**66a–c**).

Hump Nose

This is due to an excess of the bony or cartilaginous nasal skeleton. Usually, it does not cause marked functional disturbance.

Treatment. Rhinoplasty is performed with removal of the hump and narrowing of the nasal bridge. The principles of the procedure are shown in Figure 2.**58a–c**.

Saddle Nose

This condition is often due to trauma, operation, or infection (e. g., syphilis, tuberculosis) or may be congenital. There is a characteristic defect of the

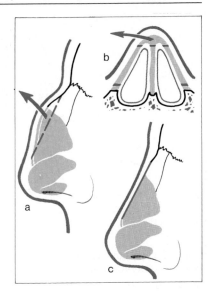

Fig. 2.**58a–c** Correction of a hump nose. **(a)** Subcutaneous removal of the hump, **(b)** osteotomy, **(c)** final result.

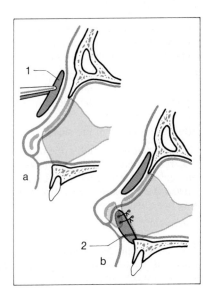

Fig. 2.**59 and b** Correction of a saddle nose. **(a)** Assessing the implant (1); **(b)** introduction of the implant. A further implant has been introduced into the nasal columella (2) to elevate the nasal tip.

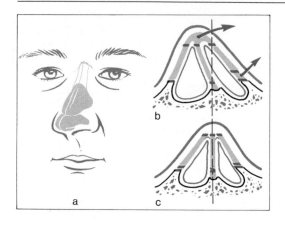

Fig. 2.**60a–c**   Correction of a scoliotic nose. **(a)** Preoperative, **(b)** osteotomies and resection, **(c)** final result.

bony or cartilaginous part of the skeleton of the nasal pyramid. There is often considerable functional disturbance.

Treatment. Rhinoplasty with dorsal augmentation is indicated, possibly combined with support of the nasal columella. The principles are shown in Figure 2.**59a** and **b**.

Deviated Nose

The cartilaginous *and* bony nasal skeleton and the nasal septum are mostly affected. The cause is usually trauma, but this condition may be congenital. It usually causes considerable interference with function.

Treatment. This consists of septorhinoplasty with correction of the skeletal parts of the external nose and of the septum. The principles are shown in Figure 2.**60a–c**, and the operation on the septum in Figure 2.**43a–c**.

Other Deformities of the Nose

The *broad nose* is usually due to trauma, particularly if initial treatment is incorrect, whereas the *narrow nose,* the *large nose,* and the *long nose* are all congenital. Interference with function is to be expected, especially in the narrow nose and in the posttraumatic wide nose. The large nose and the long nose usually cause only aesthetic problems.

Treatment. Septorhinoplasty is performed.

Anomalies of the Nasal Alae

Nasal alae that are too weak and prolapse on inspiration, or that are too flared, are corrected by strengthening or reduction of the nasal cartilage.

The profile of the forehead and the chin must be included in analysis of the aesthetic appearance of the entire face in addition to the shape of the nose. On occasion a profileplasty is required, with reduction or building up of the chin or the forehead.

Basic Plastic-Reconstructive Procedures of the Head and Neck

Soft tissue and skeletal defects of the head and neck due to *trauma,* to mutilating *tumor operations,* and to congenital *anomalies* are relatively frequent and require *reconstruction for functional, aesthetic, and cosmetic reasons.* This type of operation requires special operative techniques and also thorough basic knowledge of the complex anatomy and physiology of the structures of the head and neck. They should therefore be carried out by surgeons who are well trained in this area and who are able to combine preservation of function with reconstruction. This type of *regional plastic surgery* is also indispensable in planning reconstruction preoperatively when a mutilating resection must be performed.

There are numerous reconstructive procedures available, but they can be reduced to several basic principles which may be modified and combined depending on the type and site of the defect. This applies to planning and execution of the *incision, wound closure, and wound care.*

Defects of the overlying soft tissue may be closed by several different operations depending on the site and size:

Free skin grafts of various thickness are used for cover of the superficial defects of the skin and mucosa at the various sites.

Figure 2.**61** shows the classical types.

Local flaps are developed from the tissue immediately adjacent to the defect and can be set into the final position immediately due to the intact circulation by the techniques of advancement or rotation. The principle of advancement is shown in Figure 2.**62a** and **b** and that of rotation in Figure 2.**63a** and **b**.

Transposition flaps may be *local,* e. g., single and multiple z-*plasty* (Fig. 2.**64a** and **b**). *Regional transposition flaps* are *pedicled flaps* used in different ways to close large

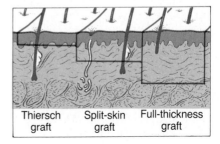

Thiersch	Split-skin	Full-thickness
graft	graft	graft

Fig. 2.**61**   Types of free skin graft.

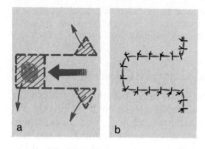

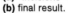

Fig. 2.**62a** and **b** Advancement flaps.
(a) Incisions with Burow's triangles,
(b) final result.

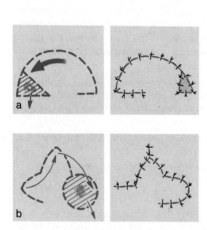

Fig. 2.**63a** and **b** Rotation flaps.
a. Simple rotation. The remaining defect
is covered with a free skin graft.
b. Bilobed flap.

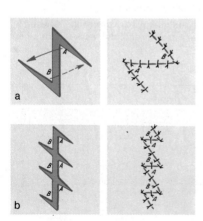

Fig. 2.**64a** and **b** Z-plasty. **(a)** Simple,
(b) multiple.

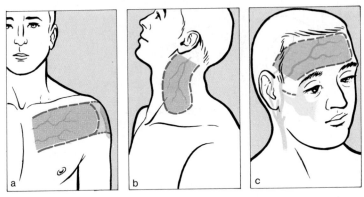

Fig. 2.**65a–c** Regional flaps. **(a)** Deltopectoral flap (the red-shaded area is an extended flap), **(b)** lateral cervical flap, **(c)** temporal flap.

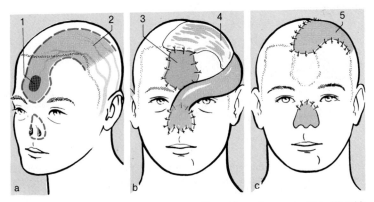

Fig. 2.**66a–c** Reconstruction of the nose. **a.** Formation of a scalp flap (2) with implanted supporting framework (1). **b.** Scalp flap attached, forehead defect covered with split skin (3), scalp defect covered temporarily with gauze (4). **c.** Nose reconstructed and remaining part of the scalp flap (5) returned.

soft tissue defects. They include the deltopectoral flap (Fig. 2.**65a**), the lateral cervical flap (Fig. 2.**65b**), and the temporal flap among others (Fig. 2.**65c**).

Figure 2.**66** shows the use of a scalp flap for reconstruction of the nose.

These flaps are also used for other purposes, e. g., reconstruction of the pharynx, cheek, oral cavity, and upper esophagus.

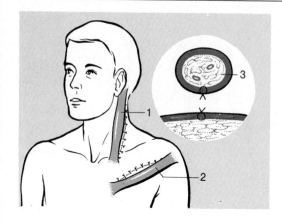

Fig. 2.**67**   Principles of a tubed pedicle. 1, Cervical flap; 2, chest flap; 3, pedicle in horizontal section.

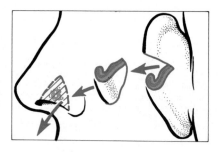

Fig. 2.**68**   Composite graft from the auricle for implantation into the nasal ala.

Distant flaps may be brought to fill a defect from other parts of the body in several stages. A classic example is the *tubed pedicle*. Typical donor sites for this type of flap are shown in Figure 2.**67**.

The various *musculocutaneous flaps,* e.g., the pectoralis major, the latissimus dorsi, and the sternomastoid, are large flaps with a generous blood supply; these flaps consist of skin and muscle. They may be used reliably for the purpose of covering large multilayered tissue defects of the cheek, the floor of the mouth, the esophagus, etc.

The blood supply, which is essential for healing of large compound flaps, may be ensured by transfer from a remote part of the body to the head and neck using microsurgery. The feeding blood vessels are exposed when the flap, e.g., from the groin, is developed, and the vessels are anastomosed to suitable local vessels at the receptor site by microvascular sutures.

Defects of compound soft tissue structures, such as the cartilaginous part of the nose, usually require reconstruction of the supporting framework to restore respiratory function. *Composite grafts* taken from the auricle are particularly suitable as they provide the three necessary layers (Fig. 2.**68**).

The bony and cartilaginous supporting framework may also be supplemented by subcutaneous implants to fill in the contour of the soft tissue defect using autologous or homologous *implants* of rib cartilage, iliac crest bone, fascia, etc. The homologous biologic implant material is kept ready in a tissue bank. If necessary, inert synthetic material such as silicone may be used under certain conditions.

Occasionally, it may be more reasonable to replace the defect by a *prosthesis* rather than to embark on multistage protracted reconstructive procedures, e.g., after total loss of the auricle or the orbital contents.

Tumors of the Nose and Sinuses

Benign Tumors

These are relatively unusual in the nasal cavity and sinuses. Aside from rare tumors, these tumors include osteoma, ossifying fibroma, papilloma, hemangioma, lymphangioma, chondroma, fibroma, and giant cell tumor.

Osteoma

This condition is relatively common in the frontal and ethmoid sinus.

Symptoms. These include headache and pressure in the head. Recurrent sinusitis or mucocele may occur due to obstruction of the drainage. Possibly displacement of the eye, and, later, possibly intracranial complications may arise.

Diagnosis. Radiographs of the nasal sinuses typically show a calcified, well-demarcated tumor. Biopsy may also be carried out.

Treatment. This consists of operative removal via a frontal sinus or ethmoid operation (see pp. 239, 240).

Ossifying Fibroma (Fibrous Dysplasia)

This occurs principally in the middle third of the face and at the base of the skull in children and adolescents.

Symptoms. These include unilateral expansion of the facial skeleton, headaches, and possibly visual field loss and lesions of other cranial nerves.

Diagnosis. Radiography shows a fairly radiopaque tumor arising from normal skeletal structures. A biopsy may also be carried out.

Treatment. Usually only partial removal is possible.

Papillomas

Papillomas are uncommon in the nasal cavity and nasal sinuses. They are of particular significance because of their tendency to undergo malignant change (particularly the inverted papilloma) and because of their tendency to recur.

Symptoms. Nasal obstruction and epistaxis are present. The tumor can be demonstrated by rhinoscopy.

Diagnosis is by biopsy.

Treatment. Because of the tendency to malignant degeneration and recurrence, a surgical excision is indicated. Papillomas are not radiosensitive.

Hemangiomas and Lymphangiomas (Capillary or Cavernous)

These are usually congenital. Ninety percent manifest themselves in the 1st year of life, and 60% occur in females. These are the most common benign tumors of childhood. Since spontaneous remission can occur, especially within the 1st year of life, treatment should be postponed if possible until the 3rd or 4th year of life.

Treatment. This is by surgery, possibly by laser or cryosurgery. Although radiotherapy is effective, removal is much preferred since radiotherapy may damage the growth of the facial skeleton and induce a later carcinoma.

Glioma

This condition is described on p. 279.

Nasopharyngeal Angiofibroma

This condition is described on p. 385.

Malignant Tumors

External Nose

Primary tumors of the external nose include *basal cell carcinoma, squamous cell carcinoma,* and *malignant melanoma. Senile keratoma* and *xeroderma pigmentosum* are to be included in the group of *precancerous lesions.* The *keratoacanthoma* is indeed benign but is often very difficult to differentiate from a squamous carcinoma.

Basal Cell Carcinoma (Rodent Ulcer)

Eighty-six percent of these tumors are localized on the head; 26% on the nose, 19% on the frontal or temporal area, 16% on the cheek, 14% on the eye, especially the medial canthus, and 11% on the auricle. Basal cell carcinoma is the most common malignant tumor of the external nose.

Symptoms. Initially, there is a small firm nodule, often with a retracted center which grows slowly. Later, it ulcerates and infiltrates superficially into the underlying tissue. There is no predilection for either sex, and the tumor usually first appears between 60 and 70 years of age. The superficially recognizable skin lesion usually has a diameter of less than 1 cm in 70% of patients, but extension into the surrounding tissue is very often *considerable,* and often the tumor occupies an area of more than 20 cm^2. A true basal cell carcinoma does not metastasize, and transition to squamous cell carcinoma is very rare. However, malignant degeneration may occur in tumors that have previously been irradiated or insufficiently excised, producing a very aggressive malignancy that may seed to other sites (e. g., the lung) via the bloodstream.

Diagnosis. The most common site is the center of the face and the auricle. Diagnosis must be confirmed by *biopsy.*

Differential diagnosis. Squamous carcinoma and precancerous lesions must be considered.

Treatment. The *initial treatment* should be generous excision with a good margin, followed by immediate reconstruction. Cryosurgery or the laser may be indicated on cosmetic grounds for *small* lesions. *Other forms of treatment* include radiotherapy and Mohs' chemosurgery.

Prognosis. This is good provided that the initial resection is generous, with histologic check on the margins and immediate further resection if necessary. This tumor does *not* metastasize, provided that is does not undergo malignant degeneration.

Keratinizing Squamous Cell Carcinoma

This is the second most common tumor of the external nose (see Color Plate **10d**).

Symptoms. This lesion begins as a precancerous lesion or as a nodular, firm, nonhealing lesion of the skin. It then grows rapidly, soon ulcerates, and forms a crater. Regional lymph node metastases occur relatively early.

Diagnosis. The most common site is the lower third of the face. Diagnosis is confirmed by biopsy.

Differential diagnosis. This includes precancerous lesions, keratoacanthoma, and basal cell carcinoma.

Treatment. If possible the primary treatment should be generous removal, including the bony and cartilaginous base. The defect is reconstructed 1 year later if there is no recurrence. *Other forms of treatment* include radiotherapy.

Prognosis. This is favorable if the tumor is removed immediately with a wide margin.

Malignant Melanoma (see Color Plate **17a** and **b**)

The most common *skin tumor,* malignant melanoma affects females with a 2:1 preponderance over males. The maximum incidence is between the 20th and 60th years of life. Ten percent of malignant melanomas occur in the head and neck, affecting the face and the scalp.

Symptoms. The tumor often arises from a pigmented mole but also may arise from apparently normal skin.

Suspicious symptoms include increase in surface area, increased prominence and darkening of color of a pigmented mole, possibly with a blackberry type of surface, formation of satellites in the neighboring tissue, or enlargement of the regional lymph nodes. *Clinical forms* include (a) superficial spreading melanoma ($\sim 45\%$), (b) malignant lentigo ($\sim 10\%$), (c) acrolentiginous malignant melanoma ($\sim 5\%$) which is rarely found on the head and neck, and (d) primary nodular malignant melanoma ($\sim 40\%$). The most unfavorable type is nodular melanoma, which grows deeply and metastasizes rapidly from the start, whereas superficial spreading melanoma, malignant lentigo, and acrolentiginous melanoma initially spread horizontally on the surface. The site is often the face, or scalp and head, or the ear and the neck. It is rare on the external nose, but more common on the anterior part of the septum. It then manifests itself by epistaxis, nasal obstruction, and formation of crusts. This tumor also may occur on the oral and pharyngeal mucosa.

Diagnosis. A dermatologic consultation is necessary. *Biopsy should be avoided* because this activates and spreads the tumor. Total removal with a wide margin of healthy tissue is indicated immediately on well-founded suspicion of malignant melanoma. Amelanotic melanomas also may occur. There are also numerous pigmented tumors which are not malignant melanoma, and an absolute diagnosis without biopsy therefore is very difficult.

Differential diagnosis. This includes juvenile melanoma, papilloma, telangiectatic granuloma, pigmented basal cell carcinoma, and blue nevus.

Note: Manipulation of a malignant melanoma should be avoided if at all possible, and immediate surgery is indicated.

Treatment. The mainstay of treatment is a rapid and extensive excision by three-dimensional surgery with a macroscopic margin of 5 cm, though this cannot always be obtained on the face. The margins should be checked by frozen section so that further resection can be undertaken if necessary. The defects should be reconstructed immediately by advancement flaps or free skin graft. Radical neck dissection is indicated, at least for the high-risk malignant melanoma on the head and neck. Its value, however, is controversial because of the occasional widespread rapid metastases. Supportive immunotherapy, chemotherapy, or endolymphatic radioisotope therapy by a dermatologist or radiotherapist may be helpful. Convincing benefit has not been shown from conventional radiotherapy, immunotherapy with bacillus Calmette-Guérin (BCG), and current chemotherapy.

Prognosis. This depends on early diagnosis and is determined by Clark's levels of growth depth and presence or absence of metastases. With adequate early operation in stage I, the 5-year survival rate is 70%, and in stage II, 30% to 40% lower. The poor prognosis depends less on the superficial extent of the lesion than on its total thickness, depth, and metastatic spread. A depth of extension of 0.76 mm marks the boundary between high- and low-risk malignant melanoma.

Nose and Nasal Sinuses

The most common tumors of the nasal cavity and nasal sinuses are *squamous cell carcinoma, adenoid cystic carcinoma,* and *adenocarcinoma.*

Mesenchymal tumors such as spindle cell sarcoma, round cell sarcoma, chondrosarcoma, osteosarcoma, and malignant lymphoma are rare. Malignancy arising within the nasal cavity or sinuses constitutes less than 1 % of all malignant tumors. Histologically, the relative incidence is as follows: squamous cell carcinoma, about 57 %; adenocarcinoma and similar forms, about 18 %; undifferentiated carcinomas, about 10 %; and mesenchymal tumors (malignant lymphoma, sarcoma, and melanoma), about 15 %.

In children, *histiocytosis X (eosinophilic granuloma)* and *rhabdomyosarcoma* are relatively common (see p. 134).

Site and extension of malignant tumors (see Color Plates **12d, 17c, d**). On clinical grounds, treatment and prognosis of tumors may be classified in relation to the three levels defined by Sébileau and in relation to Oehngren's plane (Fig. 2.**69a** and **b**). The prognosis worsens as the tumor passes from level I to level III. In a similar manner, tumors anterior to Oehngren's plane have a better prognosis (70% survival at 3 years) than those posterior to it (30% survival at 3 years). The direction of extension of these tumors, dependent on their site of origin, is shown in Figure 2.**70.** About 60% arise

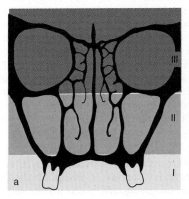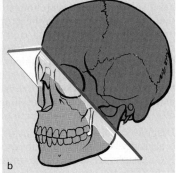

Fig. 2.**69a** and **b**   Tumor site. **(a)** Sébileau's levels; **(b)** Oehngren's plane.

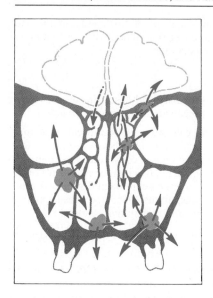

Fig. 2.**70** Typical directions of extension of tumors of the nose and sinuses.

from the antrum, 20% from the nasal cavity, 15% from the ethmoids, 4% from the nasal introitus, and about 1% from the frontal sphenoid and sinus.

Symptoms of malignant tumors of the nose or sinuses. Tumors of the nasal cavity are often clinically silent for a long period, and early diagnosis is therefore often difficult.

Suspicious symptoms, especially in persons over 50 years of age, include unilateral nasal obstruction, unilateral chronic nasal discharge, hemorrhagic nasal secretion, fetid secretion, loss of sensation of one of the branches of the trigeminal nerve, swelling of the cheek or of the medial canthus, pressure in the head or face, and a feeling of fullness in the nose. Marked headache only occurs in later stages when the tumor extends to the dura to cause pain resistant to treatment. Signs of invasion of neighboring tissue include restriction of eye movements, displacement of the eye or proptosis, swelling of the soft tissue of the medial canthus, the eyelids, the cheek, the palate, and the alveolus, loosening of the teeth, interference with mastication, cranial nerve palsies, epiphora, and regional lymphadenopathy.

Diagnosis. This rests on the history, and on inspection and palpation of the oral cavity, the nose, and the oropharynx. Endoscopy also may be used. Radiographs are taken of the sinuses and of the base of the skull in the axial view. These show a diffuse opacity destroying and obscuring the normal bony contour. CT scans are also obtained. The patient should be examined

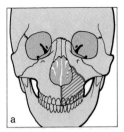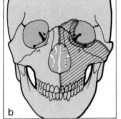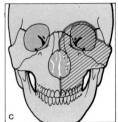

Fig. 2.**71a–c**   Resections of the upper jaw. (a) Partial resection, (b) total resection, (c) total resection with exenteration of the orbit.

by a neurologist and an ophthalmologist. If necessary, biopsy is taken after opening the suspect sinus. If invasion of the base of the skull is suspected, angiography should be carried out and the CSF examined. Regional lymph node metastases and distant metastases to the lung, skeleton, brain, and liver are looked for.

Differential diagnosis. This includes infection of the sinuses and its complications and benign tumors (see pp. 245, 289).

The *TNM system* is used for *staging* to determine treatment and prognosis and to allow recording and analysis of results (Table 2.**12**).

Principles of Treatment of Malignant Tumors of the Nose and Sinuses

Three methods of treatment are available: (1) operation, (2) radiotherapy, and (3) chemotherapy (cytostatic drugs, administered intraarterially if required).

In special situations, combinations of these three methods may be used.

Surgery. Three standard methods of removal of the tumor are used: (1) partial maxillectomy and, if necessary, resection of the frontal bone, (2) total maxillectomy, and (3) exenteration of the orbit combined with procedure (1) or (2). The principles are shown in Figure 2.**71a–c**. The operation is determined by the type, site, and size of the tumor.

The operation almost always needs to be extensive, and secondary reconstruction or provision of a prosthesis to cover both external and palatal defects therefore is necessary.

Only about 15% to 20% of these patients have a lymph node metastasis, and only 5% have a hematogenous metastasis. A radical neck dissection therefore is usually only carried out for palpable lymph node metastases or for certain other oncologic considerations.

Table 2.12 *TNM* System for the Upper Jaw and the Nose

External nose

T_1 = tumor 2 cm or less in its largest dimension, strictly superficial or exophytic

T_2 = tumor more than 2 cm but not more than 5 cm in its largest dimension or with minimal infiltration of the dermis, irrespective of size

T_3 = tumor more than 5 cm in its largest dimension or with deep infiltration of the dermis, irrespective of size

T_4 = tumor with extension to other structures such as cartilage, muscle or bone

The *nasal cavity* comprises the following areas:

1. Roof of the nose and superior turbinate
2. Lateral and nasal wall with the middle and lower turbinate
3. Nasal septum
4. Floor of the nose

The *superior sinuses* comprises the following areas:

1. Frontal sinus
2. Ethmoid sinus
3. Sphenoid sinus
4. Maxillo-ethmoid angle

T_1 = tumor affecting one area

T_2 = tumor affecting one region

T_3 = tumor extending beyond the boundaries of one region

T_4 = tumor affecting more than one neighboring region or extending beyond the limits of the organ to affect the skin, base of the skull, the nasopharynx, etc.

The *maxillary antrum* comprises the following areas:

1. Superior
2. Inferior
3. Medial
4. Lateral

The neighboring regions include:

Oral cavity with palate
Orbit

N = regional lymph node metastases
(see p. 511)

N_0 = none

N_1 = mobile homolateral nodes

N_2 = mobile contralateral or bilateral nodes

N_3 = fixed nodes

M = distant metastases

M_0 = none

M_1 = present

Staging (see also Fig. 6.**18**)

Stage I	T_1		N_0	M_0
Stage II	T_2		N_0	M_0
Stage III	T_3 or T_4		N_0	M_0
	Any T		N_1 or N_2	M_0
Stage IV	Any T		N_3	M_0
	Any T		Any N	M_1

Radiotherapy. This *may* bis used alone or before or after surgery. The survival rate for radiotherapy alone for squamous carcinoma of the nasal cavity and the sinuses is not as good as that for surgery, depending on the stage and site of the disease. Radiotherapy usually is reserved, therefore, for very radiosensitive tumors, e. g., mesenchymal tumors, and for inoperable tumors. For all other tumors, a *combination of surgery and radiotherapy,* possibly supplemented by chemotherapy, is preferred. As a rule, the operation should precede the radiotherapy, but preoperative radiotherapy may also be used, particularly for very large tumors. Sandwich treatment, half the dose of radiotherapy, then surgery, and then the second half of the radiotherapy, is also practiced. Radiotherapy is usually administered by cobalt 60 or supervoltage therapy (e. g., the Betatron) to deliver a tumor dose of 6,000 rads (60 Gy). Radiotherapy may be the treatment of choice for certain *small* tumors of the *external* nose *without* invasion of the skeleton.

Chemotherapy. At present, chemotherapy still has no established role as a primary treatment for epithelial malignancies of the face, nose, and sinuses, especially with regard to long-term results. It is useful for the palliative treatment of inoperable tumors, however.

Prognosis. With suitable treatment, 5-year survival rates of 30% to 40% may be achieved. This is only on overall figure, and it may be more or less, depending on numerous oncologic factors.

3. Mouth and Pharynx

Applied Anatomy and Physiology

Basic Anatomy

Oral Cavity

The oral cavity is bounded anteriorly by the lips, posteriorly by the anterior faucial arch, inferiorly by the floor of the mouth, and superiorly by the hard and soft palates. It is continuous with the oropharynx through the anterior faucial arch (Fig. 3.1). The faucial arch and the base of the tongue form the *faucial isthmus*. The oral cavity is divided into two parts by the upper and lower alveolar process and the teeth: first, the *vestibule of the mouth* lying between the lip and cheek on one side and the teeth and the alveolar process on the other and second, the *oral cavity proper* limited externally by the alveolar process and the teeth.

The *vestibule of the mouth* communicates directly with the oral cavity proper on both sides, even when the teeth are in apposition, between the ascending ramus of the mandible and the last molar tooth.

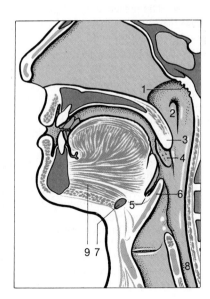

Fig. 3.1 Anatomy of the mouth and pharynx. 1, Roof of the nasopharynx; 2, ostium of the eustachian tube; 3, soft palate; 4, palatal tonsil; 5, vallecula; 6, epiglottis; 7, hyoid bone; 8, hypopharynx; 9, floor of the mouth.

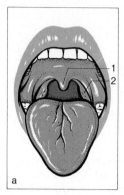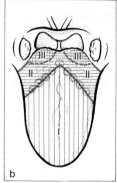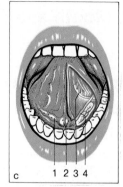

Fig. 3.**2a–c**   Tongue. **a.**From above. 1, Uvula; 2, palatine tonsils. **b.** Sensory innervation. I, Lingual nerve with chorda tympani; II, glossopharyngeal nerve; III, vagus nerve. **c.** Lower surface of tongue and floor of the mouth. 1, Plica sublingualis; 2, sublingual caruncle; 3, lingual nerve; 4, submandibular duct.

This is of practical importance, e. g., in intermaxillary wiring, because the patient can take a fluid diet making use of this communication, even when the teeth are fixed in occlusion.

The *tongue* fills the oral cavity almost completely when the mouth is closed. The presence of a slight negative pressure in the oral cavity ensures that the tongue adheres to the hard and soft palate, thus maintaining closure of the mouth.

The following parts of the tongue are distinguished: the *tip*, the *margins*, the *body*, the *base*, the *dorsum*, and the *ventral surface* (Fig. 3.**2a–c**).

The dorsum of the tongue is covered by a modified epithelium containing the filiform papillae at the tip, the fungiform papillae at the tip and margins, the foliate papillae on the posterolateral part of the tongue, and the vallate papillae on the dorsum. The boundary between the body of the tongue and the base of the tongue is formed by the V-shaped *terminal sulcus* whose central point is the foramen cecum, a remnant of the thyroglossal duct.

The base of the tongue contains the *lingual tonsil* which may be the site of inflammation and abscess due to an impacted foreign body and which may also cause mechanical difficulty in swallowing when it is hypertrophic. The base of the tongue is limited inferiorly by the edge of the *epiglottis*. The two valleculae lie in the angle between the epiglottis and the base of the tongue. On occasion they may be difficult to inspect, and they may also be the site of cysts, foreign bodies, and malignant tumors. In supine unconscious patients or patients under general anesthesia, the base of the tongue may fall backward to occlude the entrance to the larynx, and together with the epiglottis may lead to respiratory obstruction. This is pre-

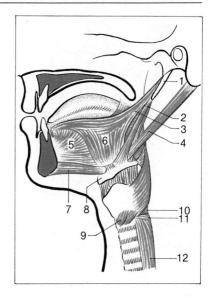

Fig. 3.3 Muscles of the tongue and pharynx. 1, Styloid process; 2, stylohyoid muscle; 3, styloglossus muscle; 4, digastric muscle; 5, genioglossus muscle; 6, hyoglossus muscle; 7, geniohyoid muscle; 8, hyoid bone; 9, cricothyroid muscle; 10, Killian's triangle; 11, inferior part of the cricopharyngeus; 12, esophagus.

vented by pulling the tongue forward and by introduction of an oropharyngeal airway.

The arrangement of the musculature of the tongue provides it with extreme mobility. Two groups of muscles may be distinguished: first, those without any bony attachments running free in the body of the tongue, i. e., the transverse, the superior, the inferior longitudinal muscles, and the vertical muscles; and second, those muscles that are attached to fixed points, i. e., the styloglossus, the genioglossus, the hyoglossus, and the palatoglossus muscles (Fig. 3.3; see Fig. 3.15a und b).

The *floor of the mouth* is formed mainly by the mylohyoid muscle which is stretched between the U-shaped mandible like a diaphragm and which is inserted into the hyoid bone and the median raphe. On the *oral surface,* with the tip of the tongue elevated, the plica sublingualis with the sublingual caruncle may be found on both sides of the *lingual frenulum* (see Fig. 3.2c).

In the caruncle and the immediate neighborhood lie the efferent ducts of the submandibular gland, the submandibular duct (Wharton's duct), and the sublingual gland and sublingual duct (Bartholin's duct). The efferent duct of the parotid gland (Stensen's duct) opens into the cheek at the level of the second upper molar and that of the anterior lingual gland (Blandin's gland) in the region of the fimbriated fold on the ventral surface of the tongue (see Fig. 3.2c).

The *mandible* consists of two separate bones at birth, but these consolidate to form *one* bone within the 1st year of life. Figure 3.4a shows the most

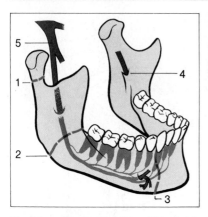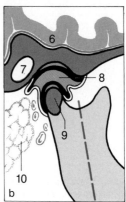

Fig. 3.**4a** and **b.**   **a.** Mandible with typical fracture lines. 1, Fracture of the neck; 2, fracture of the angle of the jaw; 3, fracture of the chin; 4, mandibular foramen; 5, mandibular nerve. **b.** Temporomandibular joint and surrounding structures. 6, Middle cranial fossa; 7, external auditory meatus; 8, articular disc; 9, head of the mandible; 10, parotid gland.

important anatomic details and the typical sites of fracture. The third branch of the trigeminal nerve runs in the body of the mandible, together with the blood vessels that supply the lower teeth. The mandibular nerve enters the mandible at the mandibular foramen and leaves it at the mental foramen.

The *temporomandibular joint* is of great clinical interest since it may be involved in dental diseases, in trauma of the facial skeleton and skull, in otologic diseases, and also in generalized arthropathies. Furthermore, it may be the cause of headache in Costen's syndrome. Figure 3.**4b** shows the anatomic relationships. The proximity to the auditory meatus and mastoid, the lateral part of the base of the skull, the parotid gland, and the lateral wall of the oropharynx and nasopharynx should be noted. The causes of trismus are given in Table 3.**6**.

The *epithelial lining of the oral cavity* consists of nonkeratinized stratified squamous epithelium which is thickened in certain points such as the alveolar edges and hard palate where it is united with the underlying periosteum to form a mucoperiosteum. Subepithelial collections of minor salivary glands are found all over the oral cavity, being more common at some parts than at others (see Fig. 7.**2**).

Vascular supply. The external carotid artery supplies the tongue via the lingual artery, the floor of the mouth via the sublingual artery, the cheek via the facial artery, and the palate via the ascending pharyngeal and descending palatine arteries. The latter arises from the internal maxillary artery. The *venous drainage* runs via the veins of the same names to the facial vein, the pterygoid venous plexus, and the

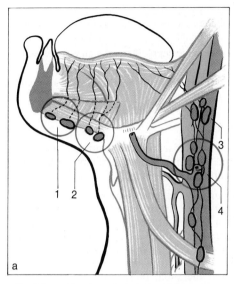
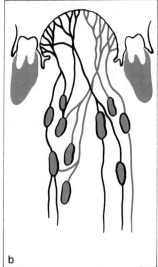

Fig. 3.**5a** and **b**.   Lymph drainage of the tongue. **a.** Groups of lymph nodes. 1, Submental; 2, submandibular; 3, upper deep cervical with lymph nodes at the superior venous angle (4). **b.** Contralateral lymphatic drainage of the tongue.

internal jugular vein. There is also a connection to the cavernous sinuses via the pterygoid plexus.

The *lymph drains* via the regional submental, submandibular, and parotid nodes to the internal jugular chain. The lymph drainage of the base of the tongue and the floor of the mouth is to the same side *and* to the opposite side (Fig. 3.**5a** and **b**). This fact is important in the formation of contralateral lymph node metastases (see pp. 484, 511 ff.).

Nerve supply. The *tongue* derives its *motor* supply from the hypoglossal nerve. Its *sensory* supply comes from the lingual nerve and the vagus nerve, which innervates the posterior part of the base of the tongue. Taste fibers come from the glossopharyngeal nerve to the base of the tongue and from the chorda tympani fibers of the VIIth cranial nerve accompanying the lingual nerve for the anterior two-thirds of the tongue (see Fig. 3.**2a** and **b**).

The *floor of the mouth* derives its *motor* supply from the mylohyoid branch of the mandibular nerve and its *sensory* supply from the trigeminal nerve. Parasympathetic secretory fibers from the salivary glands are supplied from the chorda tympani and branches of the submandibular ganglion. Sympathetic fibers for blood vessels of the glands come from the carotid plexus.

The *masticatory muscles* derive their motor supply from the mandibular branch of the trigeminal nerve, but the buccinator muscle gets its supply from the facial nerve.

The teeth of the upper jaw receive their sensory supply from the maxillary nerve and those of the lower jaw from the mandibular. These are both branches of the Vth cranial nerve.

The *temporomandibular joint* derives its nerve supply from the auriculotemporal branch of the mandibular nerve.

The *soft palate* derives its motor innervation from the glossopharyngeal, vagus, and trigeminal nerves, and probably the facial nerve also.

Naso-, Oro-, and Hypopharynx

The pharynx is a 12 to 13 cm long muscular tube in the adult; it narrows from above downward, is covered with mucosa, and is divided into *three compartments* each of which has an anterior opening (Fig. 3.**6**).

The *nasopharynx* is limited superiorly by the base of the skull, inferiorly by an imaginary plane through the soft palate, and it opens into the nasal cavity (see Color Plate **24b**). The most important anatomic *structures* are as follows: anteriorly the choanae, superiorly the floor of the sphenoid sinus, posterosuperiorly the adenoid, laterally the pharyngeal ostium of the eustachian tube and the cartilaginous torus tubarius immediately posterior to which is Rosenmueller's fossa and the tubal tonsil, and anteriorly and inferiorly the soft palate. The embryonic *pharyngeal bursa* (see Fig. 3.**7**) may persist in the posterior wall of the nasopharynx causing chronic

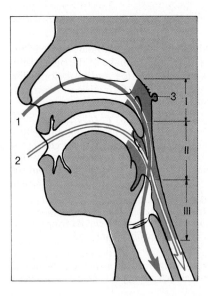

Fig. 3.**6** Divisions of the pharynx. I, Nasopharynx; II, oropharynx; III, hypopharynx. Crossing of the upper airway (1) and the upper food passage (2). Site of the pharyngeal bursa (3).

inflammation and retention of secretions. The posterior wall of the naso-pharynx is separated from the spinal column by the tough prevertebral fascia which lies on the longus capitis muscles, the deep muscles of the neck, and the arch of the first cervical vertebra.

The shape and width of the nasopharynx show marked individual varia-tion. The *epithelial lining* is respiratory ciliated and stratified squamous epithelium, with transitional epithelium at the junction with the oropha-rynx.

The *oropharynx* extends from the horizontal plane through the soft palate described above to the superior edge of the epiglottis (see Fig. 3.7) and is continuous with the oral cavity through the faucial isthmus. It contains the following important *structures:* the posterior wall consisting of the pre-vertebral fascia and the bodies of the second and third cervical vertebrae, the lateral wall containing the palatine tonsil with the anterior and poste-rior faucial pillars, and the supratonsillar fossa lying above the tonsil between the anterior and posterior faucial arches.

The valleculae (see Fig. 3.1), the base of the tongue, the anterior surface of the soft palate, and the lingual surface of the epiglottis are usually described as being part of the oropharynx.

The *epithelial lining* consists of nonkeratinizing stratified squamous epithelium.

The *hypopharynx* extends from the upper edge of the epiglottis superiorly to the inferior edge of the cricoid cartilage (see Fig. 3.6). It opens anteri-orly into the larynx. On each side of the larynx lie the funnel-shaped piri-form sinuses. Important anatomic *structures* and relations include: on the anterior wall the marginal structures of the laryngeal inlet and the poste-rior surface of the larynx; on the lateral wall the inferior constrictor mus-cle and the piriform sinus, the latter being bounded medially by the ary-epiglottic fold and laterally by the internal surface of the thyroid cartilage and the thyrohyoid membrane. Immediate relationships of the hypopha-rynx at the level of the larynx include the common carotid artery, the inter-nal jugular vein, and the vagus nerve. Relations of the posterior wall, apart from the pharyngeal constrictor muscle (see below), include the preverte-bral fascia and the bodies of the third to the sixth cervical vertebrae. Inferi-orly the hypopharynx opens into the esophagus, the boundary being the superior sphincter of the esophagus. The *epithelial lining* consists of nonke-ratinized stratified squamous epithelium.

The muscular tube of the entire pharynx consists of two layers with different func-tions:

1. A circular muscle layer consisting of the three pharyngeal constrictor muscles: the superior constrictor inserted into the base of the skull, the middle constrictor inserted into the hyoid bone, and the inferior constrictor inserted into the cricoid cartilage (see Fig. 3.3; Fig. 3.7). Each of these funnel-shaped muscular segments is

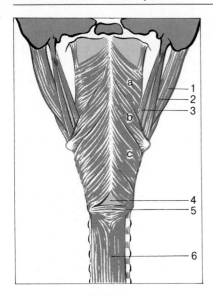

Fig. 3.7 Pharyngeal musculature. (a) Superior constrictor, (b) middle constrictor, (c) inferior constrictor. 1, Digastric muscle; 2, stylohyoid muscle; 3, stylopharyngeus muscle; 4, Killian's triangle; 5, inferior part of the cricopharyngeus muscle; 6, esophagus.

overlapped at its lower end by the segment below. All segments are inserted posteriorly into a tendinous median raphe.

The inferior constrictor muscle is of particular clinical importance. It is divided into a superior thyropharyngeal part and an inferior cricopharyngeal part. Figure 3.7 shows how the triangular dehiscence *(Killian's triangle)* is formed from the posterior wall of the hypopharynx between the superior oblique and the inferior horizontal fibers. A pharyngoesophageal pouch (Zenker's diverticulum) may develop at this weak point in the hypopharyngeal wall.

2. The raising and lowering of the pharynx is also achieved by three paired muscles radiating into the pharyngeal wall from outside. These are the stylopharyngeus, the salpingopharyngeus, and the palatopharyngeus muscles. The stylohyoid and styloglossus muscles are also responsible for elevation. A true longitudinal muscle does not occur in the pharynx and only begins at the mouth of the esophagus. The ability of the pharynx to slide over a distance of several centimeters is due to the existence of fascial spaces (parapharyngeal and retropharyngeal) filled with loose connective tissue (see p. 475). The significance of these tissue spaces in the spread of infection is described on p. 476 and in Figure 3.**17a** und **b**.

Vascular supply of the pharynx. The *arterial supply* is provided by the ascending pharyngeal artery, the ascending palatine artery, the tonsillar branches of the facial artery, branches of the maxillary artery, i.e., the descending palatine artery, and branches of the lingual artery. All these arise from the external carotid artery. The *venous drainage* is via the facial vein and the pterygoid plexus to the internal jugular vein.

The *lymphatic drainage* is either via an inconstant retropharyngeal lymph node and then to the deep jugular lymph nodes or directly to the latter group. The inferior part of the pharynx also drains to the paratracheal lymph nodes, and thus gains a connection to the lymphatic system of the thorax. See also p. 484.

Nerve supply of the pharynx. The individual pharyngeal muscles gain their motor supply from the glossopharyngeal, vagus, hypoglossal, and facial nerves. The nasopharynx derives its sensory nerve supply from the maxillary division of the trigeminal nerve, the oropharynx from the glossopharyngeal nerve, and the hypopharynx from the vagus nerve (see p. 487).

Lymphoepithelial System of the Pharynx

Note: The term lymphoepithelial tissue is used to indicate a close symbiosis of epithelial and lymphatic cells on the surface of a mucosa.

The epithelial and subepithelial tissue is loosely arranged so that lymphatic cells can enter it in large numbers ("reticulated epithelium"). The reticulohistiocytic system (RHS), more commonly named reticulo-endothelial system (RES), with its storage cells is strongly represented in lymphoepithelial tissue. Figure 3.**8** shows the principle of a lymphoepithelial unit. Solitary units of this type, solitary follicles, are found in all parts of the mucosa. The epithelium is also diffusely interspersed with lymphocytes.

A very pronounced collection of lymphoepithelial tissue, *Waldeyer's ring,* lies at the opening of the upper aerodigestive tracts. These *lymphoepithelial organs* are called *tonsils.* From above downward, the following may be distinguished:

1. The *pharyngeal tonsil,* the adenoids, which is single and lies on the roof and posterior wall of the nasopharynx
2. The *tubal tonsil,* which is paired and lies around the ostium of the eustachian tube in Rosenmueller's fossa
3. The paired *palatine tonsil,* lying between the anterior and posterior faucial pillars
4. The *lingual tonsil,* which is single and lies in the base of the tongue. Less constant and obvious are:
5. The *tubopharyngeal plicae,* lateral bands, which run almost vertically at the junction of the lateral and posterior walls of the oro- and nasopharynx
6. Lymphoepithelial collections in the laryngeal ventricle

Unlike lymph nodes, lymphoepithelial organs possess only efferent lymph vessels and do *not* have afferent vessels. The difference in pathology and

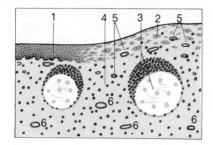

Fig. 3.**8** Lymphoepithelial   tissue. 1, Continuous squamous epithelium; 2, reticular epithelium; 3, secondary nodes with light centers and dark zone of small lymphocytes; 4, basic lymphoid tissue; 5, arterioles and venules; 6, postcapillary veins.

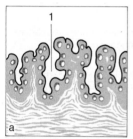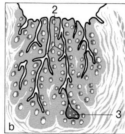

Fig. 3.**9a** and **b** Diagram of **(a)** the nasopharyngeal tonsil, the adenoids and **(b)** the palatine tonsil. 1, Tonsillar lacunae; 2, tonsillar crypts; 3, cryptic abscess.

physiology of the individual collection of lymphoid tissue rests on their different structure. Figure 3.**9a** and **b** shows the structure of a *palatine tonsil* and of the *adenoids*.

The fine structure of a *tonsil* (see Figs. 3.**8** and 3.**9a** and **b**) is in principle as follows: the soft tissue lamellae or septae arise from a basal connective tissue capsule. These serve as a supporting framework in which blood vessels, lymphatics, and nerves run. This fan-shaped supporting framework considerably increases the active surface of the tonsil since it carries the actual lymphoepithelial parenchyma. It is estimated that the epithelial surface of one palatine tonsil amounts to 300 cm². In the *palatine tonsil* the active surface is sunk within the mucosa, whereas in the *adenoids* it projects above the surface. The broad flat niches opening into the oral cavity caused by infolding are called *lacunae;* the branching clefts running throughout the entire substance of the tonsil are called *crypts.* The actual tonsil tissue consists of a collection of a very large number of the lymphoepithelial units described above (see Fig. 3.**8**). The crypts usually contain cell debris and round cells, but may also contain bacteria and colonies of fungi, collections of pus, and encapsulated microabscesses. (See p. 350 for the description of chronic tonsillitis.)

The tonsils of Waldeyer's ring are present at the embryonal stage, but they only acquire their typical structure with secondary nodes in the postnatal period, i.e., after direct contact with environmental pathogens. They begin increasing rapidly in size between the 1st and the 3rd year of life, with peaks in the 3rd and 7th year.

They involute slowly as of early puberty. Like the rest of the lymphatic system, they atrophy with increasing age.

The *arterial* blood supply of the pharyngeal tonsil is provided by various branches of the external carotid artery including the facial artery and/or the ascending palatine artery, the ascending pharyngeal and lingual arteries, and possibly direct tonsillar branches.

The *veins* of the pharyngeal tonsil usually drain via the palatal vein to the facial vein and from there to the jugulofacial venous angle of the internal jugular vein. There is also drainage via the pterygoid venous plexus to the internal jugular vein. This route provides a possible pathway of spread for infection from the tonsils to the cavernous sinus (see Figs. 3.**17a** und **b** and 3.**19**).

Physiologic and Pathophysiologic Principles

Several functional systems are collected in the mouth and pharynx including the masticatory system, the swallowing apparatus, the taste organs, the lymphoepithelial ring, pregastric digestion, and articulation. Furthermore, the respiratory and digestive tracts cross in this area (see Fig. 3.**6**). This requires a reliable reflex protective system. An important prerequisite is a well-functioning autonomic and voluntary nervous supply to this region, and also a mucosa adapted to this double function. The mouth is only involved in respiration as a *supplementary measure* (see p. 182): continuous mouth breathing causes considerable local damage and can also affect the entire body (see p. 321). Typical functional disturbances due to defects of the nervous supply are summarized in Table 3.7.

Eating, Preparation of Food, and Swallowing

Normal *feeding* requires a normal masticatory apparatus and teeth, masticatory muscles, and temporomandibular joint. The function of the cranial nerves must also be normal (see Table 3.7). The *preparation of the food* serves to reduce the size of the bolus of food by chewing, and also to moisten the food with saliva of which 1 to 1.5 liters are produced daily. The saliva lubricates the mucosa and makes the food capable of being swallowed. Furthermore, the enzymes contained in saliva (see Table 7.**3**) prepare the food by partial chemical decomposition for further digestion in the gastrointestinal tract.

The results of quantitative or qualitative defects of saliva are summarized on p. 535. Satisfactory moistening of the mucosa of the oral cavity and pharynx by saliva is also necessary for normal speech and for normal taste (see discussion of salivary function on p. 533).

The stages of the *swallowing act* are as follows (see also p. 458):

1. Displacement of the food bolus posteriorly by pressure of the tongue on the hard palate and gliding deformation of the body of the tongue.
2. Stimulation of the swallowing reflex as soon as the bolus reaches the base of the tongue. All openings not connected to the digestive tract are closed off:
   a. The nasopharynx is closed off by posterosuperior elevation of the soft palate.
   b. The larynx is drawn upward and anteriorly under the base of the tongue by muscle traction. The epiglottis lies over the laryngeal inlet.
   c. Reflex closure of the vocal cords occurs in the same phase. The bolus of food slides past the laryngeal inlet through the two piriform sinuses.
   d. When the bolus enters the hypopharynx the esophageal orifice opens. The bolus is further transported in the esophagus by serial contraction of the individual portions of the pharyngeal constrictor muscles.
   e. Autonomic peristalsis of the longitudinal and circular muscles then transports the bolus through the esophagus to the lower sphincter (the cardia) and to the stomach.

Primary, secondary, and tertiary peristalsis may be distinguished in the esophagus. Primary peristalsis is induced automatically by the swallowing act. Secondary peristalsis comes into effect when the esophageal wall is stretched by retention of food. Tertiary peristalsis is a concomitant symptom of an organic esophageal disorder, e.g., idiopathic esophageal spasm, presbyesophagus, etc. The peristaltic wave does not move in this case but is stationary.

The nervous pathways of swallowing are as follows:

Afferent pathways are supplied by the second division of the Vth, the IXth, and the Xth cranial nerves.

The center is in the medulla oblongata.

The efferent pathways are the Xth, IXth, and XIIth cranial nerves.

The pharyngeal and esophageal phases are not under voluntary control.

Pathophysiologic aspects. The closure of the laryngeal inlet by the epiglottis is not strictly necessary for normal swallowing. A patient whose epiglottis has been removed, e.g., in an operation for a tumor, usually learns to swallow without difficulty. However, the sensory nerve supply of the hypopharynx and the laryngeal inlet from the superior laryngeal branch of the vagus nerve must be intact as well as the pharyngeal constrictor for reflex protection of the laryngeal inlet. Increased tone or spasm of the cricopharyngeus is a common autonomic disorder, e.g., in thyrotoxicosis or the Plummer-Vinson syndrome. This can be the cause of the *globus* symptom of discomfort on swallowing at the level of the cricoid cartilage, of true *dysphagia* (see Table 3.7), and possibly of the development of a *hypopharyngeal diverticulum*.

Disturbances of swallowing may also occur in paralyses of one or more cranial nerves, especially the Xth but also the IXth and the XIIth, which affect the tongue, the soft palate, or the pharyngeal musculature.

Taste

The basic taste sensations are *sweet, salty, sour,* and *bitter.* All other tastes are mixed sensations in which the sense of smell is also integrated. Many foods are "tasted" by the olfactory nerve! Pure sensory nerve fibers to the tongue and oral mucosa may also be stimulated by sour or spicy foods.

The sensory organs for taste are the taste buds lying in the vallate papillae, foliate papillae, and fungiform papillae on the tongue and also on the hard palate, the anterior faucial pillar, the tonsil, the posterior pharyngal wall, the esophageal orifice, and the buccal mucosa. The fine gustatory hair cells must be bathed in saliva or other fluids to allow the sense of taste to be evoked. Figure 3.**10** shows the topical arrangement on the tongue of the sites where the different taste qualities are recognized. The sensory nerve supply is provided peripherally by two nerves in particular: the chorda tympani, arising from the VIIth cranial nerve, and accompanying the lingual nerve from the Vth cranial nerve, and the glossopharyngeal nerve, arising from the IXth cranial nerve.

The boundary of the area supplied by each individual nerve in the mouth and pharynx is still not fully agreed upon, but the following is generally accepted (see Fig. 1.**20**). The anterior half of the tongue is supplied by the ipsilateral chorda tympani via the nervus intermedius with synapse in the sensory geniculate ganglion. The posterior third of the tongue and the walls of the oral pharynx receive their sensory supply from the glossopharyngeal nerve. It is probable that the vagus nerve also has sensory contributions to the epiglottis, the laryngeal additus, the upper part of the esophagus, and possibly also a small part of the center of the base of the tongue. Gustatory sensations from the soft palate are transmitted by the palatine nerves via the pterygopalatine ganglion, the greater petrosal nerve, the geniculate ganglion, and the nervus intermedius to the medulla oblongata.

The boundary between the area supplied by the lingual nerve and the accompanying chorda tympani and the glossopharyngeal nerve is still not generally agreed upon.

Reflex reactions may affect the sense of taste as they do the sense of smell. These include: alterations in quantity and quality of salivary secretion, the

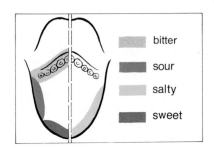

bitter

sour

salty

sweet

Fig. 3.**10**   Distribution of the qualities of taste on the tongue.

production of gastric juice, and interference with the course of the swallowing act.

Basic Pathophysiology

Classification of Disorders of Taste

Hypogeusia indicates reduced sensitivity, e. g., due to radiotherapy or in presbygeusia.

Hypergeusia is increased sensitivity and occurs, e. g., in glossopharyngeal neuralgia.

Ageusia is absence of the sense of taste. It may be *partial* due to a lesion of the chorda tympani, *total* due to toxins, or *selective* as in "taste blindness" for certain substances.

Parageusia is faulty taste and may be due to virus infection.

Cacogeusia is an unpleasant taste occurring typically in cerebral sclerosis.

In addition, *gustatory hallucinations* may occur, due to drug abuse, psychoses, and disorders of the central nervous system.

Disorders of taste occur more commonly than is generally thought. Apart from direct, accidental, inflammatory, viral, or iatrogenic causes, they may also be due to *neural lesions,* to certain *drugs* (see below), to *endocrine diseases,* and to *deficiency diseases.* They may vary in degree and involve different qualities of taste (see Table 3.1). Usually the threshold is increased, i. e., the gustatory function is reduced. Reduction of the threshold is rare but may occur in mucoviscidosis. The relation of the four senses of taste to each other may be disassociated.

Drugs with side effects on the *sense of taste* include: acetylsalicylic acid, biguanidine, carbamazepine, levodopa, ethambutal, gold, griseofulvin, lithium, methylthiouracil, oxyfedren, penicillamine, and phenylbutazone. Side effects may also occur after *local* use of ether oils, chlorhexine, and hexetidine.

Immune-Specific Functions of Waldeyer's Ring

There is now no doubt about the immune-specific function of the various lympho-epithelial organs in Waldeyer's ring and in the solitary nodes in the mucosa. Experimentally it can be shown that appropriate foreign material (also antigenic substances) in the tonsillar crypts can penetrate the reticular epithelium to reach the tonsillar parenchyma. Cellular material, including lymphocytes, segmental nuclear leukocytes, and cell debris, on the other hand, are shed in relatively large amounts from the tonsillar parenchyma and reticular epithelium into the lumen of the crypts and pass from here into the mouth. It is estimated that one hundred million round cells are shed by *one* tonsil daily into the digestive tract in this way. The specific function of the round cells passing in this way from the tonsil into the cavity is not known with certainty. They are probably intended to protect the internal surface of the body. The lymphoepithelial organs also produce immunoactive lymphocytes of the B and T series which are released into the general circulation of the blood and lymphatic vessels as from all other lymphatic organs.

Table 3.1 Disturbances of Taste

Classification	Cause
Congenital, hereditary disorders	Aplasia of the taste buds in familiar dysautonomy, "taste blindness"
Local lesions	Mucosal atrophy of the mouth and pharynx, may accompany atrophic rhinitis, glossitis, stomatitis, thrush, Sjögren's disease
Exogenous chemical toxins	Damage to the sensory endings by alcohol, nicotine, smoking, mouthwashes, acids, lyes, solutes, plant poisons Damage to the peripheral nerves by arsenic compounds, carbon disulfide, tetrachloroethane, tetrachlorocarbons Damage to the central olfactory pathway by carbon monoxide
Drug toxicity	See p. 312
Peripheral nerve lesions	Chorda tympani lesions in facial paralysis, otitis media, ear operations and injury to the lingual nerve Glossopharyngeal nerve lesions in tumors and lesions of the base of the skull, and neuralgias. After tonsillectomy very rare.
Central taste disorders	Carbon monoxide poisoning, cerebral contusion, cerebral cortical disease, cerebral arteriosclerosis, progressive paralysis
Endocrine disorders	Pregnancy, diabetes mellitus, hypothyroidism, adrenal insufficiency
Miscellaneous	Radiotherapy and chemical or mechanical damage by dentures, deficiency of zinc and copper and deficiencies of vitamins A and B_2

The present knowledge of the *function of the tonsils* may be summarized as follows:

1. The tonsils ensure controlled and protected contact of the organism with the pathogenic and antigenic environment serving the purpose of immunologic surveillance. This allows adaptation to the environment, especially in children.

2. The tonsils produce lymphocytes.

3. The tonsils expose B- and T-lymphocytes to current antigens and are instrumental in the production of specific messenger lymphocytes and memory lymphocytes.

4. The tonsils produce specific antibodies after the production of the appropriate plasma cells. All types of immunoglobulins occur in tonsillar tissue.

5. The tonsils shed topical immune-stimulated lymphocytes for both humoral and cell-mediated immunity into the oral cavity and the digestive tract.

6. The tonsils are instrumental in the production and discharge of immunoactive lymphocytes into the blood and lymphatic circulation. The information from this part of the immune system (the spleen and the lymph nodes) provides information about the present antigen situation at the beginning of the internal surface of the body ("subclinical immunity").

Basic pathophysiology. The increase of the lymphoepithelial tissue during the early years of childhood development is explained by the immunobiologic requirements. This increase of size is primarily only an expression of an active defensive function of the infantile organism to antigenic substances in the environment. *Tonsillar hyperplasia* at this period is therefore a welcome attribute and is in no way a demonstration of excess inflammation. Since the tonsils lie at a narrow point of the respiratory and digestive tract, the nasopharynx and the faucial isthmus, an increase of their volume *beyond a certain point* leads to increased narrowing of the diameter of this essential pathway, to the detriment of the rest of the body (Fig. 3.**11a** and **b**). Obstructive sleep apnea may develop in extreme cases. Removal of the tonsils and adenoids in this circumstance is therefore justified despite possible immunologic disadvantages. The *palatine tonsils alone* possess slitlike, branching, poorly drained *crypts* permeating their entire substance. As long as these clefts drain freely into the oral cavity, the function of the tonsil is not endangered. However, if the physiologic content of the crypt stagnates due to anatomic or infective stenosis, an ideal culture medium is set up for microorganisms. Colonies of bacteria or fungi are established leading to chronic suppuration (cryptitis), small abscesses in the crypts, and superficial ulceration of the surface of the crypts – that is, pathologic-

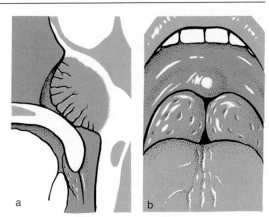

Fig. 3.**11a** and **b.**
Obstruction of the
nasopharynx by hyper-
trophied adenoid **(a)**
and of the oropharynx
by hypertrophied
palatine tonsil **(b)**.

anatomically speaking, a *chronic tonsillitis*. This is in no way related to the
size of the tonsil. Figure 3.**8** shows how the superficial tonsillar capillaries
are unprotected and run close to the lumen of the crypt, allowing relatively
unhindered access of infective or toxic contents to the general circulation.

Formation of Sound and Speech

The oral cavity and pharynx make an important contribution to the timbre
of the speech and voice because of their action as a variable resonating
space. Furthermore, the tongue, in conjunction with the palate, is necessary for the formation of consonants and vowels. Despite that, experience
of tumor surgery shows that large parts of the tongue may be removed and
yet comprehensible speech is retained.

Methods of Investigation

Inspection, Palpation, and Examination with the Mirror

Examination is carried out with good illumination from the head mirror or
head lamp using two tongue depressors (see Fig. 2.**14b** and **c**; Figs. 3.**12** and
3.**13**). The following should be observed:

- The color and the normal symmetrical mobility of the lips, the condition of the skin and mucosa, and changes in the surface, ulcerations,
  induration, and tenderness of the lips are looked for.

- The arrangement of the teeth and the occlusion are examined with the lips open, the symmetry of the contour of the jaws, the mobility of the mandible, and the function of the temporomandibular joint are also examined.
- The shape and mobility of the tongue is examined with the mouth open. In a hypoglossal paresis, the tongue deviates slightly to the *paralyzed* side. The floor of the mouth and the two caruncles are examined, using a tongue depressor, with the tongue elevated. The surface and consistency of the tongue and articulation are also assessed.
- The properties of the mucosa of the mouth and cheeks are assessed, with particular attention to color, moisture, dryness, membranes, ulceration, tumors, and disorders of sensation.
- The condition of the hard and soft palate is examined. The innervation of the two sides is compared. The uvula deviates to the *sound* side in paralysis of the palate. The innervation of the pharyngeal musculature is tested.
- The upper and lower vestibule of the oral cavity are examined with a tongue depressor.
- The parotid duct in the cheek opposite the upper second molar tooth is inspected.
- The palatine tonsils, the lingual tonsil, and the mucosa of the posterior wall of the pharynx are examined using two tongue depressors (see Fig. 3.**13**). Normally these structures should be pale yellow to pale pink, moist, and shiny. Dryness, coating, glazed crusts, and yellow streams of pus may be noted.

Examination of the tonsils. A tongue depressor is laid *carefully* with the left hand on the lateral part of the posterior part of the tongue, and the tongue is pressed gently downward. The spatula should not be placed on the base of the tongue since this elicits the gag reflex. As soon as the tonsillar cleft can be seen, the other hand is used to introduce the second tongue depressor between the ascending ramus of the mandible and the tonsil, and the edge of the tongue depressor is placed gently on the anterior faucial pillar lateral to the tonsil to dislocate it from its fossa into the oral cavity. An attempt is made to press material out of the visible crypt opening. The size of the tonsil and its connective tissue fixation to the tonsillar fossa, the color and properties of the surrounding mucosa on the faucial pillars, and the color and properties of the surface of the tonsil including any exudate and the expressed contents of the crypt are noted. Differences between the two sides are also looked for. *Palpation of the lymph nodes* now follows, paying particular attention to the nodes at the angle of the jaw and in the submandibular and submental areas (see Figs. 6.**11** and 6.**16a–e**).

Suspect areas in the oral cavity and base of the tongue should always be *palpated* also. The index finger enclosed in a fingercot or glove is used to palpate the suspected area carefully for induration, infiltration, ulceration, and tender areas. Most patients tolerate careful examination. In patients with an exaggerated gag reflex, the oral and pharyngeal mucosa, particu-

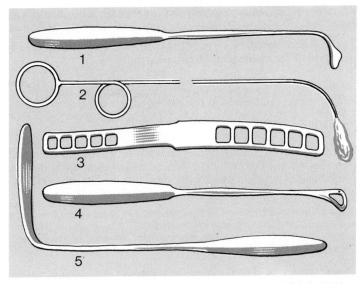

Fig. 3.12 Instruments for examination of the mouth and pharynx. 1, Reichert's hook; 2, long curved cotton applicator; 3, Bruening's tongue depressor; 4, Tuerck's tongue depressor; 5, angled tongue depressor for the base of the tongue.

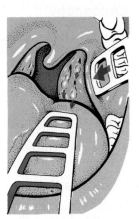

Fig. 3.13 Examination of the palatine tonsil with two tongue depressors

larly that of the soft palate, the base of the tongue, and the posterior wall of the pharynx, may first of all be made insensitive by a spray or a cotton applicator saturated with pantocaine or Xylocaine, 1 %. Local anesthesia of the pharynx is also recommended if satisfactory examination of the nasopharynx, hypopharynx, or larynx is not possible because of a marked gag reflex.

The technique described on p. 192 may be used on small children for the palpation of the mouth and the nasopharynx.

Note: Examination of the mouth with a tongue depressor or the finger must be carried out gently after explaining to the patient what is to be done. This is the only way to prevent gagging, thus allowing a satisfactory view of all the mouth and pharynx.

The nasopharynx, the hypopharynx, and the larynx are now examined with the mirror. The technique of posterior rhinoscopy is described on p. 395, that of indirect laryngoscopy on p. 395, and the introduction of the loupe endoscope on p. 202.

Indirect mirror examination of the hypopharynx may be very difficult in patients with a protruding or infiltrated base of the tongue, if it is tender, or in those with a sensitive gag reflex. These cases are best examined by *transnasal hypopharyngoscopy* using a flexible endoscope.

Note: When there is *clinical suspicion of a tumor, all* lymph node fields of the head and neck must be carefully palpated (see p. 491) and appropiate imaging studies performed (B-mode ultrasonography, CT, MRI).

Endoscopy

If the local findings cannot be elucidated clearly by examination with the mirror, various endoscopic techniques are available. Telescopic endoscopy usually requires no anesthesia (see p. 202; Fig. 2.**25**). Various other techniques can be carried out easily under local anesthesia, but are better carried out under a general endotracheal anesthesia. They include:

- Loupe endoscope
- A short straight hypopharyngoscope or esophagoscope (see p. 458; Fig. 5.**3**)
- Suspension laryngoscopy (see p. 398; Fig. 4.**8**)

Radiography

Tumors, enlarged adenoids, etc., of the *nasopharynx* are well shown in a *lateral view of the skull*. This projection is also suitable for demonstrating a *choanal atresia* after filling the nasal cavity with contrast medium.

Computed tomography, magnetic resonance imaging (MRI), and occasionally *radionuclide scanning* may also be used for demonstrating the limits of a tumor or of destruction caused by a nasopharyngeal tumor. Bilateral *carotid angiography and superselective angiography* to indentify individual branches of the carotid artery are used for the investigation of the highly vascular nasopharyngeal angiofibroma (see p. 385) in preparation for embolization (see p. 386).

The *hypopharynx* is best demonstrated after filling with a *contrast medium* such as gastrografin, barium, etc. The swallow with contrast is very useful in the diagnosis of a pharyngeal pouch, stenoses, and swallowing disorders.

Lateral views of the neck and the upper thoracic region may be used to localize the site of radiopaque foreign bodies in the hypopharynx and upper esophagus. This projection is also of great value in inflammatory soft tissue swelling and surgical emphysema of the parapharyngeal tissues due to pharyngeal injuries, pharyngeal abscess, mediastinal abscess, etc.

The radiographic demonstration of the salivary glands by sialography and scanning is described on p. 537.

Examination of the Saliva

See p. 536.

Gustometry

Taste may be tested by applying substances that represent the four taste qualities of sweet, salty, sour, and bitter in increasing concentrations to the tongue to allow determination of the lowest concentration that can be recognized.

Boernstein's concentrations are used for testing. These are as follows: glucose 4%, 10%, 40%; sodium chloride 2.5%, 7.5%, 15%; citric acid 1%, 5%, 10%; quinine 0.075%, 0.5%, 1% (stale solutions should not be used). The sensation of taste is observed 0.5 to 4 s later depending on the site which is tested, the temperature of the solution, and the size of the area tested. The test solution is applied alternatively to the right and left sides of the tongue with a pipette, or better with a small piece of blotting paper with a size of about 1 cm^2. Confirmation of the *threshold of recognition* is usually satisfactory for ordinary practice.

Electric current may also be used to stimulate the taste receptors instead of test solutions. An anode current is used with a normal threshold in adults between 2 and 7 μA. *Electrogustometry* offers numerous advantages, but is usually only used in specialist practices or clinics.

Objective gustometry may also be used in university clinics. Reflex change of the respiratory resistance of the nose or the electrical resistance of the skin are recorded simultaneously in response to a taste stimulus. Table 3.1 shows the most frequent causes of disorders of taste.

Specific Diagnostic Procedures

Bacteriologic, Mycologic, and Virologic Culture

Culture remains the basis of treatment with anti-infective chemotherapeutic agents. The diagnostic methods offered by microbiology such as culture and sensitivity should be used often.

Biopsy

Tissue must be taken for biopsy if a tumor is suspected and if abnormal findings remain unexplained. Tumors and lesions in the mouth and pharynx are easily accessible and biopsy in this area is much preferred to aspiration or cytology.

Clinical Aspects of Diseases of the Mouth and Pharynx

The *main symptoms* that indicate disease of the mouth and pharynx include:

- Pain on eating, chewing, or swallowing
- Dysphagia (see Table 3.**7**)
- Pain in the neck
- Globus symptoms (see p. 368 and Table 3.**7**)
- Burning of the tongue (see Table 3.**5**)
- Blood in the sputum
- Catarrh
- Oral fetor (see Table 3.**3**)
- Disorders of salivary secretion (see p. 534)
- Disorders of taste (see Table 3.**1**)
- Respiratory obstruction (see Table 4.**13**)
- Disorders of speech
- Swellings of the head, neck, mouth, floor of the mouth, and of the lymph nodes at the angle of the jaw (see Table 2.**11**)

Hyperplasia of the Lymphoepithelial Organs

The adenoid, the tonsil, and occasionally the lingual tonsil cause symptoms due to their size.

Hyperplasia of these organs is not of itself a disease, but only the morphologic expression of marked immunobiologic activity. A *marked increase* in size of the tonsil produces a primary mechanical obstruction of the respiratory or digestive tract and has detrimental effects on the entire body. Inflammation of neighboring organs is secondary. For that reason, tonsillar hyperplasia is here discussed separately from inflammation.

Adenoid Hyperplasia (see Color Plates **24c, 25a, b** and **c**)

Symptoms. These include nasal obstruction leading to mouth breathing, difficulty in feeding especially in small children, noisy respiration, snoring, typical adenoid facies, i. e., dull facial expression, open mouth, dilated and flattened nasolabial folds, indrawn nasal alae, protruding upper incisor teeth, enlarged lymph nodes at the angle of the jaw or in the nuchal area, the adenoid habitus, and rhinolalia clausa.

Obstruction of the nasopharynx may be responsible for:

1. *Aural diseases,* including obstruction of the eustachian tube, chronic tubal and middle ear catarrh, serous effusion, recurrent acute otitis media, formation of adhesions, also progression of chronic otitis media and conductive deafness (see p. 82)
2. Diseases of the *nose and paranasal sinuses,* including chronic purulent rhinitis or sinusitis, and even pansinusitis
3. *Disorders of the masticatory apparatus, including:* maldevelopment of the upper jaw, i.e., arched or "gothic" palate due to absence of the pressure of the tongue on the hard palate, and absence of lateral pressure on the upper jaw and alveolus by the tension of the buccinator muscle and the masticatory muscles because of the open mouth. Also including anomalies of position of the teeth, such as incorrect contact and orientation of the mandibular occlusion, and gingivitis
4. Disorders of the lower respiratory system, i.e., chronic laryngitis, tracheitis, and bronchitis
5. *Other somatic effects,* including a flat chest, round shoulders, thirst, loss of appetite, poor general development, and sensitivity to attacks of infection
6. Effects on the *intelligence and mental development* due to chronic respiratory obstruction and hypoxia during sleep; increased levels of CO_2 in the blood leading to restless, broken sleep causing tiredness during the day, apathy, dullness, poor school performance, and "pseudodementia".

Pathogenesis. The disease is caused by above-average hypertrophy of the lymphoepithelial tissue of the pharyngeal ring which is so immunobiologically active during childhood. There is probably a hereditary disposition. Endocrine and constitutional factors and the influence of diet, in particular carbohydrates, are suggested (see also p. 312 ff. and Fig. 3.**11a** and **b**).

Diagnosis. *The main symptoms* include chronic mouth breathing, snoring, and proneness to infection. Examination by posterior rhinoscopy shows the enlarged adenoid. Radiography or palpation may be needed.

Differential diagnosis. This includes choanal atresia, foreign bodies in the nose, and other causes of nasal obstruction such as nasopharyngeal angiofibroma and malignant tumors of the nasopharynx, possibly of mesenchymal origin especially in children. Dental causes should be looked for to explain the anomalies of position of the teeth and malocclusion.

Treatment. Conservative treatment by change of climate, diet, drugs, and so forth is *not* satisfactory.

Operative treatment is by adenoidectomy (Fig. 3.**14a** and **b**).

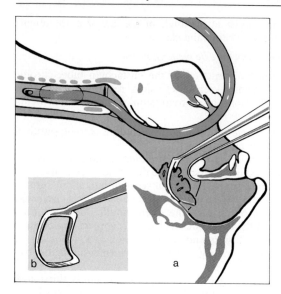

Fig. 3.**14a** and **b**
Adenoidectomy with the
head extended **(a)**,
using Beckmann's ring
curette **(b)**.

Principle of the operation. Anesthesia. Endotracheal anesthesia should be used to prevent aspiration and to guarantee optimal operating conditions. However, the operation can be carried out under a brief anesthetic without a tube, provided that the neck is extended. Adenoidectomy is usually carried out with the head in the hanging position. A *Beckman's* ring adenotome is usually used to remove the adenoid. This instrument separates the adenoid at its base.

Tonsillar Hyperplasia (see Color Plate **22a**)

Symptoms. This is usually combined with hypertrophy of the adenoid (see above). In addition, there is increased difficulty in swallowing and eating because of obstruction of the faucial isthmus. Considerable *respiratory obstruction* may also occur when only the tonsils are hyperplastic.

Diagnosis. See section on adenoid hyperplasia. The local findings are obvious.

Differential diagnosis. This is similar to that for adenoid hypertrophy. It is important to determine whether the tonsils *alone* are hypertrophic or whether there is a coexisting adenoid hypertrophy.

Note: Unilateral hyperplasia of the tonsil in an adult must always lead to suspicion of malignancy. A *rapid* hyperplasia of the lymphatic pharyngeal ring points to a disease of the entire lymphatic system.

Treatment. Tonsillectomy (technique described on p. 353) is performed, usually combined with adenoidectomy.

> *Note:* Not *every* enlargement of the tonsil or adenoid in a child is an indication for removal. There must be *considerable* hyperplasia with obvious mechanical obstruction of the naso- or oropharynx, and the appropriate *clinical effects* and disorders must be present. *Tonsillotomy,* i.e., removal of the protruding part of the tonsil, is now obsolete. Removal of part of the tonsil cuts across many of the crypts and the scarring process leads inevitably to stenosis and strictures of the lumen of the crypts and thus to the pathologic prerequisites for the development of chronic tonsillitis.

Course and prognosis. The symptoms usually resolve rapidly after removal of the mechanical obstruction. The child usually returns surprisingly rapidly to normal physical, psychological, and intellectual health. The prognosis is very good; recurrence after correctly performed adenoidectomy is unusual. *Complications* are mainly postoperative bleeding and aspiration. These are only to be feared if hemostasis is not achieved at operation, if postoperative care is inadequate, or if tissue has been left behind.

> *Note:* Because a pathologic bleeding tendency may easily be overlooked, the following investigations should be carried out *before* adenoidectomy or tonsillectomy:
>
> 1. History and family history relative to bleeding and coagulation disorders should be taken.
> 2. The bleeding time should be determined.
> 3. The partial thromboplastin time (PTT) should be determined.
> 4. The thrombocyte count should be determined.
> 5. The individual coagulation factors and the thrombocyte function should be investigated if the history and the routine tests in items (2 to 4) above indicate a disorder of hemostasis. Furthermore, analgesics or other anti-inflammatory agents should not be given for at least 3 days before the operation since they inhibit the function of thrombocytes. These drugs include salicylates, phenylbutazone, oxyfenbutazone, and Indocin.

Adenoidectomy or tonsillectomy may still be carried out in patients with manifest coagulation disorders if there are convincing indications. However, the operation should be carried out with the appropriate substitution therapy, in a special unit.

Other *postoperative complications* include a change of the sound of the voice which is usually only temporary, but occasionally rhinolalia aperta may persist. Rare complications include adhesions in the nasopharynx, injuries to the ostium of the eustachian tube, and, very rarely, injuries to the cervical spine.

Relative contraindications include cleft palate, either corrected or not. A speech therapist consultation must be obtained *before* a decision is made for surgery.

Hyperplasia of the lingual tonsil rarely occurs in children, but may occur occasionally in adults.

Symptoms. These include a feeling of pressure in the throat, especially on swallowing, and occasionally recurrent inflammation of the base of the tongue.

Treatment. If necessary, the lymphoepithelial tissue may be partially removed. The cryoprobe or the laser are particularly suitable for this.

Inflammatory Diseases

Labial, Oral, and Pharyngeal Mucosa

Internal or dermatologic diseases often present on the lips, the oral mucosa, the gingiva, and the tongue. Table 3.2 gives an overview of the most common and most important of these disorders. Since changes of the mucosa of the lips, mouth, or pharynx may occur in many disorders, the following description will be confined to the most common.

Rhagades of the commissures along with slight bleeding and pain of the commissures accompanying opening of the mouth. Causes include ill-fitting false teeth, mycotic infection, poor general resistance, diabetes, iron deficiency anemia, nonspecific pyogenic infections, and syphilis. If possible, the cause should be confirmed and dealt with before treatment is attempted. Carcinoma of the commissure may also simulate rhagades in the early phases. Nonspecific local treatment includes 1% to 5% silver nitrate solution or 1% to 2% Pyoktannin solution and steroid creams.

Cheilitis may be solitary and acute due to trauma, thermal injury (hot food), chemical injury (smoke), actinic damage (sunburn), or exposure to radiation.

Cheilitis granulomatosa, Miescher's disease, is a chronic recurring disease which is usually ushered in with a complete *Melkersson-Rosenthal syndrome* of cheilitis, granulomatous glossitis, and facial paralysis. The pathogenesis of this triad is unknown, and the treatment is the same as that of idiopathic facial paralysis (see p. 163).

Herpes labialis (see p. 328)

Although *tuberculosis* or *syphilis,* primary or secondary, may occur on the lips, a chronic or recurrent erosive or hyperkeratotic lesion of the labial mucosa must always be suspected of being premalignant (leukoplakia, Bowen's disease, etc.). Numerous diseases affecting the oral mucosa also affect the lips.

Stomatitis often combined with *gingivitis* or *inflammation of the buccal mucosa* may be a primary disease of many different causes or may be secondary to other diseases. Clinical symptoms and prognosis are thus extremely variable.

Table 3.2 Common Lesions of the Oral Mucosa in Generalized and Dermatologic Diseases

	Cause
Dryness	Febrile infectious diseases, uremia, polyglobulinemia, cachexia, atropine poisoning, Sjögren's syndrome and other sialadenoses, vitamin A deficiency, occasionally diabetes mellitus and hyperthyroidism, Plummer-Vinson disease (iron deficiency), hypertension, prolonged use of certain drugs such as phenothiazines, belladonna and psychotropic drugs
Alterations of pigmentation	
Pallid	Anemia
Cyanotic	Pulmonary congestion
Intense red	Polycythemia rubra vera, reactive polyglobulinemia
Reddish-violet	Right heart insufficiency
Yellow	Jaundice, often as an initial symptom, hepatic congestion, megaloblastic anemia
Red, like lipstick	Hepatic insufficiency
Whitish patches like leukoplakia with dry mucosa	Vitamin A deficiency
Greyish-violet staining of the gingival mucosa	Argyrosis
Greyish-blue to brownish discoloration of the gingiva	Bismuth and lead intoxication
Spotted hyperpigmentation	Oral contraceptives

Table 3.2 Continuation	
	Cause
Punctate or striated, occasionally diffuse pigmentation of the lips, cheeks, gingiva, tongue and palate	Addison's disease of which it is often the first symptom
Bleeding Bleeding from the gingiva, with a dard-red discoloration and swelling of the inter-dental papillae	Scurvy
Bleeding from cavernous angiectasia on the vermillion and on the oral mucosa	Rendu-Osler's disease
Punctate lesions White spots surrounded by an erythematous zone. The site of predilection is the buccal mucosa opposite the molar teeth, Koplik's spots	Measles
Reticular or striated bluish-white membrane and edematous red spots mainly on the lips, but also on the tongue	Lupus erythematosus
Opalescent plaques often with superficial ulceration	Secondary syphilis
Membranes on the oral mucosa Whitish, striated, nonadherent membrane brilliant white punctate spots in infants	Candidiasis
Vesicles, erosions, and cysts	Varicella (the vesicles are the size of hempseed and lie mainly on the palate), erythema multiforme, herpes simplex, herpes zoster, hereditary epidermolysis bullosa dystrophica, pemphigus vulgaris, mucosal pemphigus, AIDS

Table 3.2 Continuation	
	Cause
Aphthous ulcers	Aphthosis and Behçet's disease
Stomatitis and necrotic ulcers	Pellagra, agranulocytosis, thrombocytopenia, panmyelophthisis, leukemia, mercury intoxication
Gingival hyperplasia	Pregnancy, possibly the contraceptive pill and hydantoin
Atrophic lesions	
Induration, sclerosis, narrow pale lips, shortened frenulum, microglossia	Progressive scleroderma

* Modified from Bohnstedt.

Ulceromembranous Stomatitis

Symptoms. The disease usually begins on the gingival margins with redness, swelling, and sensitivity to pressure. Swelling of the buccal and lingual mucosa, stomatitis simplex, may also occur. The disease often progresses to ulceration with severe pain, presenting with superficial, and occasionally deep, mucosal ulcers with a dirty-grey fibrinous membrane. There are marked constitutional symptoms: oral fetor, sialorrhea, possibly cloudy or purulent saliva, loss of taste, difficulty in eating, and high fever in the initial stages. The disease may spread to the pharynx, and the regional lymph nodes may be enlarged and painful.

Pathogenesis. This includes poor oral hygiene, reduced general resistance, infections from cutlery, dental damage, virus infections with possible secondary bacterial infection, mucosal rhagades, gingival pockets, and dental calculus.

Diagnosis. Bacteriologic culture is necessary, and often shows spiral and fusiform rods as in Vincent's angina (see p. 349).

Differential diagnosis. This consists of mucosal mycosis, excluded by culture, virus infection (herpes simplex, aphthous stomatitis, and herpes zoster), syphilis, tuberculosis, AIDS, hematologic diseases including agranulocytosis and leukemia which may be excluded by a differential white count, and carcinoma which requires a biopsy.

Treatment. This includes appropriate oral and dental hygiene, 1% gentian violet, 1% to 2% Pyoktannin solution, or Dynexan. Antibiotics are given if indicated by culture and sensitivity tests. Local and general antimycotic therapy is given for fungal infections.

Course and prognosis. Both are good if the cause is treated appropriately.

Herpes Simplex Stomatitis and Gingivitis (see Color Plate **10a**)

Symptoms. These include a burning sensation in the mouth, difficulty in eating, a feeling of being unwell, fever in the early stages, and lentil-sized, clear vesicles at the mucocutaneous junctions of the lip and the nasal introitus, and also in the entire mouth. The vesicles may progress to superficial circular or oval ulcers with a red center. The disease often occurs in conjunction with febrile general infections or overexposure to sunlight. There is marked oral tenderness, oral fetor, sialorrhea, and painful regional lymphadenopathy. The disease is contagious. Serial crops of fresh vesicles may occur. Children are most at risk.

Pathogenesis. The cause is infection with the herpes simplex virus and occurs first, usually, in childhood. The first infection often causes no symptoms. The disease is very infectious: 90% of the population are said to be carriers of the virus, but clinical manifestations in the form of herpes labialis or stomatitis herpetiformis only occur in 1%.

Diagnosis. This is made by exclusion. An attempt may be made to isolate the virus from the contents of the vesicle, if possible within the first 24 h of the vesicular stage. The material is inoculated in the rabbit cornea.

Differential diagnosis. Chronic recurrent aphthous stomatitis, varicella, the acute infectious exanthems, herpangina, foot and mouth disease, Behçet's disease, pemphigus, and mycoses must all be considered.

Treatment. Only symptomatic treatment is available including ointments, local application of 1% to 2% Pyoktannin solution, 1% gentian violet solution, oral irrigations, and bland fluid diet. Steroids must *not* be given. Recently, antigen therapy and also chemotherapy (acyclovir) have been tried.

Course and prognosis. This disease is usually harmless and lasts 1 to 2 weeks. The vesicles heal to form crusts but do not form scars. Recurrence is frequent, but herpetic sepsis and herpetic encephalitis are very rare.

Infectious aphthae may also be caused by viruses of the picorna group (Coxsackie, Echo) and rarely of the variola group.

Metal stomatitis. A stomatitis with discoloration of the gingiva may be caused by either medical or occupational exposure to *mercury* or *bismuth*. This also applies to *workers in lead*. The *use of gold* in the treatment of arthritis may cause a gingival stomatitis. Finally, the mucosa may be damaged by arsenic, chlorine, chromium, fluoride, copper, manganese, nickel, sulfur, thallium, zinc, organic substances, e.g., benzol, dimethyl sulfate, tetrachlorocarbons, tetrachloroethyl, and mixed substances such as corrosive agents, synthetic resins, synthetic materials, enamels, etc., as well as by wood, dyes, hops, wool, and insecticides.

Stomatitis due to drugs. This may be observed particularly after the use of bromides, iodides, salicylates, antibiotics, and sulfonamides, psycho-active drugs that dry the mouth, and antiepileptic agents, and after pyramidone, barbiturates, laxatives such as phenolphthalein, and the contraceptive pill.

Allergic stomatitis. Hypersensitivity reactions on the oral mucosa and the lips with varying severity, with or without angioneurotic edema, may be observed in response to almost all drugs, dental material, mouthwashes, toothpaste, cosmetics, chewing gum, and also to some foods such as fruit, fish, protein, and milk. The diagnosis may be established by tests, and if the allergen is found it should be withdrawn. Otherwise, antiallergic or local symptomatic treatment are given.

Stomatitis and Mycoses

Symptoms. Burning in the mouth and tongue, superficial white foci, and exudates on the mucosa are symptomatic. The exudate can be wiped off with mild pressur (see Color Plate **18b**).

Pathogenesis. The cause is infection by fungi. In Europe this is usually a *Candida albicans;* aspergillosis is less common. Mycoses affect subjects with reduced resistance, and after long administration of antibiotics, chemotherapy, steroids, the contraceptive pill, and after radiotherapy.

Diagnosis. This is made on the characteristic membranous white or grey exudates and very inflamed mucosa. Superficial ulceration occurs. A specimen is taken for culture for fungi.

Differential diagnosis is diphtheria.

Treatment. This includes intensive oral hygiene, painting with borax-glycerine or 2% Pyoktannin, Nystatin, and local or systemic Moronal.

Course. Prognosis is good if the general resistance is good or can be restored, and if antimycotics are given in satisfactory doses over a long period with weekly cultures. Otherwise, there is a danger of generalization of the mycosis by hematogenous or intraluminal spread.

Herpes Zoster

Symptoms. Unilateral rapidly progressive vesicles are quickly followed by fibrinous superficial epithelial defects, affecting the segments of the face innervated by the second and third divisions of the trigeminal nerve. The disease is very painful. Mucosal lesions may occur in the same stage and may be partially confluent and arranged in groups.

Pathogenesis. This is neurotropic infection with a virus which cannot be distinguished from the varicella virus.

Diagnosis. The typical segmental arrangement, the severe pain, and culture of the contents of the vesicle secure the diagnosis.

Differential diagnosis. This includes herpes simplex and recurrent aphthous stomatitis.

Treatment. Causal treatment is not possible. Symptomatic treatment includes supportive antibiotics, vitamin B complex, gamma globulin, and acyclovir (Zovirax).

The disease is often followed by obstinent and severe neuralgias which may persist for months after resolution of the mucosal lesion. Occasionally, other regions and internal organs may be simultaneously involved. The generalized form in older patients suggests a systemic malignancy.

Acquired Immune Deficiency Syndrome (AIDS, HIV Syndrome)

Symptoms. Approximately 35% to 40% of HIV infections produce otorhinolaryngologic manifestations, including such *early* symptoms as *Kaposi's sarcoma* and *hairy leukoplakia* of the tongue (see Color Plates **20a, b** and **38d**). HIV infection has a relatively high association with cervical lymphadenopathies, candidiasis, herpes simplex, and herpes zoster. Other potential manifestations of HIV infection include sinusitis, tonsillitis, gingivitis, pharyngitis, esophagitis, tracheitis, sudden hearing loss, facial paralysis, and facial pain. General accompanying features are fever, anorexia, headache, muscle and joint pain, transient or persistent lymph node enlargement, diarrhea, and profound weight loss.

Pathogenesis. Infection with the human immunodeficiency retrovirus (HIV).

Diagnosis. HIV infection is diagnosed by the detection of HIV antibodies in the serum in a screening test (e. g., ELISA) followed by a *confirmatory blot test.*

Differential diagnosis. See list of symptoms above. HIV infection should be suspected whenever a "classic" disease exhibits an *unusual location and presentation,* runs an *atypical course,* and presents in an *atypical age group,* especially if the patient is in a high-risk population (male homosexuals, intravenous drug users, etc.).

Treatment. A treatment specific for the infecting organism is not yet available. Management centers on prophylaxis, especially in known high-risk populations, and on symptomatic therapy.

Chronic Recurrent Aphthae

Symptoms. *Single* aphtha, 1–5 mm in size, occur intermittently, affecting the buccal mucosa, the tongue, the palate, and the gingiva. They are very painful. The regional lymph nodes are swollen, and a concomitant stomatitis is possible.

Pathogenesis. The cause is unknown, but the disease is suspected *not* to be due to a virus infection but to be due to a trophoneurotic disturbance especially in children and young adults with a labile autonomic system. The outbreak is stimulated by infections, hormonal factors such as menstruation, and certain foods.

Diagnosis. This is made on the long history and tendency to recurrence. There is *no* sialorrhea, *no* oral fetor, and *no* fever.

Differential diagnosis. Herpes simplex, which occurs with fever, fetor, sialorrhea, a general malaise, and a large number of vesicles which are confluent and arranged in groups must be considered.

Treatment. Causal or prophylactic treatment are not possible. Symptomatic treatment includes local 2% Pyoktannin, steroid creams, 3% borax-glycerin, Glyceromerfen, and Dynexan.

Course. The lesions heal without scarring in 1 to 3 weeks but early recurrence is possible. The course may extend over decades, and familial occurrences are known.

Behçet's Disease

Symptoms. Aphthae occur in crops in the mouth and on the genitals. *Eye symptoms* which may occur are usually monocular and undulating, including hypopyon iritis which is often fleeting, and later papilledema, involvement of the retina, and blindness. Rheumatic symptoms and renal involvement may also occur.

Pathogenesis. The cause is unknown. It may be a generalized vasculitis, an autoimmune event, or virus infection.

Diagnosis. The main, and often the first symptom is involvement of the eye. Acute cochleovestibular disturbances may also occur.

Treatment. Therapy includes blood transfusion, gamma globulin, iron preparations, fever cures, immunosuppressive agents, and long-term steroids.

Course. The disease is often fatal over a period of years.

Tuberculosis

Symptoms. Mucosal lesions may take the form of a *mucosal lupus* or exudative ulcerative *mucosal tuberculosis*. Round nodules occur in groups in mucosal lupus, and they demonstrate yellowish-brown flecks in the oral mucosa on pressure with a glass spatula. They are not painful. Flat, dirty, exudative, painful ulceration with undermined edges and lymph node involvement is found in ulcerative mucosal tuberculosis (see p. 496).

Pathogenesis. The oral cavity is nowadays almost never a primary site of manifestation of tuberculosis. The disease is usually due to hematogenous or intraluminal spread from the primary site, usually the lung.

Diagnosis. This is made by biopsy and culture, and chest radiography. *The disease is reportable to public health authorities.*

Differential diagnosis. Syphilis, mycoses, and carcinoma must be excluded.

Treatment. The original focus in the lung is treated by tuberculostatic drugs. At the present time, triple therapy is usually given consisting of isoniazid, rifampicin, and ethambutol supervised by a chest physician.

Course. This depends on the outcome of the primary lesion. However, the prognosis for mucosal lesions is good with general antituberculous therapy.

Syphilis

Symptoms. All stages of syphilis may occur in the mouth. *Stage 1:* primary chancre occur on the lips, the tonsil, the anterior part of the tongue, the commissure, the gingiva, and the buccal mucosa. A sharply limited nodule 2 to 3 mm in diameter grows to the size of a penny. After a few days, a painless ulcer forms with a very hard edge and painless regional lymphadenopathy in the submandibular or jugulodigastric area. The primary lesion regresses spontaneously after 3 to 6 weeks.

Stage 2: Eight to 10 weeks after the infection, i. e., 5 to 7 weeks after the appearance of the primary chancre, and at the same time or before the the skin lesions, a superficial exanthem develops in the entire oral cavity. Dark-red mucosal spots a few millimeters in size form with a tendency to merge. The lesions are of varying severity and last for several weeks. Dark-red papules form gradually, and also flat areas with a cloudy epithelial surface. The surface of the tongue looks like sugar icing with areas of loss of papillae. A very firm indolent lymphadenopathy develops.

Stage 3: A gumma develops on average 15 years after the primary infection. The sites of predilection in the mouth are the lips, the hard palate, the tongue, and the tonsils. There is diffuse nodular infiltrate with liquefaction of the center, fetor, a sharp punched-out ulcer, and radiating scars.

Symptoms. See under *congenital syphilis,* p. 206.

Pathogenesis. This infection is caused by *Treponema pallidum.* The *pathway of infection* is either genital or extragenital. The *incubation period* is on average $3^{1}/_{2}$ weeks.

Diagnosis. Demonstration of the organism by culture and dark ground illumination is used in stages 1 and 2. Serologic tests become positive from the 4th week. The treponema immobilization test (Nelson's test) only becomes positive in the 9th week. In stage 3, serologic reactions are positive and the disease can be demonstrated by histology. *The disease is reportable to public health authorities.*

Differential diagnosis. In stage 1 tumors, tuberculosis, mycoses, and herpes are to be considered; in stage 2, erythema multiforme and tuberculosis; in stage 3, malignant tumors and leukemia.

Treatment. Penicillin should be administered by a dermatologist or a specialist in venereal diseases.

Hyperkeratosis and Leukoplakia (see Color Plate **21b**)

Symptoms. These include a velvety or nodular, usually sharply circumscribed epithelial tumor, hyperkeratosis, a flat epithelial plaque or white thickening which cannot be wiped off, leukoplakia, usually occurring on the lips, the floor of the mouth, or the buccal mucosa.

Pathogenesis. This is an epithelial disease with many different causes including exogenous irritative factors such as chronic mechanical irritation by the irregular edge of teeth, pressure from a denture, smoking, excess alcohol consumption, lichen planus, syphilis, and erythematoses. There may be no recognizable cause.

Two groups of leukoplakia may be distinguished depending on the color and surface:

1. *Simple leukoplakia* with sharp edges occurring in about 50 % of cases. This is only rarely premalignant.
2. *Patchy leukoplakia* which may be divided into (a) *verrucous leukoplakia* (about 25 % of cases) which shows an irregular wrinkled greyish-red speckled surface and which can be premalignant and (b) *erosive leukoplakia* (about 25 % of cases) with a reddish erosive lesion and often an irregular nodular surface – this form becomes malignant in about 35 % of cases and is very similar to Bowen's disease.

The probability of malignant degeneration depends largely on the degree of histo-logic dysplasia. The frequency of progression of a leukoplakia to carcinoma increases with the degree of the dysplasia (see also p. 422).

> *Note:* Leukoplakia should be regarded as being potentially premalignant and should therefore be investigated and followed up carefully.

Diagnosis. This is made by histology. The lesion should be entirely removed, if possible with a clear margin.

Differential diagnosis. Ulcerative stomatitis, mycoses, lichen ruber planus, lupus erythematosus, and pemphigus must be considered.

Treatment. This is by generous surgical removal, preferably at the time of biopsy and avoidance of possible causative agents.

Bowen's Disease (Erythroplasia, Erythroplakia)

This is regarded as a premalignant lesion or carcinoma in situ. It is an intraepidermal prickle cell "carcinoma" with an intact basal membrane; the tumor has not yet invaded the cutis or the subepithelial layer. It occurs on the skin or mucosa.

Symptoms. Sharply demarcated full red foci of varying sizes with a smooth surface that occur on the mucosa of the cheek or tongue. It may also take the form of white patches of leukoplakia or verrucous vegetative papilloma-tous lesions the size of a hazelnut. *Morbidity.* The disease occurs mainly in men in the 4th to 7th decade of life. Progression to true squamous cell carcinoma is possible at any time and is very common.

Diagnosis. Biopsy distinguishes the lesion from other precancerous lesions of the mucosa such as leukoplakia and pure hyperplasia.

Treatment. The lesion must be excised with a healthy margin.

Inflammations of the Oral Mucosa in Dermatoses

Pemphigus (see also p. 419)

Symptoms. The first symptom is often in the mouth and takes the form of flat soft or tense vesicles. These give way to superficial epithelial erosions with a fibrin layer and epithelial tags at the edge. The course is episodic and several stages may be present at any one time. There is oral fetor, often regional lymphadenopathy, and a bullous eruption on the skin. The disease usually begins between the 40th and 60th years of life.

Pathogenesis. This is probably an autoimmune disease.

Diagnosis. This is made by biopsy and cytology (Tzanck test).

Differential diagnosis. This includes stomatitis, hereditary epidermolysis bullosa, erythema multiforme, lichen planus, and mucosal pemphigoid.

Treatment. Steroids are administered under the supervision of a dermatologist.

Erythema Multiforme

Symptoms. This disease occurs most commonly in adolescent males. Fibrinous exudate, crust, and vesicles form on the lips and oral mucosa. There are simultaneous skin and joint lesions, and fever. The symptoms are those of a severe acute infection, with oral fetor, sialorrhea, pains, and regional lymphadenopathy. The course is episodic.

Pathogenesis. Many causes have been discussed; it is probable that several different antigens are involved such as antibiotics, laxatives, tranquilizers, bacteria, viruses, and fungi.

Diagnosis. This is made from the picture of the generalized disease, and possibly by biopsy.

Differential diagnosis. Pemphigus, lichen planus, and the enanthem of drug reactions must be excluded.

Treatment. If possible the cause should be confirmed. Steroids are given, and local mucosal treatment initiated. Parenteral feeding may be necessary.

Prognosis. This is serious.

Lichen Planus

Symptoms. Whitish nodules are arranged in groups or in a network on the buccal mucosa, the gingiva, and the tongue. Grey or bluish smooth plaques the size of a lentil are also found on the dorsum of the tongue. The lesions cannot be wiped off and are firm and flat. There is no pain. Similar pruritic, dry brownish-red to rose-colored papules 2 to 3 mm in diameter occur on the flexor surface of the arm and the wrist.

Pathogenesis. The etiology is unknown, but it may be a neurogenic disturbance.

Diagnosis. This is made from the entire clinical picture, at times supported by biopsy. Lichen planus is a potentially premalignant disease.

Differential diagnosis. This includes leukoplakia, hyperkeratosis, Bowen's disease, mycosis, the enanthem of drug reactions, and lupus erythematosus.

Table 3.3 Oral Fetor	
Site of Origin	Cause
Teeth, gingiva and mouth	Dental caries, parodontosis, gingivitis, stomatitis, erythema multiforme, pemphigus, neglected false teeth, abscesses of the floor of the mouth, ulcerating tumors
Pharynx	Acute tonsillitis, Vincent's angina, mononucleosis, peripharyngeal and retropharyngeal abscess, pharyngeal diphtheria, chronic tonsillitis and pharyngitis, foreign body in the nasopharynx, stage 3 syphilis
Airway	Atrophic rhinitis, ozena, purulent rhinitis, sinusitis, bronchitis, bronchiectasis, bronchial foreign body, lung abscess, and pneumonia
Digestive tract	Hypopharyngeal or esophageal diverticulum, hiatus hernia, esophagitis, diseases of the stomach and the intestines with or without hiccup and vomiting
Generalized disorders	Diabetes mellitus with ketosis (acetone), renal failure (urine) and liver coma which gives a sweet aromatic smell

Treatment. Possible toxic agents such as the sun, tobacco, and chemical agents should be excluded. Steroid oral ointments may be used. Vitamin A preparations may be given. *Careful follow-up is needed because this is a premalignant lesion.*

Other rare inflammatory lesions of the oral cavity include scleroma, leprosy, and sarcoidosis (see p. 206), as well as AIDS (Acquired Immune Deficiency Syndrome – infection by retrovirus with T-cell tropism). See also pp. 330, 496.

An overview of the common causes of oral fetor is given in Table 3.**3.**

Tongue

The inflammatory diseases described above usually manifest themselves also on the tongue. The following inflammatory disorders *affect the tongue primarily:*

Glossitis

Symptoms. These include burning of the tongue especially at its tip and edges, and often parageusia or hypergeusia. On the tongue itself only minimal mucosal lesions can be demonstrated such as circumscribed inflammation or loss of papillae.

Pathogenesis. The cause may lie in mechanical irritation by sharp teeth, dental calculi, pressure from dentures, intolerance to dental materials,

e. g., the material for making dentures, or the use of metal which is electrically noninert, mouthwashes, drug sensitivity, vitamin B deficiency, megaloblastic anemia, iron deficiency anemia, diabetes, and gastrointestinal diseases including cirrhosis and mycoses.

Diagnosis. This rests on the demonstration or exclusion of the mechanical irritation, sensitivity reactions, diabetes, gastrointestinal or hematologic diseases, and also on the mycologic findings. Finally, the diagnosis may be made by exclusion of all other causes.

Differential diagnosis. This includes allergic glossitis or depressed immunologic response.

Treatment. The cause should be eliminated if possible. Symptomatic treatment includes irrigation with Kavosan, Dynexan, Volon A ointment, etc., and a bland diet.

Allergic Glossitis

Symptoms. The signs are similar to those of nonspecific glossitis, except that the disease begins suddenly with swelling and redness of the tongue with swelling and pain progressing to itching. There is a danger of respiratory obstruction if the reaction progresses to edema.

Pathogenesis. This is an allergic reaction localized to the tongue. Many substances are possible allergens, including serum injections, antibiotics, drugs such as phenothiazine, barbiturates, Pyrazolon, sulfonamide, aspirin, local anesthetics, and foods such as fruits, fish, protein, nuts, etc. (see Color Plate **19a**).

Diagnosis. This is based on the clinical picture of a sudden onset with marked symptoms, and on demonstration of the allergen.

Differential diagnosis. Acute infectious enanthem, mycosis, intoxication, local chemical damage, and nonspecific glossitis must be considered.

Treatment. This is both symptomatic and antiallergic. Allergen tests can be done and an allergen-free diet prescribed.

The tongue is also affected by the following *specific or chronic* inflammations: tuberculosis, syphilis, mycoses, actinomycosis, dermatomyositis, Sjögren's disease, and progressive scleroderma.

Surface lesions of the tongue that encourage infection include:

1. *Geographic tongue.* The dorsum of the tongue is covered with smooth red patches which resemble a map and which can gradually change position. The cause is unknown, but this is a harmless condition which does not require treatment (see Color Plate **18a**).
2. *Fissured tongue.* In this disease, there are clefts and folds of varying depth forming islands on the mucosa of the dorsal surface of the tongue. This appears to be a simple dominant hereditary disease. It is one of the aspects of the Melkersson-Rosenthal syndrome of facial paralysis, edema of the face and lips, and fissured

tongue (see p. 324). It occurs frequently in mongolism (trisomy 21 or Down's syndrome). Harmless inflammation may occur due to penetration of foreign material into the clefts. The treatment is symptomatic.

The common causes for a coated, red, or fissured tongue are summarized in Table 3.**4**, and the causes for burning of the tongue in Table 3.**5**.

Abscess of the Floor of the Mouth (see Color Plate **20c**)

Symptoms. These include swelling and limitation of movement of the tongue, increasing pain, difficulty in articulation progressing to complete loss of speech, protrusion and induration of the floor of the mouth with marked sensitivity to pressure, severe difficulty in swallowing, and finally complete inability to eat, limitation of movement of the temporomandibular joint with trismus, fever, severe generalized symptoms, and occasionally stridor.

Pathogenesis. Infected material enters via rhagades of the tongue or the oral mucosa. The infection advances in the loose musculature of the tongue

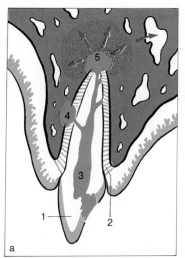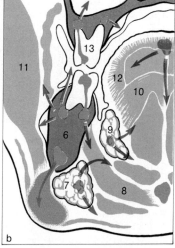

Fig. 3.**15a** and **b**   Dental infections and infections in the floor of the mouth. **a.** Infections in and around the teeth. 1, Carious incisor tooth; 2, alveolar periosteum; 3, pulpitis; 4, periapical abscess; 5, apical granuloma. **b.** Sites of origin of inflammations of the floor of the mouth. 6, Mandibular arising from the teeth or osteomyelitis; 7, submandibular gland, due to inflammation or a stone; 8, musculature of the floor of the mouth; 9, sublingual gland, inflammation or retention; 10, tongue musculature; 11, muscles of the cheek; 12, abscess of the body of the tongue; 13, apical granuloma of one of the upper teeth extending to the antrum.

Table 3.4	Surface Lesions of the Tongue		
Type of Lesion	Basic Disease	Clinical Symptoms	Details
Red tongue	Pernicious anemia	Initially dark red, later caramel-colored spots and striae on the dorsum of the tongue. The surface of the tongue is red, smooth, and shiny, Hunter's glossitis (see Color Plate **19b**)	Dysgeusia, paresthesia, xerostomia; the oral mucosa is also affected
	Scarlet fever	Strawberry tongue (see Color Plate **19c**)	Protrusion of papillae
	Hepatic cirrhosis	Glazed, shiny smooth red dry tongue with blue spots, "liver tongue"	Generalized symptoms prominent, glazed lips, yellow staining of the oral mucosa, brownish pallid face
	Sjögren's syndrome	Dry smooth, red glazed tongue	Swelling of the salivary glands, and salivary stones
	Median rhomboid glossitis	A raised or slightly sunken red area free of papillae in the center of the middle third of the tongue in the midline	A harmless lesion confined to the tongue causing no symptoms
	Vascular congestion	Red-violet swollen tongue	Right heart failure, hepatic cirrhosis and malignant tumors
	Hypertension	Pink to carmine red	Hypertension, myocardial insufficiency, left heart failure, valvular heart disease, local allergic reaction and shock
	Allergy	Strawberry or raspberry red, edema	Occurs in local allergic reaction and also in shock

Grey smooth tongue	Vitamin A deficiency	Bluish matt epithelial protrusions and bluish staining of the lips	Xerostomia, dysphagia
	Radiotherapy	Oral mucosal is sensitive to heat, circumscribed mucosal atrophy, mucosal induration	Ageusia, xerostoma
	Lichen planus	Milky bluish striae, spider web leukoplakia, papillae are retained and there is no membrane	Also affects the oral mucosa
	Progressive scleroderma	Dry tongue, limited mobility, initially edema of the tongue, later atrophy of the tongue and increasing rigidity	Dysphagia, interference with speech, mouth is too small, sialopenia
Black hairy tongue	Antibiotics	Hairy, greenish-black membrane, long black cornified papillae	Also occurs in mycosis.
Fissured tongue	Lingua plicata	Surface of the tongue is furrowed and fissured	A benign normal hereditary variant
	Melkersson-Rosenthal syndrome	Folded tongue	Periodic swellings of the lips, tongue, and cheeks, and intermittent facial paralysis

Table 3.4 Continuation

Type of Lesion	Basic Disease	Clinical Symptoms	Details
Coated tongue	Nonspecific oral infection	Whitish coat (horny scales)	Connected with reduced food intake in gastritis and enteritis and in feverish infections
	Oral thrush	Whitish membranous adherent plaques with red edges	*Candida albicans* demonstrated on culture
	AIDS	Commonly associated with oral candidiasis and hairy leukoplakia of the tongue	Multifocal symptoms are typical. Diagnosis see p. 330
	Scarlet fever	Dirty-white coating with reddended tip and edges to tongue	Pharyngitis, exanthems; betahemolytic streptococci found on culture
	Diphtheria	Greyish-white membranous coat, smells sweet and nasty	Adherent membrane, the underlying bed bleeds slightly, generalized symptoms
	Typhus	Greyish-white tongue with very red edges	Infection by Salmonella typhi, generalized symptoms
	Uremia	Brownish plaques	Renal insufficiency

Table 3.5   Burning of the Tongue

Basic Disease	Clinical Symptoms	Details
Lingua exfoliativa areata	Burning of the tongue with red-spotted tongue, absence of filiform papillae	
Toxic stomatitis	Burning of the tongue and greyish-blue discoloration of the gingiva by bismuth and lead, reddened edematous mucosa in mercury poisoning	
Stomach and intestinal disorders of various causes	Manifest or latent symptoms, depending on the site of the cause	
Patterson-Brown-Kelly syndrome, Plummer-Vinson syndrome (see p. 364)	Dry tongue, considerable dysphagia. Rhagades of the commissures, atrophic mucosa	Almost exclusively in women, dry pale skin, koilonychia, dry mucous membranes
Sjögren's disease	Xerostomia, tough sticky saliva, papillary atrophy, smooth glazed tongue, dysphagia (see Color Plate **38c**)	Dryness affecting the mucosa of the oral cavity, the pharynx, larynx, and trachea; swelling of the major salivary glands
Moeller-Hunter glossitis in megaloblastic anemia	Burning of the tongue, dysgeusia, parasthesia, dryness, spotted tongue with purple-red areas in striae alternating with bluish areas, smooth surface but not papillary atrophy, partially swollen papillae	May involve the entire oral mucosa

Table 3.5 Continuation

Basic Disease	Clinical Symptoms	Details
Diabetes mellitus	Intermittent marked burning of the tongue with dry surface	Tendency to oral infections and mycoses
Food allergy and contact allergy	Begins suddenly; marked swelling and redness; burning of the tongue increasing to cause pain and feeling of tension	Typical history or evidence of allergic cause, involvement of the rest of the oral mucosa
Pellagra, niacin deficiency	Hypoesthesia of the tongue, salty taste, feeling of a "chapped" tongue, red swollen and occasionally coated tongue, later chessboard tongue with marked fissuring, and finally atrophy	Inflammation of the remaining oral mucosa, sialorrhea is more common than sialopenia
Mucoviscidosis	Dry, burning tongue, tough glutinous secretion	Increased sodium and chloride ions in mucus and saliva
Psychogenic glossodynia	Burning of the tongue without any demonstrable organic cause	Frequent in latent depression

and in the numerous connective tissue spaces (Fig. 3.**15b**). The base of the tongue, the lingual tonsil, or a carious tooth are also possible portals of infection (see Fig. 3.**15a**). The causal organism is usually common pathogenic bacteria. Penetration of small foreign bodies such as fish bones, bone splinters, kernels of corn, etc. are also possible causes. The infection may arise primarily in the sublingual or submandibular glands lying in the floor of the mouth. An abscess of the floor of the mouth is termed a *Ludwig's angina.*

Diagnosis. This is made on the clinical picture of an inflammatory swelling of the floor of the mouth, severe pain, and a progressive course.

Differential diagnosis is hematoma, gumma, tuberculosis, and malignancy.

Treatment. Therapy should be initiated at the onset of symptoms with high doses of broad-spectrum antibiotics, combined with alcohol soaks. If this does not induce remission, the antibiotic must be changed. If there is evidence of liquefaction, the abscess is aspirated and then opened widely along the aspiration needle by an external incision parallel to the tongue. Adequate diet and fluid intake must be ensured, if necessary by a nasogastric tube or parenteral feeding. A tracheotomy is indicated for respiratory obstruction. If *Ludwig's angina* develops, the infected area is opened widely because of the danger of involvement of the larynx or mediastinum.

Course and prognosis. These are favorable provided that suppuration occurs quickly so that the abscess may be drained. Extension of the abscess to the deeper soft tissues of the neck (see Fig. 3.**17a** and **b**) and to the mediastinum is a life-threatening situation.

Actinomycosis is also a possible differential diagnosis, but it is now becoming very rare. This disease has an indolent course, causes relatively slight pain, but formation of multiple hard infiltrates with formation of abscesses and fistulae. It is mainly localized to the head and neck (98% of cases). The organisms are usually *Actinomyces israelii* and accompanying bacteria. Actinomyces agglomerations can be demonstrated in the pus from the abscess and in tissue specimens. A needle biopsy may be taken, and a specimen of pus is sent for bacteriologic identification. Serologic tests include agglutination and complement fixation. Precipitation tests and intracutaneous tests are not reliable. Treatment is with penicillin in the early phases, sulfonamides in the long term, and incision of any abscesses.

Inflammations of the Pharynx

Because of their particular pathophysiologic situation and clinical significance, infections of the lymphoepithelial pharyngeal ring will be treated separately, although many of these diseases may affect the rest of the pharynx (and vice versa).

Waldeyer's Ring

Acute Inflammations of the Tonsil

Acute infection of the lymphoepithelial tissue of the faucial isthmus, the palatine tonsil, is known as tonsillitis. The main symptoms relate to the tonsil.

Acute Tonsillitis (see Color Plate 22c)

Symptoms. The disease usually begins with high temperature and possibly chills, especially in children. The patient complains of a burning sensation in the throat, persistent pain in the oropharynx, pain on swallowing, and pain irradiating to the ear on swallowing. Opening the mouth is often difficult and painful, the tongue is coated, and there is oral fetor. The patient also complains of headaches, thick speech, marked feeling of malaise, and swelling and tenderness of the regional lymph nodes. *Both* tonsils and the surrounding area including the posterior pharyngeal wall are deep-red and swollen, but in catarrhal tonsillitis there is no exudate on the tonsil. Later, yellow spots corresponding to the lymphatic follicles form on the tonsils, hence the name *follicular tonsillitis*. Alternatively, yellow spots occur over the openings of the crypts, hence the name *lacunar tonsillitis*. A membrane occurs in *pneumococcal tonsillitis,* but is seldom confluent and rarely spreads beyond the tonsil. There is also swelling of the neighboring organs such as the faucial pillars, the uvula, and the base of the tongue. The patient also complains of sialorrhea and difficulty in eating.

Pathogenesis. The most common organism is the beta-hemolytic streptococcus. Staphylococci, pneumococci, mixed flora, hemophilus influenza, and *E. coli* are much less common. If the symptoms worsen and multifocal symptoms occur, a *generalized disorder* expressing itself particularly in the lymphoepithelial organs should be suspected. On the other hand, there are also tonsillar infections in which the generalized symptoms are minimal and only the local changes can be recognized. Virus infections are particularly important in this respect, e. g., herpangina (see p. 346). The tonsillar parenchyma is infiltrated with leukocytes in tonsillitis, causing small abscesses in the parenchyma and in the crypts. In addition, a fibrinous exudate is formed and there are marked changes in the parenchyma and the epithelium.

Note: Bacteria are constantly present in the mouth and pharynx. These saprophytic organisms include: saprophytic streptococcus viridans, pneumococci, fusiform bacteria, leptothrix, neisseria, lactobacteria, staphylococci, sarcina, and fungi.

These saprophytic organisms may become pathogenic due to a change in environment.

A virus infection may prepare the way for secondary bacterial infection.

Diagnosis. This is made from the clinical picture of an acute onset with high fever, pains in the neck and on swallowing, redness and exudate on the tonsils, and from general investigations of the blood picture, the erythrocyte sedimentation rate (ESR), the heart and circulation, and the urine. Appropriate tests or even cultures are carried out if diphtheria is suspected, and blood tests are done for mononucleosis.

Differential diagnosis. This includes scarlet fever, diphtheria, infectious mononucleosis, agranulocytosis, leukemia, hyperkeratosis of the tonsils, stage 2 syphilis, and in *unilateral* disease, ulceromembranous tonsillitis, peritonsillar cellulitis or abscess, tuberculosis, and tonsillar tumors (see below).

Treatment. This consists of bed rest, analgesics, bland fluid diet, ice packs, high-dose penicillin for 10 days, and observation for complications. Local care should include oral toilet and dental hygiene. Local antibiotics should not be given, but disinfectant and analgesic mouthwashes may be used. Moist neck dressings and a sweat pack may be used in the early phases.

Course. Tonsillitis usually resolves within 1 week. On the other hand, *complications* may occur such as respiratory obstruction due to laryngeal edema, otitis media, or rhinosinusitis; sequelae may occur (see p. 354).

Note: The following laboratory investigations should be done in tonsillitis:

1. Smear and culture to exclude diphtheria and determine causative bacteria
2. Urinalysis to exclude nephritis
3. Differential blood count to exclude mononucleosis and leukemia

Nasopharyngitis. The symptoms are as described above but are localized mainly or exclusively to the adenoid. Differential diagnosis includes viral nasopharyngitis.

Infection of the lingual tonsil. This is similar with symptoms localized to the base of the tongue. Ipsilateral involvement of the larynx or abscess formation in the tongue are possible.

Other types of tonsillitis:

1. Simple tonsillitis caused by nonspecific organisms
2. Tonsillitis in infectious diseases
3. Tonsillitis in hematologic diseases
4. Ulceromembranous tonsillitis

Infection of the Lateral Bands

This is a specific form of infection of the lateral, tubopharyngeal bands, especially in patients who have had their tonsils removed. It may be a "substitute" infection in the absence of tonsils. There is swelling, redness, and yellow spots around the lateral bands, and also in the solitary follicles on the posterior pharyngeal wall.

Treatment. As for tonsillitis one administers penicillin since complications *may* also occur in this disease. If the disease recurs frequently, the area should be cauterized with 2% to 5% silver nitrate solution; the cryoprobe may also be used carefully.

Herpangina

This disease causes marked generalized symptoms such as high fever, headache, pains in the neck, and loss of appetite and mainly affects children up to the age of 15. Vesicles form initially, particularly on the anterior faucial pillar, but are very fleeting, and therefore are not often seen. The tonsils are often *only slightly* red and swollen. Occasionally, they are covered in milky white vesicles up to the size of a lentil arranged like a chain of pearls or there are small flat ulcerations of the tonsil. Similar eruptions may occur on the palate or buccal mucosa.

Microbiology. The organism is the Coxsackie A virus which has an incubation period of 4 to 6 days.

Diagnosis. This is decided by the presence of vesicles, the minimal lesions of the tonsils, and the benign rapid course over several days.

Treatment is by oral hygiene.

Scarlet Fever

The tonsils and pharyngeal mucosa are deep red, there is pain on swallowing, severe malaise, progression to lacunar tonsillitis, and a regional lymphadenopathy. After about 24 h, a typical exanthem appears, beginning on the upper part of the body. At the same time, a definite reddening of the tip of the tongue and the edges of the tongue appears, extending later to the entire tongue, the strawberry tongue. The reddening of the face spares the perioral skin. It should be noted that the exanthem may not appear. Desquamation of the skin begins about the 8th day.

Microbiology. The type A hemolytic streptococcus is responsible.

Diagnosis. This is made from the clinical appearances of redness and swelling of the tonsil, the strawberry tongue, the small erythematous spots on the soft palate, and the Rumpel-Leede phenomenon of petechiae. The blood picture shows a leukocytosis and a left shift, and eosinophilia from the 5th day.

Differential diagnosis. This includes diphtheria, which is excluded by smear and/or culture.

Treatment is by penicillin and oral hygiene.

Diphtheria

Symptoms. There is a mild prodromal illness; the temperature is usually in the region of 38 °C and not more than 39 °C. There is slight pain on swallowing and often a very high pulse rate. The tonsils are moderately reddened and swollen with a white or grey velvety membrane which becomes confluent, extends beyond the boundaries of the tonsil to the faucial pillars and the soft palate, and which is fixed firmly to its base. The membrane can only be wiped off with difficulty and it then leaves a bleeding surface behind. The jugulodigastric lymph nodes are very swollen, tender, and often hard. There is a characteristic smell of acetone on the breath. Sixty percent of cases are localized to the pharynx including the tonsils, and in 8 % the larynx is involved in addition. Albuminuria is common.

Microbiology. The infection is due to the diphtheria bacillus, corynebacterium diphtheriae. The disease is transmitted from man to man by contact, droplets, or contamination by oral or nasal secretions. The incubation period is 3 to 5 days. In localized forms, the disease is restricted to the tonsil, the nose, the larynx, or a wound. The generalized form is progressive and toxic.

Diagnosis. This rests on: (1) bacteriologic smear from the tonsils and pharynx; Gram staining of a smear from the pseudomembrane provides the result within 1 h; (2) culture provides the answer at the earliest after 10 h; (3) isolation of the organism confirms the diagnosis in 2 to 8 days; (4) there is a membrane which is firmly adherent and which extends beyond the tonsil. *The disease is reportable to public health authorities.*

Differential diagnosis. This includes nonspecific tonsillitis, infectious mononucleosis, Vincent's angina, candidiasis, agranulocytosis, leukemia, and syphilis.

Treatment. At the earliest reasonable *suspicion* of diphtheria (possibly *before* bacteriologic confirmation), the patient should be isolated and treated with antiserum given intramuscularly in a dose of 200−500 IU/kg. In severe cases a high dose of 1,000 IU/kg may be given accompanied by antibiotic cover. Treatment also includes bed rest, oral hygiene, neck dressings changed several times a day, and steam inhalation. Diphtheria immunization by diphtheria toxoid is protective but does not become effective for several weeks.

Complications. These include general toxicity, failure of the heart and circulation, hemorrhagic nephritis or nephrosis, palatal paralysis due to polyneuritis, airway obstruction, and danger of asphyxia. A proportion of the population are silent carriers of the disease.

Normally, excretion of virulent diphtheria bacteria ceases after several weeks. However, carriers may remain a source of infection for months or even years. Cultures are therefore necessary until three cultures at weekly intervals are negative.

Long-term carriers should be treated by local and parenteral antibiotics and local disinfection. If this does not eradicate the organism, it may be necessary to carry out tonsillectomy, accompanied by adenoidectomy in children, to remove the source.

Syphilitic Tonsillitis (Stage 2)

Eight to ten weeks after the primary infection, white hazy mucosal enanthems, (plaques opalines), appear on the tonsils, the faucial pillars, and the soft palate. The hard palate is usually spared. Later they progress to dark-red papules. Signs of stage 2 infection are usually present in other parts of the body.

Diagnosis is made by dark-field illumination and serology.

Tonsillar Tuberculosis

This disease causes a superficial erosive ulcer with a necrotic slough (see p. 331).

Infectious Mononucleosis (see Color Plate **22b**)

Symptoms. These include fever, 38 ° to 39 °C, and marked lymphadenopathy of the jugulodigastric group and the deep cervical chain, later becoming generalized. The lymph nodes are moderately tender. The tonsil is very swollen and covered with a fibrinous exudate or membrane. The patient has a rhinopharyngitis, hepatosplenomegaly, pain in the neck on swallowing, and a marked feeling of being unwell. There is pain in the head and limbs. The blood picture initially shows a leukopenia, and then a leukocytosis of 20,000 to 30,000 or more of which 80% to 90% are mononuclear cells and atypical lymphocytes.

Microbiology. The causative organism is the Epstein-Barr virus, which chiefly affects children and adolescents. The disease is probably spread by droplet infection. The incubation period is 7 to 9 days.

Diagnosis. This is made from the picture of generalized lymphadenopathy and tonsillitis, the characteristic blood picture, a monospot test, the Paul-Bunnell test (demonstration of heterophile antibodies in the serum. A positive titer is > 1:28).

Differential diagnosis. This includes diphtheria (by culture), Vincent's angina, scarlet fever, syphilis, rubella, acute leukemia, toxoplasma, listeriosis, and tularemia.

Treatment. Symptomatic treatment includes oral hygiene and measures to reduce fever. Antibiotics may be given against secondary bacterial infection if there is marked ulceration. An allergic-like rash can occur in response to drugs such as ampicillin. Tonsillectomy may be indicated for *severe* local symptoms such as respiratory obstruction and, dysphagia, and persistent fever.

Complications. The course may be protracted with cranial nerve paralyses affecting the VIIth and Xth cranial nerves, serous meningitis and encephalitis, myocarditis (cardiologic supervision), hemolytic anemia, hemorrhagic complications in the gastrointestinal tract, the pharynx, and the skin, hematuria, obstruction of the airway, and danger of asphyxia. Tracheotomy should only be carried out in extreme emergency.

Note: If penicillin does not induce a rapid fall in fever in a patient with supposed tonsillitis, he probably suffers from infectious mononucleosis.

Agranulocytosis

Symptoms. The generalized symptoms are prominent and include high fever and chills. The patient feels very sick and has a typical blood picture. The disease occurs mainly in older subjects. There is ulceration and necrosis of the tonsils and the pharynx with a blackish exudate, severe pain in the neck and on swallowing, sialorrhea, and oral fetor. There is no regional lymphadenopathy.

Pathogenesis. Severe injury to the leukopoetic system may be caused by drugs, or by occupational or other toxins.

Differential diagnosis. This includes diphtheria, infectious mononucleosis, Vincent's angina, and acute leukemia.

Treatment. This consists of elimination of all possibly leukotoxic drugs, avoidance of other sources of injury, and prevention of secondary infection by high-dose penicillin, blood transfusion, and careful oral hygiene. The patient should be under the care of a hematologist.

Vincent's Angina (Angina ulceromembranacea) (see Color Plate **23a**)

The patient usually complains of *unilateral* pain on swallowing, and there is ipsilateral swelling of the jugulodigastric nodes. There is an ulcer, which is often deep, on *one* tonsil with a whitish exudate, whose site of predilection is the upper pole. The local findings are often impressive in contrast to the symptoms, which are often slight. There may only be a feeling of a foreign body in the throat, and the patient also has a characteristic oral fetor. Usually there is *no* fever. The exudate which can be easily wiped off may extend to the palate, buccal mucosa, and gingiva.

Microbiology. There is an obligatory symbiosis of a spirochete and fusiform rods.

Diagnosis. This is made on the clinical picture of a typical infection usually of *one* tonsil, with unilateral lymphadenopathy, and on the results of bacterial culture.

Differential diagnosis. This includes diphtheria, tuberculosis, syphilis, tonsillar neoplasms, acute leukemia, agranulocytosis, and infectious mononucleosis.

Treatment. Penicillin is given for 3 to 6 days. The course is usually short and the prognosis good.

Candidiasis (see Color Plate **18b**)

A white superficial punctate exudate forms which can be wiped off and which later becomes confluent. There is usually only slight redness of the surrounding mucosa. The tonsils, the palate, the posterior pharyngeal wall, and the buccal mucosa may be affected. Subjective symptoms are few.

Treatment is by antimycotic agents (see p. 329).

Differential Diagnoses of Interest

Hyperkeratosis of the tonsil is a typical yellowish-brown or white, flat or somewhat nodular prominent hyperkeratotic process on the tonsillar surface which *cannot* be wiped off. It is often diagnosed mistakenly as tonsillitis. The cause is a benign circumscribed keratinization of the tonsil, especially of the epithelium of the crypt. No treatment is necessary.

Chronic Tonsillitis

Chronic tonsillitis requires particular attention on diagnostic grounds because it is difficult to differentiate from a normal tonsil. It may also be a focus of infection with effects on the entire body.

Symptoms. The history usually shows recurrent attacks of tonsillitis, but this is not always the case. There is often little or no pain in the neck or difficulty on swallowing. There is a halitosis and a bad taste in the mouth. The jugulodigastric lymph nodes are often enlarged. Chronic tonsillitis often remains more or less symptomless. The systemic effect may declare itself by lowering of resistance, tiredness, tendency to catch colds, unexplained high temperature, and loss of appetite.

Pathogenesis. The organisms are usually a mixed flora of aerobic and anaerobic bacteria in which streptococci predominate. Group A beta-hemolytic streptococci are especially likely to cause focal symptoms. Poor drainage of the branching crypts leads to retention of cell debris which forms a good culture medium for bacteria (see p. 308). From such crypt abscesses, the infection extends via the epithelial defects of the reticular epithelium into the tonsillar parenchyma to form a cryptic parenchymatous tonsillitis. Alternatively it penetrates into the capillaries surrounding the crypts, allowing intermittent or continuous penetration of toxins and organisms into the general circulation. In the long term, the tonsillar parenchyma undergoes fibrosis and atrophy.

Diagnosis

a) History shows recurrent acute or subacute attacks of tonsillitis.

b) Local Findings

- The tonsils are more or less fixed to their bed as shown by the depressor test (see Fig. 3.**13**)
- The tonsillar surface is fissured or scarred
- *Watery* pus and greyish-yellow material may be pressed out of the opening of the crypts by a tongue depressor (see Fig. 3.**13**)
- Reddening of the anterior faucial pillar is present
- Peritonsillar tenderness is present
- Lymphadenopathy of the jugulodigastric group is found

c) General Findings

- History shows recurrent tonsillitis, unexplained high temperature, lowering of resistance, etc.
- Blood picture: there is increased ESR and antistreptolysin titer (see below)

Note: Fixed yellow concrements noted when pressure is exerted on the crypts with a tongue depressor do *not* signify chronic tonsillitis but are a physiologic phenomenon (tonsillar plugs). The size of the tonsil is also *not* a criterion for the presence of chronic tonsillitis. This disease can occur in large hyperplastic tonsils, but it more common in small and medium-sized tonsils. It is not always possible to make the diagnosis of chronic tonsillitis from the local findings. The history and general findings must also be assessed critically. The judgment and experience of the axaminer is often decisive. Immunology has so far not proven to be of any practical diagnostic value.

Besides its irritative effect on adjacent tissues and organs, chronic tonsillitis is of special clinical interest due to the possibility of a focal infection. *Is there or is there not a focal infection?* This remains a controversial issue, with opinions ranging from rigorous denial of the "focal" concept to enthusiastic acceptance of the focal-infection hypothesis as a basis for treatment. Although some skepticism is justified, it must be granted that clinical experience affirms the plausibility of causal relationships, say, between chronic tonsillitis (or an apical dental granuloma, etc.) and concomitant inflammatory diseases of other organs and structures, and that there are at least some instances in which such relationships obviously exist. Again, this is a controversial issue even among experts, and there is no point in substituting medical empiricism for medical doctrine in this situation. The individual physician should be familiar with the pro-and-con arguments so that he can define his own position and apply it to therapeutic decision making. It is with this in mind that we present the following considerations on the "focal process" issue:

1. A "focus" is any local change within the body that is capable of producing remote pathologic effects beyond its immediate surroundings.
2. As previously shown (see p. 308), the structure of the palatine tonsil with its arborizing system of narrow-necked crypts, spongy epithelium, and relatively unprotected blood vessels creates conditions ideal for the dissemination of pathologic material (microorganisms, inflammatory products, toxins) into the bloodstream.
3. Theories on the potential pathogenic mechanisms of focal disease are highly diverse (clinically subthreshold "sepsis" in which bacteria and/or toxins are swept into the systemic circulation; antigen stimulation by exogenous (microbial) proteins at the focus as a mechanism for inciting or perpetuating the disease; allergic-hyperergic reactions evoked by endogenous protein breakdown products from the focus [autoallergic or autoaggressive mechanism], etc.).
4. The difficulty in critically evaluating a presumed focal process is that while clinical experience tends to support this pathogenic mechanism (e. g., by the "eradication of foci"), experimental research in focal infection has not yet produced satisfactory results.

The *diseases that may be based on a focal process* according to clinical experience include the following:

- Rheumatic fever (acute, febrile joint and muscle disease)
- Glomerulonephritis and focal nephritis
- Localized pustular psoriasis
- Eruptive psoriasis (in children)
- Chronic urticaria
- Endo-, myo- and pericarditis
- Polyserositis
- Inflammatory disorders of the nerves and eyes (iridocyclitis)
- Vascular diseases (e. g., recurrent thromboangiitis, nodular vasculitis)

Treatment. Chronic tonsillitis requires treatment whenever it satisfies the conditions of a local pathologic process outlined above (see pp. 350ff.). Conservative measures such as gargling, painting, and suctioning are of no benefit. Even antibiotics can at best favorably influence the local process and risk of dissemination during the course of treatment. Once the antibiotic is withdrawn, the pathogenic mechanism will be rekindled because the anatomic situation has not changed.

It appears, then, that *tonsillectomy* is the only definitive treatment to be considered for chronic tonsillitis. This applies even to patients with a coexisting coagulation disorder, which will necessitate appropriate replacement measures prior to surgery, special operative techniques (e. g., "sealing" of the wound surface with fibrin glue and collagen fleece), and meticulous local supervision for a period of several days.

Tonsillectomy is indicated for the following diseases:

- Chronic tonsillitis
- Recurrent tonsillitis
- Peritonsillar abscess
- Tonsillogenic septicemia
- Tonsillogenic or posttonsillitis focal symptoms
- Marked hypertrophy of the tonsil causing mechanical obstruction
- If a tonsillar tumor is suspected

Relative indications include:

- Resistant carriers of diphtheria bacilli
- Stubborn oral fetor as a result of excess production of tonsillar plugs
- Tuberculous cervical lymph nodes (of bovine type) in which the tonsil is a possible portal of entry (see p. 496)

Contraindications include pharyngitis sicca, leukemia, agranulocytosis, serious generalized disorders such as tuberculosis or diabetes, and ulcerative or destructive processes extending beyond the tonsil if the diagnosis has not been confirmed. In some cases cleft palate also represents a contraindication.

The *age of the patient* is *no* contraindication in doubtful cases.

> *Note:* Conservative, i.e., medical, treatment of chronic tonsillitis is illogical. The previously popular tonsillotomy has now become obsolete because of the danger of postoperative development of foci in the remaining scarred tonsillar remnant. This is also true for procedures such as incising the tonsil, tonsillar irrigation, aspiration of the tonsil, electrocoagulation, and radiotherapy.
>
> The decision to advise tonsillectomy should not be taken lightly. Much critical experience is required.

The balance between immunobiologic considerations and the local pathologic findings must be weighed carefully before advising tonsillectomy, particularly in children.

Principles of Tonsillectomy

The operation may be carried out either under local or general intubation anesthesia.

Tonsillectomy is usually carried out under intubation anesthesia with the head extended (Fig. 3.**16a** and **b**). An incision is made in the anterior faucial pillar, and the connective tissue layer between the tonsillar parenchyma and the pharyngeal constrictor muscles is demonstrated. The tonsil is then freed by combined blunt and sharp dissection proceeding from the upper pole to the base of the tongue, preserving the faucial pillars. The *entire* tonsillar tissue must be removed. Hemostasis is secured by pressure, ligatures, or electrocautery. The same procedure is then carried out on the opposite side.

Complications include hemorrhage which may occur up to the 14th postoperative day. See also p.323.

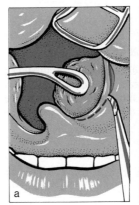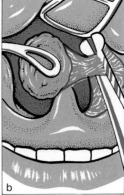

Fig. 3.**16a** and **b**   Tonsillectomy with the head extended. The tongus is above, the upper incisors are below. **(a)** Incision, **(b)** dissection and removal of the tonsil.

In countries where there is *risk of infection by poliomyelitis,* tonsillectomy should not be carried out during the warmer season of the year. Tonsillectomy should also not be carried out during epidemics of other infectious diseases.

The following questions are often asked about tonsillectomy:

1. *The tonsils are obviously protective organs. Is it not a disadvantage for the entire body if they are removed?* The tonsils ought to be removed only if they are the site of irreversible inflammatory disease, if they are acting as a focus of infection, or if they impede breathing or swallowing by their size. In these cases, the pathologic properties of the tonsils are predominant, and their original protective function is reduced or lost. This protective, immunologic function can certainly be taken over satisfactorily by the remaining lymphoepithelial organs and structures of the pharynx. The removal of irreversibly diseased or very enlarged tonsils, and those suspected of carrying a focus of infection, is thus not a disadvantage, but a prerequisite for good health.

2. *Is the tendency to upper respiratory infections increased after tonsillectomy?* A distinction must be made between pharyngitis and tonsillitis. The susceptibility to pharyngitis is not improved by tonsillectomy itself, but may improve if the tonsillectomy causes the airway to be restored to normal, e. g., in tonsillar hypertrophy, and the flora of the mouth and pharynx are restored to normal, e. g., in chronic tonsillitis. Simple pharyngitis may thus occur with the same frequency after tonsillectomy as before, but tonsillitis can no longer occur nor can the dangerous intratonsillar abscess, focal symptoms, and tonsillogenic complications.

3. *What is the best age and the best time of year to carry out tonsillectomy?* The operation may be carried out at any age and at any time of year, but the operation should only be done for the strictest indications under the age of 4 and after the age of 60.

4. *Does tonsillectomy have any deleterious effect on the voice and speech?* Tonsillectomy, if carried out by a careful conservative technique, usually has no deleterious effects on the voice and speech. Great care should be taken, however, before advising the operation in a patient with an open, corrected, or occult cleft palate. Reinforcement of the palatal insufficiency is described on p. 374ff. In singers the resonating space may be changed, although usually only temporarily, and care is advised in these patients.

Complications During and After Tonsillitis

Posttonsillitis complications include rheumatic fever, often with a symptom-free interval of 4 to 6 weeks, and endo-, myo-, or pericarditis. Acute glomerulonephritis and focal nephritis, which require urinalysis after resolution of the tonsillitis, are diseases secondary to streptococcal infection (see p. 344).

Local Complications

Peritonsillar Abscess (Supra- or Retrotonsillar Abscess) (see Color Plate **23b**)

Symptoms. Rapidly increasing difficulty in swallowing occurs after a symptomfree interval of a few days after tonsillitis. The pain usually irradiates to the ear, and opening of the mouth is difficult due to trismus. The speech is thick and indistinct. The pain is so severe that the patient often refuses to eat, the head is held over to the diseased side, and rapid head movements are avoided. The patient has sialorrhea and oral fetor, swelling of the regional lymph nodes, increase of fever with high temperatures of 39° to 40°C, and the general condition deteriorates rapidly. He also has an intolerable feeling of pressure in the neck, obstruction of the laryngeal inlet, and increasing respiratory obstruction. However, the symptoms may on occasion be only mild. Simultaneous bilateral abscesses may occur.

Pathogenesis. Inflammation spreads from the tonsillar parenchyma to the surrounding tissue, peritonsillitis, and forms an abscess within a few days. The pharyngeal constrictor muscle is usually an effective barrier against further spread. (See Fig. 3.**17a**).

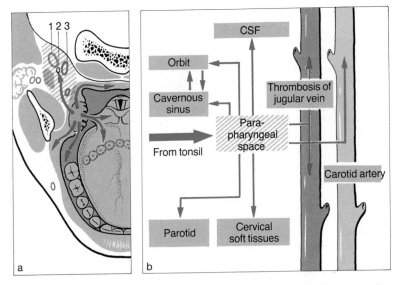

Fig. 3.**17a** and **b** Tonsillogenic complications. **a.** Extension to the immediate surrounding tissues. The red-shaded area shows the parapharyngeal space. 1, Internal jugular vein; 2, vagus nerve; 3, internal carotid artery. **b.** Further possible directions of spread of tonsillogenic infection.

Table 3.6 Trismus

Trismus is divided into three grades depending on the distance between the edges of the upper and lower incisors: grade 1: 4–2.5 cm; grade 2: 2.5–1 cm; grade 3: less than 1 cm. Total trismus indicates complete loss of mobility of the mandible.

Group	Individual Cause
Inflammation of the teeth or mandible	Unerupted dentition, stomatitis, pulpitis, osteomyelitis of the upper or lower jaw, peri- and submandibular abscess, temporomandibular arthritis, arthrosis deformans of the temporomandibular joint, chronic polyarthritis
Acute inflammation around the temporomandibular joint	Peritonsillitis and peritonsillar abscess, sialadenitis and sialolithiasis of the parotid and submandibular glands, otitis externa and meatal furuncle, parapharyngeal soft tissue abscess
Trauma	Fracture of the temporomandibular joint, fracture of the zygoma and zygomatic arch, mandibular fracture, dislocation of the temporomandibular joint, posttraumatic scarring
Muscle spasm	Epilepsy, spasticity by central nervous lesions (cerebral tumors), meningitis, tetanus, tetany and hysteria
Tumors	Benign or malignant tumors around the temporomandibular joint, results of tumor resection, scarring after radiotherapy
Miscellaneous	Congenital ankylosis of the temporomandibular joint

Diagnosis. This is made on the clinical picture of swelling, redness, and protrusion of the tonsil, the faucial arch, the palate, and the uvula. The uvula is pushed to the healthy side, and there is marked tenderness of the tonsillar area. Inspection of the pharynx may be difficult because of severe trismus (Table 3.6). The jugulodigastric nodes are tender. There is an exudate on the tongue, rarely on the tonsils and palate. The blood picture and ESR are typical of an acute infection. When the swelling is fluctuant, it may be possible to aspirate its contents for diagnosis.

Differential diagnosis. This includes peritonsillar phlegmon, tonsillogenic sepsis (see below), allergic swelling of the pharynx without fever (angioneurotic edema), malignant diphtheria, agranulocytosis, specific tonsillar infections (tuberculosis and syphilis), and nonulcerating tumors of the tonsil or neighboring tissues (malignant lymphoma, lymphoepithelial tumor, anaplastic carcinoma, or leukemia).

The differential diagnosis also includes dental infections such as peritonsillar abscess due to impacted wisdom teeth and aneurysms of the internal carotid artery (pulsation). The absence of acute local signs of infection and of fever and a prolonged course suggest that a diagnosis of peritonsillar abscess is *wrong*.

Treatment. *Conservative.* High doses of antibiotics, e.g., penicillin or cephalosporin, etc. for 1 week at least, can only prevent the formation of an abscess in the *early* stages of infiltration of the peritonsillar tissues. Analgesics, a fluid diet, cold foods, an ice pack to the neck, and mouthwashes are prescribed. Gargling should be *forbidden*.

Operative Treatment

1. *Abscess tonsillectomy* which is carried out under general endotracheal anesthesia (see p. 353). This procedure may be performed on all patients who are fit for operation, particularly those with a recurrent peritonsillar abscess. It prevents further recurrence, the patient must endure only one course of treatment and time is saved.

2. *Drainage of the abscess* followed by tonsillectomy 3 to 4 days later under general anesthesia.

Principles of drainage of the abscess. Local anesthesia is induced carefully with 1% topical Xylocaine, and infiltration anesthesia with 1% Xylocaine plus 1:200,000 epinephrine is used at the site of the intended incision. Pus often drains from the puncture site when the anesthetic agents is introduced. The anesthetic must be allowed approximately 5 min to act before incision. Endotracheal anesthesia is usually more acceptable to the patient.

The site of incision. This is made at the point of maximum protrusion, usually between the uvula and the second upper molar tooth (Fig. 3.**18**). A test aspiration may be made on occasion before the incision. A long-handled pointed scalpel is used for the incision. All but 1.5 to 2 cm of the point is wrapped in sterile adhesive tape (see Fig. 3.**18**) to prevent the point of the scalpel from penetrating too deeply and injuring the major vessels of the neck. The incision is made parallel to the ascending ramus of the mandible and must not pass externally since the internal carotid artery and internal jugular vein are immediate relations (see Fig. 3.**17a**). If the diagnosis is correct, pus gushes out and must be removed with a powerful aspirator to prevent aspiration into the trachea. After the abscess has drained, a hemostat is introduced into the abscess cavity and opened widely usually producing a further gush of pus. The abscess cavity must be opened up daily until pus no longer drains from it.

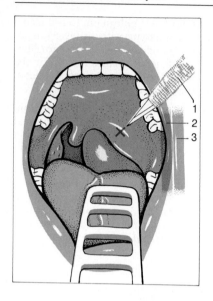

Fig. 3.**18** Peritonsillar abscess.
1, Guarded scalpel; 2, internal carotid artery; 3, internal jugular vein. X is the midpoint between the uvula and the last molar and is the typical site for incision.

Note: An incision should not be made until the abcess is "ripe," i.e., fluctuation can be shown or is probable.

Interval tonsillectomy can be performed after a delay of 1 to 2 months to prevent recurrence of the abscess.

Course and prognosis. Regression of the inflammation and prevention of an abscess is possible with timely administration of antibiotics. An abscess may also drain spontaneously and heal. However, distressing pain and difficulty in eating usually require active drainage. If tonsillectomy is not carried out, there is a high risk of recurrent abscess in the paratonsillar scar tissue.

Complications and dangers. These include extension of the inflammatory swelling and edema to the laryngeal inlet with increasing *respiratory obstruction* and possibly *danger of asphyxia*. The abscess may also rupture into the parapharyngeal space (see Fig. 3.**17a**). From here it may extend as:

- A descending internal cervical phlegmon
- A parapharyngeal abscess
- An ascending involvement of the orbit or the cranial cavity causing meningitis, cavernous sinus thrombosis, and brain abscess

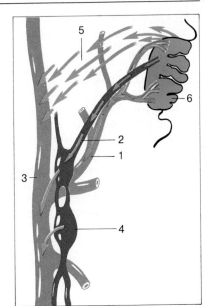

Fig. 3.**19** Genesis of tonsillogenic sepsis. 1, Extension by veins; 2 extension by lymph vessels; 3, internal jugular vein; 4, regional lymph nodes around the internal jugular vein; 5, extension in continuity via the cervical soft tissues to the internal jugular vein; 6, palatine tonsil.

- Thrombosis of the internal jugular vein
- Erosion of the carotid artery or its branches (rarely)
- Invasion of the parotid (purulent parotitis)

General Complications

Septicemia During or After Tonsillitis, Tonsillogenic Sepsis

Symptoms. These include chills with a septic temperature chart, tenderness along the internal jugular vein which appears as a tender firm cord under the anterior edge of the sternocleidomastoid muscle, or tenderness of the jugulodigastric lymph nodes. There is often simultaneous reddening of the tonsillar area but this is not essential. The patient has severe constitutional upset, a left shift in the blood picture with leukocytosis, a splenomegaly, possibly metastases to the lung, skin, or liver, dry tongue, and a weak rapid pulse.

Pathogenesis. Bacteria enter the bloodstream from the tonsil or a neighboring focus of pus.

Three different pathways are possible (Fig. 3.**19**):

1. *Hematogenous* via the tonsillar veins and the facial vein to the internal jugular vein. Thrombophlebitis develops in the vein, and infected thrombi enter the pulmonary or general circulation.

2. *Lymphogenous* via efferent lymphatics of the tonsil to the regional lymph nodes of the jugulodigastric group and along the internal jugular vein. From there the internal jugular vein becomes infected, and the disease then progresses as in paragraph (1) above.
3. *Direct spread* of the abscess in or around the tonsil with rupture into the parapharyngeal space or into the cervical soft tissue with involvement of the internal jugular vein.

Many organisms may be responsible for tonsillogenic septicemia; they can often be demonstrated in the blood if a specimen is taken during a rigor. Mixed infections are also frequent.

Diagnosis. This is made from the picture of chills and symptoms of septicemia due to continuous or intermittent bacteremia. There is a history of tonsillitis and symptoms of chronic tonsillitis (see p. 350); the ESR *increases rapidly,* and there is a rapidly rising leukocytosis. There is tenderness of the jugulodigastric lymph nodes or the internal jugular vein. Defensive spasm of the cervical soft tissues occurs with relieving posture of head and neck. The organism may be demonstrated in the blood.

Treatment. If severe sepsis is suspected, high-dose penicillin or broad-spectrum antibiotics are started immediately to protect the body from metastases. Other *obligatory* measures include:

1. *Tonsillectomy* to eliminate the focus
2. *Ligature of the internal jugular vein* inferior to the thrombus and resection of the diseased segment if the internal jugular vein is involved
3. *Wide opening and drainage* of an abscess of the cervical soft tissues

Course and prognosis. This is a life-threatening disease, but the prognosis is good if treatment by antibiotics and surgery is instituted *promptly*.

The following conditions are rare:

Tonsillogenic cavernous sinus thrombosis transmitted via the pterygoid venous plexus or the internal jugular vein to the inferior ophthalmic vein. Symptoms are described on p. 250.

Bleeding due to erosion, secondary to tonsillitis. The external and internal carotid artery may be involved in a similar manner to the cervical veins by an abscess in the parapharyngeal space. Symptoms include severe hemorrhage from the tonsil, usually after a small prodromal bleed.

> *Note:* An *immediate* tonsillectomy must be carried out under massive antibiotic cover at the first suspicion of tonsillogenic septicemia with recurrent chills.

Rare abscesses in the pharyngeal area include

Retropharyngeal Abscess in Children

An abscess may form by breaking down of lymphadenitis of the retropharyngeal lymph nodes after pharyngeal infection in children especially in the first 2 years of life.

Symptoms. These include swelling of the posterior pharyngeal wall, difficulty in swallowing, thick speech, difficulty in eating, elevated temperature, relieving posture of the neck (differential diagnosis: torticollis), leakage of food through the nose, possibly nasal obstruction, croup, and laryngeal edema.

Differential diagnosis. Benign and malignant prevertebral tumors must be considered.

Treatment. This is by paramedian incision and drainage with the head hanging if fluctuation occurs. The patient must be protected from aspiration and is given antibiotic cover.

Retropharyngeal Abscess in Adults

This is usually a descending prevertebral cold abscess originating from tuberculous caries of a cervical vertebra or of suppuration in osteomyelitis of the temporal bone, e. g., petrositis, and in mastoiditis.

Symptoms. These include pressure in the neck, attacks of coughing, difficulty in swallowing, mild dysphagia, stiffness of the neck, and typical lesions of the cervical spine on radiographs.

Differential diagnosis is benign and malignant tumors and spondylosis of the cervical spine.

Treatment. A test aspiration is made. If a cold abscess is present it is drained, if possible to the lateral part of the neck and not into the oropharynx. Antituberculous treatment is given, and the patient is referred to an orthopedic surgeon.

Other Pharyngeal Inflammations

Acute Catarrhal Pharyngitis

Symptoms. These include pain on swallowing, possibly radiating to the ear, a feeling of dryness, heat, and soreness in the pharynx, itching, scratching, burning, clearing the throat, and attacks of coughing. The patient usually feels sick. The entire pharynx (naso-, oro-, and hypopharynx), is usually involved in the infection. Fever occurs, especially in children. In viral infections, the course is often intermittent over several weeks.

Pathogenesis. This is usually a primary virus infection often with later secondary bacterial infection. Less often it is a primary bacterial infection due to streptococci, hemophilus influenza, or pneumococci. There are prodomal symptoms on acute infection such as measles, scarlet fever, and rubella. An acute pharyngitis may also be rhinogenic and/or sinugenic, or it may be caused by physical or chemical injury, scalds, caustics, etc.

Diagnosis. The mucosa appears red and thickened. The palatal and pharyngeal mucosa are dry with a glazed surface. Mucus is produced which is

initially colorless but later tenacious and yellow. Deep-red, solitary follicles are usually prominent, and there is a regional lymphadenopathy with
swelling and tenderness, especially in children. Tonsillitis often occurs, or
if the tonsils have been removed there is infection of the lateral bands (see
p. 345).

Treatment. Symptomatic treatment includes hot milk and honey, cold or
warm cervical dressings, pharyngeal irrigation, and steam inhalations.
Smoking is forbidden, and anesthetic and disinfectant lozenges are given.
Local antibiotics must *not* be given, and parenteral antibiotics are only
given for severe bacterial infections. Bed rest is advised for fever.

Chronic Pharyngitis

This is a comprehensive term for several chronic irritative or inflammatory
conditions of the pharyngeal mucosa.

Symptoms. There are *several* forms:

1. *Simple chronic pharyngitis.* This causes a globus sensation, constant
   throat cleaning, bouts of coughing, a feeling of dryness or phlegm in
   the throat, pain in the neck and on swallowing of varying degree, and
   tenacious secretion. The course is intermittent, and there is *no* generalized upset and no fever.
2. *Chronic hyperplastic pharyngitis.* The mucosa of the posterior pharyngeal wall is thickened and granular with prominent solitary follicles. It
   is a smooth red to greyish-red in color, possibly with venous telangiec-
   tasis and secretion of stringy colorless mucus. There is usually a very
   disturbing, strange sensation in the pharynx with compulsive throat-
   clearing and swallowing, gagging, and even vomiting.
3. *Chronic atrophic pharyngitis.* The posterior pharyngeal wall is dry,
   glazed often with dry, tough crusts of secretion. The mucosa is smooth,
   pink, often very tender and transparent, but may also be red and thickened. Simultaneous atrophic rhinitis and laryngitis sicca may occur.
   The patient is constantly obliged to spit out the stringy secretion. At
   night there is a feeling of choking and disturbance of sleep. Continuous clearing of the throat may produce slight mucosal hemorrhage.
   The disease depends on climatic or temperature conditions, and the
   symptoms resolve at the seaside but are worse in hot dry air. Older
   people are more often affected.

Pathogenesis. The patient often has a constitutionally determined functional weakness of the mucosa. On the other hand, the disease may be due
to chronic exogenous damage from dust, chemicals, heat (e. g., at work),
marked changes in temperature, and working in drafty and smoky conditions (butchers and restaurant personnel), and dry or incorrectly air-condi-
tioned atmosphere, marked nicotine and alcohol abuse, mouth breathing,
nasal obstruction, abuse of nose drops, chronic sinusitis, and adenoidal

hypertrophy. Other causes include endocrine disorders (menopause, hypothyroidism), avitaminosis A and general disorders (heart and kidney malfunction, diabetes, pulmonary insufficiency, chronic bronchial diseases). Finally, mucosal allergy and incorrect use of the voice in professional speakers such as teachers, politicians, and singers may be responsible.

Diagnosis. The local findings are typical. The disease lasts for years with an intermittent course. There is often a discrepancy between the unremarkable local findings and the marked symptoms.

Differential diagnosis. This includes Sjögren's syndrome (see pp. 535, 543, and Color Plate **38a** and **c**), Plummer-Vinson syndrome (see p. 364), and malignancy of any part of the pharynx or esophagus. The latter requires careful endoscopy. The disease must be distinguished from chronic tonsillitis and sinusitis, specific pharyngitis, tuberculosis or syphilis, cervical spondylosis and deficient antibody syndrome, diagnosed by serum electrophoresis, Thornwaldt's bursa (see below), elongated styloid process syndrome (see p. 364), enlarged posterior ends of the nasal turbinates, choanal polyp, and psychoneurosis.

Treatment. The above-named local or distant causes are looked for and eliminated.

Symptomatic treatment includes moisturizing of the pharyngeal mucosa by steam inhalations. Nicotine and alcohol must be avoided. Local measures are described on p. 369 and include oily preparations to provide a protective film for the dry mucosa. A change of climate is advised, and the air humidity at work is tested. The patient may even have to change his job or place of residence.

Thornwaldt's Disease, Pharyngeal Bursitis

Symptoms. These include foul-smelling drainage from the nasopharynx, particularly in the mornings.

Pathogenesis. The cause of this disease lies in persistence of the central groove of the adenoid or formation of a pouch in the roof of the pharynx as an anatomic variant (see Fig. 3.6) or on the posterior wall of the nasopharynx which retains yellowish-brown secretion and debris with and without accompanying inflammation. Gradual closure and formation of a cyst is possible. The symptoms are then intermittent. This is a rare disorder.

Diagnosis. This is made by careful endoscopic examination of the entire nasopharynx.

Differential diagnosis. Sinusitis, especially sphenoid or ethmoidal, or early neoplasm in the nasopharynx must be considered.

Treatment. Operative obliteration of the cyst is performed.

Ulceromembranous Pharyngitis (see pp. 327, 349)

Plummer-Vinson Syndrome, Patterson-Brown-Kelly Syndrome

Symptoms. This disease occurs almost exclusively in women from 40 to 70 years of age and may occasionally cause marked, painful dysphagia. The mucosa of the tongue and of the pharynx is atrophic; the skin is dry, pale, and flaccid; the mucous membranes are dry; the patient also has koilonychia and complains of burning of the tongue.

Pathogenesis. The basic cause is probably an iron deficiency. Promoting factors include achlorhydria and avitaminosis and chronic atrophic mucosal inflammation with subepithelial fibrosis.

Diagnosis. The dysphagia worsens so that ultimately only small amounts can be swallowed. The fingernails are curved, there are rhagades at the corners of the mouth, weight loss, hypochromic anemia, extremely low values of serum iron, aniso- and microcytosis, radiologic evidence of spasm of the esophageal opening with a notch at the level of the cricoid, and possibly also a web within the esophageal lumen at that level. Endoscopy should be carried out.

Differential diagnosis. This includes postcricoid carcinoma, hypopharyngeal carcinoma, and functional dysphagia.

Treatment. Therapy consists of iron and vitamin B, a bland diet, and possibly endoscopic dilatation of the stenosis.

Pharyngeal diphtheria. See p. 346.

Tuberculosis, syphilis, leprosy, and sarcoid of the pharyngeal mucosa are described on pp. 206, 207, 220, 498 respectively.

Lesions of the pharyngeal mucosa occur in blood disorders such as agranulocytosis, panmyelophthisis, acute leukemia, and chronic lymphatic and chronic myeloid leukemia.

Other Diseases Simulating Infections

Styloid Process Syndrome (Stylalgia; Eagle-Syndrome)

Symptoms include neuralgia or dysphagia, usually on one side, maximal in the tonsillar region or behind the angle of the jaw. Pain may irradiate to the ear or the temporal region. Pain may occur on swallowing or on certain movements of the cervical spine. The symptoms are reproducible by palpation of the tonsillar cleft.

Pathogenesis (Fig. 3.**20**) is mechanical irritation of the nerves and vessels close to the styloid process due to its excess length (normal length is about 3 cm). Neighboring nerves are the IXth, Xth, XIth, and XIIth cranial nerves, and the neighboring vessels are the internal and external carotid artery. An elongated styloid is not common.

Diagnosis is based of palpation of the tonsillar cleft which produces the typical symptoms at this point, and by radiography.

Differential diagnosis is neuralgias of the IXth and Xth cranial nerves (see below), and spondylosis of the cervical spine.

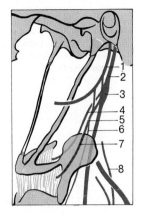

Fig. 3.**20**   The stylohyoid syndrome. 1, Glossopharyngeal nerve; 2, vagus nerve; 3, nodose ganglion of the vagus nerve; 4, pharyngeal branches of the IXth and Xth cranial nerves; 5, superior laryngeal nerve with external branch (6) and internal branch (7); 8, phrenic nerve. The red area is a persistent embryonal hyoid bone chain.

Treatment is by removal of the styloid process from the mouth via a tonsillectomy or an external approach.

Stylokeratohyoid syndrome (see Fig. 3.**20**). This syndrome is due to failure of the derivatives of the second branchial arch to atrophy, and to extensive calcification of these structures. The disease is rare.

Symptoms are similar to those of the styloid process syndrome, but are more variable and include unilateral neuralgia on the lateral side of the head and neck, unilateral pain on swallowing, a feeling of a foreign body on swallowing, a temporary feeling of dizziness, and attacks of sweating. Brief loss of consciousness in certain positions of the head and neck, tinnitus, or paralysis of the recurrent laryngeal nerve are all possible. The diaphragm may be elevated due to paralysis of the phrenic nerve, and the VIIth, IXth, Xth, XIth, and XIIth cranial nerves may be affected in different combinations.

Diganosis is made by radiography.

Differential diagnosis is as for the stylohyoid syndrome and the subclavian steal syndrome, as well as cervical rib, and stenosis of the carotid or vertebral arteries.

Treatment is operative removal of the abnormal bone.

Cervical rib syndrome, see p. 504.

Subclavian steal syndrome, see p. 483.

Stenosis of the internal carotid artery, see p. 482.

Stenosis of the vertebral artery, see p. 483.

Glossopharyngeal neuralgia (IX)

Symptoms. This is usually a disease of the older age groups. There is sudden tearing pain of one side of the tongue or the neck irradiating to the ear accompanied by discharge of tenacious saliva. Pain is induced by swallowing food, chewing, and also

Table 3.7 Dysphagia	
Site	Causal Disease
Oropharyngeal	*Inflammatory:* glossitis, abscess of the floor of the mouth, specific and nonspecific pharyngitis, tonsillitis, peritonsillar abscess, retropharyngeal and hypopharyngeal abscess, edema of the uvula and angioneurotic edema *Neural:* lesions of vagus, hypoglossal and glossopharyngeal nerves, glossopharyngeal and vagus neuralgia *Mechanical obstruction:* foreign body, hypopharyngeal diverticulum, pharyngeal stricture, styloid process syndrome, benign and malignant tumors *Congenital anomalies:* macroglossia, clefts of the lip and jaw and palate, cysts of the base of the tongue, lingual thyroid, hyoid anomalies, cervical cysts and fistulae (median and lateral) *Miscellaneous:* results of radiotherapy, xerostomia, humidifying disorders, sialedonitis, fractures of the upper and lower jaw and the hyoid, lesions of the masticatory muscles, burns and scalds, results of surgery
Laryngeal	*Inflammatory:* epiglottitis, specific and nonspecific laryngitis, perichondritis of the larynx *Neural:* neuralgia of the superior laryngeal nerve, paralysis of the superior laryngeal nerve *Miscellaneous:* laryngeal trauma (contusion, distortion, fracture), results of radiotherapy, laryngocele, benign and malignant tumor, foreign bodies, and results of surgery
Esophageal	*Inflammatory or traumatic:* esophagitis including reflux esophagitis, esophageal mycosis, esophageal trauma, caustic burns, results of trauma and surgery, strictures and stenoses, esophageal foreign bodies and esophageal perforation

	Disorders of motility: esophageal spasm, "upper achalasia" (spasm of the cricopharyngeus muscle), external compression by goiter, aortic aneurysm or tumors of the lung and mediastinum, achalasia (cardiospasm), scleroderma, results of vagotomy, esophageal varices, presbyesophagus *Neighboring organs:* goiter *Congenital anomalies:* diverticulum, megaesophagus, hiatus hernia, congenital esophageal stenosis, vascular abnormalities *Tumors:* benign or malignant esophageal tumors (the latter are more common)
Diseases of the cervical spine	Arthritis of the cervical spine, subluxation of the cervical spine, dislocation of the cervical spine, prolapsed disc, spondylolisthesis, cervical rib
Neurologic disorders	Amyotrophic lateral sclerosis, bulbar paralysis, pseudobulbar paralysis, bulbar poliomyelitis, polyneuritis, multiple sclerosis, syringomyelia, cerebral and cerebellar ischemia, thrombosis of the posterior inferior cerebellar artery or basilar artery, brain tumors and brain stem tumors, disorders of CSF circulation, vertebrobasilar insufficiency, myasthenia gravis, chorea (Huntington-Sydenham disease), Parkinson's disease, tabes dorsalis, diabetic and alcoholic neuropathy, Wallenburg's syndrome, lead intoxication
General diseases	Infections, botulism, iron deficiency anemia (Patterson-Brown-Kelley syndrome or Plummer-Vinson syndrome), megaloblastic anemia, agranulocytosis, tetany, tetanus, goiter, thyroiditis, hypocalcemia, leukemia, vitamin A and B_2 deficiency, mitral valve disease, aortic aneurysms
Skin diseases	Scleroderma, urticaria, erythematoses, erythema multiforme, pemphigus, recurrent aphthous ulcers, hereditary epidermolysis bullosa, dermatomyositis
Autonomic dysphagia	Autonomic dysfunction, psychogenic overlay (globus hystericus)

by speaking and yawning. As a result the patient eats extremely carefully and often with the head in a typical position.

Diagnosis is made by inducing local anesthesia of the trigger zones, the base of the tongue, the lower pole of the tonsil, which breaks the attacks of pain for a brief period.

Differential diagnosis is neuralgia of the nervus intermedius (Ramsay-Hunt neuralgia), neuralgia of the trigeminal or the auriculotemporal nerves, and the stylohyoid syndrome (see Table 2.**7**).

Treatment. *Conservative.* Tegretal (carbamazapine) should be tried. *Operative treatment* is division of the IXth nerve in the posterior cranial fossa.

Neuralgia of the Vagus Nerve (X)

1. *Neuralgia of the superior laryngeal nerve* (see also p. 408). There is intermittent episodic violent pain irradiating into the lateral part of the neck from the ear to the thyroid gland with a pressure point over the greater horn of the hyoid bone and at the point of entry of the nerve into the thyrohyoid membrane.
2. *Neuralgia of the auricular branch of the vagus,* causes intermittent very severe pain in the retroauricular and suboccipital areas, and in the shoulder. Combination of (1) and (2) is possible.

Diagnosis. The pressure point is the long process of the hyoid, the thyrohyoid membrane, or the musculature around the mastoid process.

Differential diagnosis is Ramsey-Hunt neuralgia of the nervus intermedius and geniculate ganglion, and auriculotemporal neuralgia (see Table 2.**7**).

Treatment. Conservative treatment should be tried first including warm local applications, poultices, and exposure to infrared light. Surgical treatment includes divison of the superior laryngeal nerve or injection of absolute alcohol (0.3–0.5–1.0 ml) at the entrance of the nerve into the thyrohyoid membrane (see Fig. 4.**18**).

Globus Hystericus (Functional dysphagia)

Globus hystericus is a symptom complex which requires investigation even when accompanying a pharyngitis.

Symptoms include an intermittent or continuous feeling of a foreign body stuck in the throat which cannot be dislodged despite swallowing. Occasionally there is also pain in the throat or irradiating to the ears. Swallowing is *not* affected. Organic lesions are absent.

Pathogenesis is an incorrect psychosomatic response to stress and possibly a tendency to spasm of the muscles of the esophageal inlet.

Diagnosis rests on the typical tenderness in the midline at the level of the cricoid arch. Radiography is normal as is esophagoscopy. Other autonomic disturbances are often present also.

Differential diagnosis. See Table 3.**7**. A benign or malignant tumor of the mouth, the pharynx, or the esophagus must be excluded.

Treatment. The patient often has a cancer phobia and this must be dealt with by counseling. Sedatives are given, and the patient is removed from the stressful situation. If organic causes are found, they are eliminated if possible, otherwise the suspected cause is explained to the patient.

Basics of Conservative Treatment of Disease of the Mouth and Pharynx

Local applications for mucosal diseases of the mouth and pharynx include *sprays, cold and warm inhalations, painting,* and lozenges. *Mouthwashes* may also be very useful. A gargle usually maintains direct contact only with the mucosa of the anterior part of the oral cavity and does not reach the faucial pillars, the tonsil, the posterior pharyngeal wall, or the hypopharynx because this will stimulate the gag reflex. Occasionally solutions that have been used for gargling reach these regions via saliva.

The substances used in the mouth and pharynx include especially the *anti-inflammatory agents, antiseptics, anesthetics* (e.g., 1% pantocaine or Xylocaine), *vitamin solutions,* iodine glycerine solutions, and *steroid preparations.* Antibiotics should not be used locally because the concentration is too low, and resistance and allergy can develop. Saline solutions or oily preparations are used for dry mucosa, and mucolytics are used to soften tenacious mucus. Pharmacologic influence on the formation of saliva is also possible (see Table 7.4).

Enteric or parenteral medication is indicated in many diseases of the mouth and pharynx. However, it must always be remembered that mucosal disorders may have been caused by drugs in the first place, e.g., by antibiotics.

Trauma of the Mouth and Pharynx

Alkali and Acid Burns and Scalds

Scalds occur in children especially. Alkali and acid burns due to mistaking the contents of a bottle (lye, vinegar essence, cleaning fluids, etc. kept in empty bottles) or to suicidal attempts (hydrochloric acid, caustic soda, vinegar essence, sulfuric acid) occur principally in adults.

Symptoms. These are dramatic. There is severe pain in the mouth and pharynx, sialorrhea, difficulty in swallowing, redness and vesicle formation on the affected part of the mucosa, and later a flat white membrane with deep red edges and mucosal edema appears. Caustic substances are usually swallowed so that the mucosa of the esophagus, the stomach, and the intestine may also be involved (see p. 463). The patient may be in shock.

Diagnosis. The history and local findings in the mouth, pharynx, and perioral tissues form the basis for the diagnosis. Involvement of the stomach and esophagus must be assessed as rapidly as possible by careful endoscopy, at the latest within 8 days. The type of fluid and the amount must be determined, and if possible the ingested fluid should be tested.

Treatment. This includes drinking large amounts of water or, even better, milk. The acids are neutralized by sodium bicarbonate or magnesium salts. Lyes are neutralized by diluted vinegar or lemon juice (see p. 464). Treatment of shock may be needed. Local treatment of the mouth and pharynx includes lozenges or ice cubes, lukewarm mouthwashes possibly with Xylocaine supplements, analgesics, cool liquid diet, feeding by a nasogastric tube, or parenteral nutrition in severe cases, antibiotics, and steroids, depending on local findings (see p. 464).

Foreign Bodies

These are less common in the mouth and pharynx than in the esophagus (see p. 465). Small pointed foreign bodies, such as splinters of bone, fish bones, bristles from a toothbrush, needles, nails, or bits of wood and glass, impact in the tonsil, the base of the tongue, the vallecula, or the lateral wall of the pharynx. Larger foreign bodies, e. g., bits of toys, flat bones, coins, buttons, large fish bones, bits of false teeth, etc. often impact in the piriform sinus or hypopharynx before entering the esophagus (see Color Plate **35a**).

Symptoms. There is pain of varying severity which is worse on swallowing, and swallowing may be completely obstructed.

Diagnosis. This is based on the history. If the material is suspected to be radiopaque, radiography is carried out. Radiographically, a swallow is also carried out with a contrast medium using a colorless medium, such as gastrografin (not barium!) which will not influence assessment of the mucosa at subsequent endoscopy. Endoscopy is then carried out. Small impacted foreign bodies in the tonsil or base of the tongue are often felt with the finger. Small foreign bodies in the *upper* pharynx are best removed without endoscopy, using grasping forceps under direct vision.

Treatment. Instrumental extraction of the foreign body is performed as quickly as possible because of the danger of pressure necrosis or mucosal injury causing abscess or mediastinitis.

Note: If a foreign body is suspected, endoscopy should be carried out as quickly as possible using an open rigid esophagoscope. The search must be continued until the foreign body is found or until it is certain that no foreign body is present. Attempts to dislodge foreign bodies by eating foods such as salads, bread, etc. is *not* justifiable because this often leads to delay and allows complications to develop.

Mucosal Injuries of the Mouth and Pharynx due to Foreign Bodies and Trauma

Because of the good healing properties of this area, suture of mucosal injuries, unless they are extensive, is only rarely required; however, antibiotic cover may be indicated.

Penetrating soft tissue injuries of the mouth and pharynx, bullet wounds, stab wounds, and wounds due to traffic accidents, must be assessed immediately from within outward, along with *injuries to the soft and related bony tissues,* mandible, maxilla, hyoid, teeth, and cervical spine. The injured structures should be debrided, repositioned, fixed, and sutured in layers. Antibiotic cover is given. Entry of air into the cervical soft tissue causes surgical emphysema.

Impalement injuries of the palate and the posterior of the wall of the pharynx usually occur in children due to falling on pointed objects. Immediate expert examination and suture of the wound are usually necessary.

Tongue bites usually heal spontaneously if the damage is slight and superficial. Penetrating bite wounds require exploration and possibly suture because of the danger of infection from carious teeth. If a portion of the tongue is completely divided, it should be reimplanted. The result depends on the speed of the reconstruction, the condition of the wound, and the arterial blood supply.

Insect bites caused by swallowing a living insect (bees, etc.) with food cause considerable edema of the pharynx, and thus respiratory obstruction.

Treatment. High-dose steroids are administered intravenously, ice packs are applied to the neck, calcium, and tracheotomy is performed if necessary.

Neurogenic Disorders

Motor Paralyses of the Pharynx

Symptoms. These include absence of the pharyngeal reflex, choking, rhinolalia aperta due to palatal paralysis, difficulty in swallowing fluids, and escape of fluids through the nose during swallowing. It is impossible to suck, or to blow out the cheeks. The soft palate deviates to the healthy nonparalyzed side.

Pathogenesis. Causes include cerebrovascular accidents, tumors of the base of the skull, jugular foramen syndrome affecting the IXth to XIth cranial nerves, or of the brain, pseudobulbar palsy, syringobulbia, and herpes zoster. In *bulbar paralysis,* the motor cranial nerve centers in the medulla oblongata degenerate gradually, causing muscle atrophy, fibrillation of the tongue, and inability to swallow. Difficulty in swallowing also occurs in *pseudobulbar palsy* due to bilateral lesions of the supranuclear pathways for the lower motor cranial nerves, but *without* muscle atrophy and fibrillation.

Differential diagnosis. Stenosing lesions in the upper digestive tract must be considered.

Treatment. Nutrition must be ensured by a nasogastric tube; a pharyngostomy or a gastrostomy may be needed. Pneumonia must be prevented by frequent aspiration, and a tracheotomy may even be needed.

Prognosis. This depends on the basic disease and the course.

Pharyngeal Spasm

The patient finds it very difficult or impossible to swallow. He has tonic spasm or vomits swallowed food. He also has pain behind the sternum.

Pathogenesis may be a prodrome preceding complete paralysis of any of the neurologic syndromes named above, but may also be a hysterical phenomenon. See also *globus hystericus* (p. 368).

The results of the paralyses of the posterior cranial nerve are summarized in Table 3.**7**.

Hypopharyngeal Diverticulum (Synonyms: Zenker's Diverticulum, Pharyngeal Pouch)

(see Fig. 3.**21** and Color Plate **36a**)

This is often incorrectly called an esophageal diverticulum, but the pouch lies immediately *above* the esophageal opening. Men are affected three times more commonly than women.

Symptoms. *Small* pouches cause a feeling of a foreign body or pressure in the throat during and after eating and irritation in the neck. *Larger* pouches cause sticking or regurgitation of food, frothy saliva, a gurgling noise on pressure on the neck, oral fetor, and attacks of coughing especially at night when the contents of the pouch may empty into the larynx. There may be associated "heartburn" and reflux esophagitis. The disease mainly affects middle-aged and elderly persons. If the pouch increases in size, the swallowing becomes progressively worse until eventually dehydration, electrolyte disturbances, and cachexia develop due to mechanical obstruction of the esophagus.

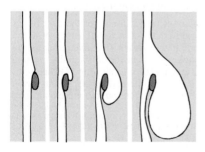

Fig. 3.**21**   Genesis of a hypopharyngeal pulsion diverticulum. The red area is the inferior part of the cricopharyngeus muscle.

Pathogenesis. The site of predilection is Killian's triangle (see Figs. 3.**3** and 3.**7**). Weakness of the wall in the cricopharyngeal area between the cricopharyngeus and the thyropharyngeus initially favors temporary bulging and later persistent and increasing herniation of the mucosa and submucosa of the posterior wall of the pharynx. The pouch passes between the pharynx and the prevertebral fascia (see Fig. 3.**21**). Suspected causes include spasm of the entrance of the esophagus, eating too quickly, or incoordination of the pharyngeal phase of swallowing with the opening of the esophagus. Formation of scars at this level may also play a part.

Diagnosis. This is made from the typical history and symptoms, especially regurgitation of undigested food, and occasionally of food eaten several days earlier. Examination with the mirror often shows frothy secretions in the piriform sinus. A barium swallow (see Fig. 5.**2a–k**) demonstrates the lesion. An esophagoscopy must be carried out.

Differential diagnosis. This includes globus hystericus, malignant tumors of the hypopharynx, esophagus, or stomach, hiatus hernia, achalasia, high esophageal strictures, and congenital vascular rings (see p. 471).

Treatment. Surgery is performed. There are two alternatives:

1. *External removal of the sac* is the method of choice.

Principle of the operation. General or local anesthesia may be used. Access is gained via an incision along the anterior border of the left sternocleidomastoid muscle. Dissection is continued between the larynx and the carotid sheath at the lateral edge of the cricoid plate. The sac of the pouch is isolated, lying between the esophagus and the prevertebral fascia. The cricopharyngeus muscle which forms the bar at the entrance to the diverticulum is identified and divided. The pouch is then resected and the hypopharynx and cervical soft tissues are closed in several layers. Complications include damage to the recurrent laryngeal nerve.

2. In very old patients who are only fit for limited procedures, *endoscopic division of the spur* may be carried out by Seiffert's method.

Principle of the operation. The procedure is carried out under general endotracheal anesthesia using a rigid esophagoscope. The spur is isolated and divided by special endoscopic scissors, by diathermy, or by the laser.

Complications include damage to large vessels running in the spur and opening of the mediastinum causing mediastinitis.

Congenital Anomalies of the Mouth and Pharynx

Congenital anomalies of the tongue such as cleft tongue, microglossia, aglossia, congenital stenosis of the junction between the nasopharynx and the oropharynx, or stenosis at the junction of the hypopharynx and the esophagus are rare. Macroglossia is much more common and is treated by surgery. Ankyloglossia is caused by a frenulum that is too short; it is corrected by a z-plasty (see p. 285 ff.).

Median Cervical Cysts and Fistulae

See p. 504.

Clefts of the Lip, Jaw, and Palate

One in a thousand of the white races suffer a congenital cleft of the lip, upper jaw, or palate; the incidence is considerably lower in the black races, but higher in the mongoloid races. Clefts of the lip, upper jaw, and palate are more common in boys, whereas pure cleft palates are more common in girls. The following types may be distinguished: *cleft lip,* (hare lip), *cleft lip and upper jaw, and cleft palate,* and these may be unilateral, bilateral, incomplete, or complete. Complete *clefts of the lip, upper jaw, and palate* may occur, total cleft, and if this is bilateral it causes the socalled wolf's nose (Fig. 3.**22a–c**).

Symptoms. The appearances are typical. In infants, there is considerable difficulty in nursing since it is not possible to close the lips and shut off the palate. Food escapes through the nose, and the child tends to aspirate milk into the trachea.

Infections of the upper and lower airways occur due to disordered swallowing and respiratory physiology. Abnormal tubal function leads to serous otitis media, chronic otitis media, and conductive deafness. The speech is affected with rhinolalia aperta, lisping, abnormal articulation, and velopharyngeal insufficiency. There are anomalies of occlusion and position of the teeth. The nose is almost always involved in clefts of the lips and palate.

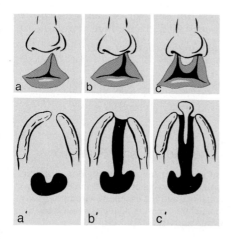

Fig. 3.**22a–c** Typical cleft formations. **(a)** Cleft lip; **(b)** cleft lip and upper jaw; **(c)** bilateral cleft of lip, upper jaw, and palate; **(a')** cleft upper jaw; **(b')** cleft upper jaw and palate; **(c')** bilateral cleft of lip, upper jaw, and palate.

Pathogenesis. The cause is probably multifactorial. Embryonic damage is caused by hypoxia, embryopathy, virus infections of the mother, toxins, and genetic lesions. There is familial clustering which is irregularly dominant.

Diagnosis. This is made from the typical facial appearance and examination with the laryngeal mirror.

A *submucous cleft palate* is often overlooked. The clue is a *slight* speech disorder. It is diagnosed by palpation which shows a bony dehiscence under an intact palatal mucosa.

Complete assessment requires the combined efforts of an ear, nose, and throat surgeon with training in plastic surgery, a phoniatrician, a dentist, an oral surgeon, and an orthodontist so that all the important aspects and defects may be detected and a common plan of treatment decided upon.

Treatment. *Operative treatment* is multilayered closure of the defect to form a solid floor of the nose and to correct the nasal deformity. Often many corrective operations and orthodontic and phoniatric assessments and treatments are necessary depending on the type and extent of the defect.

Time Schedule for Correction of Clefts

Cleft lips are corrected between the 4th and 6th (–8th) months of life by a cheiloplasty with final correction between the 14th and 16th years of life if necessary.

Cleft lip and maxilla are corrected between the 4th and 6th (–8th) months of life by an operation on the lip and nostril. Final correction may be carried out between the 14th and 16th years of life. Orthodontic measures begin as necessary from the 5th year of life.

Cleft lip, maxilla, and palate are corrected between the 4th to 6th (–8th) months of life by primary veloplasty and cheiloplasty. The remaining cleft is closed between the 12th and 14th years of life, and a final correction of lip and nose is carried out around the age of 16 years. Speech therapy begins at the age of 4 years, and orthodontic management with an obturator for the remaining cleft from the age of 6 years.

Cleft palate is treated between the 5th and 8th months of life by a primary veloplasty. Speech therapy begins at 4 years, and orthodontic management with an obturator for the remaining cleft from the age of 6 years. The remaining cleft is closed between the 12th and 14th years of life.

Plastic Procedures to Improve the Speech

Plastic closure of the cleft is intended to improve the speech and articulation and is successful in about 70% of cases. Tissue available for the repair may be inadequate so that *velopharyngeal insufficiency* persists in some cases and further procedures are necessary. Several reconstructive procedures are available to narrow the pharynx. The principle of a pharyngoplasty is to return the function of the short, immobile insufficient soft palate to as near normal as possible.

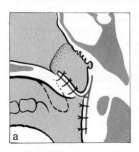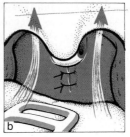

Fig. 3.**23a** and **b**   Pharyngoplasty. **(a)** Principle of bridging by a flap pedicled above, **(b)** view from the mouth.

1. Pharyngoplasty is performed with formation of a velopharyngeal flap (Fig. 3.**23a** and **b**). The soft palate is brought into contact with the posterior pharyngeal wall by a soft tissue flap (the Schoenborn-Rosenthal or Sanvenero-Rosselli method).
2. Protrusion of the posterior wall of the pharynx by implantation of autogenous or synthetic material is done to supplement Passavant's bar and to form a mucosal bolster.
3. Posterior displacement, push back, of the soft palate is performed.

Tumors of the Mouth and Pharynx

Benign Tumors of the Oral Cavity Including the Tongue and the Oropharynx

In theory all types of benign tumors can occur in this region but they are rare.

Some arise from the teeth and teeth-bearing organs and are thus the province of the oral surgeon. The more common *connective tissue* benign tumors include fibromas, lipomas, myxomas, chondromas, hemangiomas, lymphangiomas, neurinomas, and irritation fibromas, e.g., in malocclusion or absent teeth.

The more common *epithelial* benign tumors include papilloma, keratoacanthoma, true adenoma, and pleomorphic adenoma.

The diagnosis is made by biopsy. The treatment is by the appropriate operation if the size of the tumor, its histologic appearances, its growth tendency, or other properties make this advisable.

Specific Tumors

1. Hemangiomas and lymphangiomas are usually congenital and 90% affect girls. The sites of predilection are the tongue, cheek, and the parotid regions. The tumor may be so large as to threaten life due to recurrent bleeding, airway obstruction, or obstruction to feeding. These tumors often resolve spontaneously within the first 2 years of life, and surgical removal should therefore be delayed if possible until the 3rd or 4th year. Radiotherapy is not indicated because of the danger of inhibition of growth of the facial skeleton and of a later induced carcinoma. If the tumor grows quickly, embolization of the feeding vessel arising from the external carotid artery may be tried or stilbestrol may be given for a limited period.

2. Papillomas in the mouth usually cause no symptoms. Treatment is only necessary if the lesions extend to the pharynx or the larynx (see p. 421).

3. Lingual thyroid tumors, see p. 523.

4. *Tumors of neighboring organs* may extend into the mouth and oropharynx. The most frequent are tumors of the parotid gland which penetrate into the oropharynx via the retromandibular space, displacing the lateral pharyngeal wall, tonsil, or soft palate, e.g., a pleomorphic adenoma, see p. 548. Vascular tumors of the neck, e.g., carotid body tumors, can also cause similar pharyngeal displacement. Intrusion on the oral cavity by benign tumors of neighboring organs, e.g., tumors of the soft tissues of the cheek, the nasopharynx, and the maxillary sinus, is rare. On the other hand, extension of *a malignant tumor* from neighboring organs to the oral cavity is more frequent than to the oropharynx.

Malignant Tumors of the Oral Cavity (Including the Lip and Tongue) and the Oropharynx

The great majority are keratinizing squamous cell carcinomas. Nonkeratinizing and anaplastic carcinomas and adenoid cystic carcinomas are unusual and adenocarcinomas rare. This group forms about 5% of all malignant tumors. The lymphoepithelioma (Schminke tumor) is a unique tumor which today is regarded as an anaplastic carcinoma.

Connective tissue tumors may rarely arise in the oral cavity and on the tongue, especially the spindle cell sarcoma, myxosarcoma, malignant lymphoma, Hodgkin's disease, plasmacytoma, malignant giant cell tumor, rhabdomyosarcoma, hemangioendothelioma, and malignant melanoma (see Color Plate **23c**).

The prognosis varies enormously depending on the site, extent, and histologic differentiation, even if *carcinomas* alone are compared. The TNM classification is used for documentation, choice of treatment, and prognosis. Table 3.**8** summarizes the division into stages for carcinomas of the lip, oral cavity, and pharynx.

Malignant skin tumors on the upper lip are usually basal cell cancers, and those on the lower lip are mostly squamous cell carcinomas.

Symptoms. Any ulcer that does not heal rapidly and any hyperkeratotic area should be suspected of being an early malignancy. In the early stages there is little or no pain (see Color Plates **21b, c** and **24a**).

There is also a malignant form of *basal cell carcinoma* of the lips, the basisquamous carcinoma. This should be taken into account in treatment.

With increasing size of the tumor, the patient complains of pain, induration, and infiltration of the underlying tissues and a regional lymphadenopathy affecting the nodes in the submandibular triangle, the jugulodigastric, and deep cervical groups.

Table 3.8 *TNM* System for the Lips, Oral Cavity and Pharynx

Lips 1. Upper lip 2. Lower lip 3. Commissures	T_{is} = carcinoma in situ T_0 = no evidence of primary tumor T_1 = tumor 2 cm or less in its greatest dimension T_2 = tumor more than 2 cm but nor more than 4 cm in its greatest dimension T_3 = tumor more than 4 cm in its greatest dimension T_4 = tumor extending beyond the lip to neighboring structures

Oral cavity
1. Buccal mucosa
  a. Mucosal surfaces of the upper and lower lips
  b. Mucosal surface of the cheeks
  c. Retromolar areas
  d. Buccoalveolar sulci, upper and lower
2. Upper alveolus and gingiva
3. Lower alveolus and gingiva
4. Hard palate
5. Tongue
  a. Dorsal surface and lateral borders anterior to circumvallate papillae, anterior two thirds
  b. Inferior surface
6. Floor of mouth
	T_{is} = preinvasive carcinoma (carcinoma in situ)
	T_0 = no evidence of primary tumor
	T_1 = tumor 2 cm or less in its greatest dimension
	T_3 = tumor more than 2 cm but not more than 4 cm in its greatest dimension
	T_4 = tumor with extension to bone, muscle, skin, antrum, neck, etc.

Oropharynx
1. Anterior wall, glossoepiglottic area
  a. Tongue posterior to the vallate, papillae, base of tongue or posterior third
  b. Vallecula
  c. Anterior, lingual, surface of epiglottis
	T_{is} = carcinoma in situ
	T_0 = no evidence of primary tumor
	T_1 = tumor 2 cm or less in its greatest dimension
	T_2 = tumor more than 2 cm but not more than 4 cm in its greatest dimension

2. Lateral wall
  a. Tonsil
  b. tonsillar fossa and faucial pillars
  c. Glossotonsillar sulci
3. Posterior wall
4. Superior wall: inferior surface of the soft palate and uvula
	T_3 = tumor more than 4 cm in its greatest dimension
	T_4 = tumor with extension to bone, muscle, skin, antrum, neck, etc.

Nasopharynx 1. Posterosuperior wall: extends from the level of the junction of the hard and soft palates to the base of the skull 2. Lateral wall including the fossa of the Rosenmuller 3. Inferior wall: consists of the superior surface of the soft palate	T_{is} = carcinoma in situ T_0 = no evidence of primary tumor T_1 = tumor confined to one site T_2 = tumor involving two sites T_3 = tumor with extension beyond the nasopharynx or oropharynx without bone involvement T_4 = tumor with extension to base of skull and/or cranial nerve(s).
Hypopharynx 1. Piriform sinus 2. Postcricoid area 3. Posterior pharyngeal wall	T_{is} = preinvasive carcinoma, carcinoma in situ T_0 = no evidence of primary tumor T_1 = tumor confined to the piriform sinus without fixation of adjacent structures. For (2.) on the postcricoid surface; for (3.) on the posterior hypopharyngeal wall. T_2 = tumor of the piriform sinus extending to the posterior hypopharyngeal wall or postcricoid surface without fixation of adjacent structures. T_3 = tumor extending beyond the anatomic boundaries with fixation of adjacent structures T_4 = extensive tumor of the hypopharynx and surrounding structures

N classification, *M* classification, and staging are shown in Table 2.**12**, and Figure 6.**18**.

Frequency. The lower lip and tongue account for about 50% of carcinomas in this area, the floor of the mouth for about 10%, the buccal mucosa for about 10%, the palate for about 10%, and the mandible and maxilla for about 10%. From 10% to 15% of malignant intraoral tumors develop in the tonsils.

The symptoms of a carcinoma in the oral cavity affecting the *floor of the mouth or the tongue* are initially minimal so that the diagnosis is often delayed. Later symptoms include an ulcer with raised edges, bleeding and increasing pain irradiating to the ear and neck, interference with speaking and swallowing, oral fetor, and sialorrhea. Late symptoms include involvement of the regional lymph nodes and finally loss of weight because of increasing difficulty in eating. In the tongue, the most frequent site is the lateral margin. Tumors of the floor of the mouth around the opening of the submandibular duct are only slightly less frequent. Often the first symptom noticed by the patient is that his false teeth do not fit well.

Tumors of the oropharynx *(base of the tongue* and *tonsils)* cause symptoms earlier. These include increasingly severe pain on swallowing, which is often initially *unilateral,* thick indistinct speech, an ulcer on the tonsil, and increasing size of the tonsil, though this is not essential. Palpation shows induration of the tonsil or the base of the tongue. There is oral fetor, bleeding, or bloodstained sputum. The tongue is fixed, the patient has trismus, thickening of the neck and floor of the mouth, loses weight, and often has a typical pallor.

Note: Assessment of a tumor in this region requires palpation with the finger in addition to examination with the mirror.

Diagnosis. The possibility of a carcinoma must always be borne in mind in any patient with a palpable tissue induration in the oral cavity or on the tongue or with a mucosal ulcer that does not heal rapidly. A biopsy should always be taken. Palpation of the lymph nodes is described on p. 491. If the diagnosis remains uncertain, radiography and direct endoscopy should be undertaken. The *TNM* classification is shown in Table 3.**8.**

Note: Any mucosal lesion persisting for more than 3 weeks with a roughened surface, change in color, ulceration, etc. should be suspected of being an early malignancy and requires biopsy for diagnosis. If the clinical suspicion of malignancy persists, a negative biopsy should not be accepted because the material may have been taken away from the edge of the tumor or from tumor-free tissue. The biopsy should be repeated therefore until a satisfactory histologic explanation is found for the clinical appearances.

Differential diagnosis. This includes stage 3 syphilis, tuberculosis, Vincent's angina, and agranulocytosis.

Treatment. This is determined by the site and stage of the tumor (the details are described below). A neck dissection (see p. 519) must be carried out on both sides if the patient has bilateral node metastases which is common with these types of tumor. The possible methods of simultaneous or delayed bilateral neck dissection are described on p. 519 ff.

Details of Tumors at Specific Sites

1. Carcinoma of the Lip (see Color Plate **15c**)

This tumor is much more common in whites than in blacks. The male/ female ratio is 30:1, and the average age is 60 to 65 years. The lower lip is affected in the large majority of patients. Exposure to ultraviolet irradiation is an important etiologic factor. Other factors are poor oral hygiene, smoking of cigarettes or pipes, and excessive alcohol consumption. Up to 95% of tumors of the lower lip are well-differentiated squamous carcinomas. Basal cell carcinomas are more common on the upper lip than squamous cell carcinomas. About 85% of malignant squamous carcinomas occur on the lower lip, 5% on the upper lip, and 5% affect both lips. Carcinoma of the *lower* lip usually grows very slowly to begin with and does not metastasize in the early stages. The prognosis is much less favorable in carcinoma of the *upper* lip.

Treatment. Surgery is slightly better than radiotherapy with a 5-year survival of approximately 85% compared to approximately 80% for irradiation. The *principle of the operation* is wedge excision of required extent followed by primary wound closure or reconstruction by various plastic procedures, e. g., an Abbe-Estlander flap (Fig. 3.**24a−d**). A complete or suprahyoid neck dissection (see p. 519) may also be necessary depending on the tumor stage.

Results. The 5-year survival for carcinoma of the lower lip treated by surgery and radiotherapy taken together is as follows:

For small carcinomas less than 2 cm in diameter: about 90%
For carcinomas greater than 2 cm in diameter: about 60%
For large carcinomas greater than 3 cm in diameter: about 40%

2. Carcinomas of the Oral Cavity and of the Body of the Tongue (see Color Plates **18c** and **21c**)

This is a fairly frequent site for carcinoma. The male/female ratio is 70:30, but it depends on the site and race. The average age is 50 to 60 years. There is a statistically significant history of smoking and alcohol abuse in these patients, about 85% with this history and only 15% without this combination. Further suspected etiologic factors include poor dental care and poor oral hygiene. Ninety-five percent are well-differentiated squamous carcinomas. Seventy-five percent are located in the gutter between

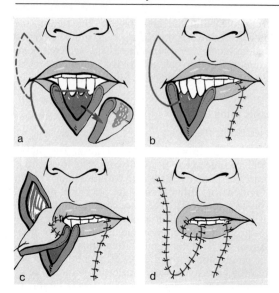

Fig. 3.**24a–d** Excision of a carcinoma of the lower lip and reconstruction. **(a)** Excision of the tumor, **(b)** creation of a modified Abbe-Estlander flap, **(c)** rotation of this flap into the defect of the lower lip, **(d)** provisional final result. A commissuroplasty is carried out later.

the lower alveolus and the lateral border of the tongue, the so-called drainage area of the mouth. The lateral border is the part of the tongue most frequently affected (in 50% of patients), and 90% of these tumors infiltrate and show superficial ulceration. There is a very high rate of lymph node metastases depending on the site of the primary tumor. More than 50% of tongue tumors produce lymph node metastases, but only 10% of tumors of the hard palate do so. Bilateral lymph node metastases can occur, especially in tumors of the tongue and the anterior part of the floor of the mouth.

Treatment. In the early stage, T_1 (see Table 3.**8**), surgery and radiotherapy are equally effective. Surgery is to be preferred for larger tumors (T_2 and T_3) or when lymph node metastases are present. The prognosis is unfavorable in cases of stage T_3, or of bone invasion, where combinations of surgery and radiotherapy, possibly combined with chemotherapy, are certain to produce the best results. *Principles of surgery.* Various routes of access are available depending on the site of the tumor (Fig. 3.**25**). The tumor must be removed with a wide margin in three dimensions. Several techniques are available for a tongue carcinoma depending on its extent including partial or subtotal glossectomy with partial mandibulectomy. A radical neck dissection is carried out. Temporary median division of the lower lip and mandible is often necessary to provide satisfactory access. The resulting soft tissue defect is closed with pedicled regional flaps from the forehead, the

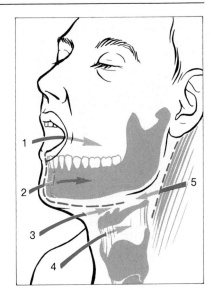

Fig. 3.**25** Routes of access for tumors of the mouth and pharynx. 1, Transoral; 2, temporary mandibulotomy; 3, suprahyoid median pharyngotomy; 4, subhyoid median pharyngotomy; 5, lateral pharyngotomy.

chest, or the neck, or also myocutaneous flaps. The mandibular defect is repaired with an autologous bone from the iliac crest or combined flaps, consisting of bone and soft tissues.

Results. The 5-year survival for 1,500 carcinomas of the tongue collected by the American Joint Committee was as follows: stage I, 90%; stage II, 64%; stage III, 34%; stage IV, 6%.

If regional lymph node metastases are present initially, the survival rates in carcinoma of the tongue and floor of the mouth falls considerably, to less than 20% for the tongue and less than 10% for the floor of the mouth.

Patients with tumors of this site often require *postoperative care* for the many attendant problems such as difficulty with speech, mastication, swallowing, tube feeding, and difficulties with false teeth.

3. Carcinoma of the Tonsil or Base of the Tongue (see Color Plate **24a**)

These are relatively frequent tumors with a male/female incidence of 4:1. The age of predilection is 50 to 70 years. The history also often shows combined alcohol abuse and smoking. Ninety percent are squamous cell carcinomas and are more often well than poorly differentiated. Sixty percent have lymph node metastases, of which 15% are bilateral. Seven

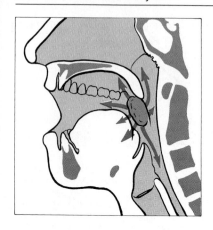

Fig. 3.**26**   Directions of spread of a malignant tumor of the tonsil.

percent have distant metastases affecting the lung, skeleton, and liver. A *second carcinoma* affecting some other part of the upper aerodigestive tract, either at the same time or later, is relatively frequent. The pathways of spread of this tumor are shown in Figure 3.**26**.

Treatment. If possible radiotherapy is combined with surgery. *Principles of surgery.* Surgery is carried out either *before* or immediately after radiotherapy, to a dose of 6,000 to 8,000 rads (= 60–80 Gy), and requires removal of the tonsil, the base of the tongue, the wall of the hypopharynx, the soft palate, and the ascending ramus of the mandible, with a good margin, if these structures are affected or suspicious. A radical neck dissection is also carried out. The soft tissue defect is repaired with a pedicled regional flap from the forehead, the neck, or the chest.

Results. Five-year survival after radiotherapy alone is about 30%, after surgery about 35%, and after combinations of radiotherapy, chemotherapy, and surgery 40% to 45%.

If the base of the tongue is involved, the prognosis falls to about 20%, and if there are bilateral lymph node metastases, it falls to about 10%.

Current experience shows that *chemotherapy* may produce surprising remissions. It is given *before,* or simultaneous to, radiotherapy especially for exophytic tumors of the floor of the mouth, the tongue, and the tonsil. Positive results have been obtained with the intraarterial or intravenous combination of bleomycin and methotrexate or cisplatin, although to date there are very few reports of definitive *cures. Disadvantages* of chemotherapy include bone marrow depression, pulmonary fibrosis, alopecia, and severe mucosal ulceration. Chemotherapy for tumors of this site has so far been regarded as palliative. A combination of chemotherapy and radiotherapy in the so-called *cell kinetic* regimes has not been shown to produce convincingly better results.

Mesenchymal tumors in this region are usually radiosensitive as are the lymphoepithelial tumors and anaplastic carcinomas. These tumors are therefore not suitable for surgery (see Color Plate **23c**).

Benign Tumors of the Nasopharynx

Benign tumors of the nasopharynx are rare. The most frequent is the *nasopharyngeal angiofibroma* (see Color Plate **25d**). This occurs exclusively in the male, beginning about the age of 10 years. This tumor is said to resolve spontaneously after the age of 20−25, but this is *not* true of all cases.

Symptoms. These include increasing nasal obstruction, purulent rhinosinusitis due to obstruction of the nasopharynx, severe spontaneous bleeding from the nose or pharynx, rhinolalia clausa, headaches, obstruction of the ostium of the eustachian tube causing conductive deafness, middle ear catarrh, and purulent otitis media. Posterior rhinoscopy shows occlusion of the nasopharynx by a smooth greyish-red tumor which may be lobulated and have offshoots penetrating the choana or Rosenmüller's fossa. The surface of the tumor often shows pronounced vessels. In later stages there is swelling of the lateral part and the face of the nasal skeleton, protrusion of the cheek, and possibly exophthalmos. Finally the child has difficulty in eating. The tumor is very hard to palpation. Palpation should be carried out carefully because damage to the surface of the tumor with the fingernail may cause extensive bleeding.

Pathogenesis. The typical nasopharyngeal fibroma is histologically benign but clinically malignant because of its expansive growth. It is a *very coarse* angiofibroma rich in fibrous tissue which arises from the roof of the nasopharynx or within the pterygoid fossa. The tumor usually has a broad base from the body of the sphenoid bone and is attached very firmly. It grows relatively quickly. After filling the nasopharynx, the tumor sends offshoots into the nasal sinuses, the upper jaw, the sphenoid sinus, the pterygopalatine fossa, the cheek, the ethmoid sinuses, and the orbit. Finally, it may extend into the cranial cavity after eroding the base of the skull.

Diagnosis. This is made by palpation, examination with the mirror and the nasopharyngoscope loupe endoscope (see p. 202), and computed tomography. Bilateral external carotid and internal carotid artery angiograms are indicated for an extensive tumor. Superselective angiography of the branches of the carotid is carried out to allow therapeutic embolization (see below).

Differential diagnosis. This includes hypertrophied adenoids, choanal polyp (which is soft and does not bleed), lymphoma, chordoma, and teratoma.

> *Note:* Care should be taken in carrying out a biopsy: this can cause massive bleeding. A nasopharyngeal tumor in an individual between the ages of 10 and 25 years and which is suspected as being a juvenile nasopharyngeal angiofibroma should only be submitted to biopsy in a hospital, and preparation should be made to proceed immediately to further surgery if massive bleeding occurs. However, an angiogram provides a characteristic picture and is quite sufficient to allow the diagnosis to be made.

Treatment. Response to radiotherapy is not to be expected because of the histologic type of the tumor. Radiotherapy with above-average dose is therefore only to be considered as a palliative measure, e. g., for massive extension of the tumor into the middle cranial fossa, or where the risk of operation is too high.

The method of choice is operative removal by combined transpalatal and transmaxillary access possibly combined with lateral rhinotomy. Immediate preoperative therapeutic embolization of the supplying vessels may be undertaken in large tumors. This reduces the otherwise massive bleeding during the operation, but there is a definite risk of undesirable results of embolization. Feeding branches from the external carotid artery identified by radiography may be ligated as a preliminary step, often on both sides. There is a high risk of recurrence, in about 20% of patients.

Rare Benign Nasopharyngeal Tumors

Chordoma. This develops from the notochord and occurs mainly in men between 20 and 50 years of age. It grows very slowly and erodes the base of the skull causing lesions of the cranial nerves, and it may also extend into the sphenoid sinus.

Treatment. Surgery should be performed if possible, but there is a considerable risk of recurrence. Radiotherapy is only palliative. Metastases to the neck are said to occur.

Other types of tumor include teratoma, dermoid, fibroma, and lipoma.

Treatment. Surgery should be undertaken if the patient has symptoms.

Malignant Tumors of the Nasopharynx (see Color Plate 26c)

The most frequent of these relatively rare tumors is the squamous cell carcinoma together with the lymphoepithelial tumor which is now regarded as an anaplastic tumor. These two together constitute 75% of tumors of this region. Tumors of children include lymphoma, plasmacytoma, and Burkitt's lymphoma in certain parts of Africa. This is thought to be due to the Epstein-Barr virus (see p. 348). Nasopharyngeal tumors affect men twice as commonly as women.

Symptoms. These include nasal obstruction, disorders of tubal aeration causing unilateral conductive deafness, middle ear discharge, middle ear effusion, bloodstained purulent nasal discharge, and headaches felt deep within the skull. Lymph node metastases are frequent and widespread in 90% of cases. Enlarged jugulodigastric lymph nodes on one or both sides are often the first symptom that brings the patient to the doctor. Lymph node metastases may also be retropharyngeal and in the nuchal area. The primary tumor may remain undiscovered despite careful endoscopic search because it grows concealed beneath the mucosa. There is gradual protrusion and loss of mobility of the soft palate and increasing, often unilateral pain in the head and the face (trigeminal nerve). Exophthalmos, oculomotor paralyses of the IIIrd, IVth, and VIth cranial nerves, involvement also of the Vth, IXth, Xth, XIth, and XIIth cranial nerves, oral fetor, and massive nosebleeds occur. Blood-borne metastases to the lung, the liver, and the skeleton are quite common.

Diagnosis. This is made by rhinoscopy, nasopharyngoscopy, palpation, retraction of the soft palate, and biopsy. Tomograms in the anterior, posterior, and lateral views and CT scans elucidate involvement of the base of the skull. Angiograms may also be needed. The roof of the nasopharynx and Rosenmüller's fossa require particular attention because these are often the site of origin of this tumor. Demonstration of Epstein-Barr viral antigens and antibodies has assumed major clinical importance, permitting, for example, the early detection of an asymptomatic recurrence and its early treatment by afterloading or by laser surgery (holmium-YAG laser).

Treatment. Radiotherapy is the method of choice for mesenchymal tumors and anaplastic carcinomas as they are very radiosensitive. It may be combined with chemotherapy. Surgery should only be considered for very small circumscribed nasopharyngeal tumors, combined with electrocoagulation, if it can be shown that the tumor does not extend into the eustachian tube or the base of the skull. Postoperative radiotherapy should be used. Advanced carcinomas are treated solely by radiotherapy, at times combined with chemotherapy for the primary tumor. Regional lymph node metastases may be treated by therapeutic neck dissection provided that the primary tumor has been destroyed.

Prognosis. The 5-year survival in carcinoma of the nasopharynx is about 15%, although the 5-year survival for stage I may be 30% or better. Unfortunately, patients are seldom seen at this stage.

Tumors of the Hypopharynx

See p. 432.

4. Larynx, Hypopharynx, and Trachea

Larynx
Applied Anatomy and Physiology
Basic Anatomy and Physiology

Embryology

The *larynx* develops from a two-part anlage: *the supraglottis develops from a buccopharyngeal bud, the glottis and subglottis from a tracheobronchial bud. This fact has clinical significance in the postnatal period. The nerves of the pharyngeal arches are branches of the vagus nerve.*

In the course of life, the larynx descends from about the level of the second vertebra at birth depending on sex to about the level of the fifth cervical vertebra in the adult.

Anatomy

The laryngeal skeleton consists of the thyroid, cricoid, and arytenoid cartilages, which are hyaline cartilage, the epiglottis, which is fibrous cartilage, and the fibroelastic accessory cartilages of Santorini and Wrisburg, which have no function.

Calcification and ossification of the thyroid cartilage begin at the time of puberty. Ossification of the cricoid and arytenoid cartilage follows somewhat later. The female larynx calcifies later than that of the male. *The calcified parts of the laryngeal framework are often difficult to distinguish by radiography from bony foreign bodies.*

Internal and external ligaments and membranes unite the cartilages and stabilize the soft tissue covering.

The laryngeal cavity is divided for clinical purposes into three compartments (Fig. 4.1 and Table 4.1):

- Supraglottis
- Glottis
- Subglottis

The *vocal cord* includes the vocal ligament, the vocalis muscle, and the mucosal covering (Fig. 4.2). The length of the vocal cord is 0.7 cm in the newborn, 1.6 to 2 cm in women, and 2 to 2.4 cm in men.

The *glottis* is formed by the free edges of the true vocal cords. The *transglottic space* is illustrated in Figure 4.1 and described in Table 4.1 (see also Color Plate **27a** and **b**).

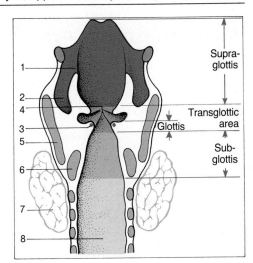

Fig. 4.1 Compartments and individual structures of the larynx. 1, Aryepiglottic fold forming the boundary between the larynx and the hypopharynx; 2, piriform sinus which belongs to the hypopharynx; 3, vocal ligament; 4, anterior commissure; 5, thyroid cartilage; 6, cricoid cartilage; 7, thyroid gland; 8, trachea.

Table 4.1	Classification and Terminology of the Laryngeal Cavity
Supraglottic space	Epilarynx = laryngeal surface of the epiglottis + aryepiglottic fold + arytenoid Vestibule = the petiolus of the epiglottis + the vestibular folds + the ventricle as far as the upper surface of the vocal cords Epilarynx + vestibule = aditus
Glottic space	Vocal cords and 1 cm inferiorly
Subglottic space	Down to the lower border of the cricoid cartilage
"Transglottic space"	Glottis + ventricle + vestibular folds

Note: Carcinoma occurs almost exclusively in the intermembranous part of the glottis, whereas intubation granuloma and contact ulcer caused by vocal abuse mainly affect the intercartilaginous part (see p. 410, and Color Plate **29b** and **c**).

Superiorly, the larynx is limited by the free edge of the epiglottis, the aryepiglottic fold, and the interarytenoid notch. *Inferiorly,* the lower edge of the cricoid cartilage marks the junction with the trachea (see Fig. 4.**1**).

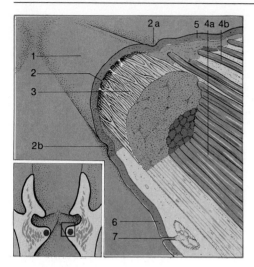

Fig. 4.2 Frontal step section through the vocal cord. The oblique three-dimensional section is through the glottis. The red area in the overview of the glottis in the inset on the lower left corresponds to the red area in the larger picture 1. Stratified squamous epithelium; 2, Reinke's space: 2a, superior arcuate line; 2b, inferior arcuate line; 3, vocal ligament; 4a, medial part of the thyroarytenoid muscle, i. e., the vocalis muscle; 4b, lateral part of the thyroarytenoid muscle; 5, epithelium of Morgagni's space consisting of cylindrical ciliated epithelium and islets of squamous epithelial cells; 6, subglottic respiratory cylindrical ciliated epithelial zone; 7, mucous gland. (Adapted from Lanz and Wachsmuth).

The *thyroid cartilage* is united by a joint to the *cricoid cartilage*. Rocking and slight gliding movements occur at this joint. The *muscles, ligaments, and membranes* between the cartilages allow the functionally important movements between different parts of the larynx.

The *external ligaments and connective tissue membranes* anchor the larynx to the surrounding structures.

The most important membranes include:

- The thyrohyoid membrane has the opening for the superior laryngeal artery and vein and for the internal branch of the superior laryngeal nerve which supplies sensation to the larynx above the vocal cords.
- The cricothyroid membrane is the point where the airway comes closest to the skin; it is the site of *laryngotomy* (see pp. 447 ff.).
- The cricotracheal ligament provides attachment to the trachea.

The *internal ligaments and connective tissue membranes,* e.g., the conus elasticus and the thyroepiglottic ligament, connect the cartilaginous parts of the larynx to each other.

The *internal muscles and the one external muscle* act synergistically and antagonistically to control the functions of the larynx. They open and close the glottis and put the vocal cords under tension (Fig. 4.3).

This interplay explains the different positions of the vocal cords in paraly-

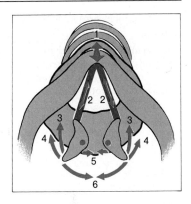

Fig. 4.3 Directions of pull of laryngeal musculature. 1, The pull of the internal laryngeal muscles and the cricothyroid muscle [the anticus muscle]; 2, medial part of the thyroarytenoid muscle (the vocalis muscle); 3, lateral part of the thyroarytenoid muscle; 4, lateral cricoarytenoid muscle (lateralis muscle); 5, interarytenoid or transversus muscle; 6, posterior cricoarytenoid muscle (posticus muscle).

Table 4.2 Functions of the Laryngeal Musculature	
Opening of the glottis, abduction of the vocal cords	Posterior cricoarytenoid muscle (posticus muscle)
Closure of the glottis, adduction of the vocal cords	Lateral cricoarytenoid muscle (lateralis muscle) Transverse arytenoid muscle (transversus muscle) Thyroarytenoid muscle, lateral part
Tension of the vocal cords	Cricothyroid muscle (anticus muscle) Thyroarytenoid muscle, medial part (vocalis muscle)

sis of the recurrent laryngeal nerve or of the external branch of the superior laryngeal nerve (Table 4.2).

Note: There is only *one* muscle which opens the glottis, the "posticus". The muscles that close it are clearly in the majority. The ratio of their relative power is 1:3. Only the interarytenoid muscle with a pars obliqua and a pars transversa is unpaired; all other muscles are paired.

The **nerve supply** of the larynx is provided by the superior laryngeal nerve and by the recurrent laryngeal nerves that arise from the vagus nerve (see Fig. 4.10).

The *superior laryngeal nerve* divides into a *sensory internal branch,* which supplies the interior of the larynx down into the glottis, and an *external branch,* which provides the *motor supply* to the external cricothyroid muscle.

The *recurrent laryngeal nerve* provides *motor supply* to the rest of the ipsilateral *internal* laryngeal musculature and to the contralateral interarytenoid muscle. In addition, it provides *sensation* to the laryngeal mucosa *inferior* to the glottic cleft.

The left recurrent laryngeal nerve loops around the aortic arch to reach the larynx in the groove between the trachea and the esophagus. The right recurrent laryngeal nerve passes around the subclavian artery and then runs upward between the trachea and the esophagus.

Both recurrent laryngeal nerves enter the larynx at the inferior cornu of the thyroid cartilage. The relations of this nerve to the inferior thyroid artery and thyroid gland are important in surgical anatomy (see p. 522).

In the diagnosis of recurrent laryngeal paralysis the cervical course of the nerve and possible intrathoracic and mediastinal disorders must be considered. Causes of recurrent paralysis include metastases, malignant lymphoma, malignant goiter, esophageal carcinoma, tuberculous lymphadenopathy, aortic aneurysm, and pulmonary hypertension.

The **blood supply of the larynx** is divided by the glottis into two areas.

The supraglottic blood supply from the superior laryngeal artery originates from the external carotid artery, whereas the subglottic vessels, the inferior laryngeal artery, derive from the thyrocervical trunk of the subclavian artery.

The *venous drainage* passes superiorly via the superior thyroid artery to the internal jugular vein and inferiorly via the inferior thyroid vein to the brachiocephalic vein.

The **lymphatic drainage** of the larynx is of great clinical importance.

The *vocal cord,* consisting of elastic fibers, has *no lymphatic capillaries.* Sparse lymphatics begin only at the fibromuscular junction with the vocalis fold and become more dense from before backward.

The *supraglottic space* on the other hand has a *rich lymphatic network.* A very dense and partly multilayered capillary network is to be found in the ventricular fold and the ventricle. The *supraglottic* lymphatic pathway converges on the anterior insertion of the aryepiglottic fold and leaves in smaller collections of vessels along the neurovascular bundle of the larynx. Submucous and preepiglottic *horizontal anastomoses* are to be found in the midline of the larynx and are responsible for bilateral and contralateral metastases in carcinoma.

The *subglottic* capillary network is not as dense as the supraglottic. Bilateral and contralateral invasion of the lymph nodes is again possible via the pre- and paratracheal lymph nodes. *The additional drainage to the peritracheal and mediastinal lymph nodes is of clinical importance.*

The laryngeal lymph is ultimately collected into the superior and inferior deep cervical lymph nodes.

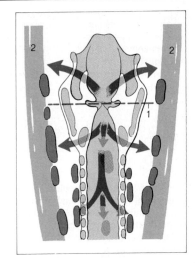

Fig. 4.**4**   Glottic lymph barrier which produces a supraglottic and a subglottic lymph flow. The first supraglottic lymph node stations are the inconstant prelaryngeal node and the upper deep cervical nodes. The first subglottic lymph node station is the pre- and paratracheal and lower deep jugular lymph nodes. 1, Glottic lymph barrier; 2, internal jugular vein.

The **mucosal lining** of the larynx is adapted to its special position at the junction of the respiratory and digestive tracts. Stratified squamous epithelium, partially keratinized, covers the laryngeal surface of the epiglottis, the vestibular folds, the vestibule of the larynx, and the vocal cords. Ciliated columnar epithelium covers the remaining parts of the mucosal surface.

Reinke's space is a closed cleft beneath the epithelium of the vocal cord with no glands or lymphatic capillaries. It is of clinical significance in *Reinke's edema* (see p. 420).

Physiology

Phonation. The tone formed by the larynx is modified by the movements of the pharynx, tongue, and lips to form speech.

The vocal function, vocal range, tone amplification, timbre, and resonance are described on p. 315.

Hoarseness is the result of noise formed by endolaryngeal turbulence of the airstream and irregularities of the normally periodic vibrations of the vocal cords.

During respiration. The vocal cords are in the respiratory position, i. e., the glottis is open and is under reflex control which depends on gas exchange and acid-base balance.

The **sphincteric function** is the oldest phylogenetic function of the larynx (see Table 4.**3**).

Table 4.3 Functions of the Larynx		
Phonation		
Respiration		
Protection of the lower airway	Closure of the aditus Closure of the glottis Reflex respiratory arrest Cough reflex	} on swallowing
Glottic closure with thoracic fixation and Valsalva maneuver, e.g., during lifting of heavy loads.		

Protection of the lower respiratory tract. The base of the tongue, the posterior pharyngeal wall, and the faucial pillars are involved in swallowing. The swallowing *reflex* transmitted in the glossopharyngeal nerve ensures *cessation of respiration* and contraction of the aryepiglottic folds, the vocal cords, and the vestibular folds, and tilting of the epiglottis by the thyroepiglottic muscle.

Simultaneously, the suprahyoid musculature contracts drawing the larynx anteriorly and superiorly by 2 to 3 cm.

Experience with surgical removal of the epiglottis shows that this structure is only of limited necessity for protection of the larynx. An intact sensory nerve supply to the mucosa of the laryngeal aditus from the internal branch of the superior laryngeal nerve is much more important. It controls reflex muscular contraction.

The *cough reflex* is stimulated by particles of food penetrating within the larynx. It consists of a deep reflex inspiration with the larynx open. The glottis closes with a rising intrathoracic pressure and then opens suddenly with an explosive expiratory stream, and the foreign body is coughed out.

Note: The larynx is the receptor field for other *vasovagal reflexes*. Mechanical irritation of the internal surface of the larynx can induce arrhythmia, bradycardia, and cardiac arrest. Satisfactory mucosal anesthesia must be ensured during endolaryngeal procedures. Particular care is necessary during repeated attempts at intubation, prolonged laryngoscopy, and laryngotracheal obstruction by foreign bodies, etc.
The vagal reflex can be blocked by atropine and increased by opiates. Reflex irritability is increased in smokers.

Thoracic fixation. The respiratory system is closed off by the glottis to provide mechanical assistance during several bodily functions, notably, coughing, defecation, micturition, vomiting, and parturition. Furthermore, the pectoral muscles are supplemented when doing chin-ups, while digging, and breathing during asthma attacks.

Methods of Investigation

These provide information about:

- The position of the larynx and its relation to neighboring anatomic structures in the neck
- The external and internal shape of the larynx
- The type, site, and extent of lesions within and outside of the larynx
- Functional disorders

Inspection

Normally, the thyroid prominence can only be seen in men. It moves upward on swallowing; absence of this movement indicates fixation of the larynx by infection or tumor.

Indrawing of the suprasternal notch on inspiration combined with inspiratory stridor points to laryngotracheal obstruction by foreign body, tumor, edema, etc.

Palpation

The laryngeal skeleton and neighboring structures are palpated during respiration and swallowing, paying attention to the following:

- The thyroid cartilage
- The cricothyroid membrane and the cricoid cartilage
- The carotid artery with the carotid bulb which must not be confused with neighboring cervical lymph nodes; the palpating finger picks up pulsations
- The thyroid gland lying inferior and lateral to the thyroid and cricoid cartilages
- The simultaneous movement of the larynx and thyroid gland on swallowing

Indirect Laryngoscopy

The larynx is inspected by means of a mirror and the unaided eye or by a telescopic system.

The technique of examination is shown in Figures 4.5–4.7 (Color Plate **27a** and **b**). The tongue is grasped with the thumb and middle finger of the left hand so that the thumb lies on the tongue. The index finger is used to push back the upper lip. The tongue must be drawn forward carefully to prevent damage to the frenulum by the lower teeth. The light from the mirror is directed toward the uvula. The laryngeal mirror is

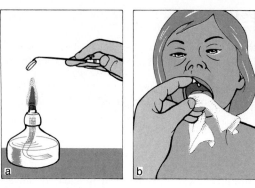
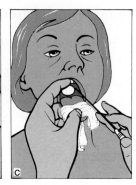

Fig. 4.**5a–c**   Indirect laryngoscopy.

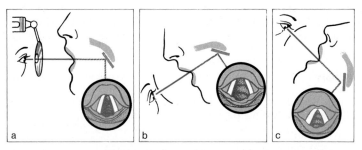

Fig. 4.**6a–c**   Indirect laryngoscopy. **(a)** Normal direction of light and vision; **(b)** Killian's position producing a better view of the posterior commissure; **(c)** Tuerck's position which produces a better view of the anterior commissure.

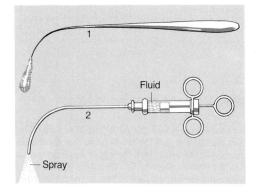

Fig. 4.**7**   Instruments for mucosal anesthesia of the larynx. 1, curved metal cotton applicator; 2, curved cannula.

warmed on its glass surface and its temperature is tested with the examiner's own hand. It is then introduced along the palate until it reaches the uvula.

Stimulation of the base of the tongue and posterior pharyngeal wall is to be avoided since this can provoke the gag reflex. The posterior surface of the mirror is used to lift the uvula and push it upward and backward. The posterior part of the tongue, the pharynx, and part of the larynx are now visible in the mirror. The patient is asked to say "e" to bring the epiglottis into a more upright position and thus give a better view of the larynx. In a patient with a sensitive gag reflex, it may be necessary to spray the pharynx first with a topical anesthetic, e.g., Pontocaine, before this examination can be carried out (Fig. 4.7).

Killian's position in which the examiner sits in front of the standing patient provides a better view of the *posterior commissure. Tuerck's* position in which the examiner stands in front of the sitting patient gives a better view of the *anterior commissure* (see Fig. 4.6b and c).

Telescopic Laryngoscopy

Telescopic laryngoscopes have become very useful in practice. These light, rigid endoscopes with wide angle lenses supplement or may replace indirect laryngoscopy with the mirror. (See also section on nasoendoscopy, p. 202, and Fig. 2.25.)

The advantages of this procedure are that it provides variable magnification and a good view of hidden, areas and that photographic documentation of conscious patients is possible.

Note: Biopsies may be taken and polyps removed under indirect laryngoscopy using topical anesthesia applied by a cotton probe or spray (see Fig. 4.7). However, microlaryngoscopy is preferable.

Direct Laryngoscopy

Table 4.4 Summary of Areas to be Examined on Laryngoscopy	
Oropharynx	Base of tongue, both valleculae, lingual surface of the epiglottis
Hypopharynx	Piriform sinus
Boundaries between the hypopharynx and the larynx	Glossoepiglottic and aryepiglottic folds
Larynx	Epiglottis, arytenoid cartilage, vestibular folds, vocal cords and ventricle
Subglottis	

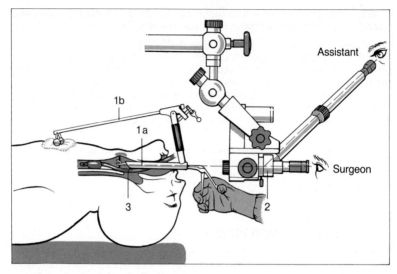

Fig. 4.**8** Microlaryngoscopy showing the laryngoscope (1a) introduced and held by a chest support and articulated lever arm (1b) supported on the patient's sternum; 2, operating microscope with assistant's eyepiece; 3, endotracheal tube.

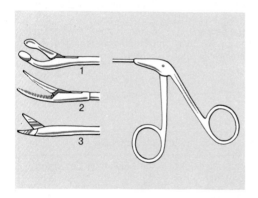

Fig. 4.**9** Typical instruments used in endolaryngeal microsurgery (magnified x3). 1, Double-cupped forceps; 2, grasping forceps; 3, scissors.

Microlaryngoscopy

The larynx and the hypopharynx may be examined directly with a rigid laryngoscope supported via a lever arm on the patient's sternum. *Microlaryngoscopy* consists of the addition of the binocular operating microscope and a suitable set of instruments (Figs. 4.**8** and 4.**9**). Anesthesia is achieved by intubation endotracheal anesthesia or injection respiration without intubation. This procedure has been a considerable advance in diagnostic and endolaryngeal microsurgery. Microlaryngoscopy provides excellent illumination of the larynx, the upper trachea, and the hypopharynx including all hidden areas. Some endolaryngeal surgical procedures may also be carried out (Table 4.**4**).

The following features are looked for: the color of the mucosa, abnormal tissue, the appearance of local or diffuse lesions, smooth, rough, ulcerated, exophytic, etc., the movement of the vocal cords, the lumen of the trachea, and the shape of the hypopharynx.

Radiography

Plain views in the sagittal or lateral plane have limited value because of superimposition of the numerous soft tissue and bony shadows. However, it is a relatively easy radiographic technique to augment.

Laryngography in which the larynx and hypopharynx are coated with a contrast medium provides information about the laryngeal surface and thus about the extent of the tumor. This technique is seldom practiced today.

Conventional tomograms and xerotomograms, particularly high-resolution computed tomography, provide accurate assessment of the site and extent of stenoses and tumors and the destruction of local, laryngeal, and neighboring structures.

Magnetic resonance imaging (MRI) expands diagnostic imaging capabilities in the larynx and adjacent regions.

Special techniques include:

Stroboscopy

High-frequency movies, allowing scientific analysis of the laryngeal function, especially that of the vocal cords

Electromyography

Clinical Aspects

Congenital Anomalies

Congenital laryngeal anomalies appear clinically with three cardinal symptoms: *dyspnea, dysphonia, and dysphagia* (Table 4.**5**).

Laryngomalacia

Symptoms. Inspiratory stridor begins immediately or within the first few weeks postpartum, in severe cases accompanied by cyanosis. The symptoms worsen during feeding.

Table 4.5 Frequency of Congenital Laryngeal Anomalies

Laryngomalacia	About 75%
Neurological disorders	About 10%
	unilateral or bilateral recurrent nerve paralysis

Seldom
  Atresia and membranes
  Cysts and laryngoceles
  Subglottic stenoses
  Hemangioma

Very rare
  Clefts

Pathogenesis. The cause lies in abnormal calcium metabolism causing unusual weakness of the supraglottic laryngeal skeleton, particularly the epiglottis.

Diagnosis. This rests on direct laryngoscopy and bronchoscopy. The epiglottis is usually omega-shaped and soft and folds over the laryngeal inlet on inspiration. The arytenoid eminences or aryepiglottic folds may be drawn in on inspiration. The form and function of the vocal cords is normal.

Treatment. Treatment consists of careful observation of the child and reassurance of the parents. The cartilage becomes stiffer within the course of weeks or months so that the symptoms slowly disappear. Feedings should be divided into fractions with a pause after every two or three swallows. If necessary, tube feeding should be used. Tracheotomy is only exceptionally required, and severe temporary dyspnea may be managed by intubation.

Neurogenic Disorders

Symptoms. If unilateral there is squealing and a weak cry. Bilateral lesions cause inspiratory stridor.

Pathogenesis. Some cases are idiopathic and some are due to congenital or cardiovascular anomalies or stretching of the neck during birth.

Diagnosis. This is made by direct laryngoscopy which shows one or both vocal cords to be in the paramedian position. An intermediate position of the cords is considerably rarer.

Treatment. Unilateral lesions do not require treatment. A large proportion of recurrent paralyses recover spontaneously. Bilateral lesions initially require intubation and a later tracheotomy for persistent obstruction.

Atresias and Webs

Symptoms. *Atresias* cause powerful, useless attempts at respiration, cyanosis, and inability to cry immediately after birth which leads rapidly to death. *Webs* cause respiratory obstruction of variable degrees.

Diagnosis. This is made by direct laryngoscopy which shows an atresia or a (subtotal) web of the glottis (Color Plate **27c**).

Treatment. Asphyxia in severe cases of dyspnea is only prevented by endoscopic division of the web or tracheotomy in the immediate postpartum period. This may be done by incision or endolaryngeal laser surgery and may be repeated if necessary.

Laryngoceles

Internal laryngoceles lie within the larynx in the vestibular fold (see Color Plate **29a**).

External laryngoceles are a prolongation of the ventricle through the thyrohyoid membrane to form a palpable cystic mass in the neck.

Combinations of both forms and bilateral laryngoceles are rare.

Symptoms. Dyspnea and dysphonia are accompanied by a foreign-body sensation in the throat.

Pathogenesis. This is a congenital or acquired expansion of the laryngeal saccule, i.e., a blind sac of the ventricle, filled with air or mucus.

Diagnosis. This is made by laryngoscopy, palpation, and tomography. The smooth swelling increases in size on puffing, straining, and on playing wind instruments.

Treatment. If severe dyspnea is not present treatment is expectant. Later, the sac may be exposed and removed via an external incision. Small internal laryngoceles may be removed endoscopically.

Subglottic Stenoses

Symptoms. Inspiratory *and* expiratory stridor are present but usually no abnormality of the voice. Recurrent pseudocroup may also occur.

Pathogenesis. The cause is usually an anomaly of the cricoid cartilage.

Diagnosis is made by direct laryngoscopy and tracheoscopy and by imaging procedures.

Treatment. Tracheotomy may be necessary in severe respiratory obstruction. The child is then observed until laryngotracheoplasty becomes possible.

Hemangioma

Symptoms. These depend on the site; these tumors may cause hoarseness or respiratory obstruction. Spontaneous bleeding with aspiration of blood can lead to an acutely dangerous condition.

Diagnosis. Direct laryngoscopy and microlaryngoscopy.

Treatment. Occasionally because of increase in respiratory obstruction or spontaneous bleeding, it may not be possible to wait for spontaneous regression of the hemangioma. Cryosurgery or laser surgery is indicated. Tracheotomy is usually unnecessary.

Functional Disorders

These are based on nervous, myogenic, or articular causes, e. g., laryngospasm. They are characterized by voice disorders such as dysphonia, aphonia, or dyspnea; see Table 4.**6**.

Dysphonia. Atypical vibrations of the vocal cords or abnormally increased or decreased passage of air through the glottis causes increased hoarseness rather than a clear tone. It is analyzed by endoscopy, stroboscopy, high-speed cinematography, and phoniatry.

Dyspnea. Audible stridor (shortness of breath, at times accompanied by cyanosis) occurs when the diameter of the respiratory tract is reduced by at least one third. The anoxia can increase dramatically during physical exercise.

> *Note:* A 1–mm mucosal swelling in an infant narrows the lumen by more than 50 %. Edema must be 3 mm thick in the adult to produce the same effect.

Neurogenic functional disorders due to causes in the cortical or subcortical areas mainly cause bilateral abnormalities of vocal cord movement. Bilateral, but more often unilateral disorders of vocal cord function, usually combined with lesions of the vagus, glossopharyngeal, and hypoglossal nerves, are localized to the medulla oblongata. A combination of paralyses in older people occurring suddenly indicates cerebral ischemia or bleeding in the area of the brainstem. Ninety percent of *isolated defects* of the vagus nerve or its branches occur in the region between the nucleus ambiguous and the inferior ganglion centrally and the laryngeal musculature. Typical vocal cord palsies result from damage to the vagus nerve inferior to the inferior ganglion (Fig. 4.**10**).

The vocal cords take up different positions during function or in paralyses relative to the imaginary reference line of the sagittal glottic axis (Fig. 4.**11**).

Functional Positions

The median position is adopted in phonation (see Color Plate **27b**). The lateral position of extreme abduction occurs on inspiration (see Color Plate **27a**).

Vocal Cord Positions in the Most Common Pareses (see Fig. 4.**11**)

● Paramedian is seen in recurrent nerve paralysis, posticus paralysis.

Table 4.6	Unilateral or Bilateral Recurrent Nerve Paralysis
Causes	Details
Thyroidectomy	Most frequent cause of a laryngeal muscle paralysis
Malignant goiter	
Bronchial carcinoma	Particularly common in tumors arising from the left upper and middle lobes and with involvement of the mediastinal lymph node metastases
Esophageal carcinoma	Particularly of the upper third
Mediastinal diseases	Lymphogranulomas, non-Hodgkin's lymphoma, metastases, mediastinitis
Aneurysms of the aorta or the subclavian artery	Congenital or syphilitic
Ductus operations	
Operations on the hypopharynx or the esophagus	Failure to display the course of the nerve during resection of the hypopharyngeal diverticulum
Cardiomegaly of various causes	May also occur in Ortner's syndrome
Pulmonary tuberculosis	
Pleural plaques	
Blunt or sharp cervical trauma	
Infective-toxic	Influenza; herpes zoster; rheumatism; syphilis; tissue toxins such as lead, arsenic, or organic solvents; streptomycin; quinine
Intubation anesthesia	Stretching of the recurrent nerve by incorrect position of the patient or pressure of the tube
Neurologic diseases	Wallenberg's syndrome, poliomyelitis, bulbar paralysis, multiple sclerosis, cerebral tumors
Idiopathic	It should be noted that a diagnosis of idiopathic recurrent nerve paralysis should only be made after all other causes have been excluded. In the great majority of these patients spontaneous recovery occurs within 2 to 3 months. After a longer period the chances of recovery become less
Cervical metastases near the skull base	Commonly associated with other cranial neuro-pathies.

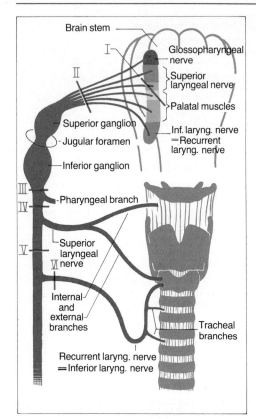

Fig. 4.**10**   Vagus nerve and its branches with sites of possible lesions (I to VI) and effects on the larynx (modified from Burian et al.).

I.   A lesion in the nucleus ambiguous produces paralysis in the intermediate or paramedian position.

II. Division of the roots of the vagus nerve causing several different types of paralysis: paramedian position, intermediate position, and simultaneous paralysis of the soft palate.

III. Loss of continuity in the jugular foramen or inferior ganglion causes paralysis of the superior laryngeal nerve and of the recurrent laryngeal nerve. The vocal cord is in the intermediate position, and the soft palate is paralyzed. Lesions in and around the jugular foramen may be accompanied by paralysis of the glossopharyngeal, accessory, and hypoglossal nerves.

IV. A lesion between the pharyngeal branches and the superior laryngeal nerve. The vocal cord is in the intermediate position and there is also loss of sensation.

V. Interruption of the vagus nerve at the superior laryngeal nerve caused a loss of tone of the cricothyroid muscle and loss of tension of the vocal cord.

VI. Division of the recurrent nerve causes a vocal cord paralysis in the paramedian position.

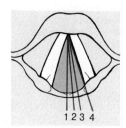

Fig. 4.**11**   Positions of the vocal cord. 1, Median or phonatory position; 2, paramedian position; 3, intermediate position; 4, lateral or respiratory position.

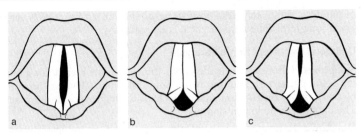

Fig. 4.**12a–c**   Myogenic abnormalities of position of the vocal cords. **(a)** Weakness of the internus muscle, **(b)** weakness of the transversus muscle, **(c)** combined type.

- Intermediate is seen in complete paralysis of the superior and inferior laryngeal nerve which thus paralyzes all internal and external laryngeal muscles.
- The cadaveric position is an incorrect term since it has no relationship to the vocal cord position in the corpse. It is rather an intermediate position similar to the position of the vocal cords in flaccid paralysis or in the end stage of a vocal cord paralysis with bowing of the vocal cords due to disuse atrophy of the vocalis muscle and with the arytenoid cartilage tilted anteriorly.

Other anomalies of position combined with hyper- or hypokinetic dysphonia include:

Internus weakness. The glottic chink is elliptical on phonation due to absent tension of the vocalis muscle as a result of atrophy, e. g., in senile dysphonia.

Transversus weakness. A triangular gap remains open posteriorly on phonation.

Combinations of both forms of inadequate closure may occur (Fig. 4.**12a–c**).

It is not always possible to predict the final position of the vocal cords after damage to the superior and recurrent laryngeal nerves because of partial recovery of residual function. Furthermore, atypical positions may be adopted because of fibrosis of the muscle or ankylosis of the arytenoid joint.

Recurrent Laryngeal Nerve Paralysis (Unilateral or Bilateral)

All the internal laryngeal musculature is *paralyzed* on the affected side. Since the external cricothyroid muscle supplied by the external branch of the superior laryngeal nerve still puts the paralyzed vocal cord under tension, the *paramedian position* is adopted. In incomplete paralysis of the adductors, the single abductor of the vocal cords (the *posterior* cricoarytenoid muscle) is functionally predominant. This unilateral or bilateral form of paralysis is thus termed a *posticus paralysis*. The stroboscope is very useful in long-term follow-up of vocal cord paralyses.

Unilateral Recurrent Nerve Paralysis

Symptoms. Often noted incidentally, the symptoms include dysphonia in the acute phase with later improvement in the voice. There is no appreciable respiratory obstruction except perhaps during severe physical activity. The patient can no longer sing.

Diagnosis. Laryngoscopy shows the vocal cord to be immobile in the paramedian position on one side. Thorough laryngologic, phoniatric, neurologic, and radiologic investigation is indicated, whose objective is shown in Table 4.**6** on page 401.

Treatment. If the causal disease cannot be treated satisfactorily, the patient is given speech therapy (electrotherapy) to achieve compensatory vocal cord closure by the action of the still-functioning vocal cord.

Bilateral Recurrent Paralysis

Symptoms. (1) *Dyspnea* occurs with the possibility of asphyxia due to narrowing of the glottic chink. Inspiratory *stridor* is particularly loud during sleep or physical activity. (2) Initially, there is *dysphonia* which lasts for a variable period, depending on the cause, and thereafter a weak, but only slightly hoarse voice. (3) Feeble cough is also symptomatic.

Pathogenesis. See Table 4.**6**.

Diagnosis. This is based on laryngoscopic findings. In bilateral paralysis the vocal cords are in the paramedian position.

Treatment

1. Relief of the airway takes first priority. Immediate tracheotomy is often necessary. The patient can later be provided with a *speaking valve* (tracheotomy inner tube).
2. If spontaneous remission does not occur, an operation to widen the glottis is indicated at the earliest 10 to 12 months later if the patient wishes to be rid of his speaking valve.

Principles of surgery. An arytenoidectomy is carried out, and one of the paralyzed vocal cords is moved laterally or superolaterally. The operation is done endoscopically with a CO_2-Laser (Fig. 4.**13a–c**).

Today a better and simpler procedure is chordotomy using the Kashima technique. This involves separating one vocal cord from the vocal process, creating a posterior gap for respiration and maintaining anterior vocal cord contact for phonation.

> *Note:* The wider the glottic opening after operation the more unsatisfactory is the voice.

Speech therapy is used to supplement the operation.

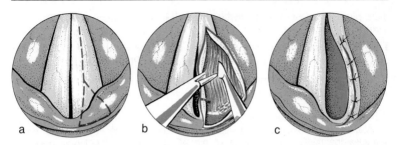

Fig. 4.**13a–c** Endoscopic operations, to widen the glottis. **a.** Arytenoidectomy and laterofixation of the vocal cord. The incision is shown by a dotted line. **b.** The arytenoid cartilage is removed and the vocalis muscle is grasped with a forceps. It is then dissected free with a round knife from the muscles. **c.** The vocal cord is then displaced laterally and sutured.

Unilateral or Bilateral Paralysis of the Superior Laryngeal Nerve

Symptoms. These include aspiration of food and drink, loss of power of the voice, and inability to sing in the higher part of the range, particularly in a bilateral paralysis. Breathing is scarcely affected.

Pathogenesis. The paralysis affects the function of the cricothyroid muscle as well as the sensory nerve supply to the supraglottic part of the larynx. The paralysis is due to mechanical lesions of the nerve particularly after thyroid gland operations, tumors, and viral infections.

Diagnosis. Laryngoscopy shows that the tension of the vocal cords is reduced so that the glottis does not close completely on phonation. In unilateral paralysis, the ipsilateral vocal cord is often shortened and lies lower than the nonparalyzed side.

Treatment. Corticosteroids should be tried and speech therapy prescribed.

Combined Lesions of the Laryngeal Nerves

Included are lesions of the superior laryngeal and recurrent laryngeal nerves (see Fig. 4.**10**).

Symptoms. *Unilateral paralysis* includes dysphonia and breathy voice due to air loss. The healthy vocal cord compensates later. Aspiration occurs because of absence of the sensory protection. In *bilateral paralysis,* there is dysphonia or aphonia and almost always good respiration at rest. There is also aspiration and a marked feeling of shortage of breath during bodily exertion.

Pathogenesis. The basic cause is central or peripheral damage to the vagus nerve causing a flaccid paralysis with immobility of the affected vocal cord in the intermediate position. There is bilateral flaccid paralysis with bilateral lesions (see Fig. 4.**10**).

Diagnosis. Laryngoscopy shows one or both of the vocal cords to be bowed and paralyzed in the intermediate position (Color Plate **32a** and **b**).

Treatment. It is seldom possible to treat the cause of this paralysis, and the mainstay of treatment is speech therapy.

> *Note:* If speech therapy for a unilateral atrophic vocal cord paralysis does not succeed in producing compensation by movement of the healthy vocal cord across the midline, the volume of the affected side of the larynx may be supplement to produce a satisfactory voice by injection of the affected vocal cord with collagen preparations or by subperichondrial implantation of autologous cartilage.

Neuralgia of the Superior Laryngeal Nerve

This is one of the localized or mononeural pain syndromes of the head and neck such as trigeminal neuralgia or occipital neuralgia (see Table 2.7).

Symptoms. These include episodic stabbing pain usually on one side radiating to the upper part of the thyroid cartilage, the angle of the jaw, or the lower part of the ear. Pain on pressure is experienced at the level of the greater cornu of the hyoid or in the region of the thyrohyoid membrane.

Pathogenesis. The cause is unknown but may relate to viral infection, previous trauma (or surgery), or mechanical-morphologic factors (e. g., hyoid bone variations). The disease occurs between the 40th and 60th years of life. The trigger zone lies in the piriform sinus and is set off by swallowing, speaking, and coughing.

Treatment. Repeated anesthetic block of the superior laryngeal nerve should be tried. The site of injection lies between the greater cornu of the hyoid and the superior cornu of the thyroid cartilage (Fig. 4.**14**). Medical treatment with carbamazepine (Tegretol) may also be tried.

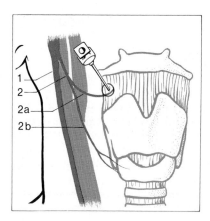

Fig. 4.**14** Infiltration anesthesia of the superior laryngeal nerve. 1, Vagus nerve; 2, superior laryngeal nerve. (2a) Internal branch; (2b) external branch.

Traumatology

The function of the larynx may be affected by vocal abuse, intubation injury, external trauma, chemical toxins, and foreign bodies.

The **symptoms** are dictated by the abnormal laryngeal function and include voice disorders, respiratory obstruction, coughing, and surgical emphysema of the neck.

The appropriate endoscopic and radiologic procedures must be used to diagnose and localize the lesion (see pp. 395 ff.).

Vocal Abuse

Acute

Symptoms. These include dysphonia, or even aphonia, and pain on speaking.

Pathogenesis. This is caused by extreme overuse of the voice in sporting spectators, politicians, market traders, and disco habitués.

Diagnosis. Indirect or direct laryngoscopy which shows hyperemia or swelling of the vocal cords and subepithelial bleeding.

Treatment. Strict voice rest and inhalations are required. If polyps form, they are removed by microlaryngoscopy.

Chronic

Symptoms. The voice is hoarse and croaking or disappears under stress. Singing is difficult or impossible.

Pathogenesis. *Screamer's or singer's nodules* develop because of chronic overuse or misuse of the voice.

Screamer's nodules occur in children and are frequent in mothers of large families and in teachers who must talk a lot.

Singer's nodes are due to unsatisfactory singing technique.

Diagnosis. Direct or indirect laryngoscopy shows the nodules on the typical site at the junction between the anterior and middle thirds of the vocal cords which is the point of maximal amplitude of the vibrations of the vocal cords. They are usually bilateral (see Color Plate **30b**).

Treatment. Once the nodules progress beyond a certain size, they become fibrotic, and voice rest and speech therapy are no longer successful. Most patients then require endolaryngeal microsurgery with postoperative speech therapy.

Contact Ulcer

Symptoms. These include dysphonia and pain in the larynx on speaking.

Pathogenesis. Almost all patients have a history of psychological stress. Vocal abuse causes the arytenoid cartilages to impinge sharply against each other.

Diagnosis. Indirect or direct laryngoscopy typically shows a hollow depression with a pronounced border over the vocal process on one side and a reactive pachydermia on the other side (see Color Plate **29c**).

Differential diagnosis. This includes ulceration or granulation due to intubation, tumors, and tuberculosis.

Treatment. The patients are usually hyperactive and do not persist with voice rest or speech therapy. Treatment centers on psychosomatic exploration and counseling. Excision is useful only for the histologic exclusion of malignancy.

Intubation Injury

Acute

Symptoms. Immediately or shortly after removal of the tube the patient complains of dysphonia, attacks of coughing, and hemoptysis. He also has pain in the larynx and neck.

Pathogenesis. Injury is caused by repeated or incorrect intubation, intermittent positive pressure respiration, a protruding guide wire, a wrong-sized tube, insufficient relaxation, overextension, and pressure of the tube cuff. These factors lead to a myogenic or neurologic paralysis. Drying of the mucosa by the premedication can exacerbate the mucosal injury. Laryngeal complications may be expected after less than 48 h of intubation in adults and after 3−7 days in young children, who tend to develop subglottic mucosal injuries.

Diagnosis. Laryngoscopy shows a subepithelial hematoma, superficial and deep mucosal injuries, and rarely a tear of the vocal cord or subluxation of the arytenoid cartilage. An intubation granuloma is usually bilateral and lies on the vocal process (see Color Plate **30a**).

Treatment. A hematoma or a superficial mucosal lesion can heal spontaneously within a few days. Pressure paralysis of the recurrent laryngeal nerve is also capable of spontaneous resolution, but tears of the vocal cord or subluxation of the arytenoid cartilage require surgery.

Chronic

Symptoms. Dysphonia or laryngeal dyspnea develop 2 to 8 weeks after intubation anesthesia or prolonged intubation.

Pathogenesis. Incorrect intubation, a tube that is too large or too rigid, incorrect (endolaryngeal or subglottic) position of the cuff, or prolonged intubation can all cause damage. The general condition of the patient including factors such as shock, retching, and vomiting are additional factors.

Note: The *early lesions* including endolaryngeal or subglottic hyperemia and edema, ischemic mucosal defects with fibrinous membrane, necrosis and ulceration lead to *late injuries.* The latter include ulceration, granulation, perichondritis, cartilaginous necrosis, synechiae, and strictures.

Diagnosis. This is made by laryngoscopy, tomography, and pulmonary function studies (see Color Plate **29b.**)

Treatment. *Granulomas* are removed by endolaryngeal microsurgery or laser. Postoperative speech therapy is indicated, but there is a tendency for recurrence (see below).

Laryngotracheal Stenoses and Synechiae

These often require several operations over a long period. The operations include excision or splitting of the scar tissue, and, if necessary, of the cricoid cartilage, with mucosal or cartilaginous grafts. A stent must be worn in the reconstructed larynx for several weeks until the patency of the lumen is assured (see p. 443; Fig. 4.**35a** and **b**).

External Trauma

Blunt and penetrating injuries, and open and closed injuries, occur and must be diagnosed.

Symptoms. These include immediate or increasing dyspnea, even complete respiratory obstruction due to hematoma, edema, and dislocation of cartilage fragments, bleeding, and dysphonia. Dysphagia and pain occur when the esophagus is affected.

Pathogenesis. These injuries are particularly common in traffic accidents, especially due to impact with the steering wheel and dashboard (Fig. 4.**15a−c**). Other causes include athletic injuries, karate blows, fighting, and attempting strangulation. In addition to the direct trauma resulting in subluxation and disruption of the laryngeal framework, the blow may force the larynx against the vertebral column causing endolaryngeal mucosal tears and vertical, horizontal, or combined fractures. Subluxation of the larynx from the trachea can occur. Perforations or contusions in the neighboring hypopharynx and upper esophagus lead to tracheoesophageal or laryngoesophageal fistulas. The neighboring nerves and vessels may also be injured (Fig. 4.**16** and Color Plate **31a**).

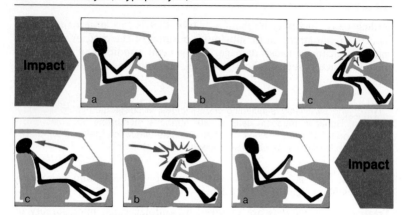

Fig. 4.**15a–c** Laryngeal trauma due to a traffic accident involving a rear-end or frontal collision.

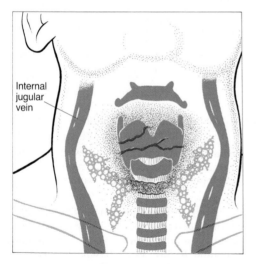

Internal jugular vein

Fig. 4.**16** Laryngeal trauma showing transverse laryngeal fracture and tear of the trachea, escape of air into the surrounding tissues, and congestion due to compression of the large cervical veins caused by hematoma, edema, and surgical emphysema.

Diagnosis. Inspection, palpation, and laryngoscopy demonstrate fractures, crepitation, or displacement of laryngeal fragments and surgical emphysema of the neck. Tomography and pulmonary function tests should also be carried out.

Table 4.7 Type and Treatment of Laryngeal Trauma	
Type of Injury	Treatment
Basic principle is to secure a free airway	
Hematoma and edema. Small tears of the mucosa.	Voice rest, steroids, tracheotomy if necessary
Extensive soft tissue injuries of the neck, exposed cartilage with otherwise intact or easily reconstructable laryngeal skeleton	Open exploration and reconstruction. A silicone keel should always be used in the anterior commissure to prevent scars.
Loss of thyroid cartilage and mucosa	Mucosal grafts and stenting of the inside of the larynx
Laryngeal fractures, vertical or horizontal	Suturing of the fragments with or without stenting
Laryngotracheal subluxation	End-to-end anastomosis of the stumps
Late stenosis	Open exploration, excision of scar, mucosal and cartilaginous grafts and stenting

Treatment. Preservation of the airway is the most important measure, if necessary by bronchoscopy, tracheotomy, or intubation (see Table 4.**14**). Emergency bronchoscopy may be used with bronchoscopes of the appropriate size. Distressing attacks of coughing are suppressed with antitussive medication. Some patients may require admission to the intensive care unit, e. g., for treatment of shock, for infusions, or transfusions, etc. Further procedures are shown in Table 4.**7**.

Inhalational Trauma by Chemical Toxins

Symptoms. *Acute* symptoms include severe attacks of coughing, a feeling of burning and asphyxia, and epiphora. *Chronic* symptoms include hoarseness, a feeling of dryness, clearing the throat, and coughing attacks.

Pathogenesis. The cause is escaping gases or steam after industrial explosions and the effect of smoke in fires. The most common chronic toxin is inhalation of tobacco smoke.

Diagnosis. Laryngoscopy shows redness, mucosal maceration, and edema.

Treatment. Voice rest, abstinence from smoking, humidification of the air, corticosteroids for edema, inhalation therapy, and laryngoscopic follow-up are indicated. Antibiotics are given as required. Intubation in case of acute respiratory insufficiency (p. 446).

Foreign Bodies

Symptoms. The initial symptoms are attacks of coughing, stabbing pains in the larynx, and dysphagia which occur during eating. Dyspnea may occur especially because of the tendency of the infant's mucosa to produce edema. Large, especially vegetable foreign bodies may cause asphyxia due to their swelling properties.

Pathogenesis. Laryngeal foreign bodies are rarer than tracheal or bronchial foreign bodies. Sharp-edged, pointed, or large foreign bodies may remain impacted within the larynx. The danger of foreign body aspiration is particularly great in sudden fright, laughing, or absence of the sensory innervation of the larynx.

Diagnosis. This is made by indirect laryngoscopy. Laryngotracheobronchoscopy should also be carried out in all suspect cases. Edema may overlie an impacted foreign body. Only radiopaque, especially metallic foreign bodies can be detected by radiography.

Treatment. The foreign body is removed carefully using the rigid endoscope, taking care to preserve the mucosa. A tracheotomy may be necessary before the removal of large impacted foreign bodies in the larynx with associated edema.

A laryngeal foreign body may occasionally be coughed out, but it is more often aspirated into the tracheobronchial tree.

Course. The mucosa tends to produce reactive edema, particularly in children. Steroids are then indicated and preparations made for intubation should severe dyspnea develop after removal of the foreign body.

Inflammation

Acute Laryngitis

Symptoms. These include hoarseness, aphonia, pain in the larynx, and coughing attacks. In children there is a danger of airway obstruction. Acute laryngitis is usually due to ascending or descending infections from other parts of the airway.

Pathogenesis. The cause is viral or bacterial infection.

Diagnosis. Laryngoscopy shows the vocal cords to be red and swollen. Depending on the underlying disease, the neighboring pharyngeal or tracheal mucosa may also be inflamed (see Color Plate **28a**).

Treatment. Since viral infections are often followed by secondary bacterial infection, antibiotics are indicated. Steroids are also indicated for marked edema. General measures include fluids by mouth, aspirin, and steam inhalation.

Note: Oil-containing inhalations should not be used. Only aerosols of a particle size of 30 (± 20) μm precipitate in the larynx.

Voice rest is indicated, and smoking should be forbidden. Chemicals such as certain dyestuffs or artificial products and allergic toxins such as hair sprays, shellfish, and crustaceans should be eliminated.

Note: If the symptoms do not improve considerably or resolve within 3 weeks, telescopic or microlaryngoscopy is indicated to exclude other laryngeal diseases. Ulceration, proliferation, and exudate are not typical of uncomplicated nonspecific laryngitis, and specific diseases, premalignant lesions, and tumors must be excluded.

Croup Syndromes

Diphtheritic croup, beginning with laryngeal membranes and obstruction, is presently rare. However, occasional endemic foci still persist in Western Europe. *Diphtheritic* laryngitis with greyish-white membranes occurring in isolation is becoming less and less common. It is more commonly combined with lesions of the oropharynx. Tracheotomy is required for increasing dyspnea.

The term *pseudocroup* includes a group of acute laryngotracheal diseases mainly affecting children:

● Acute Subglottic Laryngitis

Symptoms. There is a previous common cold followed by dry barking cough rapidly becoming worse, hoarseness, and inspiratory, expiratory, or mixed stridor leading to severe respiratory obstruction depending on swelling of the mucosa and site. There is indrawing of the suprasternal notch and intercostal spaces on inspiration, cyanosis, perioral pallor, and worsening of the symptoms due to a fear of asphyxia in children.

Pathogenesis. This is a very serious acute disease of early infancy, most common between the 1st and 5th years of life. In a short time, life-threatening narrowing of the child's airway can develop due to inflammatory mucosal swelling of the conus elasticus in the subglottic space. The disease is basically due to a viral infection with accompanying secondary bacterial infection. Cool, damp, and foggy autumn and winter weather appear to increase the morbidity. *However, recurrent infections in the nasopharynx and nasal obstruction due to chronically inflamed hypertrophied adenoids and tonsils are important in the etiology.* Whether air

Table 4.8 Treatment of Acute Subglottic Laryngitis
Basic Principle: relief of both obstruction and distressing cough which impedes circulation
Sedation of child (avoid respiratory depressive drugs) Steroids Antibiotics to prevent secondary infection Administration of fluids Croup tent

pollution plays an important role in the pathogenesis of this disease remains uncertain.

Diagnosis. The clinical picture is usually very typical. Laryngoscopy shows glottic mucosal edema and redness, possibly with crust formation.

Treatment. Mild cases, assessed on the degree of respiratory obstruction, may be managed by the family practitioner or pediatrician. Close observation by a physician must be provided to confirm the efficacy of treatment (Table 4.**8**).

If these measures fail and there is increasing dyspnea, the child must be admitted to the hospital as an emergency. There he is treated with oxygen therapy and endotracheal intubation depending on the degree of dyspnea and the results of blood gas analysis. Tracheostomy is carried out for severe obstruction and when there is a progressive sicca-type crust formation.

● **Acute Epiglottitis**

Symptoms. These include severe pain on swallowing so that food is refused which may lead to dehydration and the possibility of circulatory collapse. Inspiratory stridor usually forces the patient to sit upright in bed. The speech is thick and the temperature elevated.

Pathogenesis. The main causative organisms is *Hemophilus influenzae.* The disease is sometimes caused by mucosal damage by swallowing sharp-edged food allowing entry of pathogenic organisms. The disease mainly affects children up to 10 years of age, but adults are also affected.

Diagnosis. The diagnosis is "epiglottitis acutissima" if the course is particularly fulminant. Laryngoscopy or examination with a tongue depressor shows a thick, swollen, red epiglottic rim (see Color Plate **31b**). A lateral radiograph shows the epiglottic swelling.

Differential diagnosis. Pseudocroup may also be caused by congenital anomalies, impacted foreign bodies, angioneurotic edema of the larynx, hypocalcemic laryngospasm, tumors, and infected epiglottic cysts.

Treatment. The child is admitted to hospital and treated with intravenous steroids, broad-spectrum antibiotics in high doses, also intravenously. The airway is ensured by nasotracheal intubation for life-threatening dyspnea. Tracheotomy is now rarely required because of the usually short course of the illness.

Note: In patients with respiratory obstruction, particularly children, diagnostic procedures may lead to complete obstruction. Preparations for intubation or tracheotomy must therefore be made *before* the investigation. The patient should be referred to a hospital if the diagnosis of epiglottitis is suspected.

Prognosis and course. The disease usually improves rapidly within a few days. Possible complications include epiglottic abscess and perichondritis.

Chronic Laryngitis

Chronic nonspecific laryngitis must be distinguished from the group of specific forms such as tuberculosis, amyloid, etc. Chronic nonspecific laryngitis requires assessment and treatment by the otolaryngologist.

Chronic Nonspecific Laryngitis

Symptoms. These persist for weeks or months in contrast to those of acute laryngitis. They include hoarseness, deepening of the voice, and sometimes a dry cough. The voice is less able to withstand stress, there is a globus sensation in the larynx, a feeling of a need to clear the throat, but little or no pain.

Pathogenesis. This disease is mainly due to exogenous toxins such as cigarette smoking, occupational air pollution, and climatic influences. Another cause is vocal abuse in bartenders, construction workers, long-distance truck drivers, and professional speakers. Nasal obstruction is also an important factor in pathogenesis.

Note: Laryngopathia gravidarum due to vocal cord edema with dysphonia and deepening of the voice is sometimes observed in the second half of pregnancy. The hoarseness almost always resolves spontaneously after delivery.

The administration of male sex hormones and anabolic steroids causes voice change in women including deepening of the tone, disorders of the singing voice, and reduction of the carrying power of the speaking voice. These disorders persist because of the virilization of the laryngeal structures.

Diagnosis. Laryngoscopy shows the vocal cords to be thick and red with rough edges (see Color Plate **28c**). There is tenacious mucus and the rest of the laryngeal mucosa often shows similar appearance. Microlaryngoscopy should always be performed, and malignancy should be excluded by biopsy.

Treatment. The duration of treatment is protracted. Elimination of exogenous toxins such as tobacco is the mainstay of treatment. Voice rest is prescribed and if necessary a deviated nasal septum is corrected to restore normal nasal respiration. Antibiotics are given for accompanying inflammation, and a short course of steroids, saline inhalations, and mucolytic agents are given (see p. 415). Refractory cases may require decortication of the vocal folds.

Note: Regular laryngoscopic follow-ups are advisable in chronic laryngitis because of the possibility of dysplasia. Microlaryngoscopy and biopsy should be performed in every *doubtful case.* This is the only method of early detection of malignancy.

Specific Forms of Chronic Laryngitis

Laryngeal Tuberculosis

Symptoms. These include hoarseness and coughing persisting for several months and pain on swallowing radiating to the ear.

Pathogenesis. Tuberculous laryngitis is almost always secondary to active pulmonary tuberculosis. The infection is transmitted to the larynx by bacillae contained in the sputum. The posterior part of the larynx, the interarytenoid area, and the epiglottis are those most commonly affected. There is a danger of perichondritis. Monocorditis may also be caused by a miliary tuberculous deposit.

Diagnosis. Microlaryngoscopy in fresh cases initially shows reddish-brown submucous nodules which are partly confluent. Later ulcerations or granulations develop. *Monocorditis* is characterized by redness and thickening, occasionally with small ulcerations of *one* vocal cord. Other investigations include histology, culture, radiography, and examination by an internist.

Differential diagnosis. This includes vasomotor monocorditis, nonspecific chronic laryngitis, and carcinoma.

Treatment. Antituberculous treatment is given in cooperation with an internist. Pain is treated by blocking the superior laryngeal nerve (see Fig. 4.**14**). Isolation of the patient is rarely necessary owing to available chemotherapeutic options, but contacts should be investigated. *The disease is reportable.*

Course and prognosis. Laryngeal tuberculosis is infectious. Mucosal lesions often heal with no permanent effects on laryngeal function, but if the tuberculosis has affected the laryngeal cartilaginous framework defects arise during healing. The prognosis currently is good.

Laryngeal Sarcoid

Laryngeal sarcoid as an extrapulmonary manifestation is nowadays rare. Dysphonia and a globus sensation are caused by sarcoid deposits in the larynx.

Biopsy, if necessary combined with prescalene lymph node biopsy (see p. 517 and Fig. 6.**20a** and **b**), is necessary to establish the diagnosis.

In contrast to tuberculosis, the epithelioid cell nodules do not caseate or ulcerate. Radiography is a supplementary investigation. The disease is treated by an internist.

Laryngeal Syphilis

Isolated laryngeal syphilis is unusual, and it is much more often a manifestation of oropharyngeal syphilis in the secondary generalized stage of the disease.

Mucous plaques or hazy, smoke-colored mucosal lesions occur in the larynx similar to those of syphilitic pharyngitis (see p. 332). The patient is also hoarse. *The disease is reportable.*

Respiratory obstruction only occurs in the presence of marked mucosal swelling. The cartilage is destroyed in a gumma in stage III. The differential diagnosis from carcinoma is difficult to make.

Scleroma of the Larynx

Pale-red swellings and granulations with crusts develop mainly in the subglottic space. Subglottic, laryngeal, and intratracheal stenoses occur in stage III causing hoarseness, cough, and increasing stridor.

Diagnosis. This is established by microlaryngoscopy, histopathology, and culture.

Treatment. Tracheotomy followed by appropriate operative treatment of laryngo-tracheal stenosis is necessary for respiratory stridor.

Pemphigus Vulgaris and Pemphigoid Vesicles

Both affect the epiglottis preferentially and are often incidental findings. The vesicles are usually painless, but may occasionally cause a globus sensation and can lead to stenosis due to extensive scarring (may also affect the adjacent pharynx). Paraneoplastic symptoms may be present. Treatment is directed toward the underlying disease.

Generalized Rheumatoid Arthritis

The *cricoarytenoid joint* is often affected, causing hoarseness, stridor, and pain on swallowing radiating to the ear.

Laryngeal Amyloid

Tumorous, polypoid lesions covered by smooth mucosa and pale-waxy in appearance may develop in the larynx in this dysproteinemia. The sites of predilection are the vocal cords and the subglottic space. Surgical removal is required for severe hoarseness and respiratory obstruction.

Laryngeal Perichondritis

Symptoms. These include pain in the larynx, increasing on swallowing or external pressure, hoarseness, and dyspnea.

Pathogenesis. Surgical and accidental trauma, infiltration of cartilage by tumor, infection, e.g., tuberculosis, and irradiation can all be causes. Provided that the cartilage is not invaded by tumor, it usually tolerates radiation up to 6,000 rad. The usual clinical problem is chondroradioneurosis with inflammation of the overlying mucosa.

Diagnosis and findings. The laryngoscopic picture of radiogenic pallid mucosal edema particularly on the epiglottis and the arytenoid cartilages is, together with the history, very typical. There is intra- and extralaryngeal swelling, fistulae, and sequestration of necrotic bits of cartilage.

Treatment. Sequestrated or exposed cartilage must be removed. Broad-spectrum antibiotics are given in high doses combined with steroids (see Color Plate **28b**).

Note: Radiation edema is very difficult to treat and often disguises persistent or recurrent tumor.

Tumors

Benign Tumors

Vocal Cord Polyps

Symptoms. These include hoarseness, aphonia, and attacks of coughing. Dyspnea occurs with large polyps. If the polyp has a pedicle and is floating between the cords, the voice may return to normal for short intervals.

Pathogenesis. This is the most common benign tumor of the vocal cords, mainly affecting men between 30 and 50 years of age. It is often initiated by agents causing laryngeal inflammation. Hyperkinetic voice disorders and vocal abuse are important.

Diagnosis. Laryngoscopy (see Color Plate **30c**) shows the polyp usually lying on the free edge of the vocal cord either on a pedicle or sessile. It is seroedematous and occasionally hemorrhagic. Older polyps appear firm due to fibrosis and thickening of the overlying epithelium.

Treatment. The polyp is removed by endolaryngeal microsurgery, with preservation of the vocal ligament and vocalis muscle. The patient is advised to rest his voice until the defect epithelializes.

Note: The polyp should always be examined histologically to establish the diagnosis.

Reinke's Edema

Symptoms. These include hoarseness and deepening of the voice, or diplophonia. Stridor may occur particularly on exertion if the edema is marked.

Pathogenesis. The edema is almost always bilateral and broad-based. It develops in Reinke's space. The edema usually affects high-demand professional speakers and smokers.

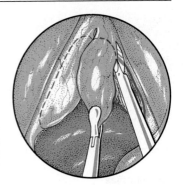

Fig. 4.**17** Decortication of the vocal cords for Reinke's edema. The dotted line shows the limits of excision. The anterior commissure is spared because of the danger of web formation.

Diagnosis. Laryngoscopy shows a bilateral broad-based edematous mass on the vocal cords.

Treatment. The mucosa is removed by decortication or stripping with microsurgery, preserving the vocalis muscle (Fig. 4.**17**). If the anterior commissure is involved, the cords must be stripped in two separate sittings to prevent adhesions anteriorly (CO_2-Laser).

Papillomas

Symptoms. Depending on the site and extent of the lesions, these include hoarseness which is often severe and respiratory obstruction.

Pathogenesis. The etiology is viral. Some juvenile papillomas resolve spontaneously about the time of puberty. Papillomas present in adults since early childhood are not uncommon and are considered potentially precancerous.

Diagnosis. This is made by direct laryngoscopy and histologic examination. Papillomas may be pedicled, solitary, or widespread. Their surface is pale-yellow to red, granular, villous, and often has a raspberry appearance.

Other areas of papillomatosis may lie in the oropharynx and the subglottic space (see Color Plate **31c**).

Treatment. Spontaneous regression rarely occurs. The effects of immunologic and antiviral treatment and vaccines have not been reproducible. *Today there is no alternative to surgery*. Microsurgery is being progressively replaced by the laser, although the overall recurrence rate is high. Tracheotomy is strictly contraindicated, as it tends to provoke rapid spread to the tracheobronchial mucosa.

Note: Papillomas in adults tend to undergo malignant degeneration.

Retention Cysts

These are glazed, white, or occasionally blue cysts derived from mucosal glands. They are localized to the vestibular fold, the ventricle, the epiglottis, the aryepiglottic folds, and the valleculae.

Small cysts are sometimes found accidentally; larger cysts can cause a globus sensation, dysphonia, and dyspnea.

Treatment is removal by microsurgery.

Chondromas

Symptoms. These include hoarseness, dyspnea, dysphagia, or globus depending on the site.

Pathogenesis. The tumors grow slowly and often arise from the cricoid cartilage.

Diagnosis. Laryngoscopy usually shows a subglottic tumor covered with smooth mucosa. The tumor is sometimes palpable externally. Tomography demonstrates the site and extent of the tumor.

Treatment. Treatment is surgical. Chondromas are radioresistant.

Leukoplakia, Dysplasia, and Carcinoma In Situ of the Laryngeal Mucosa

Leukoplakia is a clinical term covering lesions of various different histologic grades. A leukoplakic lesion may signify a premalignant or malignant process and therefore requires histologic investigation. Histomorphologic definitions of the grades of dysplasia serve to eliminate ambiguous terminologies and facilitate prognostic assessment:

Grade I: *Simple dysplasia*, i. e., an epithelial hyperplasia without nuclear atypia, without disturbances of maturation or stratification of the squamous epithelium. This is a clinically benign disease.

Grade II: *Middle-grade epithelial dysplasia* with basal cell hyperplasia, loss of basal cell polarity, moderate cell polymorphism, slightly increased mitotic rate, and occasional dyskeratosis. This is to be regarded clinically as a premalignant lesion.

Grade III: *High-grade dysplasia* with basal cell hyperplasia, loss of basal cell polarity, cell polymorphism, increased mitotic rate, numerous dyskeratoses, and abnormalities of epithelial stratification. Transition to carcinoma in situ is shown by intensification of high-grade dysplasia, loss of epithelial stratification, but no invasion of the stroma. Carcinoma in situ may be a *forerunner* of a carcinoma, an intraepithelial offshoot, or an isolated satellite focus.

Note: Squamous cell carcinomas of the larynx arise from a precancerous change with a varied length of history and may be diagnosed at this stage by the appropriate steps. Complete removal in the preinvasive stage not only establishes the diagnosis, but is also the definitive treatment.

Symptoms. These include hoarseness, feeling of a foreign body in the throat, and a desire to clear the throat.

Pathogenesis. This includes exogenous toxins, e.g., smoking and irradiation.

Diagnosis. Microlaryngoscopy shows the mucosa of the larynx or the vocal cords to be rough, thickened, occasionally deepened by scar tissue, and occasionally altered in color.

Treatment. The histologic classification determines the type and extent of treatment. Lesions confined entirely to the vocal cords are treated by decortication, i.e., removal of the epithelium of the vocal cord by microlaryngoscopy. Obvious etiologic agents should be eliminated. Laser therapy is assuming increasing importance.

Malignant Tumors (see Color Plates **32c** and **33a−c**)

Laryngeal Carcinoma

Laryngeal carcinoma accounts for approximately 40% of carcinomas of the head and neck. It is most common between the ages of 45 and 75 years. At the present time men are ten times more frequently affected than women, although in the last few decades the number of female patients in Europe and the United States has increased due to increased incidence of smoking in women.

Symptoms. Hoarseness is the first and main symptom when the tumor affects the glottis. Further symptoms, which may occur alone or in combination depending upon site and extent, include a feeling of a foreign body, clearing the throat, pain in the throat or referred elsewhere, dyspnea, dysphagia, cough, and hemoptysis. Regional lymph node metastases may also occur.

Note: Hoarseness persisting for more than 2 to 3 weeks must always be investigated by a specialist, and omission of this step is dangerous.

Pathogenesis. Invasive carcinoma may develop from epithelial dysplasia especially from carcinoma in situ. More than 90% of laryngeal carcinomas are keratinizing or nonkeratinizing squamous cell carcinomas. Rare malignant forms include verrucous carcinoma, adenocarcinoma, carcinosarcoma, fibrosarcoma, and chondrosarcoma.

Most patients with squamous carcinoma of the larynx were or are heavy cigarette smokers and, in addition, often heavy drinkers. Chronic exposure to irritation with heavy metals such as chromium, nickel, uranium, or asbestos, and irradiation are rarer causes.

There are racial differences in the frequency of site distribution within the larynx. For example, supraglottic carcinoma is commoner in Spain and in parts of South America than in the Federal Republic of Germany.

Laryngeal carcinoma infiltrates locally in the mucosa and beneath the mucosa and metastasizes via the lymphatics and the bloodstream. The limits of vascular spread are embryologically determined (see p. 392 and Fig. 4.4). Thus, supraglottic carcinomas usually remain confined to the supraglottic space and spread anteriorly into the preepiglottic space, whereas glottic carcinomas seldom spread into the supraglottic area but rather into the subglottic space. A *transglottic carcinoma* is a glottic carcinoma involving the ventricle and the vestibular folds in which the site of origin can no longer be recognized (see Color Plate **33b**). *The characteristics of the intralaryngeal lymphatics* (see p. 392) *influence the frequency of regional lymph node metastases*. Other factors influencing the frequency of metastases are the duration of the symptoms, the histologic differentiation, and the size and site of the tumor. Lymph node metastases at the time of presentation are rare in carcinomas of the vocal cord, but are found in about 20% of subglottic carcinomas, about 40% of supraglottic carcinomas, and in about 40% of transglottic carcinomas.

Contralateral metastases are unusual in unilateral glottic tumors. *Bilateral metastases* become more common if the carcinoma crosses the midline, e. g., at the anterior or posterior commissure or in the trachea, or if the tumor arises primarily in the supraglottic space.

Distant hematogenous metastases are relatively unusual in laryngeal carcinoma at the time the patient is first seen. *Second primary carcinomas* of the respiratory and digestive tracts (synchronous or metachronous) also occur.

Diagnosis. The clinical diagnosis rests initially on the findings of indirect laryngoscopy and telescopic laryngoscopy. The site and extent of the tumor and the mobility of the vocal cord must be assessed (Table 4.9). It is very important to carry out microlaryngoscopy (see Fig. 4.8 and 4.9). This allows accurate evaluation of the site and extent of the tumor, provides a view of hidden angles such as the ventricle and the piriform sinus, and allows assessment of the superficial characteristics such as nodular, exophytic, granulomatous, ulcerating, etc. (see Color Plate **33a−c**). Increasingly, CT and MRI are used to acquire data on the depth of involvement.

Differential diagnosis. This includes chronic laryngitis and its specific forms, and benign laryngeal tumors.

Table 4.**9**   Classification and involvement of Larnygeal Carcinomas According to the *TNM* System*

Glottis (80%)	T_{is} = preinvasive carcinoma, carcinoma in situ
	T_1 = tumor confined to the glottis with normal cord movement
	    T_{1a} = one cord
	    T_{1b} = both cords
	T_2 = cord tumor with extension subglottically or supraglottically with normal or slightly impaired cord mobility (see Color Plate **33a**)
	T_3 = tumor confined to the larynx with fixation of one or both cords (see Color Plate **33b**)
	T_4 = tumor extending beyond the larynx, e.g., extending into the thyroid cartilage, piriform sinus, postcricoid region or into adjacent skin

Subglottis (5%)	T_{is} = preinvasive carcinoma, carcinoma in situ
	T_1 = tumor of the subglottic region with normal cord mobility
	    T_{1a} = one side subglottis
	    T_{1b} = both subglottis areas
	T_2 = tumor of the subglottic region with extension to one or both cords
	T_3 = tumor confined to the larynx with fixation of one or both cords
	T_4 = tumor extending beyond the larynx, e.g. into the postcricoid region, trachea or skin

Supraglottis (15%)	T_{is} = preinvasive carcinoma, carcinoma in situ
	T_1 = tumor confined to the supraglottic area with normal cord mobility
	    T_{1a} = tumor confined to the laryngeal surface of the epiglottis, one aryepiglottic fold, one ventricle, or one false cord
	    T_{1b} = tumor of epiglottis involvement of one ventricle or false cord
	T_2 = tumor of the epiglottis, ventricle or false cord extending to the cord without fixation
	T_3 = tumor confined to the larynx with vocal cord fixation and destruction or other signs of deep infiltration
	T_4 = tumor extending beyond the limits of the larynx with involvement of the piriform sinus, postcricoid region, vallecula or tongue base

* see Figure 6.**18**.

Treatment. If untreated, laryngeal carcinoma leads to death within an average of 12 months by asphyxia, bleeding, metastases, infection, or cachexia. The existence of cardiovascular or pulmonary diseases and diabetes mellitus determines the course of treatment and the course of the disease. The indications for *radiotherapy or surgery* for laryngeal carcinoma vary depending on the site and stage of the tumor. They are often used in combination. *Chemotherapy* alone has so far proved to be useless for this type of tumor. *Radiotherapy* is mainly given as telecobalt megavoltage radiation. *Except for $T_1 N_0$ glottic tumors and for some $T_2 N_0$ tumors, and especially if lymph node metastases are present, surgery is clearly superior to radiotherapy.*

Radiotherapy is appropriate for patients with inoperable tumors, patients who refuse cancer surgery, and laryngeal tumor manifestations that are not amenable to surgical palliation. Extension of laryngeal carcinoma to the hypopharynx is another possible indication for radiotherapy.

The combination of surgery and postoperative radiotherapy appears to yield the best results for selected patients in advanced stages.

Complications after radiotherapy include persistent edema which makes it difficult to assess the local appearances and detect a recurrence. The edema is usually due to chondroradionecrosis leading to cartilaginous necrosis and which may require laryngectomy. Other complications include dysphagia, ageusia, xerostomia and the sicca syndrome. If surgery must be undertaken after a full course of radiotherapy, the wound healing and prognosis are considerably worse.

Surgical Procedures for Laryngeal Carcinoma

1. *Microsurgical decortication of the vocal cord* is indicated for severe dysplasia and some carcinomas in situ.

2. *Cordectomy* is indicated for a vocal cord carcinoma with a mobile vocal cord ($T_1 N_0, T_2 N_0$).

Principle of the operation (Fig. 4.**18a−c**). The thyroid cartilage is split by a thyrotomy, the affected vocal cord is excised, and the thyroid cartilage is closed again. The breathing is normal after this operation. The voice is rough or hoarse postoperatively, but may return to normal after several months as scar tissue forms a pseudocord. Decortication and chordectomy can be performed by endoscopic laser surgery in selected cases.

3. *Vertical or horizontal partial laryngectomies* are used for carcinomas for which a cordectomy is not suitable because of the extent or site of the tumor, but for which total laryngectomy is not necessary. Partial laryngectomies *preserve the vocal function and a normal airway.* The prerequisites for success are careful assessment and good surgical judgment to ensure that the tumor is removed completely.

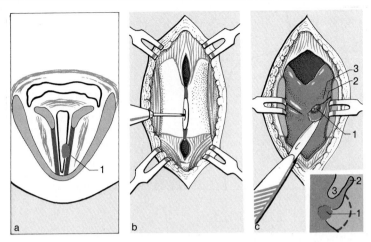

Fig. 4.**18a–c**   Cordectomy. **a.** Carcinoma in the center of the vocal cord. **b.** Thyrotomy: division of the thyroid cartilage with a rotating saw. In the diagram the incision into the conus elasticus and into the superior thyrohyoid membrane has already been undertaken. **c.** Excision of the affected part of the vocal cord with a good margin. 1, Vocal cord with tumor; 2, ventricle; 3, vestibular fold.

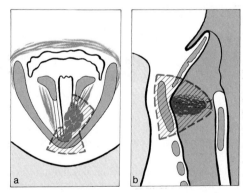

Fig. 4.**19a** and **b**   Vertical frontolateral partial resection. The area to be resected is shown in red, and the limits of resection by the dashed line.

Vertical partial laryngectomy. *Principle of the operation* (Fig. 4.**19a** and **b**). Several methods are available, but the principle common to all of them is that a wide vertical segment of the thyroid cartilage and, occasionally the cricoid cartilage, is removed together with the laryngeal soft tissues and the tumor. A *hemilaryngectomy,* removal of half of the larynx, may be carried out for a tumor limited strictly to one side.

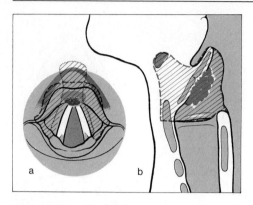

Fig. 4.**20a** and **b**   Horizontal supraglottic partial resection. The area to be resected is shaded, and the limits of resection are shown by the dashed line. The *dotted* line indicates the area to be resected not clinically visible by laryngoscopy.

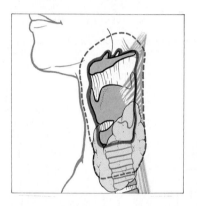

Fig. 4.**21**   Area resected in laryngectomy. The boundaries to be resected may be extended for involvement of the tongue, the hypopharynx, the upper trachea, and the thyroid gland (shown by the dashed line).

Horizontal partial laryngectomy. *Principle of the operation* (Fig. 4.**20a** and **b**). The supraglottic space is completely removed, with retention of the vocal cords and the arytenoid cartilage.

After a partial resection, the functional results are good and the airway is normal as is the vocal function, but the latter depends on the type of resection, the results of which are variable. The patient may have temporary difficulty in swallowing, which may persist in elderly patients. There is a danger of recurrence at the excisional margins if the tumor was incorrectly evaluated preoperatively or if the technique was inadequate.

4. *Total laryngectomy* may on occasion be combined with removal of the hypopharynx. This technique is indicated for tumors that cannot be removed by cordectomy or partial laryngectomy and for tumors that have spread to neighboring structures such as the tongue, the hypopharyx, the

Fig. 4.**22**   Laryngectomy.
A U-shaped incision is made
and the skin-platysma flap
turned superiorly over the
chin. The larynx together with
the hyoid bone (dashed line
above) is freed from its connection with the surrounding
soft tissue and from the trachea and is divided from the
trachea inferiorly. It is also
divided from the esophagus
below and the hypopharynx.
The excision may also proceed from above downward.
The feeding tube can be seen
in the open hypopharynx. The
thyroid gland, which is divided
and sutured laterally, can be
recognized in the lower part
of the diagram.

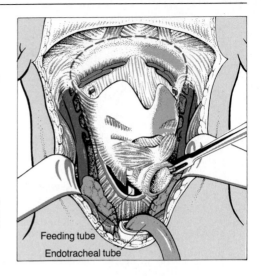

Feeding tube

Endotracheal tube

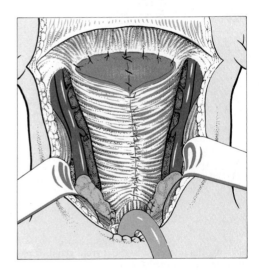

Fig. 4.**23**   Situation after
removal of the larynx and
closure of the pharyngeal
mucosa in layers.

thyroid gland, and the trachea. Total laryngectomy is also indicated for
tumors that have recurred after radiotherapy or partial procedures.

Operative technique (Figs. 4.**21** to 4.**24**). The entire larynx is removed from the base
of the tongue to the trachea, if necessary with removal of parts of the tongue, the

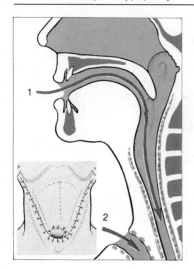

Fig. 4.**24**   Appearance after conclusion of laryngectomy. The replaced U-shaped skin flap covers the newly repaired pharynx. The T-shaped pharyngeal suture line is shown by the dotted line in the left inset. 1, Food passage reconstructed. Normal swallowing may be resumed after healing. 2, Tracheostomy for a new airway.

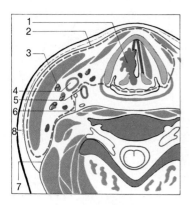

Fig. 4.**25**   Laryngectomy with radical neck dissection. The area to be resected is shown by the dashed line. 1, Larynx with the tumor; 2, superficial cervical fascia which coincides with the limits of radical neck dissection; 3, cervical lymph nodes; 4, internal jugular vein; 5, carotid artery; 6, vagus nerve; 7, deep cervical fascia; 8, platysma.

pharynx, the trachea, and the thyroid gland. If part of the tongue or the pharynx is removed, reconstructive procedures must be undertaken at the same time. After this operation *breathing* is only possible via the tracheostomy. *Swallowing* is almost normal once the wound has healed, and *voice* is produced either by esophageal speech (see below) or by means of an external electronic larynx.

Complications after laryngectomy include pharyngocutaneous fistula and recurrent tracheobronchitis.

Table 4.10 Five Year Survival in Laryngeal Carcinoma*		
Type of Tumor	%	Treatment
Glottic carcinoma		
T_1N_0	> 90	Surgery or radiotherapy
T_2N_0	70–80	Surgery or radiotherapy
T_3	60–70	Surgery or combined surgery and radiotherapy
T_4	< 50	Surgery or combined surgery and radiotherapy
Supraglottic carcinoma		
T_1 and T_2	80	Surgery or combined surgery and radiotherapy
T_3 and T_4	50–60	Surgery or combined surgery and radiotherapy
Subglottic carcinoma	< 40	Surgery or combined surgery and radiotherapy
Transglottic carcinoma	< 50	Surgery or combined surgery and radiotherapy

* The presence of a regional *lymph node metastasis* reduces the above figures *considerably*. If the nodes are fixed the survival rate is markedly reduced (see p. 511 ff.).

Note: Removal of the primary tumor by a partial or total laryngectomy should be combined with a curative neck dissection en bloc if lymph node metastases are present (see Fig. 4.25). If there is a known high risk of lymphatic metastases for a tumor at a particular site, many surgeons carry out a *modified neck dissection* even if lymph node metastases cannot be palpated.
The results of treatment are summarized in Table 4.10.

Rehabilitation of the Laryngectomee

1. *Voice and Speech*

a. Approximately 85% of laryngectomees can learn esophageal speech under the direction of a speech therapist. The esophagus is used as the air source and the mouth of the esophagus as the pseudoglottis.

b. An alternative is surgical creation of a fistula between the tracheal stump and the pharynx or esophagus, the neoglottis procedure, with or without a supplementary mechanical device. At the moment these procedures have numerous functional disadvantages.

c. An electronic device may be used to produce sound. This device delivers externally produced vibrations to the pharyngeal wall or the floor of the mouth.

2. *Tracheostomy*

a. Since it is possible to breathe only via the tracheostomy, problems arise during showering, bathing, and swimming. However, these can be overcome by a device like a snorkel.

b. Once the tracheostomy has stabilized it is usually unnecessary to use a tracheostomy tube. If the tracheostomy tends to stenose, a short individually fitted stoma button may be used, or it may be necessary to widen the stoma surgically.

c. There is often a tendency to develop tracheitis with crusts, particularly in the spring and autumn, because of the absence of the air-conditioning mechanism of the nose. Treatment is described under "Trachea".

3. *Social Reintegration*

The patient and his relatives need thorough instruction *before* the operation about future functional defects. Medical and psychological training is necessary *after* the operation. The patient is encouraged to join a laryngectomee club.

Hypopharynx

Anatomy. See pp. 372 and 373.

The most important diseases are foreign bodies (see Color Plate **35a**), pulsion diverticulum (see p. 306), and *carcinoma* (see Color Plate **33d**).

Hypopharyngeal Carcinoma

The *TNM* classification distinguishes three regions (see Fig. 4.**26**):

- Piriform sinus (see Color Plate **33d**)
- Posterior pharyngeal wall
- Postcricoid region (see Color Plate **34a**)

The T staging is as follows:

- T_1 is a tumor that is confined to one region
- T_2 is a tumor that involves two regions
- T_3 is a tumor that extends beyond the borders of the hypopharynx, larynx, esophagus, and cervical soft tissues

Symptoms. In more than 40% of cases the patient presents because of lymph node metastases. The typical site is at the angle of the jaw under the sternocleidomastoid muscle. The patient also has dysphagia and pain irradiating to the ear. Hoarseness and difficulty in breathing occur when the tumor extends to the larynx or paralyzes the recurrent laryngeal nerve. Oral fetor (degenerating tumor) and bloodstained sputum also may occur.

Pathogenesis. The previous term of extrinsic laryngeal carcinoma is no longer tenable on anatomic or clinical grounds.

In recent years the peak age incidence has fallen because of alcohol and nicotine abuse. The ratio of men to women in the Federal Republic of Germany is now 4:1. In the Scandinavian countries the tumor occurs more frequently in women, especially postcricoid carcinoma. The disease is said to be related to the Plummer-Vinson syndrome. About 50% of patients have T_3 N_{1-2} tumors when first seen. Carcinomas of the posterolateral pharyngeal wall and of the postcricoid region have a particularly high rate of metastases, often bilateral in the latter lesions. Distant metastases at the time of diagnosis are found in 10% of cases in the lung, liver, and skeleton, and in as many as 80% of patients at autopsy. Virtually all tumors are poorly differentiated squamous carcinomas.

Order of frequency of the sites of occurrence of hypopharyngeal carcinoma. Tumors of the piriform sinus are the most common followed by lesions of the posterior pharyngeal wall. Postcricoid tumors are rare (Fig. 4.**26**).

Diagnosis. The early symptoms of interference with swallowing and cervical lymph node metastases are often misinterpreted by both the patient and the doctor so that diagnosis is delayed. The time interval between the early symptoms and the first examination by a specialist is further increased by the difficulty of examining the hypopharynx with the mirror. Endoscopic examination should always be carried out if a hypopharyngeal carcinoma is suspected. The tumor may be ulcerating or exophytic in type, often surrounded by edema and covered with retained saliva and food remnants.

Note: Cervical lymph node metastases with an unknown primary tumor require special investigation of the hypopharynx.

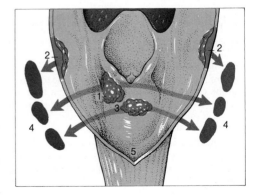

Fig. 4.**26**   The sites of carcinomas of the hypopharynx (1, 2, 3) and pathways of lymphatic metastases. The hypopharynx has been opened posteriorly. The esophageal orifice (5) lies inferiorly. 1, Piriform sinus; 2, posterior pharyngeal wall; 3, postcricoid region; 4, chain of deep cervical nodes along internal jugular vein.

Treatment. Surgery is only justifiable in a limited number of patients depending on the site and extent of the tumor and the presence of lymphatic or blood-borne metastases. If surgery is possible, it consists of pharyngectomy, or pharyngolaryngectomy if the larynx is involved.

A neck dissection is indicated on one or both sides because of the very high rate of metastases to the cervical lymph nodes. Reconstruction of the pharynx and upper esophagus by musculocutaneous flaps from the neck or chest wall is often necessary.

All therapeutic measures are limited by the advanced stage of the disease and the associated poor general condition of the patient. In early stages, surgery supplemented by radiotherapy achieves a 5-year survival rate of approximately 50%. In T_3 carcinomas with cervical lymph node metastases, the 5-year survival rate for surgery or radiotherapy is significantly poorer.

Tracheobronchial Tree

Study of the tracheobronchial system is common to several disciplines. The trachea is largely localized to the neck and is a continuation of the larynx so that diseases of one organ often affect the other. The tracheobronchial system is therefore of interest to the otolaryngologist. Furthermore, endoscopic diagnosis and treatment (bronchoscopy) was developed by ear, nose, and throat surgeons and is still practiced by them although other specialists in bronchial diseases such as chest physicians and thoracic surgeons practice diagnostic bronchoscopy. The following overview is presented from the otolaryngologist's point of view and illustrates relations with associated disciplines.

Applied Anatomy and Physiology

Basic Anatomy

The *trachea* is attached to the cricoid cartilage which is the most narrow rigid element of the airway and moves in response to movements of the floor of the mouth and the cervical muscles. It is 10 to 13 cm long in the adult and its lumen is held open by 16 to 20 horseshoe-shaped cartilaginous rings. The posterior part of the tube is formed by the membranous part which lies in contact with the anterior esophageal wall.

The carina, i.e., the origin of the two main bronchi, lies at the level of the sixth thoracic vertebra. It has an angle of 55° open inferiorly. The right main bronchus lies at an angle of about 17° to the midline and the left bronchus at an angle of about 35° (Fig. 4.**27**).

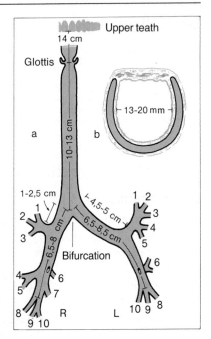

Fig. 4.**27** Tracheobronchial tree (a) and cross-section of the trachea (b). Nomenclature of the segmental bronchi. *Right.* 1, Apical; 2, posterior; 3, anterior; 4, lateral; 5, medial; 6, apical; 7, cardiac; 8, anterobasal; 9, laterobasal; 10, posterobasal (1+2+3 = the upper lobe; 4+5 = the middle lobe; 6+7+8+9 +10 = the lower lobe). *Left.* 1, Apical; 2, posterior; 3, anterior; 4, superior; 5, inferior; 6, apical; 8, anterobasal; 9, laterobasal; 10, posterobasal. (1+2 +3+[4+5 = lingula] = upper lobe; 6+8+9+10 = lower lobe).

The *bronchial tree* has an extra- and an intrapulmonary course. The horseshoe-shaped cartilaginous rings of the bronchial wall gradually become complete rings, encircling the bronchus fully in the more peripheral parts. The bronchioles do not possess cartilaginous elements in the wall but only a spiral muscle. Changes in the lumen are produced by the bronchial musculature and additionally in the middle and small bronchi by the bronchial veins.

The trachea and bronchi are lined by respiratory mucosa which becomes flatter toward the periphery and passes into a single layer of cubical epithelium in the bronchioles.

Vascular supply. The trachea is mainly supplied by the inferior thyroid artery, but there are also connections with the superior thyroid artery. The bronchi and the carina derive their blood supply directly from the aorta through bronchial arteries. There are numerous anastomoses with the pulmonary arteries for the lung tissue.

Lymphatic drainage. The trachea mainly drains to the lymphatic network of the neck but also connects with the thoracic lymph system which is important in the spread of metastases.

Nerve supply. This is provided by the vagus nerve and the sympathetic trunk.

The anatomy of the central parts of the bronchial tree is shown in Figure 4.**27**.

Basic Physiology

The self-cleaning mechanism and secretions, etc. are described on pp. 183ff. The mucociliary apparatus works in the direction of the larynx. Warming, humidification, and cleaning of the inspired air begin in the nose and are completed in the lower airway so that under normal anatomic conditions the intratracheal air temperature is maintained between 36 °C at an external temperature above 0 °C. These temperatures are considerably lower during mouth breathing. The relative humidity of the intratracheal air is 99% in normal breathing but considerably lower during mouth breathing.

Methods of Investigation

Bronchoscopy

Two methods of bronchoscopy are available.

1. The *rigid endoscope* (Fig. 4.28a–d) is historically the older method. It remains in universal use, is more productive, and has the greatest number of indications.

2. The *flexible fiberscope* (Fig. 4.29) is preferred in some special circumstances. Both methods supplement each other.

Rigid bronchoscopes are tubes of different caliber with a proximal cold light source (see Fig. 4.28a–d). Since bronchoscopy is usually carried out under general anesthesia, the bronchoscope has a direct connection to the anesthetic apparatus, *respiration bronchoscope,* so that it acts like an elongated rigid anesthetic tube. These bronchoscopes may be combined with instruments for aspiration, lavage for cytologic diagnosis, swabs for culture, aspiration biopsy, peribronchial needle biopsy, injection, curettage, biopsy, and foreign body extraction. They may also be used in

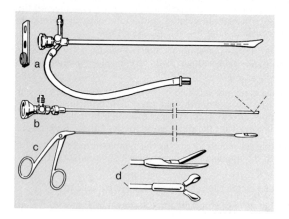

Fig. 4.**28a–d** Rigid bronchoscope.
a. Bronchoscope with anesthetic attachment, light carrier, and interchangeable window. **b.** Bronchoscopic telescope. **c.** Instrument for endoscopy used with different attachments **(d).**

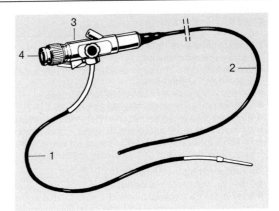

Fig. 4.**29**   Flexible fiberoptic bronchoscope.
1, cold light cable;
2, flexible fiberglass
telescope; 3, handlegrip
with control; 4, tele-
scope.

combination with catheters for bronchography or catheter aspiration biopsy and with
telescopes of various angles. The simultaneous combination of bronchoscopy and
radiographic screening is especially useful for an aspiration biopsy, manipulation of a
catheter, and the extraction of a foreign body which is a common indication for
bronchoscopy, especially in children.

The laser may be used via a rigid endoscope for a relatively bloodless removal of
benign tumors. The rigid bronchoscope may also be used for photographic, movie,
and television documentation.

Indications for the use of the rigid bronchoscope are given in Table 4.**11**.

Flexible bronchoscopes (see Fig. 4.**29**) have a diameter of 4 to 5 mm and are thinner
than rigid bronchoscopes. Their distal end can be controlled externally so that they
can be introduced into lobe bronchi, segmental bronchi, and even into the subseg-
mental bronchi. The instrument may be introduced via the nose or the mouth or a
tracheostomy if one is present. A flexible telescope may be combined with fine
flexible instruments or with simultaneous fluoroscopic monitoring.

Flexible bronchoscopy may be carried out under local anesthesia with the patient
sitting or lying, or under general anesthesia. In the latter case, the endoscope is
introduced through the endotracheal tube. Indications are shown in Table 4.**11**.

Mediastinoscopy is described on p. 518.

Clinical Aspects

Stenoses

Acute and chronic stenoses must be distinguished depending on the site of
origin in the trachea or bronchi. Furthermore, stenoses originating within

Table 4.**11** Indications for Bronchoscopy

Bronchoscopy with rigid tube
As a therapeutic measure:
- Emergency bronchoscopy as a temporary measure in sudden obstructive respiratory insufficiency
- Removal of tracheal or bronchial foreign bodies
- Arrest of bleeding in the trachea or bronchi
- Removal of retained secretions in obstructive disease of the lung or trachea
- Aspiration of tuberculous lymph nodes at the carina and of lung abscess
- To allow the use of the laser to remove a benign endotracheal or endobronchial tumor or a cicatricial membrane

As a diagnostic procedure in:
- Tracheal and bronchial stenoses
- Suspicion of a tracheal tumor or a tumor in the surrounding tissue. The elasticity of the tracheal wall and its mobility should be assessed.
- Suspicion of a bronchial tumor
- Unexplained persistent attacks of coughing and wheezing
- Hemoptysis of uncertain cause
- Suspicion of tracheal or bronchial trauma
- Transtracheal or transbronchial aspiration of a lymph node or a central tumor
- To allow a specimen to be taken for biopsy
- Bronchial lavage
- Brochiectasis or bronchography (currently rarely indicated)

Advantages: Very versatile procedure, which allows endoscopic overview, can also be used in bleeding and in the extraction of a foreign body. It gives an excellent visualization.

Disadvantages: Technically difficult in the presence of abnormal anatomy such as kyphoscoliosis. Limited access to the periphery and more discomfort to the patient than the fiberoptic bronchoscope.

Bronchoscopy with a flexible endoscope
Used as a *diagnostic measure* in:
- Suspicion of peripheral bronchial tumors, i.e., distal to the segmental ostia
- Hemoptysis of uncertain cause after the bleeding has stopped
- Undiagnosed disorders of the lung parenchyma
- Pleural effusion of uncertain cause
- Unresolved pneumonia, interstitial pneumopathy
- Middle lobe syndrome

Advantages: This endoscope can be introduced far into the periphery as far as the fifth-generation bronchi. It therefore complements the rigid endoscope. It can also be used with local anesthesia which is less troublesome to the patient.

Disadvantages: It has a very narrow working radius and cannot be used for large foreign bodies or in the presence of bleeding, atelectasis, or respiratory failure. The image obtained is not as good as with a rigid endoscope.

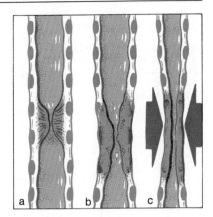

Fig. 4.**30a–c** Typical tracheal stenoses: (a) of the internal lining alone, (b) affecting all elements of the wall, (c) tracheomalacia, compression stenosis.

the wall of the trachea, *intramural,* or outside it, *extramural,* may be distinguished, as may those affecting the internal lining, *endoluminal.* Finally, there are those that affect the mucosa and the supporting elements of the wall, *compression stenoses and tracheomalacia* (Fig. 4.**30a–c**).

Tracheal stenoses usually require urgent treatment since there is no possibility of compensation, and the consequence is the danger of asphyxia.

Acute Stenoses

Symptoms. The main symptom is inspiratory stridor, in addition accompanied by restlessness, coughing attacks, fear of imminent death, cyanosis, and choking (Tables 4.**12** and 4.**13**).

Pathogenesis. The cause is sudden narrowing of the tracheal lumen by more than 50% by blunt trauma, an aspirated foreign body, edema, swelling, bleeding, infection, crusts, etc.

Diagnosis. The considerable inspiratory and often expiratory stridor also indicates an urgent situation. The history usually indicates the cause. The level of the obstruction may be localized by auscultation. Bronchoscopy is carried out using the rigid bronchoscope with preparations for immediate tracheostomy. Radiographs are taken only if delay carries no risk.

Differential diagnosis. This includes laryngeal stenoses, bronchial stenoses lying near the carina, pulmonary emboli and edema, and an asthmatic attack, which does not cause *inspiratory* stridor (see Tables 4.**12** and 4.**13**).

Treatment. Rigid bronchoscopy is performed and, if necessary, tracheotomy is performed for a high-sited stenosis, with respiration assured by leaving the bronchoscope in place. Foreign bodies are extracted if present. Otherwise the patient is intubated.

Table 4.12 Inspiratory Stridor		
Site of the Stenosis	Disease	Details
Oro- and hypopharynx	Diphtheria	Typical local findings, including a membrane
	Peritonsillar abscess	Swelling o Waldeyer's ring, pain on swallowing, trismus
	Infectious mono-nucleosis	Fever, local findings, enlarged lymph nodes
	Retropharyngeal abscess	Swelling of the posterior pharyngeal wall
	Angioneurotic edema	Typical local findings, sudden onset
	Posterior displacement of the tongue in unconscious patients	
	Obstructive sleep apnea	Symptoms occur only during sleep
	Abscess of the base of tongue	Marked dysphagia, thick speech
	Lingual thyroid	Thick speech, long history
	Benign and malignant tumors	Fetor, typical local findings, possibly pain and bleeding in malignant tumors
Larynx	Congenital stridor	Indrawing of the epiglottis on inspiration, congenital webs or flaccid epiglottis. Occurs in early infancy (see Table 4.**5**)
	Epiglottis and epiglottic abscess	Typical local findings
	Glottic edema	Typical laryngoscopic findings
	Vocal cord paralysis	Bilateral abductor paralysis
	Laryngeal spasm	Sudden life-threatening symptom, history often shows a previous tendency to glottic spasm
	Pseudocroup (subglottic laryngitis)	Typical laryngeal findings, affects small children
	Laryngeal diphtheria	Typical laryngoscopic findings (membrane)

Site of the Stenosis	Disease	Details
	Foreign body	History, attacks of coughing, variable symptoms
	Benign tumors such as cysts and celes	Usually slowly worsening symptoms
	Malignant tumors	Hoarseness, gradually worsening symptoms, pain, possibly hemoptysis
	Results of trauma	History
Trachea and bronchial tree	Tracheitis or bronchitis with stenosis or crusts	History of infection, possibly history of an operation on the trachea
	Foreign body	History
	External compression, e.g., by goiter or bleeding into a goiter	Gradually increasing symptoms; in addition, symptoms of disease of neighboring organs
	Tracheomalacia	History of goiter or trauma
	Cicatricial stenosis	History shows trauma or intubation
	Traumatic tracheal subluxation	History
	Intratracheal tumor or bronchial tumors lying close to the carina	Long history, tomograms, endoscopic findings
	Complications during and after tracheostomy	See p. 448

Initial diagnostic measures include:

1. History
2. Examination with a tongue depressor
3. Indirect laryngoscopy
4. Direct endoscopy of the larynx, trachea, and bronchi
5. Radiography
If sufficient time is available, (5) is carried out before (4).

Table 4.**13** Dyspnea

Type	Characteristic Symptoms
Obstructive respiratory insufficiency	Inspiratory stridor. If the stenosis lies distal to the bifurcation there may also be an expiratory stridor. Indrawing of the suprasternal notch, and the supraclavicular and intercostal areas on inspiration Restlessness, anxiety, loss of orientation, loss of consciousness, increased pulse rate Respiratory rate usually slowed. Inspiration longer than expiration Auscultation shows the stridor to be loudest over the stenosed area. A slapping noise is heard with mobile foreign bodies. Skin color initially pale, later cyanosed Tiredness, increasing exhaustion, anxious facies
Restrictive respiratory insufficiency, e. g. pneumonia, pneumothorax and pleuritis	Respiratory rate increased, shallow superficial breathing, vital capacity restricted Both inspiration and expiration shortened Additional abnormal findings in the lung or pleura Patient prefers to lie flat
Bronchial asthma	Respiratory rate decreased, typical wheezing noise or rhonchi noise on expiration Expiration clearly longer than inspiration Leaning on the arms on breathing to supplement the auxiliary muscles of respiration Typical findings on auscultation over the lung Shortage of breath in paroxysmal attacks
Cardiac respiratory insufficiency	Respiratory rate increased No stridor, free air passage Skin pale or cyanotic, blue lips, the patient is sweaty The patient prefers to sit upright Attacks of shortness of breath at night, cardiac asthma Additional abnormal findings in the heart and the circulation
Extrathoracic respiratory insufficiency, e. g. in central respiratory paralysis, diabetes, uremic coma, conditions of increased oxygen requirement, etc.	Irregular gasping or periodic respiration Increasing disturbance of consciousness and loss of consciousness. Stridor may also occur if the tongue is allowed to fall backward.
Psychogenic respiratory insufficiency	Respiratory rate increased, hyperventilation syndrome No stridor, possibly sighing respiration Well-perfused skin and mucosa

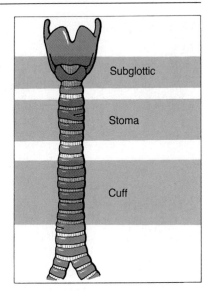

Fig. 4.**31** Typical locations of laryngo-tracheal stenoses. (1) *Subglottic:* affecting the cricoid cartilage or the first tracheal rings as a result of prolonged or incorrect intubation, incorrect tracheostomy, or trauma. (2) *Stomal:* as a result of a tracheostomy, an incorrectly carried out tracheostomy, tracheomalacia, or scar tissue. (3) *Cuff:* in the lower two thirds of the trachea due to prolonged intubation or excessive pressure on the tracheal wall during inflation of the tube.

Chronic Stenoses

Symptoms. The history shows a long period of increasing dyspnea, at times previous attacks of dyspnea, and a weak voice. The degree of severity of the respiratory obstruction often depends on the position of the head. In acute exacerbations, the cause of the respiratory obstruction is usually already known because of previous diagnostic measures. The head is held forward with the chin downward. The patient prefers to have the body upright.

Pathogenesis includes trauma, scarring due to injury, incorrect or prolonged intubation causing injury to the tracheal wall (see p. 450 and Fig. 4.**31**), incorrect tracheotomy (see p. 446 and Fig. 4.**31**), intratracheal tumors, goiter, malignant thyroid, bronchial and esophageal tumors, lymphadenopathies, tracheomalacia, tracheopathia chondroosteoplastica (see Color Plate **34b**), tuberculosis, syphilis, scleroma, nonspecific infection, radiotherapy, and mediastinal causes such as dermoid cysts, emphysema, tumors, abscess, and aortic aneurysm.

Diagnosis is made by radiography of the chest and by conventional or computed tomography of the trachea, perhaps aided by electronic reconstruction of the organ images. Other options are thyroid scans, pulmonary function tests, bronchoscopy, and biopsy.

Differential diagnosis is shown in Tables 4.**12** and 4.**13**, and Figure 4.**31**.

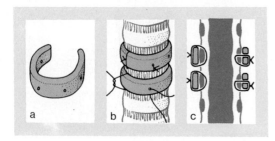

Fig. 4.**32a–c** Tracheo-pexy using extratracheal synthetic ring. **(a)** Synthetic ring, **(b)** two rings in position, **(c)** fixation of the ring to the tracheal wall by sutures.

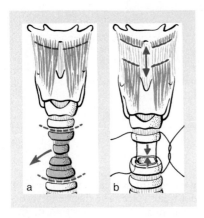

Fig. 4.**33a** and **b** Horizontal resection of the trachea and end-to-end anastomosis. **a.** Resection of the stenosed area and incision for subhyoid laryngeal mobilization. **b.** End-to-end anastomosis of the tracheal stumps by laryngeal mobilization.

Treatment is always by surgery but varies depending on the cause.

1. *Tracheopexy* consists of holding open the tracheal lumen using retaining loop sutures e. g. in tracheomalacia, due to goiter (see Fig. 4.**30c**).

Principle of the operation. Several techniques are used:

a. Introduction of loop sutures, e., g., after thyroidectomy, into the weakened wall of the trachea and anchoring the loop to structures close to the trachea such as the muscles, the clavicle, etc.
b. Stiffening of the collapsed trachea with gold, tantalum, or synthetic rings (Fig. 4.**32a–c**).

2. *Tracheal resection* with end-to-end anastomosis for scars, strictures, and tracheal trauma is used for severe destruction of *all* elements of the tracheal wall (Fig. 4.**33a** and **b**).

Principle of the operation. The diseased segment is resected and the stumps are anastomosed end-to-end. Resection of more than 4 cm requires division of the strap muscles above or below the hyoid (supra- or subhyoid mobilization of the larynx). Mobilization of the roots of the lung may also be needed.

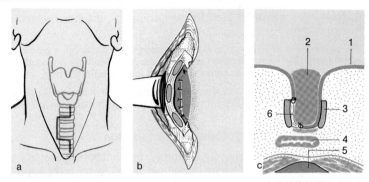

Fig. 4.**34a–c**   Partial tracheoplasty. **(a)** Incision of the overlying skin, **(b)** turning in of the soft tissue zone into the defect in the tracheal wall, **(c)** situation after reconstruction of the wall. 1, External cervical skin; 2, synthetic obturator to stabilize the new tracheal lumen; 3, lateral portions of the tracheal cartilage after median tracheofissure and excision of the stenosis; 4, esophagus; 5, vertebra; 6, half-portion of the tracheal wall with healthy mucosal lining.

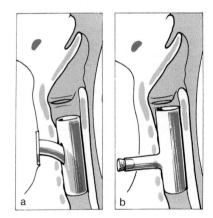

Fig. 4.**35a** and **b**   Tracheal endoprosthesis for stabilization of the reconstructed segment of the trachea. **(a)** A hollow synthetic prosthesis combined with a tracheostomy tube, **(b)** Montgomery's silicone T tube.

3. *Tracheoplasty,* with or without a previous *open gutter,* is used for long stenoses.

Figure 4.**34a–c** shows the principle of the operation. The stenosed segment is removed and the defect is covered with pedicled or free graft of cartilage and skin. Healing is achieved either by forming an open gutter which is closed secondarily or by the use of a synthetic prosthesis with the trachea closed (Fig. 4.**35a** and **b**).

Tracheal allograft material stored in a suitable chemical medium (formalin, thimerosal, acetone, etc.) can also be used to reconstruct long tracheal defects or stenoses.

4. *Endoscopic removal* is used for stenoses, webs, diaphragms, and small benign tumors.

The technique is as follows: the stenosed area is divided through a rigid broncho-scope using fine instruments or the laser without tracheotomy provided that the stenosis is not too extensive and does not affect the cartilaginous rings.

Organic bronchial stenoses are, at this time, only rarely an indication for *therapeutic* bronchoscopy, although it is possible that the laser may change this.

Tracheotomy, Laryngotomy, and Intubation

Indications. Tracheotomy, laryngotomy, and intubation are life-saving measures which must often be carried out as *emergency procedures*. Table 4.**14** summarizes the indications for tracheotomy. Tracheotomy reduces the dead space by 70 to 100 ml.

Depending on the site of tracheal entry (Fig. 4.**36a**), tracheotomy may be divided into *high* access, above the thyroid isthmus, *middle* access, after division of the isth-mus, and *low* access, below the isthmus. In urgent cases a high tracheotomy is usually carried out, although a low tracheotomy is usually carried out in children. If the isthmus is in the normal position and there is enough time, a middle tracheot-omy is preferred because of the lower complication rate.

Principle of the operation. The operation may be carried out under intubation anesthesia using an endotracheal tube or the rigid bronchoscope (see p. 434 and Fig. 4.**28a−d**) or under local anesthesia. A collar incision is made halfway between the suprasternal notch and the superior border of the thyroid cartilage, or a median vertical incision may be used. The trachea is dissected out in the midline, and an opening is created spanning from two to four tracheal rings (see Fig. 4.**36b**). Hemostasis must be secured because of the danger of valve-like aspiration of blood from disrupted vessels. A tracheotomy tube of suitable size is introduced, suturing the neck skin to the tracheal mucosa to create a mucocutaneous anastomosis.

Table 4.**14** Indications for Tracheotomy and Endotracheal Intubation

Tracheotomy

A. Mechanical airway obstruction due to

- Tumors affecting the pharynx, larynx, trachea, or esophagus
- Congenital anomalies of the upper respiratory or digestive tract
- Trauma of the larynx or trachea
- Bilateral recurrent nerve paralysis
- Trauma of the facial skeleton with soft tissue swelling or fractures, especially in the mandible
- Aspiration of a foreign body
- Inflammation causing edema of the larynx, trachea, tongue and pharynx

B. Obstruction of the airway by secretions or inadequate respiration, or both

- Retention of secretions and ineffective coughing and self during or after
  1. Thoracic or abdominal surgery
  2. Bronchopneumonia
  3. Vomiting or aspiration of stomach contents
  4. Burns of the face, neck, or respiratory tract
  5. Precoma and coma due to diabetes, liver disease, or renal insufficiency

- Alveolar respiratory insufficiency during or after
  1. Drug intoxication and poisoning
  2. Blunt thoracic trauma with fractures of the ribs
  3. Paralysis of the respiratory musculature
  4. Chronic obstructive lung diseases, such as emphysema, chronic bronchitis, bronchiectasis, asthma, and atelectasis

- Retention of secretions with alveolar respiratory insufficiency in
  1. Central nervous diseases such as a stroke, encephalitis, poliomyelitis, and tetanus
  2. Eclampsia
  3. Severe trauma to the head, neck, and thorax
  4. Postoperative neurosurgical coma
  5. Air or fat embolus

Intubation

Short-term intubation (i. e., less than 48 hours)

- For respiration of patients under muscle relaxants, e. g. intubation anesthesia

- In acute obstructive respiratory insufficiency whose cause can probably be relieved within 24–48 hours by minor operative procedures or anti-inflammatory measures such as steroids and antibiotics or which can be relieved in a short period by assisted respiration, assisted respiration as a temporary *emergency measure*
- If a tracheotomy is impossible or contraindicated

Long-term intubation, i. e., for several days or weeks

Long-term intubation should not be undertaken *in adults* because of the great danger of resulting scar tissue stenosis in the larynx or trachea. Also modern forms of tubes and cuffed tubes do not reliably prevent the development of stenosis which may only become manifest several months later. Patients with infections of the airway, those taking steroids, those with hypotension, or those under the influence of intoxicants are particularly at risk.

On the other hand, in *small children* prolonged intubation using the correct technique (transnasal-endotracheal) and inert soft materials often produces fewer complications than a tracheotomy.

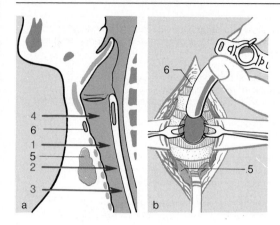

Fig. 4.**36a** and **b**
a. Operative access for tracheotomy or laryngotomy. 1, High tracheotomy; 2, middle tracheotomy; 3, low tracheotomy; 4, laryngotomy; 5, thyroid gland; 6, cricoid cartilage.
b. Introduction of a tracheostomy tube into the stoma.

The "plastic" stoma, unlike conventional stomas without a mucocutaneous anastomosis, is associated with few if any complications, although a second operation is needed to reverse the plasty once the stoma is no longer required.

Complications. *Intraoperative complications* include massive hemorrhage especially by venous congestion or by goiters or tumors overlying the trachea. *Damage to the cricoid cartilage* causes a cricoid stenosis. For this reason, the first tracheal ring should not be included in the tracheostomy if at all possible. *Damage to the pleura* causes pneumothorax which is more likely if the pleura lies higher than normal. Other complications include recurrent nerve paralysis and *sudden cardiac arrest,* or vasovagal collapse.

Postoperative complications include *secondary hemorrhage* with aspiration of blood from the wound into the trachea, *hemorrhage due to erosion* external to the trachea because of a poorly fitted tube, and *false position of the tube* outside the trachea. In children the tube may be coughed out if it is not fixed securely. Other complications include emphysema, tracheitis, cervical cellulitis, mediastinitis, pneumonia, lung abscess, esophagotracheal fistula, and difficult decannulation (see p. 452).

Figure 4.**37** shows several different types of tracheotomy tubes.

Laryngotomy

This is an *emergency procedure.* It must be revised as rapidly as possible by a regular tracheostomy because of the danger of tracheolaryngeal hermorrhage. Today this surgery is largely obsolete owing to the high availability of intubation.

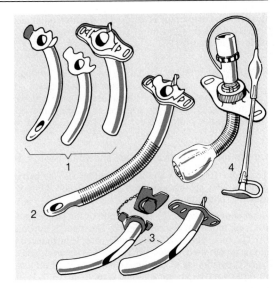

Fig. 4.37 Various types of tracheostomy tubes. 1, Metal cannula with introducing tube, inner tube, and outer tube; 2, lobster tail tube; 3, tube with speaking valve; 4, inflatable tube with cuff.

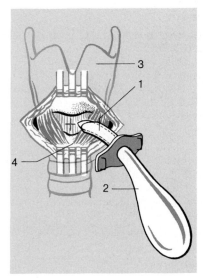

Fig. 4.38 Laryngotomy. 1, Short cannula mounted over a trocar; 2, trocar with handle; 3, thyroid gland; 4, cricoid cartilage. The cross shows the point at which the conus elasticus is opened.

Principle of the operation (Fig. 4.38). A skin incision is made just superior to the prominent arch of the cricoid cartilage with the head extended. At this point the cricothyroid ligament lies superficially under the skin, and there are no large vessels at this site. The membrane is exposed and a horizontal incision is made in it. The incision is held open with a tube or a spreading instrument. A special laryngotomy tube is shown in Figure 4.**38**.

Note: Laryngotomy should not be carried out if intubation, emergency bronchoscopy, or tracheotomy are feasible. If delay would be life-threatening laryngotomy can be carried out, if necessary even with a penknife. The incision can then be held open with a piece of rubber tube or other suitable utensil. A definitive tracheotomy must then be carried out as rapidly as possible.

Intubation. The indications are shown in Table 4.**14**.

Technique (Fig. 4.**39a** and **b**). Intubation may be carried out *without* anesthesia in patients who are already deeply unconscious. Otherwise general anesthesia with muscular relaxation is required.

Intubation technique. (1) The position of the patient must be such that the head and neck are mobile and accessible. (2) The blade is introduced and the glottis exposed. (3) The tube, stiffened with a guide wire, is introduced into the trachea through the glottis *under direct vision.* (4) The tube is secured, and the guide wire is withdrawn. Correct positioning of the tube is assessed by the air flow. The tube is connected to a respirator and fixed with adhesive tape.

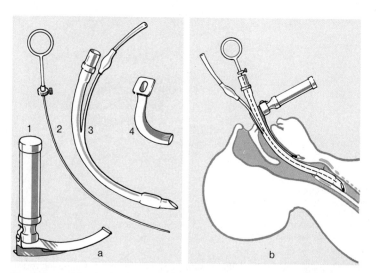

Fig. 4.**39a** and **b**   Intubation. **a.** Necessary instruments. 1, McIntosh laryngoscope; 2, stylette; 3, tube with cuff; 4, Guedel tube. **b.** Introduction of the tube.

Note: An indwelling tube to provide assisted respiration, e.g., in the intensive care unit or after cervical injuries, etc., should not be retained for longer than 24 to 48 h and certainly for no more than 72 h. Otherwise, there is a danger of endo- and peritracheal inflammation leading to tracheal stenosis. If assisted respiration is needed for longer periods, the tube should be replaced by a tracheotomy. Infants are an exception because experience has shown that a soft transnasal tube carries less risk than a treacheotomy.

Increasing respiratory obstruction due to tracheal stenosis may not manifest itself for several months.

Corticosteroids may be given when a fast-acting medication is needed to relieve edematous swelling (i.e. in pseudocroup in a child).

Practical Points for the Nursing Care of a Tracheostomy Patient

1. The tube must be cleaned-daily, or even more often when there are profuse secretions or crusts. Sterile gloves should be worn.
2. The secretions must be aspirated from the trachea several times daily using sterile technique.
3. The tube must not be left out of the trachea for too long in a conventional tracheostomy because it is then difficult to reintroduce. A rubber catheter of a caliber smaller than the lumen of the tracheostomy tube should be available which can be inserted into the tracheal lumen and used as a guide over which the tracheostomy tube can be reinserted with the aid of a lubricant. This danger does not exist when a plastic stoma has been constructed.
4. Crusting is prevented by the use of mucolytic agents and by applying ointment to the stoma.
5. Five percent saline inhalation solution is used to loosen and remove crusts. This can also be achieved by the installation of several drops of 1% to 2% saline solution with a pipette into the tracheostomy or instillation of several drops of olive oil. Suitable mucolytic agents are given by mouth.
6. A heat and moisture exchanger ("artificial nose"), may be attached to the opening of the tracheostomy.
7. The skin around the tracheostomy may be covered with aluminum-coated stoma compresses if the patient develops dermatitis ("soreness"). Once the acute phase has healed, bland fatty ointments or skin oil are used.
8. Difficulty in breathing through the tracheostomy may be due to the following causes: (a) incorrect reintroduction of the cannula; (b) crusts at the distal end of the tube in the trachea or in the tube itself; (c) granulations of the trachea at the end of the tube; (d) a tube of wrong shape or width for the individual trachea; (e) stenosis of the tracheobronchial tree beyond the tracheostomy.
9. Bleeding in a tracheostomy may have the following causes: (1) tracheitis; (2) granulations in the trachea; (3) erosive hemorrhage from the brachiocephalic trunk or other vessels surrounding the trachea, e. g., due to a decubitus ulcer caused by the end of the tube; (4) bleeding from a tumor.

Note: Immediate expert advice and assistance should be sought for difficulty in breathing or bloodstained tracheal secretion.

Difficult decannulation. Decannulation may be impossible due to incorrect construction or care of the tracheostomy. Factors include: injury to the first tracheal ring or cricoid arch leading to perichondritis of the cricoid cartilage; a hole in the tracheal wall that is too small or too large; granulations around the orifice; tracheomalacia; and extratracheal causes such as goiter or tumor. In these cases, the cause of the stenosis must be dealt with first by reconstruction procedures on the trachea or the larynx (see p. 444) or by dealing with the extratracheal cause as appropriate, e. g., by thyroidectomy.

Foreign Bodies and Trauma (see Color Plate **34c**)

Foreign Bodies

Foreign bodies in the trachea or bronchi usually occur in children, with about 80% occurring between the 1st and 3rd year of life. Typical foreign bodies include peanuts, nails, needles, buttons, coins, balls, peas, and bits of eggshell.

Symptoms. *The main symptoms* are episodes of coughing, intermittent or continuous dyspnea with cyanosis, pain, and intermittent hoarseness. Total occlusion of the airway causes sudden death. There may also be apparently symptomfree intervals of days to weeks.

Site. This depends on the size and shape of the foreign body. The most common site is the right main bronchus because of its straighter angle of origin from the trachea. If the foreign body is retained for a longer period the following occur depending on the type of foreign body and duration: accumulation of secretions; tracheitis or bronchitis with edema, swelling, and granulations; bleeding and bloodstained secretions; inspiratory and expiratory valvular stenoses; partial obstruction of the lower airway or emphysema; atelectasis or overinflation of the poststenotic part of the lung.

Pathogenesis. The cause is usually aspiration. *Rare* causes include broncholiths, i.e., calcification of retained sputum, rupture of tuberculous lymphadenopathy into the trachea, and ascarides.

Diagnosis. The history shows that the symptoms are of sudden onset often coinciding with eating. Percussion shows a dampened or hyperresonant note. Auscultation reveals a hissing stenotic noise at the level of the foreign body and rhonchi. If the bronchus is occluded, there is cessation of respiratory sounds and delayed movement of one half of the thorax on respiration. *Radiography* includes chest views, tomograms, and bronchography. Holzknecht's symptom consists of oscillation of the mediastinum in bronchial stenosis. Bronchoscopy is the most important therapeutic procedure.

Differential diagnosis. This includes diphtheria, pseudocroup, laryngeal spasm, whooping cough, bronchial asthma, intraluminal tumors, pulmonary tuberculosis, pneumonia, and laryngeal stenosis. Marked up and down movements of the larynx are absent in *tracheal stenoses.*

Treatment. Endoscopy is performed and the foreign body is extracted.

Important: Suspicion of a tracheobronchial foreign body is an absolute indication for endoscopy.

Trauma

Trauma is due to stabbing and gunshot injuries, blunt and penetrating traffic accidents, and injuries to the neck and thorax.

Symptoms. These are very variable. The history indicates the cause.

The main symptoms are dyspnea or danger of suffocation, hemoptysis, escape of air from an unusual site, surgical emphysema, pneumothorax, tension pneumothorax, and atelectasis.

Pathologic anatomy includes rupture of the trachea or bronchi, damage to the great vessels, infection of surrounding structures, and mediastinitis.

Diagnosis. This is made by auscultation, chest radiographs, tomograms, and bronchoscopy.

Treatment. Ruptures or tears of the trachea or main bronchi should be treated as rapidly as possible by exploration of the area and *immediate* repair or anastomosis. Peripheral bronchial rupture is treated by lobectomy (thoracic surgery). Scar tissue stenosis is described on p. 443.

Tracheoesophageal fistula is dealt with by separation of the two tubes and reconstruction (see p. 445; see Figs. 4.**34a−c** and 5.**2k**). This is usually a technically demanding operative procedure.

Infections

Tracheitis

Acute tracheitis is often due to spread of a laryngitis or bronchitis, but it may also occur primarily and is usually viral in origin. Chronic tracheitis may occur in chronic inflammation of associated organs such as the sinuses, larynx, and bronchi, and in broncheactasis. It may also be due to unfavorable climatic and occupational environment, neoplasms, and pulmonary cavities.

Symptoms. These include coughing, retrosternal pain, increased purulent or nonpurulent sputum, occasionally mixed with blood, and mild dyspnea. By itself this disease is not a life-threatening condition and often there is no fever.

Treatment. This is the same as for laryngitis (see p. 414).

Acute Laryngotracheobronchitis in Children, Subglottic Laryngitis, Croup (see p. 415ff.)

This occurs in infants and young children up to about the age of 3 years. It is a life-threatening disease with a barking cough, stridor, indrawing of the suprasternal notch and of the intercostal spaces, cyanosis, and a moderate fever.

Pathogenesis. Infection by viruses or bacteria produces a serious inflammation of the mucosa of the upper trachea with edema, tenacious secretions, and formation of crusts. There is cardiac and circulatory insufficiency and danger of atelectasis or suffocation.

Differential diagnosis. These include epiglottitis and diphtheria.

Treatment. Therapy consists of inhalation of oxygen, steroids, humidification of the air, and antibiotics. When severe respiratory obstruction occurs, nasotracheal intubation or tracheotomy are necessary. Sedatives are contraindicated!

Diphtheritic Tracheitis

Main symptoms. The typical signs of diphtheria are found in the larynx or the pharynx. Bits of membrane formed from secretions on the mucosol surface are expectorated.

Treatment. High-dose penicillin and antitoxic serum (see p.346) are given and tracheotomy is performed if indicated.

Tracheitis Sicca

This usually accompanies rhinitis or laryngitis sicca, (sicca syndrome). Dry crusts are coughed out, and there is an audible wheeze.

Treatment. This includes removal of the crusts, liquefying the secretions, inhalation, humidification of the air, and antibiotics.

Rare forms of tracheitis include tuberculosis, sarcoid, stage II und III syphilis, and scleroma.

Congenital and Hereditary Anomalies

These include accessory bronchi opening into the trachea, megatrachea, megabronchi, and congenital stenoses of the trachea and bronchi.

Bronchiectasis (Cylindrical or Saccular).

This is congenital or acquired, usually affecting the lower lobes on the right more often than the left. *Congenital* forms are due to weakness of the wall of the bronchi or mucoviscidosis. *Acquired* forms are due to bronchitis, emphysema, chronic destructive bronchitis, and secondary bronchial stenosis. *Kartagener's triad* consists of bronchiectasis, sinusitis and/or nasal polypi, and situs inversus.

Symptoms. The *main symptom* is chronic coughing and profuse sputum. Examination demonstrates finger clubbing. Tomograms of the chest and bronchography are carried out.

For further details, see textbooks on internal medicine and pulmonary diseases.

Tumors

Benign tumors of the trachea are very rare and include adenomas (common in the *bronchi*), fibromas, lipomas, chondromas, amyloid tumors, neurinomas, hemangiomas, papillomas, (usually accompanied by papillomas of the larynx), and pleomorphic adenomas. An added lesion is an intratracheal goiter which is thyroid tissue growing into the trachea, usually the posterior wall.

Main symptoms. These include coughing attacks, increasing dyspnea, and occasionally hemoptysis. Pains in the chest, wheezing, and expectoration are less common.

Treatment. The tumor is endoscopically removed, using the laser if possible. Otherwise, the tracheobronchial tree must be opened by the cervical or thoracic route.

Malignant Tracheal Tumors

Adenoid Cystic Carcinoma

This is relatively common in the trachea where it grows slowly especially along nerve sheaths. It extends very aggressively and tends to produce hematogenous and lymphatic metastases.

Treatment. Extensive surgery is required.

> *Note:* Vague terms such as "semimalignant", "potentially malignant", or "conditionally benign" can be fatal for the patient. These terms depend on morphologic appearances and not an the clinical course. Adenoid cystic carcinoma must *always* be treated as an extremely aggressive malignancy (see p. 552).

Carcinoma

A tumor arising in the *trachea* is relatively unusual. More often the tumor extends from a neighboring organ such as the larynx, esophagus, bronchus, mediastinum, or thyroid gland. The lower half of the trachea is the more common site.

Morphology. Squamous and adenocarcinoma have a roughly equal frequency, and both metastasize frequently.

Main symptoms. These include cough, increasing dyspnea, hemoptysis, and dysphagia. Dysphonia or aphonia occur if the recurrent laryngeal nerve is invaded.

Diagnosis. This rests on diagnostic imaging of the chest, tomograms of the trachea, bronchoscopy, which is mandatory, and biopsy.

Treatment. Tumors of the cervical trachea are treated if possible by resection and neck dissection. Tracheostomy and later reconstruction may be indicated. Otherwise the patient is irradiated. The long-term prognosis is poor whatever the type of therapy.

Bronchial Carcinoma (see Color Plate 34d)

About 80% of the lesions occur in men most commonly between the ages of 50 and 70 years.

Main symptoms. In the early phases the symptoms may be slight. They include attacks of coughing, pains in the chest, difficulty in breathing, sputum, hemoptysis, a feeling of being unwell, loss of weight, and atypical and recurrent infections of the airway with fever, pneumonia, and dyspnea.

Diagnostic procedures. These include chest imaging, bronchoscopy, biopsy, and cytology. Bronchography, possibly needle biopsy, pulmonary function tests, and exploratory thoracotomy are indicated depending on the individual lesion.

Diagnostic and therapeutic details are included in texts on internal medicine and pulmonary surgery.

5. Esophagus

Diseases of the esophagus overlap several disciplines. The following chapter presents the otorhinolaryngologic aspects, especially endoscopy and the clinical aspects and treatment of esophageal disorders.

Applied Anatomy

The esophagus begins at the level of the lower border of the cricoid cartilage, at the level of the sixth cervical vertebra, and ends at the cardia which lies at the level of the eleventh thoracic vertebra. The opening of the esophagus in the adult lies about 15 cm from the upper incisor teeth and the cardia at about (35 to) 41 cm. The entire length of the esophagus is thus approximately 26 cm.

The wall of the esophagus is capable of expanding and contracting and is resistant to considerable mechanical stress. The internal lining is of stratified nonkeratinized squamous epithelium. The external longitudinal musculature and internal circular muscle layer form separate layers of the wall (Fig. 5.1b). There are also muscle fibers running spirally.

The *esophageal musculature* is striated in the upper third, consists of mixed smooth muscle fibers and striated fibers in the middle third, and is almost exclusively smooth muscle in the lower third.

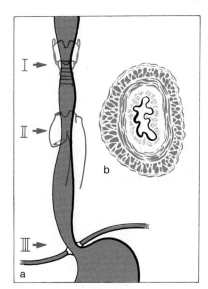

Fig. 5.**1a** and **b** Esophagus. **a.** With the zones of physiologic narrowing, I to III. **b.** Cross-section through the esophageal wall.

The esophagus has *three physiologic sphincters* (see Fig. 5.**1a**):

1. The *upper* is the opening of the esophagus formed by the cricopharyngeus muscle.
2. The *middle* is caused by the crossing of the esophagus by the aortic arch and the left main bronchus. This lies at 27 cm from the incisor teeth in the adult.
3. The *lower* lies at the level of the esophageal hiatus, the cardia.

There is a *cervical and a thoracic* portion of the esophagus.

The *blood supply* is segmental as is the lymphatic drainage.

Innervation is mixed somatic from the IXth and Xth cranial nerves and autonomic from the sympathetic nervous system.

Physiology and Pathophysiology

The esophagus possesses its own active motility and also a passive mobility due to respiration and to movement of the neighboring great vessels and the heart. The *act of swallowing* may be divided into an *oral phase* which is under voluntary control and a *pharyngeal and esophageal phase*. The latter are under reflex control depending on stimulation of the posterior pharyngeal wall and can be recognized by the elevation of the larynx (see p. 310).

The entrance of the esophagus and the cardia are usually closed. The entrance of the esophagus opens during swallowing, and the cardia opens in response to the oncoming peristaltic wave.

The sphincteric and transport functions can be investigated by the following: radiography with contrast medium, videofluorography, cineradiography, and manometry (intraluminal measurement of pressure in the esophagus; see p. 462).

Disorders of peristalsis and tone are possible in the following: (1) mechanical obstruction and narrowing and (2) paralysis of the muscles or nerves (see Table 3.7).

In *presbyesophagus* there is a disorder of coordination of the various phases of motility with increased tertiary contractions and atonic phases. This causes prolonged transit time of the food.

Methods of Investigation

Clinical Examination

Inspection and palpation of the external part of the neck shows redness, swelling, tenderness, e. g., over the carotid sheath, venous congestion, and lymphadenopathy. The course of the esophagus should be auscultated. A complete mirror examination of the nose and throat should be carried out, cranial nerve paralyses, particularly of the IXth, Xth, and XIIth cranial nerves, should be looked for, and the pharynx and larynx should be examined.

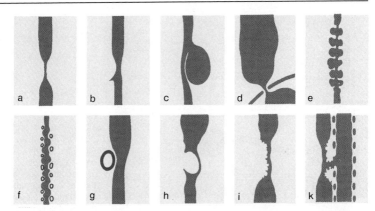

Fig. 5.**2a–k**   Typical findings on barium swallow. **(a)** Stenosis due to caustics, **(b)** traction diverticulum, **(c)** pulsion diverticulum, **(d)** achalasia with superimposed megaesophagus, **(e)** idiopathic esophageal spasm, **(f)** esophageal varices, **(g)** external compression of the esophagus, **(h)** benign intraluminal tumor, **(i)** esophageal carcinoma, **(k)** tracheoesophageal H-type fistula (adapted from Schwarz).

Radiography

Radiography includes contrast medium, tomography, cineradiography, and videofluorography for the analysis of function and other diagnostic questions. Radionuclide scanning is used to measure reflux.

A contrast swallow with gastrografin is commonly used to show the mucosa and the lumen. Typical findings are shown in Figure 5.**2a–k**.

Note: Barium must *not* be used if a perforation or a foreign body is suspected, if there is a danger of aspiration, and in the newborn with a suspected esophageal atresia. Barium masks the foreign body, adheres to the mucosa, incites a significant foreign-body reaction, and makes subsequent endoscopy more difficult. Esophagoscopy should always be preceded by radiographic investigation without a contrast medium provided that an urgent situation does not require immediate treatment.

Esophagoscopy

This procedure may be carried out with *rigid* or *flexible* esophagoscopes. These are not rival methods for investigation. Each method has its own indications, and the two may need to be combined.

Esophagoscopy with a rigid tube can be used for 95% of all endoscopic requirements in the esophagus. Figure 5.**3** shows such an instrument with its accessories.

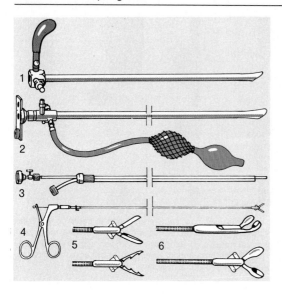

Fig. 5.3   Rigid esophagoscope. 1, Standard esophagoscope; 2, pneumatic esophagoscope sealed by interchangeable eyepiece; 3, esophageal telescope with instrument channel; 4, flexible endoscopic forceps; 5, 6, interchangeable tip attachments.

Principle. Esophagoscopy with a rigid tube is usually carried out under endotracheal anesthesia because there is less discomfort for the patient and the pharyngeal and esophageal muscles are relaxed. The esophagoscope has a high-powered light source either at the proximal or distal end of the tube. The light is transmitted via glass fibers as "cold light". An optic magnification system and continuous lavage and suction can be used. Extraction, excision, and coagulation instruments and injection needles can be introduced, and pneumatic pressure may be increased in the esophagus to expand a particular part. Lasers may also be used, and photographic and movie records may be made.

The tube is introduced with the patient relaxed in the supine position. It is introduced under visual control of the oropharynx, the hypopharynx, and the postcricoid area into the esophagus and is then advanced to the cardia (Fig. 5.4). The wide tube allows ample space for procedures within the lumen or the walls of the esophagus. It also allows assessment of the elasticity, the stiffness, and the mobility, etc. of the esophageal wall.

Indications are shown in Table 5.1.

Esophagoscopy with a flexible fiberglass endoscope is usually carried out by the gastroenterologist. Its indications are much more limited than those for a rigid tube, but it does have specific indications because of its narrow caliber and its maneuverable end (see Table 5.1). Figure 5.5 shows the fiberoptic esophagoscope.

Note: Even a fiberoscope can cause perforations.

Table 5.1 Indications for Esophagoscopy

Esophagoscopy with a rigid tube

As a therapeutic measure
- Removal of foreign bodies and impacted food remnants
- Endoscopic removal of benign tumors, e.g., polyps, fibromas, etc.
- Endoscopic division of the spur of a hypopharyngeal diverticulum
- Dilatation of the stenosis or stricture
- Injection of varices, hemostasia, occasionally combined with the laser
- Intubation of malignant esophageal tumors to maintain a food passage

As a diagnostic procedure in
- Diseases of any part of the esophagus
- Diseases of the upper or lower esophageal sphincters, e.g., spasm
- Tumors of the hypopharynx and esophagus
- Diverticulae of the hypopharynx and esophagus
- Diseases narrowing the lumen – also in infants!

Further indications include
- To allow photographic and movie documentation
- Follow-up
- Unsatisfactory or unproductive fiberoptic endoscopy, or if the latter is contraindicated

Esophagoscopy with the flexible endoscope

As a diagnostic procedure:
- If esophagoscopy with the rigid endoscope is contraindicated, e.g., in marked scoliosis, kyphosis, or rigid spinal column, mechanical obstructions; or if satisfactory anesthesia is not possible or available
- For the assessment of functional phenomena that are suppressed in the anesthetized patient, e.g., the swallowing act, and the gastroesophageal transitional zone
- If panendoscopy is indicated when the esophagus only needs to be examined en passant and the main interest is the stomach or duodenum

Advantages of esophagoscopy with a rigid tube:
It is a versatile procedure, and is the only procedure suitable for foreign body extraction. It is highly efficient for both diagnosis and treatment, and it provides good photographic documentation for permanent record-keeping.

Advantages of fiberoptic endoscopy:
There is less discomfort for the patient, simultaneous panendoscopy of the stomach and duodenum is possible, and it is a good screening instrument. However, the diagnostic success rate is lower and it cannot be used as a therapeutic procedure.

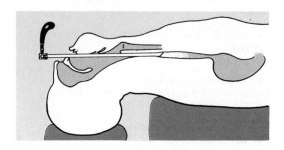

Fig. 5.4   Rigid esophagoscope introduced into the esophagus.

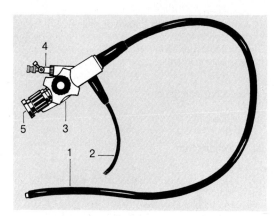

Fig. 5.5   Flexible fiberoptic esophagoscope. 1, Flexible fiberglass telescope; 2, cold light cable; 3, handgrip with angle knob; 4, attachment for suction apparatus; 5, eyepiece.

Principle of use. A fiberoscope may be introduced on patients who are only sedated and anesthetized locally. The patient lies on his left side. Gastroscopy and duodenoscopy may also be carried out at the same sitting. The indications are shown in Table 5.1.

Manometry

The intraluminal pressure in the esophagus is measured at various points, e.g., the sphincters. Various methods are in use:

1. *Three-channel manometry* is continuous recording of the pressure with three measuring catheters at separate measuring points.
2. *Pull-through manometry* is continuous recording of pressure during continuous withdrawal of the end of the catheter from the stomach into the esophagus.

3. *Radiomanometry* is a combination of radiography and manometry.
4. *Pharmacomanometry* is a combination of manometry and the action of autonomic drugs.

Clinical Aspects

Traumatology

Burns by Acid or Lye (see Color Plate **35c**)

Symptoms. There is a typical history of initially very severe pain in the mouth, the pharynx, behind the sternum, and in the epigastrium. There is retching, vomiting, sialorrhea, and at times glottic edema and dyspnea. White corrosive crusts and burned areas are to be found in the mouth and the surrounding area. Shock becomes progressive with falling blood pressure and rising pulse, cyanosis and pallor, cold sweats, and circulatory collapse. Later, perhaps in 24 to 48 h, there are increasing signs of intoxication such as renal damage, hematuria, evidence of liver damage, hemolysis, disturbance of electrolyte and water metabolism, and occasionally involvement of the central nervous system (CNS). There is increasing risk of perforation or mediastinitis, pleuritis, peritonitis, and tracheoesophageal fistula. Rapid wasting occurs. If the patient survives, dysphagia gradually sets in due to stricture formation.

Pathogenesis. The coagulation necrosis due to acids and colliquative necrosis due to lyes penetrates to varying depths. The corrosive scars in the mouth and pharynx may be minimal because of rapid passage, with *severe* degrees extending into the esophagus and possibly the stomach and intestine. The esophagus is more severely afflicted than the stomach in lye burns because of reflex cardiospasm. In acid burns the stomach is more severely affected.

The time course is as follows: (1) primary local necrosis in the mouth, pharynx, esophagus, stomach, and intestine; (2) generalized intoxication; (3) acute, subacute, and chronic corrosive esophagitis; (4) healing of the esophagitis with scarring or stricture; (5) late complications such as late or restenosis and possibly malignant degeneration. The scar tissue stenosis begins about the 3rd week.

Diagnosis. This is made from the typical history of an accident or suicide and the typical local findings. The corrosive substance must be identified. Radiographs are taken of the thorax and abdomen. If the corrosive burns appear to be mild, contrast views of the esophagus are taken and a careful esophagoscopy may be done to allow the esophagus and stomach to be examined and a feeding tube to be introduced. *Contraindications* include shock and suspected perforation. Immediate esophagoscopy is only carried out if the degree and extent of the corrosive burn are not clear.

Treatment. If possible, large quantities of fluids (water) should be drunk. The juice of citrus fruits of dilute 2% vinegar are given for lye burns; magnesium oxide and antacids are given for acid burns but must be given within 2 h. Analgesics and sedatives are given, and the patient is admitted to an intensive care unit for intravenous management of shock, administration of fluids, parenteral feeding, broad-spectrum antibiotics, and if necessary gastrostomy and tracheotomy. High-dose steroids are given intravenously, e. g., 200 to 400 mg hydrocortisone, and they are continued for at least 4 weeks, adjusting the dosage on the basis of endoscopic findings (granulations). On the other hand steroids are not indicated in mild burns and are contraindicated in severe burns because of the danger of perforation.

The first careful esophagoscopy is carried out after 6 to 8 days. Dilatation can begin at the end of the 2nd week if the radiographs and endoscopy show the formation of a stricture. Follow-up esophagoscopies are carried out at intervals of 10 days until mucosal defects are epithelialized. The patient is then checked by radiography and esophagoscopy after 1, 3, 6, and 12 months.

Technique of bouginage. Two methods are available:

Early bouginage about 8 to 12 days after the burn using a thick bougie of about 40 Fr in adults, 20 Fr in children, and 30 Fr in adolescents, increasing daily in caliber until the patient can swallow without difficulty. The intervals are then prolonged until the stenoses can no longer be demonstrated by radiography.

Late bouginage is only used if an organic stenosis forms despite steroids. This may only occur several weeks later. Bouginage must *never* be done blindly, but must always be carried out at esophagoscopy or over a thread (see below) or stylet.

Bouginage begins using the bougie of appropriate caliber *under vision* with an esophagoscope. Contrast radiographs should be taken first to localize the stricture and to exclude intraluminal neoplasms or multiple stenoses.

Bouginage over a thread (Fig. 5.6) may be carried out to save the patient daily esophagoscopy and to ensure that the bougie is correctly introduced through the stenosis and reaches the distal part of the esophagus. Fenestrated bougies are used. First, the patient swallows a perforated lead shot with several meters of silk suture fastened to it. The thread is let out daily and the metal shot reaches the intestine via the stomach and may be checked by radiography. The thread is then securely anchored. Fenestrated bougies of increasing caliber may now be introduced safely over this thread and through the stricture. Bouginage may take several weeks. When no longer needed, the end of the thread is then cut off at the mouth and the sphere and thread are passed normally.

The goal of treatment by bouginage in adults is to achieve an esophageal lumen of about 45 Fr (i. e., 15 mm diameter), about 30 to 35 Fr in children up to 10 years, and 30 to 40 Fr in adolescents.

The thread may also be brought out via a gastrostomy and *retrograde bouginage* carried out from the stomach to the mouth.

Dangers of bouginage include *perforation* of the esophageal wall. This does not

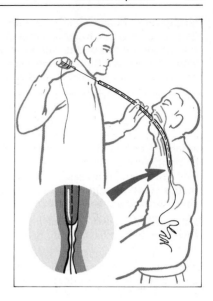

Fig. 5.6   Principle of bouginage over a thread.

occur using the bouginage over a thread. Perforations tend to occur particularly in the area of the necrotic stricture, in blind pouches, etc. and cause mediastinitis, pleuritis, or peritonitis which must be drained externally.

If treatment by bouginage is unsatisfactory, operative treatment of the stricture, partial esophageal resection and replacement by a segment of stomach or bowel, must be considered. Because of the tendency to restenosis and to malignant degeneration in old age, patients with esophageal strictures must be kept under medical supervision by radiography and endoscopy at increasing intervals.

Foreign Bodies (see Color Plate **35b**)

These are usually unintentionally swallowed objects of various types. Children, usually those younger than 3 years, swallow coins, toys, etc., whereas adults swallow bones, glass splinters, fish bones, parts of false teeth, nails, needles, large fruit stones, or even cutlery (e. g., prisoners).

Symptoms. These include considerable dysphagia (difficulty in swallowing), odynophagia (pain on swallowing), localized to the neck or retrosternal area and rarely the epigastrium, and attacks of coughing. *Lifethreatening symptoms* include severe pain in the back between the shoulder blades and behind the sternum and indicate early mediastinitis.

Pathogenesis. Foreign bodies usually stick in the upper sphincter, the esophageal orifice, and rarely at the second or third sphincters. Retained or impacted foreign bodies cause necrosis of the esophageal wall leading, depending on the site, to mediastinitis, pleuritis, or peritonitis with the formation of paraesophageal abscess and, on occasion, surgical emphysema.

Diagnosis. This is made on the history. Initially, the pain on swallowing is localized to a certain area and the neck and the cervical spine are held rigid. There may be swelling of the neck or surgical emphysema, or crepitation on palpation of the neck and the supraclavicular fossae. Lateral radiographs of the neck, the thorax, and the chest are taken to determine the position of radiopaque foreign bodies. Air shadows in the esophagus above a foreign body are also shown as is mediastinal emphysema in perforation. Gastrografin is used for a radiolucent foreign body. Esophagoscopy is carried out both to establish the diagnosis and for treatment.

Differential diagnosis. This includes persistent mucosal lesions made by a foreign body that has already been passed, and early obstructive tumor.

Treatment. Esophagoscopy is done as early as possible with a *rigid* esophagoscope under general endotracheal anesthesia to allow removal of the foreign body. If this does not succeed, a cervical esophagotomy is carried out or a thoracotomy for a more distal foreign body. Perforation is treated by suture of the defect and high-dose antibiotic cover. Paraesophagitis and abscess are treated by drainage.

Course and complications. There may be no sequelae if the foreign body is removed rapidly without complications. If it is retained for a long period, pressure necrosis occurs leading to mediastinitis whose symptoms are rapidly increasing pain behind the sternum or between the shoulder blades. Lateral neck and chest radiographs show gas emphysema (appearing as a "cloudy" prevertebral shadow), widening of the prevertebral stripe, and possible fluid levels. Oral gastrografin demonstrates the site of perforation. Many small foreign bodies that impact initially pass on into the stomach and have a 95% chance of being passed spontaneously. The stool should be checked for up to 8 days or even longer to ensure that the foreign body has been passed.

> *Note:* If a foreign body is suspected, the hypopharynx and esophagus must be inspected endoscopically even if radiographs are negative. Removal of foreign bodies with a flexible fiberscope should not be attempted.

Blunt and Penetrating Injuries, Perforations, and the Mallory-Weiss Syndrome

Blunt injuries of the esophagus occur especially in traffic accidents due to impact of the thorax on the steering wheel causing tears of the esophageal wall. Traumatic esophagotracheal fistulae, often delayed, may also occur as a result of localized necrosis of the wall.

The main symptom is coughing on swallowing. Rupture in the lower third of the esophagus is usually a result of blunt trauma to the thorax.

Open penetrating injuries usually lie in the cervical segment and are due to automobile and motorcycle accidents and suicides.

The *main symptoms* are escape of saliva or food from the wound. The Mallory-Weiss syndrome is hematemesis due to a tear of the esophageal wall in a patient with a tendency to vomit who has a hiatus hernia or gastroesophageal prolapse. Treatment is the same as for esophageal varices (see p. 470).

Iatrogenic esophageal perforation can occur due to blind exploratory probes, trauma due to feeding tubes, or perforations by a stomach tube or an endotracheal tube for anesthesia. A common cause is esophagoscopy and bouginage. The sites of predilection are the three sphincters, the stenosed area, and the piriform sinus. It is vitally important that the condition be recognized *immediately* and be treated surgically by mediastinotomy, thoracotomy, or laparotomy depending on the site of the perforation.

Spontaneous rupture of the esophagus, Boerhaave's syndrome, is caused by a sudden increase of the intraesophageal pressure due to vomiting or cicatricial stenosis and is relatively common in patients with habitual vomiting and alcohol abuse. The *symptoms* are *dramatic* and include bloodstained vomitus, hematemesis, very severe pain behind the sternum and between the shoulder blades, pain in the left upper quadrant and in the renal area, pallor, rapid fall of blood pressure, dyspnea, and rapid circulatory collapse.

Diagnosis. This is made from the simultaneous appearance of surgical emphysema of the neck and acute abdominal signs, pneumothorax, and dyspnea.

Differential diagnosis. This must include rupture of the diaphragm, incarcerated hiatus hernia, perforation of a gastric or duodenal ulcer, acute pancreatitis, and myocardial infarct.

Treatment. Thoracotomy, reparation of the defect, and drainage of the pleura must be undertaken.

Prognosis. Mortality lies between 25% and 40%.

Esophageal Diverticulum

A hypopharyngeal diverticulum is the most *common* diverticulum of the upper digestive tract (see p. 372 and Color Plate **36a**).

Diverticula of the esophagus proper are usually acquired and can affect any part of the esophagus.

Symptoms. Diverticula of the upper esophagus often cause no symptoms. Those at the level of the carina cause mild symptoms related to breathing, a retrosternal feeling of pressure, and attacks of coughing. An epiphrenic diverticulum causes pressure at the appropriate site, heartburn, epigastric pain, and dysphagia. Twenty percent are combined with a hiatus hernia.

Diagnosis. The diagnosis rests on radiography and endoscopy.

Differential diagnosis. This includes achalasia, hiatus hernia, and globus hystericus.

Treatment. This is transthoracic removal, but only if the symptoms are severe or if complications such as ulceration, bleeding, spontaneous perforation, and malignant degeneration are suspected.

Traction diverticula are due to scar tissue contracture from inflammatory paraesophageal or paratracheal (bifurcation) lymph nodes. They are demonstrated by radiography as an inverted cone arising from the wall, usually localized to the middle third of the esophagus.

Symptoms. There are no symptoms. There may be attacks of coughing and a vague retrosternal feeling of pressure and slight dysphagia.

Diagnosis. Radiography is more reliable than endoscopy, but esophagoscopy must always be done to exclude malignancy.

Treatment. There is usually not treatment necessary, but transthoracic removal may be necessary for *marked* symptoms.

Inflammations and Inflammatory Stenoses

Nonspecific acute esophagitis accompanies trauma, stenoses, or obstruction due to diverticula, achalasia, presbyesophagus, or retention esophagitis. Without additional etiologic factors, esophagitis is uncommon.

Ulcerative esophagitis may be due to tablets or capsules that are taken without sufficient fluid, e. g., doxycycline, tetracycline, clindamycin, quinidine, iron preparations, aspirin, indomethacin, etc.

Reflux esophagitis is due to gastric cardiac insufficiency allowing reflux of acid stomach content into the lower segment of the esophagus leading to erosion of the esophageal mucosa with esophagitis and peptic ulcers.

Symptoms. This is usually a disease of middle age with an episodic course, causing retrosternal heartburn or a feeling of pressure, epigastric pain, and hiccup. The symptoms are made worse by bending down or lying flat, straining, alcohol, nicotine, or fatty foods. Bleeding is uncommon.

Pathogenesis. The cause is insufficiency of the lower sphincter due to gastric operations, diabetes, neurologic disorders, scleroderma, alcohol and nicotine abuse, obesity, habitual vomiting in pregnancy, or a retained feeding tube.

The mucosa undergoes erosion, and the squamous epithelium is replaced by columnar epithelium in the lower part of the esophagus. A *hiatus hernia* or *Barrett's syndrome* may be present. The latter is metaplastic columnar epithelium with an acquired short esophagus due to peptic ulceration and stenoses. Ten percent of these cases proceed to adenocarcinoma.

Diagnosis. Manometry demonstrates the insufficiency. Esophagoscopy with biopsy is the most useful diagnostic method, but radiography is only positive when there are very severe degrees of mucosal damage.

Differential diagnosis. This includes carcinoma of the cardia, which may grow beneath the mucosa, achalasia, scleroderma, pregnancy esophagitis, and the changes produced by vagotomy. Angina pectoris must be ruled out.

Treatment. *Conservative.* The patient is advised to take frequent small meals, to eat slowly, to diet, to lose weight, and to take foods low in fat and rich in protein. Cimetidine, antacids, and anticholinergic drugs are prescribed, nicotine and alcohol are forbidden, and the patient is advised to sleep with the head of the bed elevated.

Surgical treatment is excision of the ulcerated zone and plication of the fundus. Strictures are managed by bouginage or plastic repair.

Moniliasis of the esophagus has become more common since the advent of antibiotics.

Symptoms. These are pain on swallowing, heartburn, and regurgitation of food mixed with blood.

Diagnosis. This is made by esophagoscopy with a specimen for culture and biopsy.

Treatment. Therapy consists of antimycotics.

Scar tissue stenosis is caused by corrosives, reflux postoperative esophagitis following anastomoses, by ingested foreign bodies, epidermolysis bullosa, and other dermatologic diseases.

Motility Disorders of the Esophagus

These may present as atonic or spastic dyskinesias and may be a primary disease or secondary to other organic disorders.

Idiopathic Esophageal Spasm

Symptoms. These include dysphagia varying in severity, a feeling of pressure behind the sternum, and prolongation of the act of swallowing.

Pathogenesis. This is a disorder of the autonomic innervation ("dyschalasia").

Diagnosis. Radiographic findings are characteristic showing a variable traveling constrictor ring of the esophagus on a contrast swallow (see Fig. 5.2e). Manometry is carried out with esophagoscopy to exclude organic intraesophageal diseases.

Treatment. Spasmolytic agents are prescribed, and small meals at regular intervals are advised.

Achalasia (Cardiospasm) is absence of the relaxation of the lower esophageal sphincter during swallowing. The normal peristalsis is lost. There is retention of material in the esophagus causing megaesophagus, especially in children. The age of predilection is 30 to 50 years but the disease may occur in children.

Symptoms. The symptoms are prolonged, gradually becoming more severe. There is a feeling of retention of food in the esophagus, a tendency to wash every mouthful down with fluid, and vomiting of material that does *not* smell acid since it is not mixed with gastric acid. In the late stage there is a severe loss of weight or even cachexia.

Pathogenesis. The disease is thought to be due to a neuromuscular disorder, possibly degeneration of Auerbach's plexus. Psychogenic or hormonal factors are also possible.

Diagnosis. This is made by contrast radiograph which shows the dilated atonic esophagus (see Fig. 5.**2d**), reduced peristalsis, and smooth walls. Esophagoscopy shows the esophageal lumen filled with decomposed food, and esophagitis. Endoscopy is also necessary to exclude carcinoma or other organic stenoses of the cardia. Manometry is carried out.

Differential diagnosis. This includes carcinoma of the cardia, scleroderma, and gastric disorders.

Treatment. Long-term medical treatment is useless, and dilatation of the sphincter muscle with a special dilating sound is needed. Recurrences are dealt with by extramucosal Heller's cardiomyotomy and possibly fundoplication. Malignant degeneration occurs in about 4% of patients after 15 to 20 years.

Technique of dilatation. An expandible dilator is used. Esophagoscopy should be carried out first to exclude a tumor as a cause of the stenosis. As soon as the dilating part of the instrument is in the cardia, the sphincter is dilated by rapid closure of the handgrip of the instrument. There is striking improvement in the dysphagia which often lasts for the rest of the patient's life. Dilatation of the cardia may also be carried out with a water- or air-filled balloon instead of the dilator. The pressure is checked by a manometer.

Complications. These include perforation of the esophagus especially if an intramural carcinoma of the cardia has not been recognized before.

Cricopharyngeal Achalasia

Symptoms. A globus sensation is accompanied by a "sticking" sensation during food ingestion (dysphagia).

Pathogenesis. The cause in any given case may remain unclear. The basic pathogenic mechanism is neuromyogenic impairment of upper sphincter relaxation, often combined with gastroesophageal reflux.

Diagnosis. Essential studies are upper GI contrast examination, videofluorography, and manometry.

Differential diagnosis. Differentiation is required from Zenker's diverticulum and malignant disease.

Treatment. The treatment of choice is cricopharyngeal myotomy, which is best done endoscopically (laser).

Involvement of the Esophagus by Disease of Neighboring Organs

The esophagus may be compressed or completely obstructed by goiter, osteophytes of the cervical spine, especially the fifth to the seventh cervical vertebra, marked kyphoscoliosis, tumors of the mediastinum, aortic enlargement, and hypertrophy of the left ventricle.

Esophageal Varices (Color Plate **36b**)

Symptoms. These include hematemesis which is often severe consisting of fresh clear red blood; tarry stools; and intermittent, usually mild dysphagia. The patient may bleed to death.

Pathogenesis. The cause is almost always portal hypertension. The blood from the portal venous system drains via collateral vessels because of obstructed drainage. The causes of obstruction include cirrhosis, which in 50% of cases is accompanied by varices, hepatitis, thrombosis of the portal arterial, the splenic venous, or vena caval systems, and mediastinal tumors.

Diagnosis. This is made on the findings of an internist. Esophagoscopy should be carried out and is more accurate than radiography.

Differential diagnosis. This includes pulmonary bleeding, bleeding from the nasopharynx, gastric or duodenal ulcer, and erosive gastritis.

Treatment. Emergency measures are needed for the bleeding including treatment of shock. A Sengstaken-Blakemore tube can be used to achieve immediate hemostasis. Surgical or medical treatment is also necessary. A shunt operation is carried out in a disease-free interval. The otolaryngologist may be called in to obliterate the bleeding vessel by local use of the laser or injection of sclerosing substances.

Congenital Anomalies and Fistulae

Most of these congenital anomalies lie in the field of the thoracic or pediatric surgeon. Only those will be discussed that are of interest during esophagoscopy.

Congenital Esophageal Stenosis

Symptoms. Dysphagia, coughing attacks, and possibly vomiting are symptomatic.

Diagnosis. Radiology and endoscopy.

Treatment. Bouginage or endoscopic laser removal of circumscribed webs in performed.

Short Esophagus

This is a congenital disease. Reflux symptoms are already present in about 50% of these infantile patients. The lower esophageal segment is absent.

Symptoms. See reflux esophagitis.

Diagnosis. Contrast radiogram and endoscopy which shows heterotopic gastric mucosa above the diaphragm, thoracic stomach, congenital short esophagus, or Barrett's syndrome provide the diagnosis.

Differential diagnosis. Sliding hiatus hernia must be considered.

Treatment. See reflux esophagitis.

Tracheoesophageal Fistula

This is a congenital or acquired communication between the lumen of the esophagus and the trachea. It may or may not be accompanied by atresia. An "H-fistula" is shown in Figure 5.**2k**.

Symptoms. The disease is usually recognized immediately after birth by choking attacks, dyspnea, cough, and cyanosis. The fistula may remain symptomfree for a long time due to valvular action or formation of scar tissue. The fistula may occasionally only produce symptoms in later life including coughing on eating or drinking, expectoration of food, and recurrent aspiration pneumonia.

Diagnosis. This is made by contrast radiography and endoscopy, consisting of combined bronchoscopy and esophagoscopy.

Differential diagnosis. This includes acquired tracheoesophageal fistula, e.g., due to necrosis of the esophageal wall as a result of trauma, ruptured diverticulum, or breakdown of a malignancy of the esophagus or the trachea.

Treatment. Using a cervical or thoracic approach (depending on the site), division and reconstruction of the trachea and esophagus are performed.

Dysphagia Due to Congenital Aortic Arch Anomalies

When the subclavian artery is the last vessel to arise from the aortic arch due to a congenital anomaly, it crosses over the esophagus en route to the right side, creating a mechanical impediment to swallowing. In 80% of patients the atypical artery passes between the vertebral column and the esophagus, in 15% between the trachea and the esophagus, and in 5% in front of the trachea.

Symptoms. These usually occur in middle age due to loss of the elasticity of the vessel wall causing difficulty in swallowing, impaction of food, etc.

Diagnosis. This is made by contrast radiography, arteriography, and esophagoscopy which shows a pulsating horizontal bar at a variable level in the esophageal wall.

Treatment. Division of the vessel is performed if the patient has serious symptoms.

Hiatus Hernia

Part of the cardia and the fundus of the stomach protrude through the esophageal hiatus. There are two main types:

1. *Sliding hiatus hernia* which is clinically silent in 80% of patients
2. *Paraesophageal, fixed hernia* which is symptomfree in 50% of patients

Symptoms. These are often absent, but include retrosternal pain or pressure after eating, heartburn, dysphagia, vomiting, and reflux esophagitis.

Diagnosis. Contrast radiography is used. At times it is necessary to examine the patient in Trendelenburg's position. Esophagogastroscopy with the fiberoptic endoscope is indicated.

Treatment. This is not necessary for a sliding hiatus hernia if it is not causing symptoms. A transabdominal gastropexy is carried out for paraesophageal hernia because of the danger of incarceration.

Tumors of the Esophagus

Benign tumors may be intraluminal, intramural, or periesophageal but are uncommon. The most common are leiomyomas, rhabdomyomas, fibromas, hemangiomas, lipomas, neuromas, and papillomas. Often they do not cause symptoms until they attain a considerable size, and then they cause dysphagia, stenosis, pain, pressure behind the sternum, and bleeding.

Diagnosis. This is made by contrast radiography, esophagoscopy, and biopsy.

Treatment. The tumor is removed, either endoscopically, or using a transcervical, transthoracic, or transabdominal approach depending on the type of tumor and site of origin.

Malignant Tumors (Color Plate **36c**)

The most frequent esophageal malignancy is the squamous carcinoma which is often histologically undifferentiated.

This tumor forms 40% of all gastrointestinal malignancies. It affects, almost exclusively, men over the age of 50 years. Esophageal carcinoma can develop without previous disease, but it may also arise from chronically irritated esophageal mucosa due to corrosion, diverticula, short esophagus of the Barrett's syndrome type, reflux esophagitis, hiatus hernia, achalasia, or Plummer-Vinson syndrome. It may rarely spread from neighboring organs such as the thyroid gland, the larynx, the trachea, the bronchi, or the stomach. Lymph node metastases from distant organs are also possible. Rare histologic forms include adenocarcinoma, usually affecting the lower segment of the esophagus, and sarcoma.

Symptoms. These include increasing dysphagia, initially only for solid foods, burning or a feeling of fullness behind the sternum, pain which is late and inconstant and felt behind the sternum or the back, loss of weight, hiccup, vomiting, coughing, and hoarseness due to paralysis of the recurrent laryngeal nerve. The symptoms only become obvious after 4 to 5 months on average. Later there is marked loss of weight, inability to eat, vomiting, marked thirst, and severe pain.

Diagnosis. This is often made very late. *Radiography* shows widening of the mediastinum and lateral displacement of the trachea. A *contrast radiograph* shows a filling defect or a holdup, irregular outline of the wall, and narrowing of the esophageal lumen (see Fig. 5.**2i**). Paralysis of the recurrent laryngeal nerve is sometimes the first symptom. *Esophagoscopy* with a rigid esophagoscope and biopsy is the most useful diagnostic measure.

Differential diagnosis. This includes achalasia, esophageal stricture, diverticulum, Plummer-Vinson syndrome, benign esophageal tumors, bronchial carcinoma invading the esophagus and an intraesophageal foreign body.

Treatment. Only one third of cases are operable, usually those arising in the middle and lower thirds of the esophagus. Often only palliative measures are possible such as bypass with an endoprosthesis (intubation), or gastrostomy. Radiotherapy is also of only palliative benefit. The 5-year survival rate after surgery is about 10% and is 0% to 5% after radiotherapy. For more details, see surgical and internal textbooks.

Chemotherapy is at most of palliative benefit for tumors at this site.

6. Neck (Including the Thyroid Gland)

Applied Anatomy and Physiology

The neck supports the head, allows it to move, and connects it to the trunk. The *osteomuscular part* of the neck is adapted to the upright human posture.

The *visceral part* of the neck accommodates the upper respiratory and digestive tracts: the larynx which functions as a sphincter and as the organ of voice, the thyroid gland, the carotid sheath and its contents on each side, and the cervical lymphatic system.

The upper border of the neck runs along the inferior border of the mandible through the apex of the mastoid process to the external occipital protuberance. The suprahyoid triangle of the neck belongs on clinical and surgical grounds to the neck. Inferiorly, the neck ends in a plane formed by the suprasternal notch, the clavicle, and the spinous process of the seventh cervical vertebra. Laterally, the borders of the trapezius muscle form the boundary with the posterior part of the neck (Fig. 6.1).

The external shape of the neck depends on *constitutional and sexually determined factors*. In men the larynx is angular and forms the Adam's apple, and the

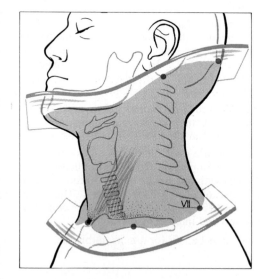

Fig. 6.1 Boundaries of the neck.

sternomastoid muscle is well developed. In women the structures are more slender and delicate.

The sternocleidomastoid muscles and the borders of the trapezius muscle on both sides, the hyoid bone, the laminae of the thyroid cartilage, and the cricoid cartilage contribute to the profile and are visible and palpable.

An *enlarged thyroid gland* (goiter) and tumor masses are readily detected visually and by palpation (see p. 523).

Basic Anatomy and Physiology

Regions

The sternocleidomastoid muscle divides the neck for clinical purposes into:

1. The median region of the neck: inferior to the hyoid is the clinically important *superior carotid triangle* (Figs. 6.2 and 6.3) whose boundaries are the anterior borders of the sternocleidomastoid muscle, the superior belly of the omohyoid muscle, and the posterior belly of the digastric; and the *small inferior carotid triangle* whose boundaries are the anterior and posterior borders of the sternocleidomastoid muscle, the medial edge of the omohyoid muscle, and the root of the neck (so-called *regio sternocleidomastoidea*).
2. The lateral region of the neck is divided into two triangles by the inferior belly of the omohyoid muscle. The lower of these is the *omoclavicular triangle* whose boundaries are the omohyoid muscle, the clavicle, and the internal jugular vein. It corresponds to the often visible supraclavicular fossa.

The *suprahyoid triangle* (see Fig. 6.2) is divided into the *submandibular triangle* and the *submental triangle*.

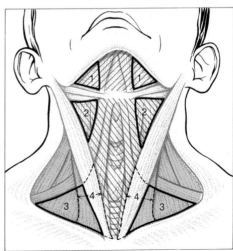

Fig. 6.2 Regions and important triangles of the neck. The red cross-hatched area is the median region of the neck with the suprahyoid and infrahyoid triangles. The lateral region of the neck is shown in red. 1, Submandibular triangle; 2, superior carotid triangle; 3, omoclavicular triangle; 4, sternocleidomastoid region; the extent is shown by black dotted line and arrow.

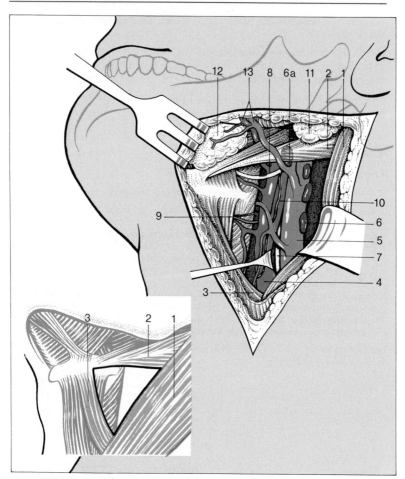

Fig. 6.3 Superior carotid triangle. 1, Sternocleidomastoid muscles; 2, posterior belly of digastric muscle; 3, superior belly of omohyoid muscle; 4, common carotid artery; 5, internal jugular vein; 6, deep cervical lymph node; 6a, lymph nodes in the jugulofacial venous angle; 7, vagus nerve; 8, hypoglossal nerve; 9, superior laryngeal neurovascular bundle; 10, ansa cervicalis; 11, lower pole of the parotid; 12, submandibular gland; 13, facial artery and vein.

Fascia

The cervical muscles, viscera, and carotid sheath (Fig. 6.4) are enclosed in a fascia which is partly tight, partly loose, and partly incomplete.

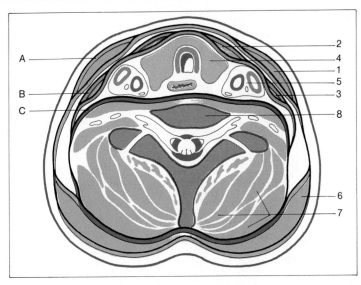

Fig. 6.4   Fascial envelopes. A, superficial cervical fascia; B, middle cervical fascia; C, deep cervical fascia. 1, Sternocleidomastoid muscle; 2, infrahyoid muscles; 3, omohyoid muscle; 4, thyroid gland; 5, carotid sheath with common carotid artery, internal jugular vein, vagus nerve, and cervical sympathetic trunk; 6, trapezius muscle; 7, deep muscles of the neck; 8, cervical vertebral body.

1. The superficial cervical fascia lies under the platysma, encloses the sternocleidomastoid and trapezius muscles, inserts onto the hyoid bone, and extends superiorly to the border of the mandible and inferiorly to the superior border of the sternum and the clavicle.
2. The medial cervical fascia is a multilocular system enclosing the entire cervical viscera, the thyroid gland, the esophagus, the trachea, the pharynx, the vessels, and the nerves. It stretches between the two omohyoid muscles, the hyoid, the clavicle, the upper part of the sternum, and the scapula.
3. The deep cervical fascia forms a tight tube around the deep cervical muscles arising from the spinous processes of the bodies of the cervical spine. The prevertebral layer is part of the fascial system running continuously from the base of the skull to the inferior end of the spinal column.

The deep cervical fascia is divided into the alar fascia and a prevertebral part lying directly on bone. The prevertebral fascial space is thus divided into two to form the "danger space" (Fig. 6.5). Infection can spread directly within it into the *posterior mediastinum*.

The contents of the carotid sheath, the common carotid artery, the external and internal carotid artery, the internal jugular vein, the vagus nerve, and the sympathetic plexus possess their own relatively thick fascial envelope consisting of parts of all three layers of the cervical fascia.

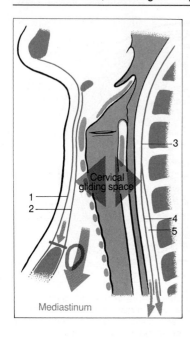

Fig. 6.5 Cervical interfascial spaces. 1, Superficial cervical fascia; 2, middle cervical fascia; 3, deep cervical fascia; 4, alar layer of the prevertebral fascia; 5, "danger space".

The interfascial spaces have great functional and clinical significance. They can change in shape and move relative to each other, thus adapting to movements of the head, vascular pulsation, chewing, swallowing, and respiration.

> *Note:* The space between the *superficial and middle* cervical fascia is closed inferiorly as a sac because of their common insertion to the sternum and clavicle. This prevents inferior extension of infection. In contrast, the space between the *middle and deep* cervical fascia communicates freely below with the mediastinum (see Fig. 6.5). This allows abscesses to track downward and allows infection due to esophageal injuries or surgical emphysema to spread.

Spaces

- The visceral space of the neck (see Fig. 6.5) allows gliding movements. It lies anterior and lateral to the middle cervical fascia and posterior to the prevertebral fascia. It encloses the retropharyngeal space which lies posterior to the pharynx but anterior to the deeper cervical fascia.
- The parapharyngeal space contains the neurovascular bundle and has areas of contact with the eustachian tube and the tonsil.
- The submandibular space with the submandibular gland is in contact with the dental alveoli.

- The sublingual space encloses the sublingual gland and is the site of abscesses of the floor of the mouth (see Fig. 3.**16a** and **b**).
- The submental space is important in Ludwig's angina (see p. 343).
- The parotid space.

> *Note:* The boundaries described on the basis of individual anatomic structures are often not respected by nonspecific and specific inflammations, primary tumors of the cervical organs, lymph node metastases, and primary and malignant lymphomas.

Blood Vessels

The *common carotid artery* is the main artery of the neck. On the right side it rises from the brachiocephalic trunk and on the left from the aortic arch. It runs superiorly lateral to the trachea and larynx without giving off any branches to reach the level of the upper border of the thyroid cartilage where it divides into the external and internal carotid artery.

The *external carotid artery* is the *anterior* branch of the common carotid artery. It runs superiorly in the carotid triangle giving off branches and runs under the posterior belly of the digastric muscle and under the stylohyoid muscle. It crosses the retromandibular fossa and then runs in front

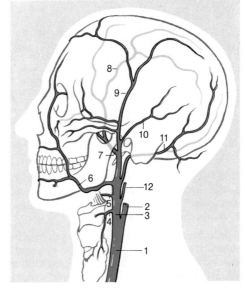

Fig. 6.**6**   The carotid artery and its branches. 1, Common carotid artery; 2, internal carotid artery; 3, external carotid artery; 4, superior thyroid artery; 5, lingual artery; 6, facial artery; 7, internal maxillary artery; 8, middle meningeal artery; 9, superficial temporal artery; 10, posterior auricular artery; 11, occipital artery; 12, ascending pharyngeal artery.

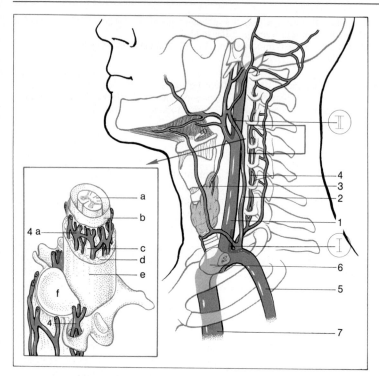

Fig. 6.**7** Cervical venous system. 1, Internal jugular vein; 2, external jugular vein; 3, anterior jugular vein; 4, vertebral veins; 4a, venous plexus in the cervical vertebral canal; 5, subclavian vein; 6, brachiocephalic vein; 7, superior vena cava. a, Cervical medulla; b, arachnoid; c, dura; d, epidural space with venous plexus and fat; e, periosteal tube; f, vertebral body. I, Greater jugulosubclavian venous angle; II, Lesser jugulofacial venous angle.

of the external ear to reach the temporal region where it divides into its final branches.

The branches of the external carotid artery are: the superior thyroid, lingual, facial, ascending pharyngeal, occipital, posterior auricular, internal maxillary, which gives off the middle meningeal artery, and the superficial temporal arteries (Fig. 6.**6**).

The *internal carotid artery* is the *posterior* branch of the common carotid artery. It supplies the brain and the eyes and runs initially, like the external carotid artery, in the carotid triangle but then runs deeper in the retromandibular fossa and through the carotid canal into the skull.

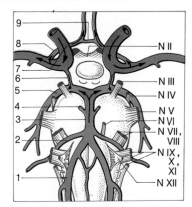

Fig. 6.8   Arteries of the base of the brain with the circle of Willis. 1, Vertebral artery; 2, anterior inferior cerebellar artery; 3, basilar artery; 4, superior cerebellar artery; 5, posterior cerebral artery; 6, posterior communicating artery; 7, internal carotid artery; 8, anterior cerebral artery; 9, anterior communicating artery.

The lower part of the neck obtains its important arterial supply from branches of the *thyrocervical trunk:* the suprascapular, inferior thyroid, and ascending and superficial cervical arteries.

The *carotid sinus* lies in the bulging part of the carotid bifurcation. It is provided with pressor receptors for blood pressure regulation.

The *carotid body* is a small body up to 5 mm in size lying in the *adventitia* of the medial wall of the bifurcation with *chemoreceptor* properties which control respiration, blood pressure, and heart rate depending on the blood levels of O_2, CO_2, and pH. It may undergo malignant degeneration as a chemodectoma (nonchromaffin paraganglioma, carotid body tumor) (see pp. 127, 128 and 506 ff.).

The *vertebral artery* does not take part in the blood supply of the soft tissue of the neck, but it gives branches for the meninges and the cervical medulla and supplies the circle of Willis. The vertebral arteries transport about 30% of the cerebral blood supply.

The *internal jugular veins* together with their main tributaries, the anterior and external jugular veins, provide the main venous drainage for the head. The *vertebral veins* and the *venous plexus in the cervical spinal canal* normally carry about 30% of the cerebral venous drainage. When one or both internal jugular veins are ligated, the vertebral venous plexuses can restore an adequate level of cerebral venous drainage (Fig. 6.7) within a few days.

A *central venous catheter* is introduced via the internal jugular vein or the subclavian vein. Indications include total parenteral alimentation, administration of drugs, and measurement of central venous pressure. The position of the catheter should be checked by radiography before the infusion begins.

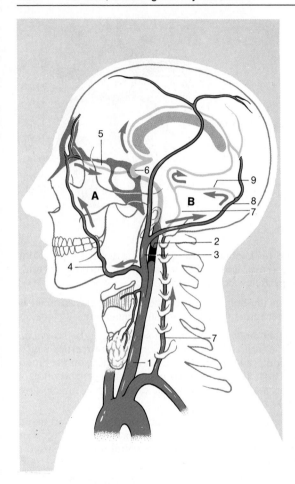

Fig. 6.9 Collateral circulation in insufficiency of the internal carotid artery. A, ophthalmic collateral; B, occipital anastomoses. 1, Common carotid artery; 2, internal carotid artery with stenosis; 3, external carotid artery; 4, facial artery; 5, ophthalmic artery; 6, carotid siphon; 7, vertebral artery; 8, occipital artery; 9, meningeal anastomoses.

Note: The *greater jugulosubclavian venous angle* lies posterior to the sternoclavicular joint at the root of the neck, and lateral and superior to it lie the supraclavicular or prescalene lymph nodes. This angle should be distinguished from the *lesser jugulofacial venous angle* which is formed by the opening of the facial vein into the internal jugular vein. There is also a collection of important lymph nodes at this point (see Fig. 6.7).

Circulatory disorders of the internal carotid artery may cause little or no symptoms provided there is *a competent collateral circulation via the circle of Willis* (Fig. 6.8) or

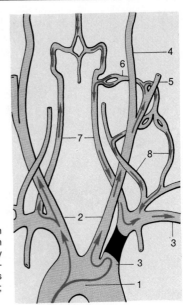

Fig. 6.**10** Bypass circulation in subclavian steal syndrome. 1, Aortic arch; 2, common carotid artery; 3, occluded subclavian artery (black); 4, internal carotid artery; 5, external carotid artery; 6, occipital anastomoses (see also Fig. 6.**9B**); 7, vertebral artery; 8, branches of the thyrocervical trunk.

from the external carotid artery: (1) via the facial, angular, and ophthalmic arteries to the carotid syphon *(ophthalmic collaterals)* (Fig. 6.**9A**) *or* (2) via the occipital, meningeal, and vertebral arteries *(occipital anastomosis)* (see Fig. 6.**9B**).

Acute occlusion of this arterial system and its collaterals causes hemiplegia and unilateral sensory deficits. If the occlusion *develops slowly* (e.g., in arteriosclerosis) ischemic cerebral attacks = drop attacks occur initially, and later generalized cerebral insufficiency.

Prior to surgery for head and neck carcinoma with cervical metastasis (N_3), it is important to test the capacity of the cerebral collateral reserve before proceeding with resection of the internal carotid artery.

Vertebrobasilar insufficiency. One of the sites of predilection for stenosis of the vertebral artery is the segment between the origin from the subclavian artery to the entry into the canal in the transverse process of the sixth cervical vertebra. Stenosis at this site causes temporary, recurrent, or prolonged attacks of dizziness, drop attacks hearing disorders, disorders of vision, and sudden syncope. A resulting chronic deficient cerebral circulation often declares itself by the oblongata or *Wallenberg's syndrome.*

The *subclavian steal syndrome* and the resulting cerebral circulatory disorders are due to occlusion of the subclavian artery between its origin from the aorta and the origin of the vertebral artery. Vascular anomalies, trauma, and arteriosclerosis cause a reverse flow in the vertebral artery in favor of the arterial supply of the ipsilateral arm and the thyrocervical trunk at the expense of the cerebral circulation (Fig. 6.**10**).

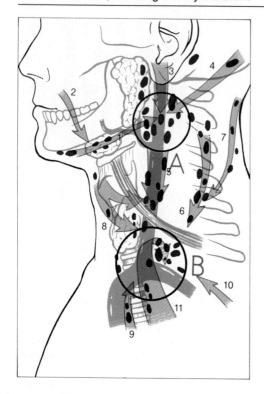

Fig. 6.**11** Lymphatic pathways in the neck. 1, Submental-submandibular; 2, facial; 3, parotid-auricular; 4, occipital; 5, along the internal jugular vein; 6, along the accessory nerve; 7, nuchal; 8, laryngotracheothyroid; 9, bronchomediastinal; 10, axillary; 11, thoracic duct; A, lymph nodes at the jugulofacial-venous angle; B, central lymph space at the base of the neck on the left side, the jugulosubclavian venous angle.

Cervical Lymphatic System

There are a total of approximately 300 lymph nodes in the adult human neck.

The cervical lymphatic system is a component of the reticuloendothelial or reticulohistiocytic system. Portals to this system include the lymphoepithelial organs of the naso- and oropharynx (see p. 307).

Note: Up to the age of about 8 or 10 years, hyperplasia of the cervical lymph nodes in the drainage area of the naso- or oropharynx due to reactive swelling of the tonsils often results from the close connection of the lymphoepithelial and reticuloendothelial systems. Newly developed *lymphadenopathy always requires investigation at any age.*

Lymph channels lead from *tributary tissue areas* to *regional lymph nodes or groups.* The lymph nodes in the neck are incorporated in a network of lymph capillaries and lymph vessels which drain on both sides into the

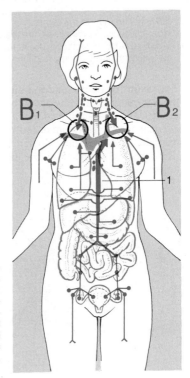

Fig. 6.**12**   A, Central lymph spaces of the body at the base of the neck on both sides and their efferents from the cranial; cervical; thoracic, e.g., mediastinal and tracheobronchial lymph nodes; abdominal, e.g., mesenteric, lumbar, inguinal, and iliac nodes; and the inferior lymph nodes. B1, Right central lymphatic space; B2, left central lymphatic space with the opening of the thoracic duct. 1, Thoracic duct.

large lower deep cervical lymph nodes from which the lymph finally flows back into the venous system (Fig. 6.**11**).

On the left side the *thoracic duct* usually ends in a delta-shaped network. On the right side the *right lymphatic duct* sinks into a 1 to 2 cm long cervical lymph trunk in the respective jugulosubclavian angle. These cervical lymph trunks receive afferents on both sides from the *cranial area* by the jugular trunks from the *axilla* by the subclavian trunks and from the *thoracic area* by the bronchomediastinal trunks.

The *main drainage of the intrathoracic lymph* is to the *right jugulosubclavian angle* with the exception of the lymph of the left upper lobe of the lung.

The lymph of the lower half of the body reaches the *left jugulosubclavian angle* via the thoracic duct. Also the lymph of the left superior lung segments flows into the venous system via the left jugulosubclavian trunk (*B* in Figs. 6.**11** and 6.**12**).

Note: *The lymph node groups in both the jugulosubclavian angles, the supraclavicular lymph nodes,* are the last stations for the lymph of the entire body (see Fig. 6.**12**). This fact explains the value of *prescalene lymph node biopsy* in clinical diagnosis (see Fig. 6.**20** and pp. 517ff.).

The chains of lymph nodes around the great veins of the neck, especially the internal jugular vein, are embryologically determined. The lymph node groups of greatest clinical significance lie between the middle and deep cervical fascia. Horizontal and vertical chains anastomose in the carotid triangle. They can be palpated below the angle of the jaw and can be demonstrated surgically in the jugulofacial venous angle in the carotid triangle (see *A* in Fig. 6.**11**).

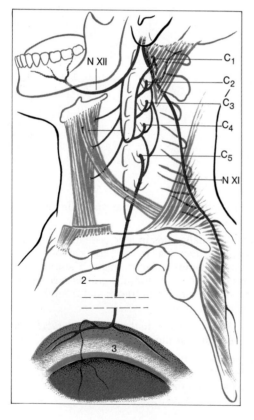

Fig. 6.**13**   Motor nerves in the neck. 1, Ansa cervicalis; 2, phrenic nerve; 3, diaphragm.

Nerves

The motor, sensory, and autonomic nerve supply of the neck is complex.

The motor supply of the cervical musculature is as follows (Fig. 6.**13**):

- The accessory nerve supplies the sternocleidomastoid and trapezius muscles.
- The hypoglossal nerve supplies the tongue.
- The ansa cervicalis supplies the infrahyoid muscles.
- Branches of the Vth, VIIth, and XIIth cranial nerves innervate the suprahyoid musculature of the floor of the mouth.

The phrenic nerve arising from C_3 to C_5 runs inferiorly over the scalenus anterior muscle to supply the diaphragm.

Sensory Nerve Supply of the External Neck

This arises from the cervical plexus, C_1 to C_4, and consists of the great auricular nerve, the greater and lesser occipital nerves, the transverse nerve of the neck, the supraclavicular nerves, and the dorsal rami over the nape.

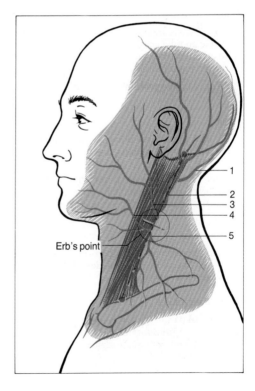

Fig. 6.**14**   Sensory nerves in the neck. 1, Occipital nerve; 2, posterior branch of the great auricular nerve; 3, anterior branch of the great auricular nerve; 4, transverse cervical nerve; 5, supraclavicular nerve.

Erb's point marks the collection of the anterior branches at the midpoint of the posterior border of the sternocleidomastoid muscle. Infiltration of Erb's point produces local anesthesia of the lateral part of the neck (Fig. 6.14).

> *Note:* The nerves of the cervical plexus, especially the great auricular nerve, are often used as a graft for reconstruction of the facial or hypoglossal nerves.

Mixed Nerves

The *vagus nerve* has much in common anatomically and functionally with the *glossopharyngeal nerve* and the cranial root of the *accessory nerve*. They can thus be described together as a *vagal system.*

These nerves leave the base of the skull through the jugular foramen and have motor, sensory, and parasympathetic functions in the neck especially for the pharynx and the larynx. The superior ganglion of the *vagus nerve* lies at the base of the skull and the inferior ganglion at the level of the hyoid bone.

Motor, Sensory, and Autonomic Parts of the Vagus System

Motor

Larynx. The recurrent laryngeal nerve curves around the subclavian artery on the right side and the aortic arch on the left side. The paired nerves then run superiorly between the trachea and the esophagus on each side. The recurrent nerves supply all the laryngeal muscles with the exception of the cricothyroid (see Fig. 4.10).

Pharynx. Motor vagal impulses reach the pharyngeal musculature via the glossopharyngeal nerve.

Sensory

In the neck these nerve branches are responsible for the sensory supply of the base of the tongue, the epiglottis, and the larynx.

> *Note:* Sensory impulses from the posterior meatal wall and the tympanic membrane run in the auricular branch of the vagus (see p. 3). The tracheal and bronchial branches of the vagus take part in the reflex control of respiration.

Autonomic

Secretory parasympathetic fibers run from the neck to the organs of the thorax and abdomen. The *secretory* regulation of the parotid gland is controlled via the glossopharyngeal nerve (see p. 532).

Sympathetic Chain

The cervical part of the sympathetic trunk lies in front of the prevertebral fascia and the transverse processes of the cervical spine. The sympathetic trunk supplies the heart, the blood vessels, the glands, the smooth muscular organs, and the accessory glands of the skin.

The superior cervical ganglion and the inconstant middle cervical ganglion arise from several segments. The inferior cervical ganglion with the upper thoracic ganglia forms the *stellate ganglion*. It lies between the transverse process of the seventh cervical vertebra and the head of the first rib. Post-ganglionic fibers from the superior ganglion run to the carotid, middle ear, salivary and lacrimal glands, and the ciliary ganglion via the IXth, Xth, and XIth cranial nerves and the upper three cervical nerves.

> *Note:* Stimulation of the superior cervical ganglion (e.g., fright) produces dilatation of the pupil and widening of the palpebral cleft, exophthalmos, sweating, and increase of vascular tone. Blockade of the stellate ganglion by drugs or tumor leads to the opposite reaction, i.e., enophthalmos, miosis, and ptosis, *Horner's syndrome.*

Blocking the stellate ganglion is *indicated* for acute vascular disorders of the inner ear, e.g., sudden hearing loss or acute vestibulopathy (see pp. 145, 146). The *mechanism of action is thought* to be a sympatheticolytic influence on the myogenic vascular elements, extending as far as the cochlear arterioles.

Technique of Transcutaneous Blockage of the Stellate Ganglion (Fig. 6.15)

Premedication with 0.5 mg atropine is advisable. The patient lies on his back with his head directed straight forward and relatively extended so that the transverse processes of the cervical spine and the heads of the ribs are more easily felt. The carotid

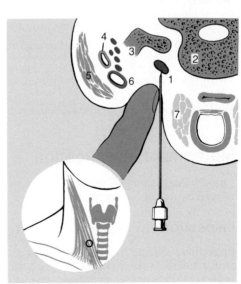

Fig. 6.15 Technique of blocking the cervical sympathetic. 1, Stellate ganglion; 2, vertebral body; 3, transverse process; 4, internal jugular vein; 5, sternocleido-mastoid muscle; 6, common carotid artery; 7, thyroid gland.

artery is palpated and pressed laterally together with the sternocleidomastoid muscle. Injection is made two fingerbreadths lateral to the midline and two fingerbreadths above the sternoclavicular joint proceeding perpendicularly in a posterior direction. The point of the needle usually reaches the head of the first rib and is then withdrawn 1 cm. Ten milliliters of 1% procaine solution is injected with frequent repeated attempts at aspiration. Initially, there is a feeling of warmth and prickling in the face on the same side, and then Horner's syndrome appears after a few minutes.

The effect of the blockade lasts about 24 h even if the Horner's syndrome disappears before this.

Dangers include penetration of the anesthetic medium into the spinal canal leading to respiratory paralysis, intravascular injection leading to generalized convulsions, pneumothorax due to pleural injuries, and damage to the brachial plexus which is usually temporary.

Basic Physiology

Swallowing and vomiting are described in Table 3.7.

Coughing. Afferent impulses running in the vagus nerve cause reflex deepening of the inspiration followed by glottic closure. The glottis opens suddenly with explosive escape of the compressed air after contraction of the expiratory thoracic muscles. High air speeds are obtained during coughing attacks which can eject mucus, crusts, and foreign bodies (see p. 370).

Straining. The thoracic and abdominal muscles are strongly contracted with voluntary closure of the glottis. The trunk is converted into a mechanically fixed unit so that the hip and shoulder muscles can respond with a coordinated brief and maximal effort, e. g., in lifting or bringing the body into the upright position.

In the **Valsalva maneuver** the thoracoabdominal muscle pump develops a high-compression pressure on the vascular system with an extrathoracic increase in venous pressure producing protrusion of the veins of the head and neck and decrease of the arterial pressure due to obstruction of the venous return to the heart. The patient may faint.

The Valsalva maneuver to open the eustachian tube is described on p. 40.

Methods of Investigation

Clinical examination of the neck by *inspection and palpation* is supplemented by *technical procedures.*

Inspection

Inspection is oriented on those structures of the neck that contribute to the profile and seeks lesions of the overlying skin (vascular signs, venous congestion, radiodermatitis, pigmented nevi, and melanoma), as well as fistulous openings in branchiogenic fistula, swellings or indurations (lymph-adenopathy, tumors, abscesses). The position and mobility of the head are examined looking for spasm of the neck muscles, e.g., in abscesses, thyroiditis, and torticollis.

Palpation

Palpation is carried out either from in front or behind, and both sides are palpated and compared. The head should be tilted slightly forward to

---

Table 6.1 Summary on Findings of Examination and Palpation of the Neck

Site	Topographic description
Form and size	Size in centimeters
Mobility	Vertically or horizontally mobile, fixed or adherent to the overlying skin
Consistency	Soft, elastic, fluctuant, firm, or hard
Pulsation, skin temperature, and color	Comparison to the surrounding tissues
Tenderness	

Table 6.2 Cervical Swellings

Causes:

Thyroid swellings

Nonspecific lymphadenopathy

Specific lymphadenopathy

Mononucleosis

Aids lymphadenopathy (on the increase)

Malignant lymphadenopathy
  Metastatic carcinoma
  Hodgkin's and Non-Hodgkin's lymphoma

Median and lateral cervical cysts

Inflammation and tumors of the submandibular gland and the cervical part of the parotid gland

Deep inflammation or abscess

Lipoma

Hemangioma, lymphangioma, cystic hygroma

Carotid body tumor

More rare tumors include sebaceous cysts, dermoid cysts, neuroma, vascular aneurysms, infective lymphadenopathy, e.g., rubella, toxoplasmosis relax the soft tissues. Palpable abnormalities mostly relate to the thyroid gland, lymph nodes, salivary glands, tumors, cysts, and abscesses (Tables 6.1 and 6.2).

Auscultation and palpation are carried out for suspected carotid body tumors, vascular aneurysms, and carotid artery stenoses.

Lymph nodes usually become palpable when their diameter is more than 1 cm. It is advisable to palpate the individual lymph node groups in a specific order, e.g., from the submental to the submandibular triangle, then along the sternocleidomastoid muscle to the omoclavicular triangle, and finally superiorly again along the course of the accessory nerve (Fig. 6.**16a–e** and Table 6.**1**).

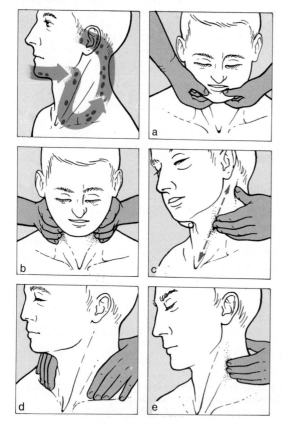

Fig. 6.**16a–e** Systematic palpation of the cervical lymph nodes. **(a)** Submental-submandibular; **(b)** and **(c)**, along the anterior border of the sternocleidomastoid muscle; **(d)** supraclavicular; **(e)** along the accessory nerve and the nuchal.

Technical Methods of Investigation

Conventional **radiographs of the cervical soft tissues** demonstrate cysts, collections of air in the tissues, tuberculous foci of calcification, sialoliths, radiopaque foreign bodies, and phleboliths.

1. *Xeroradiography* may be very helpful in many cases, particularly in demonstrating alteration in structure of the cervical soft tissues and of the tracheobronchial system, e. g., tumors.
2. *Tomography*. Conventional tomograms provide structural analysis of circumscribed bony lesions of the cervical spine and demonstrate the larynx.
3. *Computed tomography* allows greater differentiation. Vascular lesions, hematoma, tumors (especially lesions of the deep lymph nodes), and cysts are well demonstrated, including their position and extent.
4. *Radiography of the cervical spine.* Routine anteroposterior, lateral, and oblique views of the cervical spine demonstrate the position, form, and structure of the cervical spine and the relation of the bodies of the vertebrae to each other. Lesions of the intervertebral foramina are demonstrated by oblique views. Lateral views in extension and flexion and anteroposterior views with rotation to each side serve to assess the function of the cervical spine. Abnormalities are found in more than 80% of patients over 50 years old, but these are often symptomless.

Angiography. Arterial and venous angiographic procedures serve to demonstrate primary vascular diseases and also secondary vascular lesions, e. g., glomus tumors or highly vascular tumors such as nasopharyngeal angiofibromas, aneurysms, etc. Subtraction views are used to make the vessels stand out against the soft tissue and skeletal shadows.

Ultrasound. Particularly the Doppler technique is being used increasingly since it can provide information about vascular lesions. Stenoses of the cervical vessels can be detected and localized in about 90% of patients by recording changes of the echoes in the blood flow.

Cervical lymphangiography. Radiographic demonstration of the deep cervical lymph system via an exposed retroauricular lymph vessel is of little clinical value when compared with the other methods of investigation. This is also true of cervical *lymph scanning* which only provides information about the direction and extent of the lymphatic drainage. There is controversy about the results of experiments using both these techniques.

MRI is a very promising method of diagnostic imaging.

Clinical Aspects

Inflammation of the Cervical Soft Tissues

Superficial infections affecting the skin and its appendages and *deep infections* affecting the viscera must be distinguished.

Superficial infections are usually *primary* infections of the skin and its appendages by *staphylococci*. Inflammations of the cervical visceral spaces are usually secondary to necrosis or inflammation of the regional lymph nodes with and without suppuration or extend from internal organs such as the airway and the esophagus. The infection is by *mixed flora* of staphylococci, streptococci, gram-negative organisms, or tuberculous bacillae.

Superficial Infections

Furuncles or *carbuncles* on the neck are most common on the nape in men and are often found in diabetics and alcoholics.

Furuncles are treated surgically by decapping after disinfection of the skin.

Carbuncles are treated by parallel incisions and undermining of the subcutaneous septal skin, followed by drainage and concomitant antibiotic therapy.

Infected *sebaceous cysts* and subcutaneous *dermoids* may mimic a cervical abscess. They are excised completely after a course of antibiotics to suppress the local inflammation.

Abscesses

Symptoms. The site of an inflammatory process in the fascial spaces determines the clinical picture. The parapharyngeal and submandibular spaces are most commonly involved. Collections of pus lying deep in the neck often cannot be palpated. The functions of the soft tissue of the neck are restricted and deep swellings cause pain such as trismus, pain on swallowing, and muscle rigidity. Examination of the blood shows the typical signs of infection. Shivering, respiratory obstruction, or mediastinitis indicate thrombophlebitis or an early septicemia.

Pathogenesis. The cause is a soft tissue infection extending from the head, primary or secondary inflammation of the cervical lymph nodes, a purulent thyroid infection, and infected cysts. Descending specific otogenic abscesses (Bezold mastoiditis, see p. 93) are uncommon today.

Diagnosis. This rests on the history, clinical findings, special imaging studies, and microbiology.

Treatment. In severe cases broad-spectrum antibiotics are given immediately without waiting for the results of culture and sensitivity tests. The site of the abscess may be determined by aspiration. *However, antibiotics and aspiration must not be used to replace drainage of the abscess.* Definitive surgical treatment must often be carried out in a second stage because of infection of the surrounding soft tissues, the veins, arteries, and nerves.

Mediastinitis

Symptoms. These include severe malaise, fever, retrosternal or intrascapular pain, cutaneous emphysema (gas formation), and venous congestion.

Pathogenesis. The visceral space of the neck is not closed off from the superior mediastinum (see pp. 477, 478) so that an inflammatory process in the former may spread into the area of the latter. A common cause is perforation of the hypopharynx or esophagus particularly initial at its inlet during diagnostic endoscopy, removal of a foreign body, or operations on a pharyngeal pouch.

Diagnosis. This is made on the history, the clinical findings, radiographs of the thorax, if necessary contrast films using a watery medium to demonstrate the perforation, and computed tomography.

Treatment. The *posterosuperior mediastinum* is drained. An incision is made along the anterior border of the sternocleidomastoid muscle, and blunt dissection is carried down to the esophagus. The sternocleidomastoid muscle and the thyroid gland are separated by retractors, and a finger is pushed along the esophagus into the posterosuperior mediastinum. A drain is introduced once the abscess has been opened. The *anterior mediastinum* is opened through a horizontal incision above the suprasternal notch. The anterior wall of the trachea is exposed as in a low tracheotomy, and the upper mediastinum is opened by the finger. A drain is introduced.

Actinomycosis is a chronic disease causing fistulae. It is relatively painless with hard infiltrates mainly affecting the neck, but also uncommonly the cheek and the floor of the mouth. The skin undergoes livid discoloration. The infection is responsive to penicillin.

Inflammatory Cervical Lymphadenopathy

Nonspecific Lymphadenitis

Symptoms. These include acute painful swellings of the lymph nodes. If the course is subacute, induration and decreasing tenderness occur. The site of the lymphadenitis depends on the primary site of the inflammatory disease. The lymph nodes may fluctuate if treatment is inadequate or the organisms are very virulent. Fluctuation and spontaneous perforation through the skin are possible.

Pathogenesis. The *first peak of frequency* is in children up to the age of 10 years and is usually due to nasopharyngeal infection; the *second frequency peak* is in adults between 50 and 70. In these older patients, the adenitis is often an expression of inflammation accompanying malignancy.

If a nonspecific lymphadenitis is found, a careful *topographic* search must be undertaken for the primary infection. The scalp, the auricle, the meatus, the naso- and oropharynx, the oral mucosa, and teeth must all be examined.

Note: The primary focus may already have resolved, but enlarged cervical lymph nodes may persist.

Diagnosis. The primary focus of infection is looked for in the area of drainage of the lymph nodes. The enlarged and fluctuant lymph nodes may be tender. The blood picture is typical of infection. *If there is any doubt, lymph node biopsy must be undertaken.*

Differential diagnosis. This includes metastatic carcinoma, Hodgkin's and non-Hodgkin's lymphoma, cervical cysts, tuberculous lymphadenopathy, toxoplasmosis, and Acquired Immune Deficiency Syndrome: AIDS (see Color Plate **38d**).

Treatment. Broad-spectrum antibiotics are administered. If an abscess forms, it should be incised and drained. Aspiration of the abscess is not adequate treatment. The wound may be sutured but a drain must be left in. A specimen of pus is taken for culture and sensitivity tests, and any tissue removed is submitted for histology.

Note: Nonspecific cervical lymphadenitis resolves after treatment of the primary infection. Occasionally, induration of the lymph nodes persists. Persistent or recurrent lymph node swellings are not compatible with a diagnosis of nonspecific lymphadenitis. This is also true of enlarged lymph nodes not lying in the correct site for the suspected site of origin. These cases require biopsy! A sinus follwing lymphadenitis suggests a diagnosis of tuberculosis, infected branchial cyst, lymph node tumors, fluctuating lymphadenitis in cat scratch fever, or tularemia. In these doubtful cases a lymph node must be removed for histology.
Cervical lymph node swelling is a leading symptom in AIDS.

Specific Lymphadenopathy

Tuberculous Lymphadenopathy

Symptoms. Any group of lymph nodes in the cervical region may be affected and in 20% of cases the disease is bilateral. The upper jugular, supraclavicular, and nuchal lymph nodes are most often involved today. This specific lymphadenopathy is painless or only slightly painful. The lesions may be solitary, multiple, small or large, firm or fluctuant. Often in addition to acute reactivated lymph nodes possibly with reddening of the skin and fluctuation, there may be fistulae or old retracted fistulous scars (see Color plate **37a**). Since cervical lymph nodes today usually present the site of *postprimary* disease, the symptoms of pulmonary tuberculosis such as cough, sputum, which may be bloodstained, or the symptoms of tuberculosis of other organs must be sought.

Pathogenesis. Apart from occasional endemic areas, primary *oropharyngeal* disease and regional lymphadenopathy, *primary complex,* are now very unusual in Western Europe and the United States as a result of elimination of bovine tuberculosis. Lymph node tuberculosis is currently mainly a postprimary hematogenous exacerbation, usually caused by human bacillae and occasionally atypical mycobacteria. The peak incidence has thus been displaced from childhood to later years, 20 to 45. The source of infection is patients with tuberculosis and apparently healthy tuberculin-positive subjects. In the German Federal Republic, 40% of the newly registered cases occur in foreign workers.

A relative increase of new reports is observed after the age of 65 years. Women are affected more often than men of the same age. These cases are almost always due to an exacerbation on an *old* specific lymph node focus (see Color Plate **37a**).

> *Note:* Calcification of lymph nodes is not an indication that they are healed. Bacillae may survive for decades in caseous and calcified centers of lymph nodes.

Diagnosis. Points to be looked for in the history include country of origin, a family history of tuberculosis, and visits to epidemic areas in Asia, Africa, and southeastern Europe. Soft tissue radiographs of the neck showing calcification of the lymph nodes are almost always pathognomonic. Radiographs are taken of the lungs, and an intracutaneous tuberculin test is done.

The diagnosis is confirmed by the histologic appearance of the excised lymph nodes and by microbiology.

Differential diagnosis. The diagnostic value of biopsy of a suspect lymph node is shown by the proportion of incorrect diagnoses in 1,000 lymph nodes excised for a suspected diagnosis of tuberculosis. In 13% tuberculosis was not found but the patient proved to have, in decreasing order of frequency, nonspecific lymphadenitis, branchial cyst, metastatic carcinoma, Hodgkin's disease, sialadenitis, salivary tumor, non-Hodgkin's lymphoma, neurinoma, nodular goiter, dermoid cysts, and salivary stone.

Treatment. *Antituberculous treatment* is conducted in cooperation with a chest physician or an internist. A combination of three drugs is usually used consisting of isoniazide, rifampicin, and ethambutol.

Streptomycin and dihydrostreptomycin often cause vestibular disturbances and ototoxicity and are not used routinely at present. At times a short course of therapy is used perioperatively to prevent spread of infection.

Surgery consisting of removal of specifically affected lymph nodes and invaded surrounding soft tissues and cervical skin is indicated for:

- Lymph nodes 2 cm or more in diameter which show no tendency to resolve further
- Lymph nodes with calcification
- Fluctuant lymph nodes
- Fistulae
- Collarstud abscess, involvement of the lymph nodes, soft tissue abscess, and involvement of the overlying skin

In many cases, particularly for a collarstud abscess, a conservative (modified) neck dissection (see p. 519) with reconstruction of the skin defect may be necessary. Tonsillectomy to eliminate a tuberculous primary focus has now become less important in the light of present-day knowledge of epidemiology and pathogenesis.

Syphilis. See p. 332.

If the primary chancre lies on the lips, mouth, tonsils, or facial area, an indolent regional lymphadenopathy appears 1 to 2 weeks after the primary focus. Multiple cervical lymphadenopathy may also occur in stage II syphilis. Stage III syphilis only rarely causes lymphadenopathy. *The disease is reportable.*

Sarcoidosis (Boeck's Disease)

Symptoms. The *lymphadenopathy* of sarcoidosis affects the mediastinal and supraclavicular nodes in 65% to 75% of cases, the peripheral nodes in 10% to 20% of cases, and the retroperitoneal nodes also. The *eyes, lacrimal glands, and salivary glands* are affected in 5% to 25% of cases. For Heerfordt's syndrome of uveoparotitis and facial paralysis, see p. 544. The *skin* is affected in 10% to 40% of cases by erythema nodosum or lupus pernio. The *mucous membranes* of the nose and sinuses, pharynx, larynx, trachea, mouth and esophagus demonstrate pale-red granular areas.

Pathogenesis. This disease of uncertain etiology is regarded as an epithelioid cell granulomatous reaction spreading in the reticulohistiocytic system.

Differential diagnosis. Distinguishing sarcoidosis tuberculosis may be very difficult and requires the services of an internist.

Diagnosis. Radiography shows disseminated shadows resembling miliary tuberculosis or bilateral butterfly hilar lymph node enlargement. The Kveim test is positive in 80% of cases, and the tuberculin test is negative or weakly positive.

A suspect lymph node should be removed for histology.

Biopsy of a supraclavicular node often combined with *mediastinoscopy* and histologic examination of any lymph nodes removed (see p. 518) is in many cases a great help to the internist.

Treatment. Steroids are given, monitored by an internist.

Cat Scratch Fever and Tularemia

Symptoms. The pustulous primary focus, which tends to ulcerate, occurs in the skin or oral mucosa. This is followed 1 to 5 weeks later by a regional painless or almost painless lymphadenopathy. In more than one third of cases, the lymph nodes fluctuate and a fistula forms.

Pathogenesis. *Cat scratch disease* is caused by the cat scratch virus which has not yet been isolated with certainty. Chlamydia has been implicated. In most cases the infection follows a scratch or a bite from a cat, but dogs, rodents, or hedgehogs may also be carriers.

Tularemia is caused by the Pasteurella tularensis named after the county of Tulare in California. The zoonosis is widespread in rodents, particularly in hares. It is transmitted by ticks and other biting insects.

Diagnosis. History shows contact with the animals named above. Histologic examination of the involved lymph node shows reticulocytic lymphadenitis with abscess formation, both in cat scratch disease and in tularemia. An intracutaneous test is available in cat scratch disease using the Mollaret-Debré antigen.

Treatment. The necessity for surgical treatment of tularemia may be deduced from the severity and type of the lymphadenopathy. Lymphadenopathies indeed tend to heal spontaneously. Tetracyclines are the treatment of choice for tularemia.

No specific treatment is available for cat scratch fever.

Reporting both these diseases is mandatory.

Toxoplasmosis

Symptoms. Patients with the *congenital form* may present with hydrocephalus, chorioretinitis, and intracerebral calcification. Deafness or deaf mutism may be observed in rare cases. *Acquired toxoplasmosis* causes in acute or subacute cases an influenza-like illness with subfebrile temperatures. The disease lasts 6 to 8 weeks. *An important symptom is lymphadenopathy especially affecting the nuchal nodes, periauricular nodes, jugulodigastric nodes, supraclavicular nodes, and rarely the axillary and inguinal nodes.* The *chronic form* in adults causes few characteristic symptoms but may cause headache or chronic eye disease. The *blood picture* shows marked lymphocytosis.

Abortion or stillbirth is possible if the mother is first infected during her pregnancy.

Pathogenesis. Infection in man by *Toxoplasma gondii* is mainly acquired orally by eating raw beef or pork but also by contact with feline feces. There is evidence of infection in a high proportion of the population as antibodies are found in up to 70% of clinically healthy people. The great majority of postnatal infections proceed without causing characteristic clinical symptoms.

Diagnosis. Changes in the titer, e. g., the Sabin-Feldman test, are interesting but can rarely be assessed because high titers, up to 1:64,000, have usually already been reached by the time the disease declares itself. This is also true of the indirect immunofluorescence test. The complement binding reaction is a valuable supplementary method and is always positive in titers up to 1:640 in acute cases. Toxoplasma should be suspected in fresh infections by a combination of a high Sabin-Feldman titer or high immunofluorescence titer up to 1:1,000 or higher with simultaneous complement binding titer of 1:10 and higher.

Histology of lymph nodes usually shows a *Piringer-Kuchinka syndrome,* i. e., an epithelioid cell lymph node reaction with no necrosis and argyrophil granules in the protoplasm of the reticulum cells. This is a subacute form of reaction manifest mainly in the cervical lymph nodes and is caused by a number of stimulating factors, above all *toxoplasmosis.*

Differential diagnosis. The above *serologic findings* particularly *in combination with lymph node biopsy are very characteristic* of toxoplasmosis. Lymphadenopathy with similar lymphocytic changes in the blood picture also occur in infectious lymphocytosis, rubella roseola infantum, and listeriosis. Similar findings occur in lymphadenopathies in response to antiepileptic drugs, antitoxins, some antibiotics and serum injections, in the drainage area of transplanted tissues, and in mononucleosis.

Treatment. See appropriate textbooks. The preferred regimen involves a combination of pyrimethamine and sulfonamides.

Lyme Disease

Symptoms. Symptoms begin with the lesions of erythema migrans and pain at the bite site with lymphadenitis. Variable organ involvement supervenes at 3−8 weeks. Peripheral facial palsy develops in 60% of cases. The late stage is dominated by neurologic symptoms such as meningopolyradiculitis.

Pathogenesis. The disease is caused by the bacterium *Borella burgdorferi,* transmitted mainly by the bite of the tick *Ixodes ricinus.*

Diagnosis. This is established by demonstrating specific antibodies in the blood and CSF.

Differential diagnosis. Differentiation is required from spring-summer meningoencephalitis.

Treatment. Treatment consists of large parenteral doses of penicillin or tetracycline.

Prognosis. The prognosis is favorable with treatment.

Trauma

Traffic accidents are the most important cause. Other causes include stabbings and bullet wounds. Injuries of the larynx are described on p. 409ff. and Color Plate **31a,** those of the trachea on p. 453, and those of the esophagus on p. 463ff.

Blunt trauma of the soft tissues leads, with varying degrees of rapidity, to swelling due to a hematoma, which may be pulsatile, and to surgical emphysema as a result of a defect of the continuity of the subglottis, the trachea, or the hypopharynx.

Blunt trauma due to steering wheel contusions or blows received in karate or boxing can cause sudden falls in blood pressure or asystole via the pressure receptors of the carotid sinus.

The cut throat of a *suicide attempt* usually passes through the trachea and only rarely through the more posterior contents of the carotid sheath which are protected by the sternocleidomastoid muscle.

Lesions of the *cervical nerves* may develop immediately or later due to scar tissue contracture.

Open injuries of the respiratory or digestive tracts are only slightly less dramatic than a tear of the carotid artery or internal jugular vein. The danger of opening of the large *veins* is *air embolus.* If the volume of the air embolus is greater than 10 to 20 ml the result is fatal. Embolus is treated by *immediate digital compression,* laying the patient flat, and transferring him to a hospital.

Carotid artery hemorrhages are usually fatal at the site of injury because of volume deficiency shock. They are treated by *immediate digital compression* and transferred to a hospital. A high proportion of the survivors of open injuries to the common and internal carotid artery show persistent cerebral defects.

The goals of management in the hospital consist of restoration of the circulating blood volume, reconstruction of the great vessels by direct suture, by replacement by autologous vein, e.g., the long saphenous vein, or at least temporary allogenic vascular prosthesis. Intraluminal shunts may be used during operations on the common and internal carotid artery to ensure the cerebral circulation. One late result of cervical vascular injury may be *arteriovenous fistulae* between the carotid artery and the internal jugular vein. More than 8% of all arteriovenous fistulae occur in the neck.

Congenital Anomalies

Lateral Branchial Fistulae and Cysts

Embryology. Between the 3rd and 4th weeks of embryonic life, five entodermal pharyngeal pouches develop in the lateral part of the *foregut.* Four ectodermal branchial grooves develop at corresponding sites on the external surface of the embryo. Five mesodermal branchial arches develop in man between these external and internal grooves. Each contains one cartilaginous bar, one branchial arch artery, one branchial arch nerve, and branchial arch musculature (Table 6.3). In the 6th week, the second arch grows over the third and fourth arches and fuses with the neighboring caudal precardial swelling. The *cervical sinus* is thus formed from the disappearing second, third, and fourth branchial grooves. At the same time the internal third, fourth, and fifth pharyngeal pouches disappear and form the *branchiogenic organs,* the parathyroids and the thymus. Normally the cervical sinus disappears completely. *Lateral branchial cervical fistulae* are caused by persistence of the external opening of the sinus. Persistent parts of the cervical sinus with obliteration of the external opening are said to cause *lateral branchial cervical cysts.*

Lateral Cervical Fistulae (see Color Plate **37d**)

Symptoms. The cutaneous fistula opening may periodically become red and swollen. In some cases there is a noninflamed skin pit. The opening of the fistula is always at the anterior border of the sternocleidomastoid muscle either at the level of the carotid triangle if it arises from the second branchial arch, at the level of the cricoid cartilage if it arises from the third branchial arch, or close of the suprasternal notch if it arises from the fourth arch. The discharge may be milky or purulent, recurrent, or persistent. In 5% of patients the fistula is bilateral.

Pathogenesis. The cause is genetic or external toxic factors during pregnancy, e.g., hypoxemia, hypercarbia, smoking, alcohol, aspirin, urethane, thalidomide, lead,

Table 6.3 Development of the Anlage of the Branchial Arches

First branchial arch, mandibular arch

Ectodermal. Skin of the cheek, mandible, anterior half of the auricle, external meatus, trigeminal nerve, parenchyma of the salivary glands, tooth enamel, epithelial covering of the lip, the tongue as far back as the foramen cecum, tympanic membrane

Mesodermal. Masticatory muscles, anterior belly of the digastric muscle, tensor tympani muscle, articular process of the mandible, malleus, incus, tragus, crus helicis, stratum fibrosum of the tympanic membrane

Entodermal. Epithelium of the floor and lateral surfaces of the mouth, eustachian tube, and mucosa of the tympanic membrane, middle ear cavity, and mastoid

Second branchial arch, hyoid bone

Ectodermal. Skin of the posterior surface of the auricle and of the upper part of the neck, parts of the VIIth and VIIIth cranial nerves

Mesodermal. Stapedius muscle, helix-anthelix, body of the hyoid bone

Entodermal. Epithelium of the base of the tongue, the foramen cecum, the central part of the thyroid gland, the palatine tonsil

Third branchial arch

Ectodermal. Skin of the central part of the neck, parts of the IXth cranial nerve

Mesodermal. Superior part of the pharyngeal constrictor muscle, common and internal carotid artery

Entodermal. Epithelium of the pharynx, base of the tongue, epiglottis, and piriform sinus

Fourth branchial arch

Ectodermal. Xth cranial nerve

Mesodermal. Inferior part of the pharyngeal constrictor muscle, laryngeal musculature, thyroid cartilage, parts of the epiglottis, right subclavian artery, aortic arch

Entodermal. Epithelium of the base of the tongue, pharyngeal epithelium, epiglottic epithelium, parts of the thyroid gland

Fifth branchial arch

Ectodermal. Skin of the lower part of the neck, XIth cranial nerve

Mesodermal. Laryngeal musculature, arytenoid and cricoid cartilages

Entodermal. Submucosal lymphoid tissue, lungs

mercury, metabolic disturbances, or irradiation leading to incomplete obliteration of the branchial groove or to persistence of the cervical sinus.

Diagnosis. A subcutaneous cord running superiorly is often palpable arising from the fistulous opening at the anterior edge of the sternocleidomastoid muscle. Secretion can usually be expelled from the fistula by stroking in a downward direction. Introduction of a contrast medium through the fistula shows the course and branches of the fistula. If the fistula is complete with a pharyngeal ostium, the contrast medium flows into the pharynx, and the patient can taste the contrast material.

Treatment. Recurrence from epithelial remnants can only be prevented by complete excision of the fistula. *Complete dissection is made easier by the use of a binocular loupe or microscope and by injecting dye into the fistula.*

Note: The surgeon must bear in mind the variable course of a lateral cervical fistula. The most common fistulae from the second branchial arch run through the carotid bifurcation, the tonsillopharyngeal duct, whereas inferior fistulae run superiorly behind the common carotid artery, the thymopharyngeal duct.

Lateral Cervical Cysts

Symptoms. Although the anlage is congenital, these cysts are mainly noticed during childhood or early adulthood. The cyst is firm, elastic, and fluctuant but may also be fixed as a result of infection. It is usually oval, with a diameter of about 5 cm. Over the course of years, very large cystic sacs may form in patients not concerned with their health. Epipleural or mediastinal branchial cysts arising from the fifth branchial arch system may also be found rarely. Secondary infection may cause severe pain with inflammation of the overlying skin. Bilateral branchial cysts are very uncommon.

Pathogenesis. The supposition that these cysts are branchial arch rudiments is still regarded as likely, although a lymph node origin is also discussed (cystic structures formed by inswept epithelial debris).

Diagnosis. This rests on the history, palpable findings, ultrasound findings, and the site which is usually the carotid triangle (see Color Plate **37c**). In doubtful cases, the cyst may be aspirated which produces greenish-yellow stringy secretion. The cyst may then be filled with a contrast medium.

Treatment. The cyst is completely excised.

Note: Epithelial cysts may undergo malignant degeneration, but this is exceedingly rare. The diagnosis of *branchiogenic carcinoma* delays the search for an occult primary tumor. Almost without exception, malignant lymph node metastases are due to an as yet undisclosed primary tumor mainly in the clinically "silent" regions of the naso-, oro-, or hypopharynx and the thyroid gland. Bronchial carcinoma, breast carcinoma, and abdominal malignancy may also metastasize via the bloodstream to cervical lymph nodes.

Thyroglossal Duct Cysts and Fistulae

Symptoms. A firm elastic swelling the size of a cherry or an apple is found in the midline of the neck at the level of, above, or below the hyoid bone (see Color Plate **37b**).

The patient may have a globus sensation and complain of the cosmetic appearances. If a fistula is present its external opening is often inflamed.

Pathogenesis. *Thyroglossal cysts* are remnants of the thyroglossal duct.

Median cervical fistulae may be caused by perforation of the thyroglossal duct through the skin, by spontaneous perforation of median thyroglossal cysts due to infection, or by surgery.

Diagnosis. This is based on the typical site. *The cyst or fistula moves up and down when the patient swallows.* A probe may be introduced into a fistula as far as the body of the hyoid bone. The lesion can be delineated by ultrasound.

Differential diagnosis. This includes tumors of the pyramidal lobe of the thyroid gland, ectopic thyroid tissue, inflammatory or malignant lymphadenopathy, and submental dermoid cyst.

Treatment. The cyst or the fistula is removed. *It is essential to remove the body of the hyoid bone to prevent recurrence since it contains epithelial rests.* Careful hemostasis and drainage are particularly important since oozing of blood and postoperative swelling may lead to acute laryngeal obstruction and suffocation.

Musculoskeletal Defects

Klippel-Feil Syndrome

This is a congenital synostosis of the cervical spine often accompanied by a high spina bifida. The ears are set low on the head, and the patient may have a hearing defect or be totally deaf.

Goldenhar Syndrome

This is fusion or absence of a cervical vertebra, auricular tags and middle ear anomalies, occasional unilateral hypoplasia or aplasia of the ascending ramus of the mandible, a coloboma of the iris, and an epibulbar dermoid.

Cervical Rib, Costoclavicular Compression Syndrome, and Naffziger Syndrome

About 1% of the population have a cervical rib, usually arising from the seventh vertebra. Only about 10% of these cause symptoms, mainly compression of the brachial plexus or of the subclavian artery and vein: the thoracic outlet compression syndrome. Other manifestations include circulatory disorders of the forearm and hand, brachialgia, paralysis of the brachial plexus, intermittent cerebral ischemia with attacks of vertigo, occipital headache, and double vision. Surgery is only undertaken when conservative measures fail and especially for severe neurologic signs or intermittent venous thrombosis. Treatment consists of division of the scalenus anterior muscle or resection of the cervical rib.

Tumors

Vascular Tumors

Hemangiomas

Symptoms. The commonest site of predilection is the face and the nape of the neck. The symmetrical median nevus flammeus (capillary hemangioma) sometimes causes cosmetic difficulty. The asymmetrical hemangiomas are often combined with other anomalies, e.g., a Sturge-Weber syndrome, the Klippel-Trénaunay syndrome. They tend to bleed spontaneously and in response to slight trauma.

Pathogenesis. Two thirds of these are cutaneous hemangiomas which are evident at birth. The remainder lie subcutaneously or deeper with a particular tendency to penetrate the masseter muscle. They are mainly flat hemangiomas which grow rapidly in the first months of life but tend to atrophy spontaneously. If they do not atrophy, they are dealt with *surgically* in one or more stages.

Lymphangioma (Cystic Hygroma)

Symptoms. Cystic hygromas usually lie on the lateral part of the neck. They may be so large as to occupy the entire lateral part of the neck and cause stridor, cyanosis, and dysphagia due to displacement of cervical viscera. They may also cause difficulty in birth due to their size. Large hygromas cause torticollis. They may also cause a parotid swelling since a lymphangioma is the most common parotid tumor in the newborn and infants after hemangioma.

Pathogenesis. The capillary, cavernous, and cystic lymphangiomas are sequestrated parts of the embryonal lymphatic vascular anlage.

Diagnosis. This is made on the presence of a compressible swelling containing lymph, usually in the lateral cervical area but also in the parotid area.

Differential diagnosis. This includes hemangioma, branchial cyst, and solid or cystic congenital teratoma (dermoid cyst).

Treatment. Spontaneous remission is very uncommon. Aspiration is helpful if the patient is threatened with suffocation. The cystic hygroma is usually multilocular and radioresistant. *The treatment of choice is removal in one or more stages with preservation of vital structures and nerves.*

Aneurysms

Symptoms. A pulsating cervical swelling ("pseudotumors") causing a hissing noise on auscultation usually lies anterior to the sternocleidomastoid muscle. It may also be visible and palpable in the parapharyngeal area depending on its site and growth propensity.

Pathogenesis. The cause is rarely birth trauma or congenital anomalies. Acquired aneurysms are usually due to trauma or syphilis.

Diagnosis. This depends on palpation and auscultation of the neck and oropharynx.

The diagnosis can be established by angiography and by ultrasound.

Treatment. Vascular surgery is performed when indicated.

Malignant vascular tumors in the neck include the very uncommon *angiosarcoma* and the more frequent *hemangiopericytoma*. The prognosis is poor because they are usually not resectable, tend to recur, and metastasize. They are resistant to radiotherapy and chemotherapy.

Carotid Body Tumor (Chemodectoma) (see Fig. 6.**17**)

Symptoms. The tumor is usually a painless and well-defined swelling located in the carotid triangle. It grows slowly and causes no symptoms in about 70% of cases. It may cause a feeling of globus or dysphagia. About 20% of patients have Horner's syndrome. The carotid sinus syndrome includes *vertigo, tinnitus, and attacks of sweating* in about 2% of cases, particularly on turning the head. It is bilateral in 2% to 5% of patients.

Pathogenesis. The tumor of the carotid body consists of precapillary arteriovenous connections and contains a collection of chemoreceptor nonchromaffin paraganglion cells. These cells belong to a group of similar appearance in the area of distribution of the vagus and glossopharyngeal nerves: the tympanic, jugular (see p. 127), vagal, or periaortic glomus. The tumor may grow around the external or internal

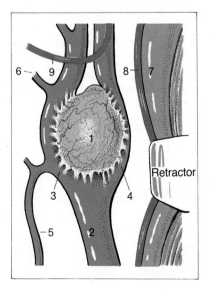

Fig. 6.**17**   The carotid body tumor and its anatomic relations. 1, Tumor of the carotid body; 2, common carotid artery; 3, external carotid artery; 4, internal carotid artery, here compressed by tumor; 5, superior thyroid artery; 6, lingual artery; 7, internal jugular vein; 8, vagus nerve; 9, hypoglossal nerve.

carotid artery and narrow it. Hypertrophy of the carotid body is observed significantly more often in persons living continuously at heights of more than 3,000 m, e.g., in Peru and Mexico City, and therefore subject to chronic oxygen deficiency. Malignant change or metastases develop in 1% to 10% of patients.

Diagnosis. All too often this tumor is only diagnosed during operation since it is not considered in the preoperative differential diagnosis. It is compressible, but *it can only be moved from side to side.* It does not move on swallowing. Auscultation occasionally shows a vascular bruit. The lateral pharyngeal wall must always be examined since the pulsating tumor can often be recognized and felt at that point beneath an intact mucosa. *Carotid angiography* is definitive, and subtraction techniques are particularly helpful since they determine the surgical strategy. Displacement of the internal and external carotid arteries by the very vascular tumor produces a typical "egg-shaped" splaying of the carotid bifurcation. The tumor can be delineated by ultrasound, CT, and MRI.

Note: Biopsy is contraindicated because of the severe danger of bleeding.

Differential diagnosis. This includes aneurysms, branchial cysts, neurogenic cervical tumors, lymph node metastases, and Hodgkin's and non-Hodgkin's lymphoma.

Treatment. The carotid body tumor is radioresistant and should be treated surgically since its future growth cannot be predicted. Tumors in persons over 60 years which are not causing symptoms should be left alone. Surgery for this tumor requires extensive experience in head and neck and vascular surgery. The technique depends on the fact that the tumor develops within the adventitia and can therefore be freed from the tunica media by careful dissection. Preoperative embolization is advised.

Postoperative neurologic deficits occur in 50% or more of cases if the common or internal carotid artery must be resected or if these vessels are damaged during dissection. A vascular prosthesis and blood for transfusion must always be ready during this procedure. Advances in vascular surgery have reduced the incidence of neurologic deficits and death. Embolization significantly reduces intraoperative bleeding and is routinely advised prior to the surgery.

Neurogenic Tumors

Neurogenic tumors occur relatively often in the neck. They arise either from the autonomic nervous system or from the sheaths of peripheral nerves. *Neurofibromas* and *schwannomas* arise from the Schwann cells of the peripheral nerves.

Von Recklinghausen's disease is a generalized *neurofibromatosis*. Solitary tumors are unusual. Twenty-five percent of all schwannomas occur in the head, acoustic neurinoma, and in the neck. The lesions in the neck arise from the sheaths of the glossopharyngeal, accessory, and hypoglossal nerves. *The most frequent site of origin is the vagus nerve* and these lesions are known as parapharyngeal neurilemmomas.

Schwannomas are firm to palpation which usually causes fairly severe pain. Their size varies from several millimeters to 20 cm. They are solitary *tumors mobile only in the horizontal plane when they arise from the vagus nerve.* They grow slowly and only rarely cause neurologic defects.

The definitive *diagnosis* is provided by histology of tissue removed at operation if necessary. The *differential diagnosis* includes paraganglioma, lymphoma, and metastases.

The rare *malignant neurogenic tumors* such as neurilemmosarcoma and sympathicoblastoma lead to symptoms arising from neighboring organs such as otalgia, dysphagia, and Horner's syndrome.

Note: An amputation neuroma must be excised to exclude persistent or recurrent tumor at the edge of the operative field.

Torticollis

Symptoms. Typically the head and neck are held to the diseased side and the chin is turned to the healthy side. It is almost always unilateral.

Pathogenesis. *Muscular* torticollis is the most common. In congenital torticollis it is assumed that there was intrauterine damage or birth trauma causing a muscle tear or hematoma so that the sternocleidomastoid muscle is shortened by fibrosis of the muscle.

All forms of torticollis in early childhood, if untreated, cause damage to the growth of the face and the base of the skull or scoliosis of the cervical spine. Congenital *bony* anomalies of the cervical spine can also cause torticollis.

Diagnosis. In muscular torticollis the sternocleidomastoid muscle is thickened, usually in its lower third, and is hard and tender. It is noticed several days or weeks after birth by the increasingly obvious incorrect position of the head.

Differential diagnosis. See Table 6.4.

Treatment. Congenital muscular torticollis should be treated before the beginning of the 2nd year of life *at the latest* if it has not undergone spontaneous remission or if conservative orthopedic measures have been unsuccessful. Several forms of tenotomy and plastic elongation of the sternocleidomastoid muscle are possible.

Cervical Lipoma

Symptoms. Simple *lipomas* may arise in all parts of the neck and may be solitary or multiple. They are subcutaneous, grow slowly, are clinically and histologically benign, and cause few symptoms. They are often removed for cosmetic reasons.

The *fatty neck* affects mainly the nuchal region. The fatty deposits may attain a great size so that the patient has to hold his head forward. The tumors of the neck are typically occipital and notched in the midline. There may be coexisting lipomas on the trunk.

Table 6.4 Torticollis	
Causes:	
Muscular	Inflammatory or cicatricial lesions, neoplastic infiltration of the sternocleidomastoid muscle and the overlying skin
	Removal of the sternocleidomastoid muscle, e. g., in radical neck dissection
	Paralysis of the accessory nerve
	Rheumatic torticollis, myogelosis
	Progressive myositis ossificans
	Neuralgic-neurovascular symptom complex in the scalene syndrome
Osseous	Atlantoepistrophealis torticollis due to inflammation radiotherapy or operations on the nasopharynx, (Grisel syndrome)
	Subluxation of a verterba due to trauma
Symptomatic	Ocular-reflex torticollis in compensation for unilateral lesions of the ocular muscles
	Stiffness of the neck in peritonsillar, retrotonsillar, or parapharyngeal abscesses
	Acute and subacute cervical inflammatory lymphadenopathy
	Otitis externa and media, particularly Bezold's mastoiditis
	Unilateral labyrinthine disorders
Psychogenetic-neurotic	

Anterior *lipomatosis* often begins as a double chin, grows slowly downward in the neck, and tends to infiltrate the muscles. It appears to affect men more frequently and it is also more common in alcoholics and is found more regularly in persons in certain occupations such as those working in the asphalt, rubber, or plastics industries. Removal in one or more stages is indicated because of inability to hold the head in the correct position and interference with function.

The malignant *liposarcoma* occurs only rarely in the head and neck.

Myogenic Tumors

The *benign leiomyoma and malignant leiomyosarcoma* may arise in the neck both from superficial and from deep smooth muscle.

Thorotrastoma with late malignant change is nowadays seldom seen since thorotrast (contrast medium) has not been used for several decades.

Neoplastic Lymphadenopathy

About 50% of nonthyroid swellings in the neck are due to enlarged lymph nodes. About 40% of the enlarged nodes are metastatic carcinomas. These are followed in frequency by malignant lymphomas and Hodgkin's disease.

Benign Lymph Node Tumors

These are very uncommon. The *localized benign lymphoma* occurs as a slowly growing lymph node tumor. Treatment consists of excision of the affected lymph nodes for biopsy.

Malignant Lymph Node Tumors

The great significance of malignant lymphomas for the general practitioner and the otolaryngologist lies in the fact that the early manifestations are present in a high proportion of cases in the cervical lymph nodes or occasionally in the mucosa of the upper aerodigestive tract. Biopsy of a lymph node or of suspicious mucosa is therefore *essential* for making an *early diagnosis* and in determining *treatment* of this malignant disease.

> *Note:* Histologic examination of affected lymph nodes including the supraclavicular nodes should be one of the *first* diagnostic steps in many cases since much time may thereby be saved.

Hodgkin's Disease

Symptoms. The generalized symptoms are often not very typical and consist of fatigue and generalized itching. Weight loss, night sweats, and fever are of prognostic and therapeutic significance.

The disease is usually localized initially but tends to metastasize. At the time of diagnosis, the cervical lymph nodes are affected in 70% ($\pm$10%) of patients. In about 10% of patients there is primary extranodal disease affecting the naso- or oropharynx, the gastrointestinal tract, the skin, or the skeleton. The *affected lymph nodes* are indolent, firm, usually mobile, and tend to occur in groups. Pain is often noticed in these lymph nodes after ingestion of alcohol. Spontaneous fluctuation in size is observed fairly commonly and can lead to an incorrect diagnosis.

Diagnosis. This depends on histologic examination of suspect lymph nodes or mucosa, biopsy of supraclavicular nodes, and mediastinoscopy. There are several different histologic types: lymphocyte predominant and nodular sclerosing which are prognostically favorable and mixed types and lympho-cytic-depleted types which have a poor prognosis. Imaging studies include isotope organ scans, ultrasound, CT, and MRI. Bone marrow aspiration with histologic examination and hematologic and laboratory investigations complete the workup.

Treatment. This depends on the histologic type and staging. Radiotherapy predominates for stages I to IIIA and chemotherapy for stages IIIB to IV.

Prognosis. The outlook has improved in the last two decades for all stages. There are correlations between the histologic picture, including cytochemical and histochemical findings, the therapeutic response, and survival rates.

Non-Hodgkin's Lymphoma

This term includes a number of lymphoreticular malignant tumors which must be distinguished clinically and morphologically from Hodgkin's disease. Their classification (Table 6.5) is important in treatment and prognosis.

Chronic lymphatic leukemia also belongs to this group of diseases.

Symptoms. Malignant lymphadenopathy most commonly in the neck, in up to 80% of cases, and extranodal manifestations in the nasopharynx, oropharynx, nose, and nasal sinuses are the most obvious manifestations. In addition to these local findings, there are also generalized radiographic, hematologic, and abnormal laboratory findings. There is a marked tendency to develop systemic disease.

Pathogenesis. Non-Hodgkin's lymphomas usually arise from the B-cell system. They are classified as neoplasms of the cells of the immune system. These tumors may have a viral etiology (see Table 6.5).

Diagnosis. The morphological classification of *excised lymph nodes* or *extranodal tissue* with respect to immunologic characteristics is the basis for tumor classification. As in Hodgkin's disease the main function of the ear, nose, and throat surgeon is early removal of suspect lymph nodes and biopsy of extranodal foci in the nasopharynx, oropharynx, nose, or sinuses.

Treatment. This usually consists of combinations of radiation and chemotherapy given in cooperation with the oncologist.

Prognosis. Patients with involvement of one lymph node group have a considerably better prognosis than those with primary extranodular mucosal or organ disease.

Lymph Node Metastases

Carcinomatous cells reach the peripheral sinus and then the trabeculae and medullary sinus of the lymph nodes via the afferent vessels.

There is reason to believe that the cytotoxic potency of the lymph node resistance, demonstrated histologically by the premetastatic changes of the parenchyma, is

Table 6.5 Entities of the Kiel classification and their equivalents in two American classifications of Non-Hodgkin's Lymphomas

Kiel classification	Lukes and Collins (1974)	Rappaport (1966)
Low-grade malignant lymphomas		
Lymphocytic		ML, lymphocytic, well differentiated, diffuse
B-CLL	B cell type, small lymphocyte (CLL)	
T-CLL		
Hairy-cell leukaemia		
Mycosis fungoides and Sézary's syndrome	T cell type, mycosis fungoides and Sézary's syndrome	
T-zone lymphoma	T cell type, immunoblastic sarcoma of T cells	
Lymphoplasmacytic/-cytoid (LP immunocytoma)	B cell type, plasmacytoid lymphocyte	ML, lymphocytic with dysproteinemia
Plasmacytic	–	–
Centrocytic	B cell type, FCC types (follicular, diffuse, follicular and diffuse, and sclerotic)	ML, lymphocytic, well differentiated, nodular or diffuse / ML, lymphocytic, poorly differentiated, nodular or diffuse
Centroblastic-centrocytic follicular ± diffuse diffuse ± sclerosis	{ small cleaved / large cleaved }	ML, lymphocytic, well differentiated / ML, lymphocytic, poorly differentiated } nodular or diffuse / ML, mixed (lymphocytic-histiocytic) / ML, histiocytic

Table 6.5 Continuation

Kiel classification	Lukes and Collins (1974)	Rappaport (1966)
High-grade malignant lymphomas		
Centroblastic	large noncleaved	{ ML, histiocytic, nodular or diffuse { ML, undifferentiated, nodular or diffuse
Lymphoblastic	small noncleaved T cell type, convoluted lymphocyte U cell (undefined cell type)	{ ML, undifferentiated, diffuse { ML, lymphocytic, poorly differentiated, diffuse

Burkitt type
convoluted-cell type
unclassified
	B cell type, immunoblastic sarcoma
	    of B cells
	T cell type, immunoblastic sarcoma
	    of T cells	

Immunoblastic		ML, histiocytic, diffuse

only maintained for a limited period. Once this resistance is overcome, the malignant cells multiply initially in the lymph node segments and then diffusely within the node. *Malignant infiltration of the capsule causes loss of mobility of the lymph nodes and adherence to surrounding tissue. The prognosis then becomes much worse* (see Table 4.**10**). The primary orthograde lymph flow containing malignant cells can flow in a retrograde direction or irregularly when the lymph nodes are obstructed. The practical effect of this is that metastases may spring up in distant lymph node groups, on the other side of the neck, or in extranodal tissue.

The regional lymph node status in patients with a tumor is recorded before treatment according to the Union Internationale Contré le Cancer (UICC) classification:

N_0 = regional lymph nodes are not palpable
N_1 = mobile, homolateral enlarged lymph nodes are present
N_2 = mobile, bilateral, or contralateral enlarged lymph nodes are present
N_3 = fixed lymph nodes are present

Further subdivisions are provided by the letter *a,* which indicates that no clinical metastases are suspected, or *b,* which indicates that metastases are suspected.

Histologic findings complement the clinical status using the symbol "-" indicating no metastases or " + " indicating histologically confirmed metastases.

The complete *TNM* classification of the tumor allows division into *stages* I to IV (Fig. 6.**18**).

The lymph nodes are placed in the lymphatic drainage area of a tumor to function as a *mechanical filter and immunologic barrier.* Important parameters of the frequency of lymph node metastases include: the histologic characteristics of the tumor, the richness of the capillary lymphatic network at the site of the tumor, delay in diagnosis, the size of the tumor, the patient's total immunologic resistance, the mobility of the organ, e. g., the oropharynx or the hypopharynx, and the stability of the tumor area.

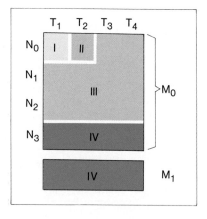

Fig. 6.**18** Stage grouping (roman numerals) based on the *TNM* classification for malignant tumors.

Table 6.6 Frequency of Clinical Lymph Node Enlargement (N_{1-3}) in Head and Neck Carcinoma at the Time of Diagnosis

Organ	%
Hypopharynx	65
Oropharynx	60
Nasopharynx	60
Oral cavity	40
Salivary glands	25
Larynx, depending on the site	0–60
Skin	15
Nose and nasal sinuses	10

The cervical lymph nodes may be affected by metastases from any primary tumor in the head and neck. Most common are initial metastases to the appropriate first regional lymph node groups. A *contralateral* metastasis is present in about 20% of carcinomas of the head and neck at the time of diagnosis (Table 6.**6**).

Bilateral cervical lymph node metastases are to be expected in midline tumors, e.g., those of the nasopharynx, base of the tongue, palate, and postcricoid region and in advanced tumors.

Typical sites of metastases are shown in Figure 6.**19a–h**.

Palpation of a lymph node does not provide *entirely reliable information* about invasion by metastases. Histologic examination has shown that about 30% of enlarged lymph nodes are free of tumor, whereas clinically nonpalpable lymph nodes contain carcinoma in 50% of patients. Fixed lymph nodes almost always contain tumor.

Note: The presence of lymph node metastases reduces the 5-year survival rate considerably, and the presence of fixed metastases reduces the chance of survival markedly.

Virchow's node can be seen or felt in the supraclavicular fossa on the left side at the site of entry of the thoracic duct into the angle between the internal jugular vein and the subclavian vein. Metastasis to the supraclavicular prescalene lymph nodes is a contraindication to surgery for abdominal, gynecologic, or thoracic malignancy.

The lymph of the neck usually passes through three lymph node stations before it reaches the venous circulation.

The methods of surgical treatment of lymph node metastases play a dominant part in surgery of this area.

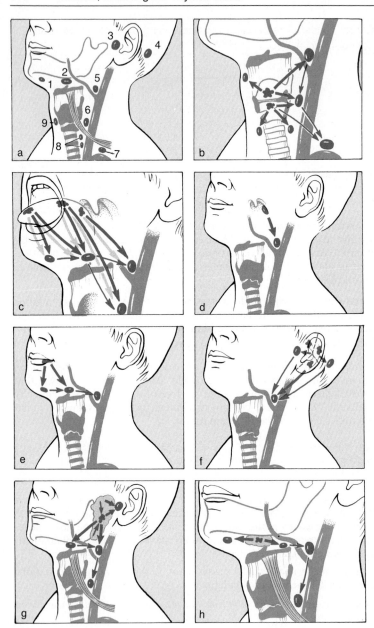

Principles of Surgery

Prescalene Node Biopsy

The lymph nodes lying in the prescalene fatty tissue anterior to the scalanus anterior muscle and in the omoclavicular triangle are of great clinical and diagnostic importance *even if they are not palpable*. Because of the central position of these lymph nodes in the entire lymphatic system, their histologic examination provides early information about the extension of malignant and inflammatory diseases. Numerically the highest proportion of positive results, about 80%, is achieved by biopsy of these lymph nodes in sarcoidosis. When epithelioid cell foci of sarcoid are found in the scalene muscles, this differentiates the lesion from tuberculosis.

About 60% positive results are obtained in Hodgkin's and non-Hodgkin's lymphoma, and between 10% and 40% of positive metastases are found in bronchial, abdominal, and gynecologic carcinomas.

Technique (Fig. 6.**20a** and **b**). The operation may be carried out under local anesthetic. A horizontal incision 3 to 4 cm long is made above the clavicle. After dividing the platysma, the posterior border of the sternocleidomastoid muscle is retracted medially and the inferior belly of the omohyoid muscle is retracted laterally and superiorly. The operative field is the prescalene omoclavicular triangle lying between the internal jugular vein, the subclavian vein, and the omohyoid muscle.

The prescalene fat pad is excised preserving the phrenic nerve and the contents of the carotid sheath, and the 8 to 15 lymph nodes are excised. This simplifies histologic examination of the nodes.

◀ Fig. 6.**19a–h**   **(a)** Typical sites of regional lymph node metastases. 1, Submental lymph nodes; 2, submandibular lymph nodes; 3, parotid and preauricular lymph nodes; 4, retroauricular lymph nodes; 5, lymph nodes of the jugulofacial venous angle; 6, deep cervical lymph nodes; 7, lymph nodes in the juguloclavicular venous angle: lower deep cervical lymph nodes and supraclavicular lymph nodes; 8, pre- and peritracheal lymph nodes; 9, prelaryngeal lymph nodes. **(b)** Laryngeal carcinoma, see Fig. 4.4, p. 393; **(c)** carcinoma of different parts of the tongue. Note the tendency to contralateral metastases. **(d)** Tonsillar carcinoma; **(e)** lower lip carcinoma; **(f)** carcinoma of the external ear. Note the segmental lymphatic efferent from the auricle. **(g)** Parotid carcinoma (note the intraglandular lymph node metastases); **(h)** submandibular gland carcinoma.

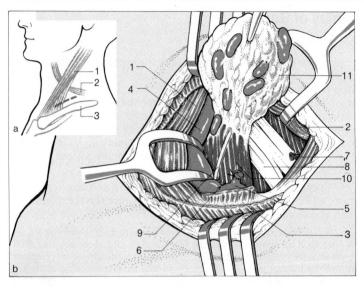

Fig. 6.**20a** and **b** Prescalene lymph node biopsy, Daniels operation. **a.** Incision and limits of dissection: border of the clavicle, omohyoid muscle, jugulosubclavian venous angle covered by the sternocleidomastoid muscle. **b.** Intraoperative appearance. 1, Sterno-cleidomastoid muscle; 2, inferior belly of the omohyoid muscle; 3, clavicle; 4, internal jugular vein; 5, subclavian vein; 6, jugulosubclavian venous angle; 7, transverse cervical artery, divided; 8, brachial plexus; 9, phrenic nerve; 10, scalene muscles; 11, presca-lene fat pad with lymph nodes.

Mediastinoscopy

Mediastinoscopy, especially combined with prescalene biopsy, is an important complement to modern imaging procedures for diagnosis of lymphadenopathy of the intrathoracic, especially the mediastinal, lymph nodes. The entire upper and paratracheal part of the superior mediastinum as far as the origin of both upper lobe bronchi can be examined. Occasionally even the pericardium lying beyond the bifurcation, when one is looking for cysts, thymomas, teratomas, intrathoracic goiters, and pneumoconioses, can be *visualized*. Of special value, however, is the ability to take a *biopsy* of paratracheal, tracheobronchial, and bronchopulmonary lymph nodes.

Indications for this procedure consist of: (1) the establishment of histologic diagnosis of metastatic carcinoma, Hodgkin's and non-Hodgkin's lymphoma, or sarcoid and tuberculous lymphadenopathy and (2) the assessment of operability of bronchial and esophageal carcinoma.

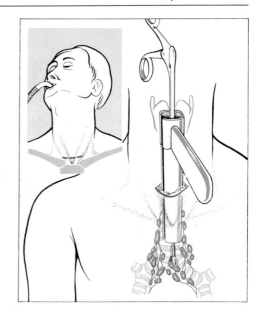

Fig. 6.**21** Mediastinoscopy, Carlens, under endotracheal anesthesia. Skin incision. Mediastinoscope with biopsy forceps.

Technique (Fig. 6.**21**). Intubation anesthesia is necessary. A 4-cm horizontal skin incision is made 2 cm above the suprasternal notch. The trachea is exposed as in tracheotomy taking care to identify and divide the pretracheal fascia horizontally.

The mediastinoscope is inserted into a pocket created by finger dissection *under* the pretracheal fascia and is pushed inferiorly along the anterior tracheal wall as far as the carina. *Needle aspiration must be carried out before a biopsy is taken to avoid serious hemorrhage* which can require thoracotomy, although this is uncommon. Further uncommon complications include recurrent nerve paralysis and pneumothorax.

The *treatment of choice* for malignant cervical lymph node metastases in head and neck malignancy is radical neck dissection (Fig. 6.**22a** and **b**). The results of radiotherapy for malignant lymph node metastases are inferior to those of surgery.

Neck Dissection

The *radical curative* neck dissection is the classic operation for confirmed extensive lymph node metastases.

The upper *boundary of the operation* is the base of the skull and the lower bondary lies at the level of the clavicle and includes the prescalene lymph node groups in the angle between the internal jugular vein and the subclavian vein. The sternocleido-

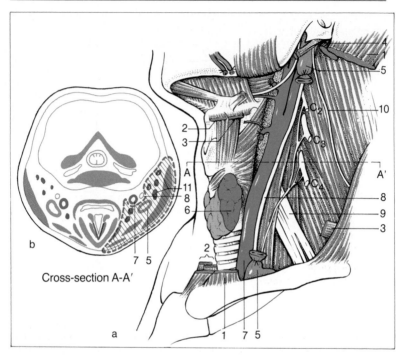

Fig. 6.**22a** and **b**   Appearance after radical neck dissection. **a.** Situation after removal of: 1, sternocleidomastoid muscle; 2, infrahyoid muscles; 3, omohyoid muscle, divided; 4, digastric muscle and stylohyoid muscle, divided; 5, stumps of the internal jugular vein; 6, partial resection of the thyroid gland. The following are retained: 7, carotid artery (the *external* carotid artery may need to be resected depending on the extent of the tumor); 8, vagus nerve; 9, brachial plexus; 10, accessory nerve (may be preserved if the accessory chain of nodes is not affected). **b.** Equivalent cross-section through the neck. The resected area between the deep and superficial cervical fascia is shown by the hatched area, plane at A-A'; 11, cervical lymph node metastases.

mastoid muscle, the internal jugular vein, and if necessary the external carotid artery are removed.

The common and internal carotid arteries are preserved though increasing experience of vascular surgery indicates that it may be possible to replace these vessels. If bilateral metastases are present, dissection of the less severely affected side can generally be performed concurrently or may be deferred for 4–6 weeks if a compelling reason exists. The vertebral venous plexus (see Fig. 6.**7**) is capable of assuring collateral cranial venous drainage after resection of one or both internal jugular veins.

Variations of the operation, e. g. for small carcinomas of the lip and the tip of the tongue, are possible in which removal of lymph nodes is restricted to the submental, submandibular, and jugulodigastric area. This is the suprahyoid neck dissection.

The goal of neck dissection is complete removal of lymph nodes and vessels between the superficial and deep cervical fascia. Depending on the site of the primary tumor, the submental, submandibular, pre- and postauricular, parotid, jugular, supraclavicular, and accessory nerve chain of nodes are removed en bloc with the fatty and connective tissue of the neck in which the lymph nodes and lymph vessels are embedded. The operative field is exposed widely by a suitable H- or Y-shaped skin incision. The incision must be made so that the blood supply of the skin is preserved to prevent flap necrosis and to ensure that the carotid arteries are protected by the flap.

The *modified neck dissection* preserves the sternocleidomastoid muscle, the internal jugular vein, the accessory nerve, and other functionally significant soft tissue structures of the neck. The decision to carry out this operation requires care. *Elective* resections of lymph node groups also may be indicated according to the oncologic situation of the primary tumor.

Prerequisites for all forms of neck *dissection* are:

- Absence of distant metastases
- Previous or simultaneous *complete removal of the primary tumor*
- Good general condition

Note: The isolated removal of lymph node metastases is contraindicated since this does not deal with the cervical metastatic pathways so that the danger of retrograde, irregular, and contralateral metastases increases.

Thyroid Gland and Otorhinolaryngology

Topographic Anatomy

The normal thyroid gland covers the lower lateral part of the thyroid cartilage on both sides. Its isthmus lies on the cricoid cartilage and the upper tracheal rings. The lobes grasp the upper cervical trachea and the thyroid cartilage to a varying extent. Fibrous connections of the gland to the cricoid and thyroid cartilage and to the upper tracheal ring explain the movement of the thyroid gland which accompanies all movement of the larynx, particularly on swallowing. A thyroid gland of normal size is not visible externally.

Often a pyramidal process is present as a remnant of the thyroglossal duct leading from the isthmus to the hyoid bone. The terms high, middle, and low tracheotomy derive from the relation of the thyroid isthmus to the tracheotomy opening (see Fig. 4.**36a**).

Note: Ear, nose, and throat symptoms caused by disease of the thyroid gland may or may not be accompanied by visible enlargement of the gland. The macroscopic findings do not reflect the function of the thyroid gland although functional disorders often accompany the formation of a goiter.

The superior thyroid artery arises from the external carotid artery and arches inferiorly to penetrate the upper pole of the gland. Shortly after its origin from the external carotid artery, the superior thyroid artery lies in fairly close relation at the level of this curve to the external branch of the superior laryngeal nerve.

The inferior thyroid arteries arise from the thyrocervical trunk, bend medially at the level of the sixth cervical vertebra, and reach the lower pole of the thyroid gland after dividing into two and occasionally more branches. The recurrent laryngeal nerves run on both sides close to the inferior thyroid artery or its branches in the region of the lower pole of the thyroid gland. More than 25 anatomic variations of the relation between the nerve and the artery have been described. However, in 25% of patients the recurrent nerve runs *anterior* to the artery, in 35% *posterior* to the artery, and in 35% *between* the branches of the artery.

Knowledge of the relations between the artery and nerve is absolutely necessary to avoid unilateral or bilateral vocal cord paralysis during operations on the thyroid gland.

On the average, a unilateral immediate vocal cord paralysis is seen in 3% of patients after *first operations* on the thyroid gland. A proportion recover spontaneously provided the nerve has not been divided. Bilateral recurrent nerve paralyses are uncommon at the first operation but are *more common at secondary operations*. The incidence in the latter case is between 7% and 10%.

Function. The thyroid gland produces two hormones, thyroxine, T_4, and triiodothyronine, T_3, in which the iodine is bound to the amino acid tyrosine. The hormone is mainly bound in follicular colloid and stored as thyroglobulin. The hormone reserves are sufficient for about 2 months. This compensates changing intake of iodine and changing biological requirements. The hormone secretion is activated by proteolytic enzymes of the thyroid-stimulating hormone (TSH), thyrotropin-releasing hormone (TRH) system.

The main functions of the thyroid are the regulation of metabolism, control of oxygen consumption, and regulation of heat, bodily growth, and mental development.

Overview of Methods of Diagnosis of Thyroid Disorders

History and general examination. Questioning is directed especially to symptoms of *thyrotoxicosis* such as nervousness, inability to sleep, sweating, loss of weight, and palpitations, or to those of *hypothyroidism* such as apathy, sensitivity to cold, somnolence, and weight gain.

Physical diagnosis. This includes palpation, inspection, measurement of the circumference of the neck, auscultation, barium swallow, and specific views of the thoracic inlet to show compression or displacement of the esophagus or trachea. Technetium 99 or other isotope scans are also carried out.

The larynx is examined by *indirect* laryngoscopy to demonstrate a recurrent nerve paralysis. *Direct* laryngoscopy and tracheoscopy may be needed if a tumor is suspected. Computerized tomography and MRI are also rewarding.

Functional diagnosis. At the present time the main screening tests are the determination of T_4 and the free T_4 index, the T_3, and TSH response to administration of TRH. The TRH test is particularly useful in the confirmation or exclusion of a functional disorder. The radioiodine test remains irreplaceable for certain indications, not least to demonstrate ectopic thyroid tissue.

Serologic tests for antibodies against thyroglobulin or microsomes are of value, especially in thyroiditis.

Histologic or cytologic diagnosis must be used in many cases, especially in the diagnosis of cold or hot nodules.

Goiter

The term goiter has been associated for many years with the endemic type of thyroid disease occurring in areas deficient in iodine. Enlargement of the thyroid may be diffuse or nodular. It is due to increase of tissue caused by increase of thyrocytes, to adenomas, or to degenerative changes with cyst formation. Other causes of goiter include malignancy and infection.

Large retrosternal goiters can cause considerable compression and displacement of the trachea or of the esophagus and thus affect breathing and swallowing. Pressure on the recurrent laryngeal nerve may affect the function of the vocal cords.

The World Health Organization (WHO) classification is as follows. In *goiter grade I* the gland is palpable but not visible, in *grade II* the gland is palpable and visible, in *grade III* the gland is clearly visible at a considerable distance with the neck free of clothing. These grades may be subdivided into (a) adenomatous or (b) diffuse.

Ectopic thyroid tissue is most often found in the region of the foramen cecum in the base of the tongue, lingual thyroid, and rarely in the neck and mediastinum.

During the embryonic period thyroid tissue may grow into the trachea or larynx and cause dyspnea in the postnatal period or in later life. Dyspnea can occur in women during menstruation as the result of an endotracheal goiter.

Hypothyroidism

Hypothyroidism may be *primary* or *secondary*.

Primary hypothyroidism is spontaneous and is due to deprivation of the thyroid after total or subtotal resection without subsequent replacement, congenital hypoplasia or aplasia, ectopic thyroid in children, or disordered synthesis of thyroid hormone.

Secondary hypothyroidism is caused by absent TSH stimulation from the pituitary.

Symptoms. *General symptoms* include mental motor inactivity, increased need for sleep, dry scaly skin, and myxedema.

Special ear, nose, and throat symptoms include a rough voice, hoarseness, deep monotonous voice, and slow speech with nasal twang. Symptoms also include difficulty in swallowing and globus sensation particularly in the presence of a goiter. Deafness and dizziness may occur in prolonged hypothyroidism.

Hypothyroidism is the most common endocrine disorder of children after diabetes mellitus. In addition to aplasia and ectopia, *Pendred's syndrome* should be mentioned. The picture includes *sensorineural deafness* combined with disorders of iodine metabolism leading to the formation of a goiter.

Pathogenesis. See special literature.

Diagnosis. See literature on nuclear medicine. Otologic diagnosis includes pedoaudiology, electric response audiometry (ERA) (see p.57), and vestibular tests.

Treatment. This consists of hormone substitution in cooperation with a pediatrician, an endocrinologist, and an expert in nuclear medicine. The management of the deafness is described on pp.155 ff.

Hyperthyroidism

The following types occur: primary thyrotoxicosis, toxic adenoma, and thyrotoxicosis factitia.

Generalized symptoms. These include loss of weight, tremor of the fingers, fluttering of the eyelids, tremor of the tongue, attacks of sweating, and sleeplessness. *Merseburger's triad,* goiter, tachycardia, and exophthalmos, is classic for primary thyrotoxicosis. Thyrotoxicosis demonstrating only *one* of these symptoms or mild symptoms is more common.

The *endocrine orbitopathy with exophthalmos,* conjunctivitis, swelling of the lids, chemosis, periocular edema, and oculomotor paralyses can occur on one or both sides and is most often accompanied by thyrotoxicosis. However, exophthalmos also occurs without evidence of abnormal function of the thyroid gland.

Note: Infections or tumors of the nose and sinuses must be excluded by special investigations. Orbital phlegmon, mucopyocele, and malignancy of the base of the skull, e. g., may cause proptosis.

Pathogenesis. An endocrine orbitopathy is caused by increased volume of the retrobulbar tissues, probably stimulated by immunologic processes or by abnormal levels of the thyrotropic hormone.

Diagnosis. This rests on palpation of a diffuse or nodular goiter, scan, radioiodine studies, serum tests with hormone determination, and a TRH test. Orbitopathy is investigated by computer tomography.

Differential diagnosis. Differentiation from Basedow's disease is accomplished by the ISH-receptor autoantibody test (IRMA).

Treatment. Thyroidectomy is performed after medical therapy or radioactive iodine is given. Malignant exophthalmos leads to blindness if untreated. In addition to specific treatment of the thyroid disorder and medical treatment of the exophthalmos by cortisone, a *transantral decompression of the orbit* may also be necessary.

Infections of the Thyroid Gland

1. *Subacute and acute infections* may be divided into purulent and nonpurulent forms.

2. Chronic thyroiditis takes the form of lymphocytic thyroiditis *(Hashimoto's disease)*, and perithyroid invasive thyroiditis *(Riedel's thyroiditis)*.

1. *Subacute and Acute Forms*

Symptoms. These include swelling and pain in the gland which appears suddenly, redness of the overlying skin, and exhaustion. *In the acute form the patient often sits up in bed with the head held forward. There is pain on swallowing radiating to the ear, fever, dyspnea, and fluctuation if an abscess forms.*

Pain on pressure in *de Quervain's subacute nonpurulent granulomatous thyroiditis* is often not so marked. The disease initially usually affects one lobe only so that local induration and adherence to the surrounding tissue can lead to an incorrect diagnosis of tumor. Typically in this form of thyroiditis the inflammatory process passes from one lobe to the other in the course of several weeks. Subacute granulomatous thyroiditis is much more frequent in areas where goiter was previously endemic.

Pathogenesis. This disease is due to virus infection (e. g., influenza), metastatic infection (typhus, paratyphus), or by extension of infection (from oropharyngeal disease, specific and nonspecific cervical lymphadenopathy, and deep cervical abscesses).

Diagnosis. The peripheral hormone values are often initially normal in subacute and acute thyroiditis. Depending on the extent of the infection, the uptake of technetium or iodine may fall during the course of the disease. Cold areas may be found on scan in circumscribed lesions. Serologic investigation of thyroid antibodies is undertaken to identify chronic lymphocytic thyroiditis. If the diagnosis from tumors or hematoma is not certain, a fine needle or open biopsy must be undertaken.

Treatment. Steroids, thyroid hormones, and anti-inflammatory measures are indicated. The rare purulent form is treated by antibiotics and incision if an abscess forms.

2. *Chronic Forms*

Hashimoto's Disease

Symptoms. The thyroid gland is fairly firm to palpation and enlarged. It often causes relatively few symptoms. The course is indolent but may lead to myxedema after many years.

Pathogenesis. This form of thyroiditis is now regarded as an autoimmune disease. The frequency of familial occurrence indicates genetic factors.

Diagnosis. This is based on demonstration of thyroglobulin and microsomal antibodies in the serum. Fine needle biopsy shows tight collections of well-differentiated lymphocytes with scattered plasma cells.

Treatment. Therapy is medical by thyroid hormones. For large goiters steroids and thyroidectomy may be necessary.

Riedel's Thyroiditis

Symptoms. A hard, often asymmetrical thyroid swelling grows into the surrounding tissues causing recurrent nerve paralysis and marked symptoms due to lateral compression of the trachea and less often of the esophagus.

Pathogenesis. The cause is said to be arteritis of the thyroid gland and the periglandular tissue. The disease appears to be related to generalized arteritis and sclerosing and fibrosing processes which occur in the orbit, the lacrimal glands, and the mediastinum.

Diagnosis. Biopsy shows severe inflammatory infiltrate especially in the periglandular tissue.

Differential diagnosis. This includes thyroid malignancy.

Treatment. *The purpose of operation is to free the trachea from the compression caused by the surrounding tumor tissue.*

Thyroid Malignancy

In Central Europe this forms about 0.5% of all tumors. Women are affected almost twice as often as men. *Cold nodules* demonstrated by scanning are *potentially malignant*. The term *hot nodule* indicates an *autonomous adenoma* with relatively slight tendency to undergo malignant degeneration.

Differentiated and anaplastic carcinomas and rare types are to be distinguished. *Differentiated* thyroid tumors include *follicular and papillary carcinoma.* Follicular thyroid carcinomas tend to rupture the capsule, invade vessels, and produce hematogenous metastases.

Papillary thyroid carcinoma *is the most frequent malignant thyroid tumor. It produces lymphatic metastases in the neck. Regional cervical lymph node metastases are often the first symptom of a primary tumor of the thyroid*

Table 6.7 Histologic Classification of Thyroid Tumors

I. Epithelial tumors

    A. Benign
        1. Follicular adenoma
        2. Others

    B. Malignant
        1. Follicular carcinoma
        2. Papillary carcinoma
        3. Squamous cell carcinoma
        4. Undifferentiated carcinoma (spindle cell, giant cell, or small cell type)
        5. Medullary carcinoma

II. Nonepithelial tumors

    A. Benign

    B. Malignant
        1. Fibrosarcoma
        2. Others

III. Miscellaneous tumors

    A. Carcinosarcoma

    B. Malignant hemangioendothelioma

    C. Malignant lymphoma

    D. Teratoma

IV. Metastases

V. Unclassifiable tumors

VI. Pseudotumors

Source: World Health Organization, 1974.

gland, particularly if it is small. In areas where goiter was previously endemic, **follicular carcinoma** *is the predominant tumor.*

Anaplastic (undifferentiated) carcinomas spread rapidly to neighboring organs and metastasize by blood and lymphatic pathways.

The **rare types** include *medullary carcinoma.* This tumor arises from the C cells (the parafollicular cells which form calcitonin) and not from thyroid cells themselves. The presence of amyloid is one of its histologic characteristics. Medullary carcinomas usually grow slowly and do not store iodine.

Symptoms. Apart from the undifferentiated thyroid carcinomas, malignant goiters usually grow slowly. They are often unilateral and present as one or more firm nodules. Occasionally the primary tumor is too small to be noticed, and the diagnosis is first made on the presence of metastases. The thyroid function as demonstrated by the peripheral level of hormones is not affected in the initial stages of the disease. When the thyroid has ruptured, the mobility of the thyroid on swallowing is reduced due to infiltration of the surrounding tissues. Globus symptoms, otalgia, or recurrent nerve paralysis may occur.

Pathogenesis. A hereditary disposition appears likely. The medullary carcinoma may be part of an autosomal-dominant syndrome. There appears to be a correlation with increased TSH stimulation in iodine deficiency in carcinomas arising from thyrocytes. Thyroid tumors thus often develop from a long-standing goiter. An increased incidence is also observed in recurrent goiter after previous surgery and in advanced Hashimoto's disease.

Diagnosis. A needle biopsy or open biopsy is carried out if the disease is suspected on the basis of palpation or a scan, particularly if a cold nodule is found. Tumor markers are very important both for diagnosis and follow-up. In medullary carcinoma there is an increased level of calcitonin, whereas an increased serum thyroglobulin level is found in both follicular and papillary carcinomas.

Treatment. Thyroidectomy is performed with preservation of the recurrent nerve and of at least one parathyroid gland. *Unilateral or bilateral neck dissection, depending on the primary tumor, is indicated particularly in papillary carcinoma.* Postoperative radioactive iodine is used in follicular carcinomas, and thyroid hormones must be administered. Percutaneous radiotherapy may be indicated.

Cooperation between the specialist in nuclear medicine, the radiotherapist, and the surgeon is indispensable.

7. Salivary Glands

There are three paired major salivary glands (Fig. 7.**1**):

1. Parotid gland
2. Submandibular gland
3. Sublingual gland

In addition there are *700 to 1,000 solitary minor salivary glands* occurring mainly in the oral and pharyngeal mucosa (Fig. 7.**2**).

Embryology, Structure, Congenital Anomalies
(Table 7.**1**)

The major salivary glands arise from solid ectodermal cell accumulations of the foregut between the 4th and 8th embryonal week. Thickening of the surrounding mesenchyme encapsulates the developing gland and also includes lymph node anlages. The ducts become patent in the 22nd week.

Aplasia of one or several glands may occur, but complete absence of all the major glands is extremely rare.

Diverticula and ectasia of the parotid duct system can predispose to parotitis.

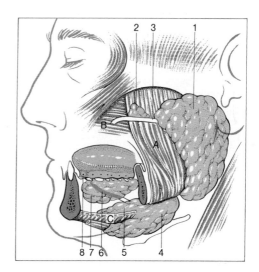

Fig. 7.**1** The major salivary glands. Parotid gland (1) with small accessory gland (2) and Stensen's duct (3). Submandibular gland (4) with uncinate process (5) and submandibular, Wharton's, duct (6). Sublingual gland (7) with sublingual caruncule (8). A, masseter muscle; B, buccinator muscle; C, mylohyoid muscle.

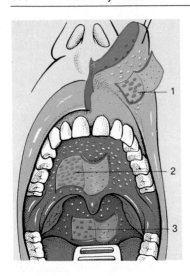

Fig. 7.**2** The minor salivary glands. 1, Labial glands; 2, palatine glands; 3, pharyngeal glands.

Table 7.1 Morphological and Functional Structure of the Salivary Glands		
Functional System	Functions	Structural Elements
Acini	Formation of the primary saliva, proteoenzymes, sialomucine	Endoplasmatic reticulum, Golgi apparatus, secretory granules, mucosal vacuoles
Salivary duct system consisting of intercalated ducts, striated ducts, and excretory ducts	Electrolyte and water regulation, formation of secretory components	Cytomembranes, mitochondria, ATP pump system
Mesenchyme	Structure stabilizer, material transport, impulse transmission, IgA formation	Connective tissue fibers, mucopolysaccharide, blood and lymphatic vessels, nerve fibers, immunocytes

Abbreviations: ATP, adenosine triphosphate; IgA, immunoglobulin A.

Abberrant salivary gland tissue may be found in the cervical lymph nodes, the middle ear, and the mandible.

Accessory glands are appendages of the major glands, most commonly the parotid, and they possess efferent ducts and are capable of function.

The theory that the parotid gland consists of two lobes lying lateral and medial to the facial nerve connected by an isthmus has been rejected as incorrect, although the terms superficial and total parotidectomy are still used (see Fig. 7.**8**).

Anatomy and Physiology of the Major and Minor Salivary Glands

Parotid Gland

The largest of the salivary glands lies in the retromandibular fossa in a subcutaneous pocket surrounded by a capsule of compressed connective tissue. This pseudocapsule is very thick, particularly laterally, and is the cause of tension pain in parotid swelling. Inferiorly there are defects in this connective tissue mantle through which infections and tumors can penetrate into the pterygopalatine fossa or parapharyngeal space.

Borders. *The superior part of the parotid glands* is limited anteriorly by the anterior border of the ascending ramus of the mandible, posteriorly by the external meatus, and above by the zygomatic arch. The inferior portion of the gland is the *cervical portion* which lies between the angle of the jaw and mastoid process. The inferior border is the anterior margin of the sternocleidomastoid muscle and the posterior belly of the digastric muscle.

Clinical significance. Pleomorphic adenomas arising in the *cervical part of the gland* may form a dumbbell tumor passing into the oropharynx with only a relatively small external tumor.

The *parotid duct* (Stensen's duct) is approximately 6 cm long. It leaves the anterior border of the gland, crosses the masseter muscle, and perforates the buccinator muscle and the buccal mucosa. The edges of its orifice are slightly elevated and are red and swollen in inflammation. The orifice lies opposite the second upper molar tooth. The *facial nerve* leaves the base of the skull through the stylomastoid foramen and enters the gland parenchyma as a short trunk 0.7 to 1.5 cm long. It divides into two or three main branches and then divides again peripherally into the terminal temporal, frontal, zygomatic buccal, and cervical branches. The zygomatic and buccal branches have numerous anastomoses with each other. The forehead branch and the marginal mandibular branch for the lower lip usually have no anastomoses to neighboring branches (see Figs. 1.**77** and 1.**8**).

The facial nerve supplies the entire mimetic musculature and the platysma. Medial to the nerve, the pes anserinus major, lie the *branches of the external carotid artery,* the transverse facial, maxillary, and retroauricular artery, which supply the parotid gland. The venous drainage is via the internal jugular vein.

Note: The safest point from which to find the facial nerve in conservative procedures, e. g., for pleomorphic adenoma, is its trunk (see Fig. 7.**8**).

Lymph drainage. There are several intra- and periglandular lymph nodes from which the lymph drains via the submandibular nodes or directly into the upper deep cervical nodes. The first regional lymph node station for the parotid lies *within* the gland, a circumstance that has major clinical significance in oncologic patients.

Autonomic control of salivary secretion. The *preganglionic* fibers originate in the inferior salivatory nucleus. They follow the glossopharyngeal nerve to the jugular foramen, leave that nerve at the inferior ganglion, and then join the tympanic nerve which forms the tympanic plexus of the middle ear and from which the lesser superficial petrosal nerve arises. The fibers finally reach the otic ganglion in which they synapse.

The *postganglionic* parasympathetic fibers run from here with the auriculotemporal nerve to the parotid gland.

The *sympathetic* fibers arise from the carotid plexus and regulate the circulation of the gland by vasoconstriction. They have less influence on salivary production.

Submandibular Gland

This is embedded in the submandibular triangle and is bordered anteriorly by the digastric muscle, posteriorly by the stylomandibular ligament, and superiorly by the mandible.

The main part of the gland lies inferior to the mylohyoid muscle and is covered by the external cervical fascia.

The *submandibular duct* (Wharton's duct) is about 5 cm long, runs anteriorly beneath the mucosa of the floor of the mouth, and opens close to the frenulum in the sublingual caruncle in the *floor of the mouth*.

Clinical significance. Infection can spread along the U-shaped body of the gland into the posterior part of the floor of the mouth causing a phlegmon or abscess in the floor of the mouth.

The duct *crosses* laterodorsally over the lingual nerve. If the duct is slit over a probe, e. g., for acute obstruction due to a sialolith, the nerve is not in danger. The very thin marginal mandibular branch of the facial nerve running between the upper pole of the gland and the mandible is in danger during operations on the submandibular gland. Injury to the lingual or hypoglossal nerves during removal of the gland for sialolithiasis or benign tumors is avoided by exposing the nerves.

Autonomic supply is from the lingual nerve with preganglionic *parasympathetic fibers* which reach it via the chorda tympani and synapse in the submandibular ganglion to give off postganglionic fibers.

Sympathetic fibers from the superior cervical ganglion control the blood supply.

Sublingual Gland

The smallest of the major glands lies under the mucosa of the floor of the mouth, and its posterior part touches the anterior end of the submandibular gland. Its duct system usually unites with that of the submandibular gland, and its innervation is the same as that of the submandibular gland.

Clinical significance. The **ranula** is a *retention cyst* caused by obliteration of one of the smaller openings, not the main opening (Beck), of the sublingual gland. Depending on its size it causes difficulty in swallowing and speaking due to interference with the mobility of the tongue. It is **treated** by removal of the ranula.

Minor Salivary Glands

These are scattered throughout the oropharyngeal, nasal, sinus, laryngeal, and tracheal mucosa. There are also accumulations on the inner surface of the lip, in the buccal mucosa, and in the palate. The minor salivary glands produce only 5% to 8% of the entire volume of saliva, but despite that they ensure satisfactory moistening of the mucosa if one or more of the major salivary glands fails. Severe xerostomia occurs if their salivary secreting function is also suppressed, e.g., after radiotherapy.

Clinical significance. Tumors of the *minor* salivary glands are often malignant (adenoid cystic carcinoma, acinic cell tumor). Benign tumors (e.g., pleomorphic adenoma) occur less frequently.

Formation and Function of Saliva

Physical, chemical, and mental factors stimulate the production of saliva. The amount produced in a day varies between 1,000 and 1,500 ml, and 99.5% of it is water. The rest is inorganic, organic, and cellular material. The individual salivary glands make a variable contribution to the quantity and quality of the whole (Tables 7.**2** and 7.**3**).

The secretion is formed in two steps: primary secretion is formed in the acini and is then partially resorbed and modified during passage through the duct system in a manner somewhat analogous to the formation of urine by the kidney.

Physiologic Functions of the Saliva

- Saliva exerts a *protective action* on the mucosa of the mouth and the upper respiratory tract by mechanical cleansing and immunologic defense via defense-carrying proteins, lysozymes and immunoglobulins, especially immunoglobulin A (IgA).
- Saliva has a *digestive function;* it lubricates the food and begins the splitting of starch by amylase.
- Saliva aids in the *excretion of autogenous and foreign material,* particularly iodine and coagulating factors, alkaloids, viruses including the Epstein-Barr, poliomyelitis, rubella, Coxsackie, cytomegaly, and hepatitis virus. The excretion of blood group substances in the saliva may be important in forensic medicine.

Table 7.2 Mixture and Quality of Saliva		
Salivary: Amount and Composition Under Nonstimulated Conditions		Salivary Quality
Parotid gland:	about 30%	Mainly serous
Submandibular gland:	55–65%	Mixed mucous and serous
Sublingual gland:	about 5%	Mainly mucous
Minor salivary glands:	5–8%	Mixed, mainly mucous
The proportion of parotid saliva increases on marked stimulation.		

Table 7.3 Composition of Human Parotid Secretion*		
	Resting Secretion	Stimulated Secretion
Secretion rate	0.03–0.1 ml/min	0.2–1.2 ml/min
Electrolytes		
Sodium	2–8 mEq/L	20–65 mEq/L
Potassium	25–30 mEq/L	20–30 mEq/L
Calcium	1–5 mEq/L	1–5 mEq/L
Total protein	2–10 mg/ml	2–10 mg/ml
Amylase	150–600 U/ml	100–700 U/ml
Immunoglobulin A	0.03–0.3 mg/ml	0.01–0.1 mg/ml
Albumin	0–0.02 mg/ml	0–0.02 mg/ml
Lysosyme	16–520 μg/ml	8–60 μg/ml
Kallikrein	8–48 mU/ml	5–20 mU/ml
Trypsin inhibitor	5–18 mU/ml	0.5–10 mU/ml

* The main anions in parotid saliva are chloride, phosphate, and bicarbonate. The main cations are magnesium, iron, copper, zinc, selenium, and lead. Other anions include floride, bromide, iodine, thiocyanate, and nitrate. Immunoglobulin G (IgG) and immunoglobulin M (IgM) are only present in trace amounts in normal parotid secretion. IgG and IgM increase in inflammatory lesions.

- Saliva aids in *protection of the teeth*. The organic and inorganic, e.g., fluorine, content of the saliva is important for the formation and maintenance of the dental enamel. It helps prevent bacterial deposition.
- Saliva helps *mediate the sense of taste* by lavage of the taste buds.

Table 7.4 Factors Affecting Salivary Production				
	Sialopenia	Sialorrhea	Serous	Mucous
Hypertension	+			
Endogenous depression augmented by psychotropic drugs, anxiety, and stage fright	+			
Acute inflammation	+			
Marasmus	+			
Radiotherapy > 1000 rad	+			
Sjögren's syndrome	+			
Vomiting		+		
Nervous disorders and excitement		+		
Pregnancy		+		
Appetite stimulants		+		
Acids in fruits		+	+	
Topical anesthetics	+			
General anesthesia, barbiturates, chlorothiazide	+			
Beta-blockers	+			+
Parasympathicomimetic drugs, (e.g., pilocarpine)		+	+	
Sympathicomimetic drugs (e.g., atropine)	+			+
Many psychotropic drugs	+			

The **composition of the saliva** depends on its flow rate, the circadian rhythm, the season of the year, sex, and nutrition. The great variability of this parameter must be taken into account during analysis (see Table 7.**3**), although it must be emphasized that salivary analysis has not assumed clinical importance.

Disturbances of secretion. *Xerostomia* is exceedingly distressing. It may be caused centrally by lesions of the autonomic nervous supply to the salivary glands, by diseases of the salivary glands, by dehydration due to diarrhea or vomiting, by radiotherapy, or by systemic diseases such as Sjögren's syndrome.

Sialorrhea indicates an increased formation of saliva. Predisposing factors are diseases of the mucosa of the mouth and tongue and of the teeth, and psychogenic factors.

Ptyalismus is abnormal dribbling of saliva from the mouth in neurologic disease, e.g., Parkinson's disease, epilepsy and paralysis of the muscles of deglutition.

The production of saliva is also influenced by generalized diseases and drugs (Table 7.**4**).

Methods of Investigation

Salivary gland diseases can often be diagnosed on the basis of the history, the patient's age, and the clinical findings. The latter include swelling, consistency, mobility, rapidity of enlargement, pain, and function of the facial nerve.

Examples of disorders of salivary gland function include:

- *Recurrent attacks of severe pain indicate sialolithiasis or recurrent parotitis.*
- *Bilateral disease indicates sialadenosis or mumps.*
- *Sex: myoepithelial sialadenitis, Sjögren's disease, occurs almost exclusively in women.*
- *Malignancy is indicated by pain, facial paralysis, regional lymph node metastases, and ulceration*

Age-Dependent Conditions

- Congenital hemangiomas and lymphangiomas occur in the newborn.
- Mumps and chronic recurrent parotitis occur in school age children.
- Adenomas and sialadenosis occur in middle age.
- The proportion of malignancy increases with increasing age.

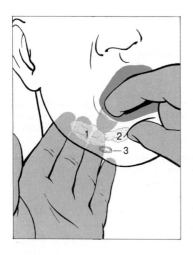

Fig. 7.**3** Bimanual palpation of the submandibular gland (1), of the sublingual gland (2), and of a periglandular lymph node or stone in the part of the submandibular duct (3) close to the submandibular gland.

Normally only the flat contour of the submandibular gland can be recognized with its soft overlying skin in the submandibular triangle. The parotid gland is not visible unless it is increased in size. Specific findings can be detected by *palpation* which should be carried out bimanually to allow both sides to be compared or bimanually intra- and extraorally (Fig. 7.**3**).

Note: Unilateral or bilateral masseteric hypertrophy is often confused with parotid disease. The parotid gland can be distinguished from the masseter muscle by asking the patient to press his teeth together firmly, which causes the muscle to stand out.

The size in centimeters, the consistency, superficial profile, mobility, tenderness, and reddening of the overlying skin should be noted. Redness and swelling of the ducts and their orifices should also be looked for, and the appearance of the expressed saliva (clear, flocculent, purulent, or bloodstained) should be noted. Stones in the ducts, particularly the submandibular, are often palpable.

Radiographic Diagnosis

Conventional plain views of the floor of the mouth with the submandibular and parotid glands in tangential and lateral views are only useful if the stone has a high calcium content. Radiotranslucent stones can often be demonstrated by **sialography** which shows a round negative contrast.

Technique of sialography. *A plastic catheter and a cannula are introduced into the duct of the parotid or submandibular gland. Contrast medium is injected slowly in small amounts. Radiographs are taken in two planes or under the image converter.*

Note: Sialography is contraindicated during acute infections.

Typical sialographic pictures are obtained in chronic recurrent sialadenitis which shows the typical "tree in leaf" appearance, i.e., ectasia of the acini and terminal and excretory ducts. In benign tumors a round space-occupying lesion displacing the ducts filled with contrast medium can often be recognized. Malignant tumors may cause duct tears, sudden changes in duct width, and extravasation of contrast medium. The findings in Sjögren's syndrome vary: initially the picture is that of a "ripe" tree with delicate branching of the duct system and an indistinct gland periphery. The appearance of a "bare tree" is found in later cases with rarefaction of the ducts and parenchymal atrophy (Fig. 7.**4a–e**).

Computed tomography of the parotid, particularly when combined with sialography, is becoming of increasing importance. It allows determination of the size and the exact extent of the depth of tumors of the parotid, particularly of the deep lobe. This method makes it easy to distinguish tumors arising from the gland itself and from those growing into the gland from other structures, e. g., metastases and parapharyngeal tumors.

The salivary glands are also accessible to *ultrasound imaging*.

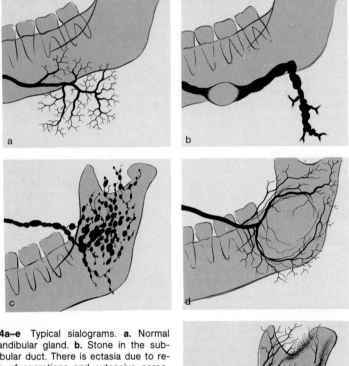

Fig. 7.**4a–e** Typical sialograms. **a.** Normal submandibular gland. **b.** Stone in the submandibular duct. There is ectasia due to retention of secretions and extensive parenchymatous atrophy. **c.** Chronic recurrent parotitis with ectasia of the acini and terminal ducts, showing the "tree in leaf" appearance. The excretory duct looks like a string of pearls. **d.** Benign tumor of the parotid gland with basket-shaped displacement around the tumor. **e.** Malignancy of the parotid gland with interruption of the ducts and extravasation of contrast medium.

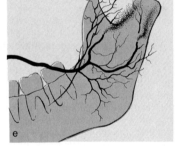

Biopsy

Histologic diagnosis is the key to all salivary gland disease. It is the basis on which the decision is made to operate or to treat the patient medically, e. g., for sialadenosis or Sjögren's disease.

Fine needle biopsy is only useful if the findings are positive. The evaluation must be done by an experienced cytologist.

Large needle biopsy, if necessary, taken in more than one direction is more useful but difficult in cystic tumors. Damage to the facial nerve can be avoided. The seeding of tumor cells along the needle track is conceivable, but its occurrence has never been documented. Biopsy of an ulcerated lesion is easy. If the skin is intact, the best approach to the parotid for biopsy is anterior to the tragus to protect the facial nerve.

If the clinical findings indicate a salivary tumor, a *superficial parotidectomy* or *excision* of the submandibular gland provides a *large biopsy* and at the same time is the correct *treatment* of benign tumors. *Intraoperative frozen section* allows the decision to be made between a partial or total parotidectomy or a more extensive procedure.

Clinical Findings

Inflammatory Diseases (See Table 7.5)

Acute Bacterial Infections

Symptoms. The gland suddenly becomes swollen and tender. If the parotid gland is infected, the auricle protrudes and this can be particularly well

---

Table 7.5 Inflammatory Salivary Disorders

Acutes:

Bacterial
Acute sialadenitis of the parotid and submandibular glands

Viral
Parotitis mumps
Cytomegalus virus
Coxsackie infection

Allergy
Reactions to drugs, food etc., very rare

Chronic:

Chronic sclerosing sialadenitis of the submandibular gland, Kuettner's tumor

Chronic recurrent parotitis

Sjögren's syndrome, myoepithelial sialadenitis

Granulomatous diseases

Epithelioid cell sialadenitis
(sarcoidosis, Heerfordt syndrome or uveoparotid fever)
Tuberculosis
Syphilis
Actinomycosis

seen from behind the patient. The overlying skin may be red, and fluctuation may be felt if there is suppuration. Infection may rupture spontaneously externally or through Santorini's cleft into the external auditory meatus. The opening of the duct is red and swollen. Pus drains spontaneously or after external massage. The patient has trismus.

> **Note:** The presence of facial paralysis places grave doubt on the diagnosis of an infective disorder, and malignant disease should be strongly suspected.

Pathogenesis. Reduction of salivary flow is an important prerequisite for bacterial infection ascending the duct. The previously common *postoperative parotitis,* especially after abdominal operations, has now become much less common due to the use of antibiotics, fluid and electrolyte replacement, and postoperative oral toilet. However, acute purulent infections still occur occasionally in uncontrolled diabetes or renal failure with electrolyte disturbances and dehydration, or in the presence of carious teeth or poor oral hygiene. Nursing home residents are predisposed.

Diagnosis. The history shows a previous disease or operation. Clinical findings are noted (external appearance, palpable findings, gross characteristics of secretions), and smears may be obtained (Color Plate **38b**).

Differential diagnosis. This includes lymphadenitis due to a meatal furuncle, abscess of the cheek of dental origin, unerupted teeth, infected sebaceous cyst, and zygomatic abscess of mastoiditis in children.

Treatment. High-dose parenteral antibiotics are given, and especially those active against gram-negative organisms, changed later if necessary depending on the results of culture and sensitivity tests. Fluid and electrolyte balance is corrected, and sialogogues are given. Pilocarpine drops 0.2%, vitamin C tablets, or lemon slices are sucked, and oral hygiene is attended to. Fan-shaped external incisions are made for an abscess, using care to avoid the facial nerve (see Fig. 1.**77**).

The same treatment is prescribed for purulent infection of the *submandibular gland.* The most common cause in this case is obstruction by stone or dental disease.

Viral Infections

Mumps

Symptoms. These include swelling of the involved gland, redness and slight swelling of the opening of the duct, and displacement of the auricle. The secretions are not purulent, and there is no fever in 30% of cases. In 75% of cases both glands are involved. The swelling of one side can precede the other by up to 5 days. The submandibular and sublingual glands may also be involved but they are only rarely affected alone without parotid involvement.

An irreversible lesion of the VIIIth cranial nerve may be caused by this neurotropic virus leading to unilateral or bilateral complete deafness. The pancreas, testes, ovaries, and central nervous system may also be affected, or one of these organs may be involved alone either at the same time or later.

Pathogenesis. The virus is one of the paramyxoma group. Local epidemics occur in kindergartens and schools. The incubation period is 20 ± 10 days. Following infection it is likely that immunity is permanent.

Diagnosis. *Direct* demonstration of the virus is only possible in the early phase of the disease, a few hours to several days.

The virus can be isolated from saliva, cerebrospinal fluid (CSF), or urine. It is demonstrated by culture in the kidneys of apes or the cells of hens or guinea pigs.

Serologic tests consist of complement-binding reaction or hemagglutination inhibition tests. The initial value is assessed and a further reading is taken 2 to 3 weeks later. A fourfold increase of the antibody titer is evidence of a mumps infection. The increase of *amylase excretion* in the blood and urine reaches its maximum on the 3rd to 4th day of the illness.

Note: Unilateral deafness if often not noticed during childhood either by the child or by the parents. Audiologic tests during the course of the illness are therefore important.

Differential diagnosis. This includes cervical lymphadenitis, purulent parotitis, chronic recurrent parotitis, and sialolithiasis. Dental infections are easy to exclude clinically or by serology.

A common faulty diagnosis is mumps in adults. There is often a tumor present.

Treatment. It is not possible to treat the cause. Mumps hyperimmunoglobulins are recommended in the early stage. Symptomatic treatment includes analgesics and if necessary anti-inflammatory drugs. Ample fluids must be given. A preventative vaccine is available.

Cytomegalus Virus

This is mainly a disease of children which manifests itself in the newborn and infants up to the age of 2 years. The congenital infection is mild and has no characteristic symptoms. Severe cases are accompanied by jaundice, petechial exanthems, hepatosplenomegaly, thrombocytopenia, hemolytic anemia, choreoretinitis, and psychomotor and mental retardation.

Acquired cytomegalous virus infection in adults usually does not cause any characteristic signs of infection.

Pathogenesis. The cytomegalious virus is transmitted across the placenta and by droplet or dirt infection. It affects the salivary glands with preference although it is a generalized disease.

Diagnosis. Serology shows antibodies. Histology shows owl eye cell nuclei and cell inclusion bodies in the salivary and urinary sediment or in tissue from the salivary glands.

Treatment. Special treatment is so far not known and must therefore be symptomatic.

Course. Mortality is high in the newborn.

Coxsackie Infection

Symptoms. These include parotid swelling and gingivitis often beginning with herpangina.

Pathogenesis. Cause of infection by a virus secreted by the pharyngeal and intestinal mucosa.

Diagnosis. This is based on epidemiology and serologic tests.

Treatment. Therapy is symptomatic and if necessary local treatment for the mucosa is given.

Chronic Inflammation

Chronic Sclerosing Sialadenitis of the Submandibular Gland (Kuettner's Tumor)

Symptoms. These include hardness and enlargement of the gland which is often difficult to differentiate from a true tumor. Pain is minimal.

Pathogenesis. Histology shows chronic inflammation of the gland with destruction of the serous acini, lymphocytic infiltration of the interstitial connective tissue, periductal sclerosis, and, in the late stage, "cirrhosis" of the salivary glands due to metaplasia of the gland parenchyma and connective tissue. The etiologic agents are so far unknown, but this is possibly an immune disease.

Diagnosis and treatment. The gland is removed for differential diagnosis and histology.

Chronic Recurrent Parotitis

Symptoms. These are mostly unilateral or alternating, but occasionally there may be a simultaneous bilateral parotid swelling which may be very painful. The disease mainly occurs in children. The saliva is milky, granular, or pure pus and tastes salty. Trismus is often present. Attacks recur at variable intervals. Between the recurrences the patient is symptomfree, but the parotid is usually indurated in the intervening interval.

Pathogenesis. The cause is not clear. It is suspected that congenital duct ectasia is a predisposing factor.

Diagnosis. This is made from the history and the clinical course. Sialography shows a "tree in leaf" appearance. Duct ectasia often presents similar to a string of pearls or a cluster of grapes (see Fig. 7.**4c**). Tissue should be taken for histology in doubtful cases.

Treatment. Measures to treat the cause are not available. Parenteral antibiotics may shorten the acute attack of pain. Instillation of antibiotics into the duct in the acute phase is painful and not recommended. The patient is taught to massage the gland himself. Oral care and sialogogues are prescribed. Ligation of the parotid duct is successful in some cases as is resection of the tympanic plexus. Finally, parotidectomy with preservation of the facial nerve may be undertaken for very painful and frequently recurring parotitis. In these cases dissection of the gland is difficult.

Course. Secretion of saliva may ultimately cease due to scar tissue obliteration of the parenchyma if the disease persists for a long time. The symptoms are then relieved. The childhood form is considerably more favorable since the symptoms resolve at puberty in many cases.

Myoepithelial Sialadenitis (Sjögren's Syndrome, Benign Lymphoepithelial Lesion) (see Color Plate **38a** and **c**)

Symptoms. These include xerostomia or the sicca syndrome of the mucosa of the upper airway. There is almost always bilateral parotid swelling and atrophy of the glands in the end stage. Other symptoms include keratoconjunctivitis sicca, chronic recurring joint disorders, rheumatic purpura, periarteritis nodosa, and scleroderma.

Pathogenesis. There is an obvious relation to the rheumatic diseases. The autoaggressive immune pathologic reaction leads to atrophy of the gland parenchyma, interstitial lymphocytic infiltration, and myoepithelial growth.

Diagnosis. The complete picture of the diagnosis is characteristic, but *abortive forms are common.* Examination by an internist is therefore recommended to look for dysproteinemia, elevated erythrocyte sedimentation rate (ESR), and lupus erythematosus. Sialography shows a picture between "the ripe tree" and "the bare tree" in the end stage. The clinical diagnosis is supplemented by histology.

Treatment. Because the etiology is unknown, treatment is difficult and requires prolonged cooperation with the internist. Artificial saliva and frequent small amounts of water or milk are prescribed for the distressing dryness of the mouth. Secretion of saliva may be stimulated by pilocarpine hydrochloride 0.2 ml made up to 2 ml with distilled water. Ten drops in one glass of water are given three times a day. The solution is first washed around the mouth and then swallowed.

Steroids may be tried as well as immunosuppressive agents in very severe cases.

Mikulicz Syndrome

The term *Mikulicz* disease which was previously used frequently is superfluous since it has no uniform pathologic basis.

This term for symmetrical swelling of the salivary and lacrimal glands may include any of the following: lymphadenopathy, chronic lymphatic leukemia, lymph node metastases from primary tumors of the base of the skull, nose, and other sinuses, hematogenous metastases, Hodgkin's and non-Hodgkin's lymphoma, or tuberculous lymphadenopathy. *Biopsy is necessary to establish the correct diagnosis.*

Epithelial Cell Sialadenitis (Heerfordt Syndrome or Uveoparotid Fever)

Symptoms. These are usually symmetrical with a parotid swelling which is occasionally painful, swelling of the lacrimal glands and uveitis, facial nerve paralysis, and meningoencephalitis. A sensorineural deafness is also observed. The flow of saliva is reduced as may be the production of amylase. Women are most often affected.

Pathogenesis. This is an extrapulmonary manifestation of sarcoid.

Diagnosis. This is made by the demonstration of sarcoid tissue changes in the gland parenchyma or in the intra- or periglandular lymph nodes and by exclusion of tuberculosis by an internist.

Treatment. Mainly steroids are given.

Tuberculosis

Symptoms. There is a relatively painless swelling, mainly in the parotid or submandibular area. The peri- and intraglandular lymph nodes are almost always the primary site of infection. Caseation, infiltration of the salivary parenchyma and surrounding tissues, external fistulae, and skin tuberculosis are now less common than previously.

Pathogenesis. Primary lymph node infection is now uncommon. The most usual form at present is a postprimary hematogenous spread to the lymph nodes of the salivary glands.

Diagnosis. *Intra- or periglandular affected lymph nodes are very difficult to distinguish by palpation from a salivary gland tumor.* Radiography may show calcification which is to be distinguished from sialoliths or extravasated material. Tuberculosis of other organs, especially the lung, must be excluded. Microscopy and culture for tuberculosis organisms are important investigations in addition to histology. The disease is reportable.

Treatment. Antituberculous drugs are given and the affected lymph nodes or the salivary gland are removed with preservation of the facial nerve.

Note: Serious errors, e.g., failure to diagnose malignancy, can only be avoided by operation and biopsy.

Radiation Sialadenitis

Symptoms. The early reaction is reduction of salivary flow followed later by the sicca syndrome often combined with hypogeusia or ageusia. In the end stage, there may be an extremely distressing xerostomia depending on the size of the field and the dose of radiation.

Pathogenesis. Membrane damage to the nuclei and intracytoplasmatic cell organelles occurs in the major and minor salivary glands during radiotherapy for malignant head and neck tumors above a dose of 1,000 to 1,500 rads, 10 to 15 Gy. This leads to interstitial fibrosis of the secretory elements. Permanent damage is to be expected above a dose of 4,000 to 5,000 rads, 40 to 50 Gy.

Diagnosis. This may be made on the history of exposure to irradiation.

Treatment. Therapy is symptomatic. An attempt may be made to stimulate the secretion by one of the following: (1) pilocarpine hydrochloride 1%, ten drops three times a day on a piece of sugar; (2) artificial saliva; (3) the patient is advised to drink frequent small quantities of water or milk.

Course. Production of saliva and the sense of taste *may* return to some extent in some cases after months or years.

Sialolithiasis

Symptoms. These are related to eating or to psychological gustatory stimulation which produce a severe, often painful swelling of the affected salivary gland, salivary colic. In many cases swelling of the salivary gland due to retention of secretion persists for variable periods of time.

Pathogenesis. Sialolithiasis is the end stage of the so-called *electrolyte sialadenitis*. It is probably due to the primary dyschylic disturbance of secretion of salivary electrolytes. Changes of the duct are caused by increase of viscosity of the saliva with mucus obstruction which potentiates the primary disorder of secretion. Lumps of secretion are formed consisting of an organic mucoproteid complex matrix. Inorganic material is deposited like onion rings around this center. Mineralization-promoting factors include mechanical causes such as dilatation of the ducts, stenoses, localized attacks of inflammation, impacted foreign bodies, e.g., bristles from a toothbrush, bits of wood, and dental calculi, and neurohumeral dysregulation.

The scale deposited around the organic center consists of calcium phosphate and calcium carbonate in the structure of apatite. The stones may be single but are more often multiple and vary in size from a pinhead to the size of a cherry stone. Sialolithiasis is more common in men (2:1) and mainly occurs in adults. In most cases only one gland is affected at any one time. *In 85% of*

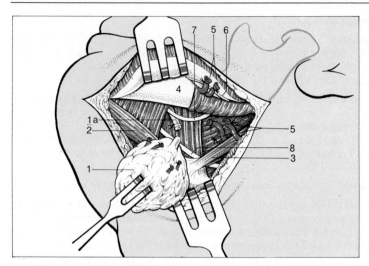

Fig. 7.5   Removal of the submandibular gland. 1, Submandibular gland; 1a, submandibular duct ligated; 2, anterior belly of the digastric muscle; 3, stylohyoid muscle
covered by posterior belly of the diagastric muscle; 4, horizontal ramus of the mandible; 5, facial artery and vein ligated; 6, marginal mandibular branch of the facial nerve
which must be preserved because it innervates the lower lip; 7, lingual nerve; 8, hypoglossal nerve.

*cases the stone lies in the submandibular gland and in 15% in the parotid
gland.* This ratio is explained by differences in flow. The submandibular
saliva flows superiorly against gravity and has a higher viscosity due to an
increased mucin content.

Diagnosis. The stone is often palpable in the floor of the mouth or the
cheek. There is a grating sensation on introducing a probe into the duct. If
the calcium content is high enough, the stones may be demonstrated on
plain X-ray views. Radiotranslucent stones are demonstrated indirectly by
the presence of a filling defect on the sialogram (Fig. 7.**4b**).

Differential diagnosis. This includes facial phlebolith, calcified tuberculous lymph node, and intraglandular tumor.

Treatment. Removal of the stone by slitting the duct over a probe provides
immediate relief of pain. The patient may then be observed for recurrences
which are common. Repeated attacks of stone formation and duct obstruction lead to irreversible chronic inflammatory parenchymal damage so that
the diseased gland should be removed (Figs. 7.**5** and 7.**8**). *Lithotripsy* can be
beneficial in patients with a short history.

Sialadenosis

Symptoms. These include recurrent or more often persistent bilateral *painless* swelling mainly of the parotid gland. *Painful* sialadenosis occurs during treatment with antihypertensive drugs.

Pathogenesis. Salivary gland disorders with acinar swelling, degenerative lesions of the myoepithelium, and hydropic swelling of axoplasm of autonomic nerve fibers can occur in *endocrine and metabolic disorders* such as diabetes, pregnancy, puberty, menopause, adrenal dysfunction, avitaminosis, protein deficiency, starvation dystrophy, alcoholism, central neurogenic and autonomic dysfunctions, and *the action of drugs,* e. g., antihypertensives.

Diagnosis. The endocrine and metabolic systems are investigated. Sialography initially is unimpressive but later shows narrowing of the ducts and "a bare tree". Histology and electron microscopy demonstrate the special lesions of the autonomic nervous system and of the gland parenchyma.

Treatment. Metabolic or endocrine disorders are treated, and the antihypertensives are stopped or changed.

Trauma

Injury to the Nerves or Ducts and Salivary Fistulae

A *damaged nerve,* i. e., the facial nerve in the parotid area or the lingual or hypoglossal nerves in the sublingual area, must be treated immediately (see pp. 165 and 166).

Injuries to the ducts. It is only necessary to repair injury of a main duct. A fine plastic catheter is introduced, and the two parts of the duct are reanastomosed using microsurgery. If part of the duct is lost, an attempt may be made to reconstruct it or to implant the shortened duct into the buccal mucosa, creating a new orifice.

Salivary fistulae. Treatment of *parenchymatous fistulae* usually causes no difficulty *provided that the main duct system is intact.* In most cases a fistula of the external parenchyma heals spontaneously. Occasionally it may be necessary to suppress the secretion temporarily by atropine or radiotherapy. If this does not succeed in closing the salivary fistula, it must be excised and the soft tissues, particularly the capsule, closed in layers.

Auriculotemporal or Frey's Syndrome (Gustatory Sweating)

Symptoms. The patient complains of sweating and reddening of the skin in the preauricular area before, during, and after eating. Pain is uncommon. Minor forms which can be demonstrated with the starchiodine test are more common than the complete picture with excessive sweating which causes great suffering for the patient. The symptoms develop slowly and often do not appear for several months after the primary traumatic or inflammatory cause.

Pathogenesis. This disease is usually due to trauma or surgery and only rarely to parotitis. There is aberrant regeneration and anastomosis of postganglionic parasympathetic nerves supplying the gland, with sympathetic autonomic fibers running in the auriculotemporal nerve supplying the skin. This causes hypersensitivity of the cutaneous sweat glands to cholinergic impulses.

Treatment. There is no satisfactory method of treatment. An ointment containing 1% glycopyronium bromide may be used on the affected area of skin, the tympanic plexus may be divided in the middle ear, or lyophilized dura or a sheet of fascia may be implanted subdermally in the affected area.

Salivary Tumors

Ninety percent of all salivary tumors are epithelial in origin. The remainder are nonepithelial tumors such as hemangioma, lymphangioma, malignant lymphoma, and periglandular tumors.

Benign Tumors

Adenoma

The frequency and histologic structure are shown in Tables 7.**6** and 7.**7**.

The clinical picture of the various adenomas is very similar. A long history, slow growth, absence of metastases, skin infiltration, and ulceration, and preservation of function of the facial nerve suggest a benign salivary tumor. The final diagnosis is provided by histologic examination of the operative specimen. All adenomas should be treated surgically. The details are discussed below.

Pleomorphic Adenoma

Symptoms. The site of predilection is the parotid where 80% of these tumors arise (see Color Plate **39a**). They are almost always unilateral. Pleomorphic adenomas grow slowly over many years. The average length of history is 5 to 7 years, but a history of 20 years is often obtained in some patients. Women are more often affected than men. The tumor is firm, often nodular, and not painful. The function of the facial nerve is retained even in very large tumors so long as they remain benign. Difficulty in swallowing due to tumor size may be caused by extension of the tumor into the pharynx or by adenomas of the minor salivary glands of the palate or pharynx.

Pathogenesis. The epithelial origin of the pleomorphic adenoma has been proved. About two thirds arise in the superficial lobe of the parotid. There is great variation in the histologic picture. Increasing experience allows *subtypes deficient in stroma* to be recognized which have a clinical tendency to malignant degeneration.

Table 7.6 Frequency of Tumors in the Individual Salivary Glands	
Parotid tumors	80% of all salivary tumors, of which 30% are malignant
Submandibular tumors	10% of all salivary tumors, of which 50% are malignant
Tumors of the minor salivary glands	10% of all salivary tumors, of which 50% are malignant
Sublingual tumors	1% of all salivary tumors, of which 80% are malignant

Table 7.7 Classification of the Benign Epithelial Salivary Tumors	
Pleomorphic adenoma, previously called mixed tumor	85%
Monomorphic adenoma Cystadenolymphoma, Warthin's tumor Oxyphil adenoma Adenomas of other types	15%

In about half the cases the adenoma possesses a capsule, otherwise there is an indistinct boundary between the tumor and the gland. A truly multilocular tumor is uncommon. Recurrent "multicentric" pleomorphic adenomas are usually the result of using the incorrect surgical procedure of enucleation of the tumor.

Diagnosis. Sialography (see Fig. 7.**4d**) and needle biopsy provide the preoperative diagnosis. Intraoperative diagnosis may be made by frozen section, but the definitive diagnosis is made by the histologic examination of the surgical specimen.

Treatment. Parotid tumors are treated by superficial parotidectomy with preservation of the facial nerve. For submandibular gland tumors, treatment is excision of the gland with the tumor and surrounding tissue. Tumors of the minor glands are treated by excision with a margin of normal tissue (see Figs. 7.**5** and 7.**8**).

Prognosis. The outlook is very good. Malignant degeneration is to be expected in 3% to 5% of pleomorphic adenomas, but the frequency of malignant degeneration is higher in recurrences, after inadequate primary surgery, and in patients with a long history.

Cystadenolymphoma (Warthin's Tumor)

Symptoms. This tumor is usually unilateral but 10% are bilateral. It causes a firm elastic, mobile, nontender swelling. Most cases occur in elderly men.

Pathogenesis. This soft cystic tumor usually develops in the inferior part of the parotid. It probably arises from segments of the salivary ducts which have been included in intra- or extraglandular lymph nodes in the embryologic phase. Histology thus shows a rich lymphoreticular stroma with lymph follicles between the epithelial glandular segments from which the term *papillary cyst adenoma lymphomatosum* is derived.

Diagnosis. There is uptake of technetium-99 on a salivary scan. Aspiration or needle biopsy is less helpful in this cystic tumor. Definitive diagnosis rests on histologic examination of the surgical specimen.

Treatment. Depending on the site of the lesion, therapy consists of excision of the parotid gland (preserving the facial nerve), or excision of the submandibular gland.

Prognosis. The outlook is very good and malignant degeneration is uncommon.

Malignant Tumors

Of all salivary tumors, 25% to 30% are malignant (Table 7.**8**).

Main symptoms indicating malignancy:

- *Rapid growth or episodes of growth (the exception is adenoid cystic carcinoma which grows very slowly)*
- *Pain*

Table 7.8 Classification of Malignant Salivary Tumors	
Acinar tumor	15%
Mucoepidermoid tumor	30%
Carcinoma	55%
Adenoid cystic carcinoma, previously called cylindroma	35%
Adenocarcinoma	10%
Squamous cell carcinoma	10%
Carcinoma in pleomorphic adenoma	20%
Other carcinomas (duct carcinoma, sebaceous carcinoma, clear cell carcinoma, undifferentiated carcinoma)	25%

Table 7.9 Frequency of Facial Paralysis in Parotid Malignancy at the Time of Presentation	
Adenoidcystic carcinoma	25%
Undifferentiated carcinoma	25%
Carcinoma in pleomorphic adenoma	15%
Adenocarcinoma	10%
Mucoepidermoid carcinoma	10%

- *Firm infiltration, occasionally ulceration of the skin or mucosa, poor mobility of the tumor*
- *Cervical lymph node metastases*
- *Facial paralysis in parotid tumors*

> **Note:**
> Survival ist reduced in patients with facial paralysis or regional lymph node metastases. As a rule, the smaller the gland of origin, the greater the clinical likelihood of malignant growth in firm salivary gland tumors.

The classification of **epithelial malignancy** is shown in Table 7.**8**.

Acinous Cell Tumors

Symptoms. These are caused by local growth of the tumor.

Diagnosis. This rests on histologic examination. The tumor cells resemble acinar cells.

Treatment. Total parotidectomy is performed since the rate of recurrence after a less extensive operation is very high. The decision to remove the facial nerve or individual branches should rest on the clinical (e. g., paralysis) or intraoperative findings. Neck dissection is advised.

Course and prognosis. These tumors are malignant, but their prognosis is better than that of carcinoma. Regional or distant metastases are uncommon and occasionally late. There is a peak age incidence between 30 and 60 years. Survival rates of 75% and 55% are attained at 5 and 15 years, respectively.

Mucoepidermoid Tumors

Symptoms. These tumors may be of low-grade malignancy and grow slowly, while those with high-grade malignancy grow very rapidly with pain, facial paralysis, and regional lymph node metastases in 40% to 50% of cases. Distant blood-borne metastases are also more common in the latter group.

Pathogenesis. *Well-differentiated tumors (low-grade malignancy, approx. 75%) must be distinguished from undifferentiated (high-grade malignancy, approx. 25%) tumors.*

The degree of malignancy is determined by the ratio between epidermoid and mucous cells. Tumors with mainly mucous cells have the better prognosis. The most common site of this tumor is the parotid gland and the minor salivary glands of the palate. The peak age incidence in between 40 and 50 years, but this tumor may also occur in children.

Diagnosis. This is made by histology.

Treatment. Parotidectomy is performed for parotid lesions, irrespective of the grade of malignancy. A neck dissection is also indicated for high-grade tumors. Facial nerve excision and reconstruction must be decided for each patient individually.

Prognosis. Five-year survival rates of about 90% are achieved in low-grade muco-epidermoid tumors but *considerably* less than this in high-grade tumors.

Adenoid Cystic Carcinoma (Cylindroma)

Symptoms

- Growth is usually slow, but fulminating growth can occasionally occur.
- Pain or paresthesia is present.
- Facial paralysis is present in about 25% of patients.
- There are cranial nerve lesions, particularly in extension to the base of the skull affecting the Vth to VIIth and the IXth to XIIth cranial nerves.
- Regional lymph node metastases are present in about 15% of patients when first diagnosed. Blood-borne distant metastases to the lung and skeleton are common, occurring in up to 20% of patients (Fig. 7.**6**).

Pathogenesis. Histologically this tumor is formed from primitive duct epithelium and myoepithelial cells which form glandular-cystic, cribriform cell nests and also solid trabecular structures. The previous term of cylindroma for this tumor has led to an underestimation of the seriousness of this tumor and for this reason is no longer used. Indeed, this tumor is to be regarded as particularly malignant because of its pattern of growth with extensive local diffuse perivascular and perineural infiltration.

Adenoid cystic carcinomas also occur relatively often in the minor salivary glands, especially those of the palate, followed by the sublingual, submandibular, and parotid glands. The average age of the patient is 55 ± 10 years.

Diagnosis. This tumor can be diagnosed with a high degree of likelihood from the clinical picture, computer tomograms, and sialographic findings. These are confirmed by histology.

Treatment. Blood-borne metastases to the lung and the skeleton must be excluded before operation. *The only chance of cure rests on a radical first*

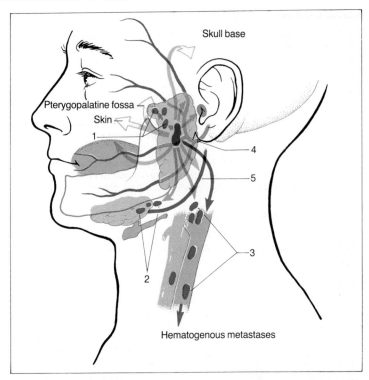

Fig. 7.6   Directions of extension of a parotid tumor showing growth in continuity (light orange arrow), lymphatic (medium orange arrow), and hematogenous (dark orange arrow) metastases. 1, Intra- and periparotid; 2, submandibular and 3, jugular lymph node metastases; 4, facial nerve; 5, hypoglossal nerve.

operation dictated by the site of the tumor. The facial nerve must be resected for an adenoid cystic carcinoma of the parotid gland. The value of *radiotherapy* for adenoid cystic carcinoma is *controversial.*

Prognosis and course (see Fig. 7.6). Poor prognosis is determined by local regional infiltration, early regional and systemic metastases to the lungs, brain, and skeleton, and insensitivity to radiotherapy and chemotherapy. A prolonged course over 10 or more years, even in the presence of distant metastases, is not exceptional. The customary calculation of 5-year survival is not relevant to the particular characteristics of the adenoid cystic carcinoma, but the outcome is almost invariably fatal.

Adenocarcinoma

Papillary and mucus-secreting carcinomas arise from the salivary duct system and infiltrate and destroy locally. The sexes are equally affected. Pain, facial paralysis, and cervical lymph node metastases are common.

Squamous Carcinoma

This infiltrating, rapidly growing tumor mainly attacks the parotid gland where it forms 5% to 10% of all parotid tumors. Regional lymph node metastases are found in about one third of patients.

> *Note:* Before accepting the diagnosis of a primary squamous cell carcinoma of the salivary gland, the possibility of metastases from other head and neck carcinomas to the salivary lymph nodes should be considered.

Carcinoma in Pleomorphic Adenoma

Symptoms. The previous history is often typical. In most cases the tumor has been present for years causing nothing more than a cosmetically unacceptable parotid swelling. This undergoes a sudden spurt of growth often with pain irradiating to the ear, total facial paralysis, or paralysis of individual branches of the nerve. In 25% of patients, regional lymph node metastases develop with infiltration of the tumor into the skin with external ulceration (see Color Plate **39c**).

Pathogenesis. A malignant pleomorphic adenoma which is malignant ab initio is very unusual. It is now thought more likely that malignant degeneration occurs after a long latent interval, particularly in the subtype of pleomorphic adenoma which is poor in stroma (see p. 548). About 3% to 5% of all pleomorphic adenomas undergo malignant degeneration, and the frequency rises with the length of the history. These patients are therefore a decade older on average than those with benign pleomorphic adenomas.

Diagnosis. This is based on *history,* the clinical findings of facial paralysis and regional lymph node metastases, frozen section during operation, and definitive histologic examination.

Treatment. Radical parotidectomy is performed with en bloc neck dissection.

Prognosis. The outlook is doubtful.

Basic Principles of Treatment of Salivary Tumors

The following recommendations can be made about treatment based on the particular tumor biology of salivary gland tumors and on clinical experience. For both benign and malignant tumors, the first operation almost always determines the success of the treatment (pleomorphic adenoma) or the chance of survival of a patient (adenoid cystic carcinoma). The treatment of benign epithelial tumors by radiation is not justified by radiation biology. The results of irradiation alone for malignant epithelial salivary tumors is inferior to that of surgery. Irradiation may, however, be indicated for inoperable tumors, carcinomas which cannot be removed completely, and especially for malignant lymphomas.

The operation is determined by the site and extent of the tumor, and especially by neighboring structures such as the facial nerve, the hypoglossal and lingual nerves, the pharynx, the contents of the carotid sheath, the external auditory meatus, the base of the skull, the facial skeleton, the lymph nodes, and the overlying skin.

Techniques for preservation or reconstruction of the facial nerve by autologous nerve grafts have been the greatest advance in parotid surgery (see also pp. 165 ff.).

Medicolegal comments. The patient should be warned of the possibility of injury to the facial nerve and its results before *any* operation on the parotid.

Note: Lymph node metastases from primary tumors of the eye such as melanoma or from other tributary areas of the head can simulate primary tumors of the major salivary glands, particularly the parotid, especially if the primary tumor, e.g., squamous carcinoma of the skin, has previously been treated by surgery or radiation and the surgical scar or radiation dermatitis is hidden by hair.

Neck dissection is indicated for adenoid cystic carcinomas, carcinomas, high-grade mucoepidermoid tumors, carcinoma in pleomorphic adenomas, and metastases to the parotid lymph nodes from the skin of the face and scalp.

The *first stations of lymph node metastases* are the intra- and periglandular parotid or submandibular nodes and next the deep cervical nodes. Bloodborne distant metastases can be demonstrated especially in adenoid cystic carcinoma relatively often.

Note: Extension by continuity, especially of adenoid cystic carcinoma along the nerves and vessels, is so extensive that the prognosis remains doubtful even after an extensive operation.

Basic Surgical Procedures

1. Superficial Parotidectomy with Preservation of the Facial Nerve for Benign Tumors (see Figs. 7.7 and 7.**8**)

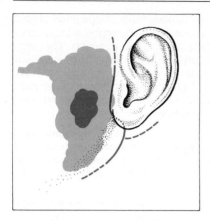

Fig. 7.7 S- or Y-shaped incision for parotidectomy.

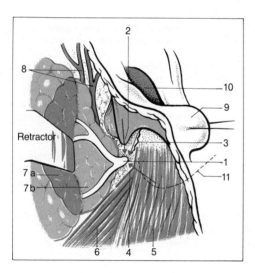

Fig. 7.8 Conservative parotidectomy. Sites for exposing the main trunk of the facial nerve (1). 2, Apex of the cartilaginous meatus, pointer. 3, The tympanomastoid fissure; 4, angle between the anterior border of the sternocleidomastoid muscle (5) and the posterior belly of the digastric (6); 7a, superficial lobe of the parotid gland; 7b, deep lobe of the parotid gland; 8, superficial temple artery and vein; 9, retracted lobe of the auricle; 10, meatal introitus; 11, mastoid apex.

An S- or Y-shaped skin incision in front of or behind the auricle is extended down to the sternocleidomastoid muscle. The main trunk of the facial nerve is sought about 5 mm below the triangular apex of the cartilaginous meatus. The trunk is followed to the branches. The trunk may also be found by beginning dissection at the tympano-mastoid fissure and dissecting 6 to 8 mm medialward. An even better technique is to expose the anterior borders of the sternocleidomastoid muscle and the posterior digastric belly; a line bisecting the angle formed by their borders points to the facial nerve trunk. The branches of the facial nerve are dissected peripherally using the loupe or the operating microscope. The nerve stimulator is very helpful for identification of the branches of the facial nerve during surgery.

The extent of this operation is determined by the size and site of the tumor. It may be necessary to carry out either a superficial or a total parotidectomy with preservation of the facial nerve.

2. Radical Parotidectomy for Malignant Tumors

The operation is determined by the site and extent of the tumor. Thus, it may be necessary to carry out mandibulectomy, petrosectomy, resection of the supra- or periglandular skin, and a neck dissection. Resection of the facial nerve is absolutely indicated in the presence of a partial or complete facial paralysis. Since the malignant cells, especially of an adenoid cystic carcinoma, penetrate the nerve sheath, removal of the nerve is almost always indicated even if there is no clinical evidence of a paralysis.

Facial paralysis after operations for malignancy can be treated by muscle grafts, fascial slings, or nerve grafts (see pp. 163–167).

3. Removal of the Submandibular Gland (see Fig. 7.5)

The skin incision is made 2 cm below and parallel to the horizontal ramus of the mandible. The dissection is carried down to the gland beginning posteriorly. The marginal mandibular branch is protected in order to preserve the nerve supply of the lower lip by elevating the facial artery and vein after they have been ligated. The hypoglossal and lingual nerves are preserved by precise dissection on the capsule of the gland and, if necessary, by exposing the nerves. The duct is ligated anteriorly after freeing the gland.

The principles described for radical parotidectomy also apply to malignant tumors of the submandibular gland.

8. Emergency and First Aid Procedures

1. *Bleeding*
   Nasal bleeding . . . . See p. 253
   Bleeding from the larynx and trachea . . . . . . See pp. 392, 411, 438
   Bleeding from the esophagus . . . . See p. 470
   Bleeding from the ear . . . . See p. 118

2. *Dyspnea*
   Differential diagnosis . . . . See Tables 4.**12** and 4.**13**
   Emergency bronchoscopy . . . . See pp. 436, 438
   Tracheotomy . . . . See p. 446
   Intubation . . . . See p. 450
   Laryngotomy . . . . See p. 448
   Care of a tracheostomy . . . . See p. 451

3. *Foreign bodies*
   In the hypopharynx and esophagus . . . . See pp. 370, 465
   In the larynx, trachea, and bronchi . . . . See pp. 414, 452
   In the nose . . . . See p. 211
   In the ear . . . . See p. 77

4. *Corrosions and scalds*
   In the mouth . . . . See p. 369
   In the esophagus . . . . See p. 463
   In the ear . . . . See p. 76

5. *Sudden deafness* . . . . See p. 145

6. *Acute vertigo*
   Vestibular failure . . . . See p. 144
   Ménière's disease . . . . See p. 139

7. *Facial paralysis* . . . . See p. 163

9. Further Reading

Authors names have been omitted as far as possible in the text to preserve the character and purpose of a pocket-sized book. Furthermore, an exhaustive literature review is not given. The following handbooks, atlases, and monographs are recommended for further information:

Alberti, P. W., R. J. Ruben: Otologic Medicine and Surgery, Vol. I & II. Churchill Livingstone New York, Edinburgh, London, Melbourne 1988

Arnold, W. J., J. A. Laissue, I. Friedmann, H. H. Naumann: Diseases of the Head and Neck. Thieme Stuttgart and New York 1987

Ballantyne, J., J. Groves: Scott-Brown's Diseases of the Ear, Nose and Throat, 5th ed., Vol. I–IV. Butterworths, London 1987

Becker, W., R. A. Buckingham, P. H. Steiner, M. P. Jaumann: Atlas of Ear, Nose and Throat Diseases, 2nd ed. Thieme, Stuttgart and Saunders, Philadelphia 1984

Nager, G. T.: Pathology of the Ear and Temporal Bone. Williams & Wilkins, Baltimore 1993

Naumann, H. H.: Differential Diagnosis in Oto-Rhino-Laryngology. Thieme Stuttgart and New York 1993

Naumann, H. H.: Head and Neck Surgery, Vol. I–IV. Thieme, Stuttgart and Saunders, Philadelphia 1980–1984

Paparella, M. M., D. A. Shumrick: Otolaryngology, 2nd ed., Vol. I–III. Saunders, Philadelphia 1980

Schuknecht, H. F.: Pathology of the Ear. Harvard University Press, Cambridge/Mass. 1974

Valvassori, G. E., G. D. Potter, W. N. Hanafee, B. L. Carter, R. A. Buckingham: Radiology of the Ear, Nose and Throat. Thieme, Stuttgart and Saunders, Philadelphia 1982

Index

Boldface numbers refer to the respective color plates

A

abscess
  brain
    otogenic, 111–12
    rhinogenic, 249–50
  cervical soft tissue, 494
  epidural, 248–9
  eyelid, **14a**
  nasal septal, 261–2
  oral/pharyngeal,
    337–43, 354,
    20c, 23b
  peritonsillar, 354–9,
    23b
  subdural, 249
  subperiosteal, 247, **14c**
achalasia
  cardiac, 469–70
  cricopharyngeal, 470
acid burns
  esophageal, 463–5
  oral/pharyngeal,
    369–70
acinous cell tumor,
    salivary, 551
acoustic agnosia, 153–4
acoustic neuroma/schwan-
    noma, 130–3,
    142, 146
acoustic trauma, acute,
    124–7
actinomycosis
  cervical soft tissue, 496
  oral/pharyngeal, 343
adenocarcinoma
  middle ear, 129
  nasal, 293
  salivary, 553
adenoid(s) (pharyngeal
    tonsils)
  anatomy, 307, 308, 309
  hyperplasia/over-
    growth, 320–2,
    24c, 25a–c
  removal, 321–2
adenoid cystic carcinoma
    (cylindroma)

nasal, 293
salivary, 552–3
tracheal, 455
adenoma, salivary gland,
    548–9, 554
  pleomorphic, 548–9,
    39a, b
    malignancy/carci-
      noma in, 549, 554
adhesive otitis media, 86,
    105, **8b**
adjustment nystagmus, 66
aerosol inhalation, 223
ageusia, 312
agnosia, acoustic, 153–4
agranulocytosis, 348–9
AIDS (HIV syndrome)
  lymphoma, 496, **38d**
  oral involvement, 330,
    341, **20a, b**
air, sound conduction by
    bone and, relation-
    ship between,
    45–8
air embolus, internal jugu-
    lar vein injury-
    associated, 500–1
airway/respiratory tract
  anatomy, 434–5
  lower
    nasal sinuses and,
      pathophysiological
      relationships,
      243–4
    obstruction,
      434–56, 442, 447
    protection, struc-
      tures involved, 394
  upper
    local conservative
      treatment, 222–5
    obstruction, 195
    post-tonsillectomy
      risk of, 354
alae, nasal, anomalies,
    284–5
alkali/lye burns
  esophageal, 463–5, **35c**

oral/pharyngeal,
    369–70
allergic glossitis, 336
allergic rhinitis, 208–10,
    213, 228
allergic stomatitis, 329
allergy, investigations, 203
Alport's syndrome, 152
alveolar respiratory
    insufficiency, 447
aminoglycosides, oto-
    toxic, 136–7
ampullofugal stimulation,
    29
ampullopetal stimulation,
    29
amyloid, laryngeal, 419
aneurysms, cervical,
    505–6
angina
  Ludwig's, **20c**
  Vincent's/ulceromem-
    branous, 349, **23a**
angiofibroma, nasopharyn-
    geal, 385
angiography, cervical,
    493, 507
angiosarcoma, cervical,
    506
angular acceleration,
    29–30
angular vein, 171
anosmia, 182, 196
  central, 182
  essential, 182
anotia, 82
antibiotics
  blood–brain barrier
    for, 108
  ototoxic, 136–7
  upper airway/digestive
    tract conditions
    treated with, 224
antituberculous drug ther-
    apy, 331, 418, 497
antritis, occult infant, 91
antroscopy, 202
antrostomy, 238

antrotomy, 91, 94
antrum
    mastoid, 6
    maxillary, *see* maxillary sinus
aortic arch anomalies, 472
apex, orbital, syndrome of, 247
aphthae, chronic recurrent, 330–1
appendages, auricular, 82, **1a**
arterial supply
    cervical, 479–81, 482–3
    laryngeal, 392
    middle ear, 8
    nasal, 170
    oral cavity, 302
    pharyngeal, 306, 309
    tracheobronchial, 435
arthritis, rheumatoid, cricoarytenoid joint in, 419
arytenoid cartilage
    injuries affecting, 410, **31a**
    prolapse, **32b**
arytenoidectomy, 406
asthma, bronchial, 442
atresia
    choanal, 280, **26b**
    laryngeal, 401, **27c**
    nostrils, 280
atrophic pharyngitis, 362
atrophic rhinitis, 218–19
audimutism, 154
audiometry, 21, 41–60
    cholesteatoma, 101
    deaf children, 159
    electric response, 57–9
    impedance, *see* impedance audiometry
    labyrinthine concussion, 121
    noise-induced deafness, 125–6, 126
    otosclerosis, 115
    pure-tone, *see* pure-tone audiometry
    speech, *see* speech
auditory cortex, 17

auditory evoked potentials, brainstem, 57, 58–9
auditory nerve, *see* vestibulocochlear nerve
auricle (pinna), 3
    amputation, partial and complete, 76
    congenital anomalies, 82
    hematoma, 3, 76, **2c, d**
    reconstructive procedures, 82
auricular neuralgia, 368
auriculotemporal neuralgia, 231
auriculotemporal syndrome, 547–8
autonomic nervous system
    cervical, 488
    dysfunction, dysphagia relating to, 367
    nasal, 179–80
    salivary gland, 532
    see also parasympathetic nervous system; sympathetic nervous system
autophony, 86
axonotmesis, facial nerve, 70, 163

B

bacterial infections
    aural, 219–21
    external ear, 73, 74, 76
    salivary gland, 539–40
    see also specific conditions/viruses and infections
balance, 10–18, 26–33, 136–9
    central connections, 17–18
    disorders, 30–3, 136–9, 160–2
        pathophysiology, 30–3
        toxin-induced, 136–8, 163
    mechanism, 12–14

organs of, 10–18
    physiology, 26–30
barbiturate intoxication, balance problems with, 163
barotrauma
    middle/inner ear, 123–4
    nasal sinus, 274–5
Barrett's esophagus, 468
basal cell carcinoma (rodent ulcer)
    external ear, 79, 81, **4a-d**
    external nose, 290–1
bat ear, 81
B cell lymphoma, 512, 513
Beck's trephine, 240
Behçet's disease, 331
Békésy audiometry, 50
Bell's palsy, 163
Besnier–Boeck–Schaumann sarcoidosis, 206
biopsy
    nasal, 203
    oral/pharyngeal, 320
    prescalene lymph node, 517
    salivary gland, 538–9
bites
    insect, oral/pharyngeal, 371
    tongue, 371
black hairy tongue, 339
blastomycosis, nasal, 221
bleeding/hemorrhage
    carotid artery, 501
    emergency/first aid procedures, 558
    esophageal variceal, 468–9, 470–1
    nasal (epistaxis), 253–60
    oral, 326
    tonsillitis complicated by, 360
blindfold gait, 60
blood–brain barrier for antibiotics, 108
blood disorders

blood, epistaxis with, 254–5, 256
  pharyngeal mucosal lesions with, 364
blood supply/drainage
  laryngeal, 392
  middle ear, 8
  nasal, 170–1, 177–8
  oral cavity, 302–3
  pharynx, 306, 309
  tracheobronchial, 435
blowout fracture, orbital, 273–4
Boeck's disease see sarcoidosis
Boerhaave's syndrome, 467
bone(s)
  disorders
    otologic manifestations, 115, 117
    sinusitis-related, 251–3
  facial, trauma, 265–78
  nasal
    anatomy, 170
    trauma, 263–5
  sound conduction by and air, relationship between, 45–8
    hearing aids employing, 136, 159
  tumors, aural, 129
  see also specific bones
bouginage, 464–5
Bowen's disease
  external ear, 79
  oral, 333
Bowman's glands, 173
brain, see abscess; blood–brain barrier, entries under cerebral and other brain structures
brainstem
  compression, infratentorial tumors with, 161
  optokinetic dysfunction with lesions of, 69

brainstem auditory evoked potentials, 57, 58–9
branchial arches, development, 501, 502
branchial fistula, 501–3
breathing and the nose, 182–3
bronchial system
  anatomy, 435
  disorders, 437–43, 452–3, 454, 455
  nasal sinuses and, pathophysiological relationships, 243–4
  see also laryngotracheobronchitis; tracheobronchial tree
bronchiectasis, 454
bronchoscopy, 436–7, 438
Bruening loupe/pneumatic otoscope, 34, 37
bullous myringitis, 74
burns
  chemical, see chemicals
  emergency/first aid procedures, 558
  thermal
    aural, 76
    nasal, 204–5
bursa, pharyngeal, 304–5
  inflammation, 363

C

cacogeusia, 312
cacosmia, 196
caisson disease, 124
calculi, see cupulolithiasis; otolith; sialolithiasis
Caldwell–Luc antrostomy, 238
caloric labyrinthine testing, 67–8
cancer, see malignancy
candidiasis/moniliasis/thrush
  esophageal, 469

oral/pharyngeal, 329, 341, 349, **18b**
capillary hemangiomas/lymphangiomas, nasal, 290
carbuncle, cervical, 494
carcinoma
  branchiogenic, 503
  bronchial, 456, **34d**
  ear
    external, 79, 81, **4a–5b**
    middle, 96, 129–30
  esophageal, 473, **36c**
  laryngeal, 423, 423–32, **32c**, **33a–c**
  nose, 293, **11d, 17c, d**
    external, 290–1
  oral/pharyngeal, 377, 380, 381–5, 432–4, **18c**, **21c**, **24a, 26c, 33d**, **34a**
  regional lymph node metastases, 516
  salivary, 550, 552–4, **39c**
  thyroid, 526–8
  tracheal, 455–6
carcinoma in situ
  laryngeal, 422–3
  oral, 333
cardiospasm, 469–70
Carhart (tone decay) test, 50
carotid artery
  common, 479
  external and internal, 479–80
    nasal supply from, 177–8
  hemorrhages, 501
  radiography, 507
carotid body, 481
  tumor, 506–7
carotid sinus, 481
  syndrome, 506
carotid triangle, 503
  inferior, 475
  superior, 475, 476
cartilage
  laryngeal, 388, 390

nasal, 170
  duckbill, 262
  see also perichondritis
  and entries under
  chondrocatarrh,
  207, 208
catarrhal pharyngitis,
  acute, 361–2
catheterization
  central venous, 481
  eustachian tube, 41
cat scratch fever, 498–9
cauliflower ear, **2d**
cautery with epistaxis,
  256–7
cavernous hemangiomas/
  lymphangiomas,
  nasal, 290
cavernous sinus thrombo-
  sis, tonsillogenic,
  360
cavernous spaces, nasal,
  179
cavity, mastoid, *see*
  antrotomy; antrum
cavity, nasal, 171–3
  anatomy, 171–3
  endoscopy, 202
  inflammation localized
    mainly in, 207–22
    acute, 207–11
    chronic, 211–22
  malignancy, 297, **12d**
  obstruction, causes, 216
cellulitis
  oral floor, **20c**
  orbital, **13c**, **14a**
central nervous system
  balance/movement and
    the, 17–18, 30,
    160–2
  disorders of, 160–2
  hearing and the, 17
    disorders of, 25–6,
    56, 151, 153–4
  olfactory disorders and
    the, 182
cephalgia, vasomotor, 229
cerebellum, balance/eye
  movements and
  the, 30, 32
cerebral abscess, oto-
  genic, 111

cerebral concussion,
  balance disorders
  with, 161
cerebrospinal fluid rhinorrhea, 276
cervical lymph nodes
  anatomy, 484–6
  biopsy, 517
  inflammatory dis-
    orders, 496–500
  lymphoid tumors affect-
    ing, 510–11
  metastases, 512–15,
    516
    from laryngeal carci-
      noma, 434
    management,
      517–21
  palpation, 31, 515
  see also lymph nodes
cervical sinus, 501
cervical syndrome, 146–7
Charlin's syndrome, 231
cheilitis, 324
chemicals
  burns due to
    esophageal, 463–5,
      35c
    oral/pharyngeal,
      369–70
  inhalation, trauma due
    to, 413
chemodectomas, 127–9
chemosis, 250, **14b**
chemotherapy
  laryngeal cancer, 426
  nasal cancer, 298
  oral cancer, 384–5
children
  deafness in, 153, 155–9
    rehabilitation, 155–9
  Hand–Schueller–
    Christian disease,
    134
  laryngotracheo-
    bronchitis, 454
  otitis media, 90–1
  retropharyngeal
    abscess, 360–1
  sinusitis, 243
  young
    hearing tests, 59–60
    otoscopy, 34

see also infants; new-
  born
choanal atresia, 280, **26b**
choanal polyps, 217
cholesteatoma, 4, 95,
  96–105, **9a–c**
  acquired, 96–105
  congenital, 98, 105
  facial nerve paralysis
    associated with,
    163
  flaccida/attic/primary,
    98, 99, 100, **9a**
  occult, 98
  tensa/secondary, 98, 99
  tympanic membrane
    perforations and,
    37
chondrodermatitis nodu-
  laris circum-
  scripta helicis, 78
chondroma, laryngeal, 422
chordoma, nasopharyn-
  geal, 386
chromosomal disorders,
  deafness with, 152
chronaxy with facial
  nerve lesions, 70
cilia
  inner ear, of sensory
    hair cells, 12, 13,
    14, 15, 22
  nasal mucosal, 184
circle of Willis, 481, 482
circulation, *see* vascular
  system
cleaning
  of air by nose, 183
  of ear, self-, 72, **6a**
clefts
  face/nose, 279
  lip/jaw/palate, 279,
    374–6
coagulation disorders,
  epistaxis with,
  254–5, 256
coated tongue, 340
cochlea, 14–16, 21–3,
  136–54
  dysfunction, clinical
    aspects, 136–54
  function, 21–3

cochlea, implants, in deaf children, 157
cochlear amplifier, frequency-specific, 23
cochleography, 57–8, 58–9
cold, common, 207–8, 212
commissures, labial, rhagades, 324
compliance, *see* tympanic membrane
computed tomography
    aural, 38
        cholesteatoma, 100
    cervical soft tissues, 493
    paranasal sinus lesions investigated via, 198
    spread of, 192
    salivary gland, 537
concussion
    cerebral, balance disorders with, 161
    labyrinthine, 121–2
conduction, sound, audiometry with disorders of, 45–8
conductive cochlear presbycusis, 148
conductive deafness, 25, 45–9, 149
    in middle ear trauma, 122
congenital conditions
    cervical soft tissue, 501–5
    ear
        external, 1, 81–2, 134–6, **1a–d**
        internal, 135, 136
        middle, 1, 105, 134–6
    esophageal, 471–2
    laryngeal, 399–402
    nose, 279–80
    oral/pharyngeal, 373–6
    tracheobronchial, 454
    see also specific conditions
conjunctivitis, 227

connective tissue membranes, laryngeal, 390
connective tissue tumor, oral/pharyngeal, 377
contact ulcer, laryngeal, 410, **29c**
cords, vocal, *see* vocal cords
corrosives, *see* chemicals
Corti, organ of
    central connections, 17
    structure, 14–16
cortical potentials, slow and late, 57
corticosteroids, *see* steroid therapy
coryza, 207–8, 212
costoclavicular compression syndrome, 504–5
coughing, 490
cough(ing) reflex, 394
coxsackie virus, parotid infection, 542
cranial fossa, anterior, frontobasal injury to, 275–8, **16a, b**
cranial nerves, *see specific nerves*
cranium/skull
    lesions
        headaches due to, 235
        olfactory disorders due to, 195
        pressure within, increased, otic tumors associated with, 130, 132
        sinus infection affecting, 251–3
        sinus infection spreading within, 248
cricoarytenoid joint in rheumatoid arthritis, 419
cricoid cartilage, 390
    injury, 448
cricopharyngeal
    achalasia, 470

cricothyroid membrane, 390
cri-du-chat syndrome, deafness in, 152
crista ampullaris, 13, 14
croup syndromes, 415–17
cryosurgery, turbinate mucosal, 216
crypts, tonsillar, 308
    disorders, 314–15
cup ear, **1b**
cupula, 13, 29
    acceleration indicators, 30
cupulolithiasis, 146
cylindroma, *see* adenoid cystic carcinoma
cyst(s)
    cervical, 494, **37b, c**
    dermoid, *see* dermoid cysts
    laryngeal retention, 422
    nasal, 244, 245, 279
    retention, *see* retention cyst
    sebaceous cervical, 494
    sublingual (ranula), 533, **21a**
    thyroglossal duct, 504, **37b**
cystadenolymphoma, 550
cystic carcinoma, *see* adenoid cystic carcinoma
cystic fibrosis, 244
cystic hygroma, 505
cytology, nasal mucosal, 202
cytomegalovirus, parotid infection, 541–2

D

dacryocystitis, **15c**
deafness, 136–59, 169
    classification based on severity of, 155–7
    complete, 157–9
        bilateral, 156
    conductive, *see* conductive deafness
    inner ear, recruitment in, 48

Ménière's disease, 140, 141
middle ear, 25, 122
noise-induced, 54, 55, 125–6
rehabilitation, 155–9
retrocochlear, 50, 56
sensorineural, *see* sensorineural deafness
simulated, 56–7
sudden, 145–6
tests, 41–60
trauma-related, 122
decibels, audiometry and, 44, 50
decompression, facial nerve, 163, 164–5
decompression sickness (caisson disease), 124
defences, *see* immune system; protection
de Quervain's thyroiditis, 525
dermatology, *see* chondrodermatitis; eczema; skin
dermoid cysts
cervical, 494
nasal, 279
development/embryology
cervical soft tissue, 501
laryngeal, 388
otological, 1–2
disorders, 1
salivary gland, 529–31
deviation
of nasal septum, 260–1, 284
of nose, 284
diabetics, cholesteatoma, 105
digestive tract, upper, local conservative treatment, 222–5
diphtheria, 219–20, 346–7
laryngeal, 415
nasal, 219–20
oral, 341, 346–7
tracheal, 454
discharge
aural, 168

nasal
causes, 212–13, 226
in sinusitis, 226
distortion products, 59
diuretics, ototoxicity, 137
diverticulum
esophageal, 467–8
Zenker's, 306, 310, 372–3, 467, **36a**
diving accidents, 124
dizziness, *see* vertigo
Doefler–Stewart test, 56–7
drainage
of middle ear spaces, 85, **7b**
disordered, 82–7
of peritonsillar abscess, 357
drop attacks, 147, 160, 483
drugs
rhinitis caused by, 217
stomatitis caused by, 329
taste affected by, 312
upper airway/digestive tract conditions treated with topical, 223–4
see also specific (types of) drugs
duckbill nose (saddlenose), 262, 281, 282–4
ducts, *see* parotid duct; submandibular duct; thoracic duct; thyroglossal duct
dyslalia, otogenic, 157
dysphagia, 310, 366–7, 472
functional, 368–9
dysphonia, 402
dysplasia
auricular, **1c**
fibrous, 289
laryngeal, 422–3
oculoauriculovertebral (Goldenhar syndrome), 504

dyspnea, 402, 442
emergency/first aid procedures, 558

E

Eagle syndrome, 364–5
ear, 1–169
anatomy, 1–20
development, *see* development
disorders/diseases, 3, 4, 25, 25–6, 30–3, 71–169, 321
headache with, 234
synopsis, 168–9
external, *see* external ear
internal, *see* internal ear
investigations, 21, 33–71
middle, *see* middle ear
eardrum, *see* tympanic membrane
eating, oral/pharyngeal aspects, 309–10
ectopic salivary gland tissue, 530
ectopic thyroid, 523
eczema
aural, 75
nasal, 203–4, 227
edema
orbital/periorbital, 246, 247
Reinke's, 393, 420–1
see also swelling
effusions, middle ear, *see* otitis media
electric response audiometry, 57–9
electrocochleography, 57–8
electrodiagnosis with facial nerve lesions, 70–1, 163–4
electrogustometry, 70, 319
electrolyte(s), inner ear disturbances of, 11–12

electrolyte sialadenitis,
    545
electromyography with
    facial nerve
    lesions, 70, 175
electroneurography with
    facial nerve
    lesions, 70–1,
    165, 173
electronystagmography,
    63
embolus, air, internal
    jugular vein
    injury-associated,
    500–1
embryology, see develop-
    ment
emergency procedures,
    558
emissions, otoacoustic,
    see otoacoustic
    emissions
empyema, epidural, 107
encephalitis, balance dis-
    orders in, 161
endocrinology, see hor-
    mones
endolymph, 11–12, 13
    in caloric labyrinthine
        testing, 67
    movement, 29
endoscopy, 318
    esophageal, 459–61,
        462, 473
    hypopharyngeal, 318
    laryngeal, 395–9, 523
        in vocal cord paraly-
            sis, therapeutic,
            406, 407
    nasopharyngeal, 192,
        202, 215, 318
    tracheobronchial,
        436–7, 438
        therapeutic, 446
endotracheal intubation,
    see intubation
eosinophilic granuloma,
    see granuloma
epidural abscess, 248–9
epidural empyema, 107
epiglottitis, 416–17, **31b**
epistaxis, 253–60

epithelial cell sialadenitis,
    544
epithelium
    nasal, 173
    oral cavity, 302
    pharyngeal, 305
    see also lym-
        phoepithelial sys-
        tem; mucosa
epitympanitis, 6
epitympanum, 5–6
Erb's points, 488
erysipelas
    external ear, 73, **3b**
    external nose, 205
erythema multiforme, 334
erythroplakia, oral, 333
erythroplasia, oral, 333
erythroprosoplagia, 229
esophagitis, 468–9
esophagoscopy, 459–61,
    462, 473
esophagus, 457–73
    anatomy, 457–8
    disorders, 463–73
        dysphagia due to,
            366–7, 472
    function, 458
        peristaltic, 310, 458
    investigation, 459–63
    see also pharyng
        (oesophag)eal
        pouch
ethmoid(al) labyrinth
    anatomy, 176
    evacuation, 201
    mucocele, **15c**
ethmoid(al) sinus
    polyps, **26a**
    radiography, 198
    sphenoid sinus surgical
        approach via, 242,
        243
ethmoid(al) sinusitis (eth-
    moiditis), 226,
    238–40, **26a**
eustachian tube, 4–5,
    40–2
    functional assessment,
        40–2
    occlusion, 83–4, 84–5
        acute, 84–5
        long-standing, 83

short-lasting, 83
    patulous, 86–7
evoked otoacoustic emis-
    sions, 59
evoked potentials, brain-
    stem auditory
    (ABR), 57, 58–9
exophthalmos
    malignant, 248
    thyroid-related, 524
exostosis, external ear,
    78, **5d**
expiration and the nose,
    182
explosions, aural trauma,
    124, 125
external ear, 3–4, 71–82,
    134–6
    anatomy, 3–4
    diseases/disorders, 3,
        4, 71–82, 134–6,
        216
        see also specific dis-
            orders
    inspection, 33
external nose
    anatomy, 170–1
    deformed shape, 281–9
    inflammation, 203–7
    inspection/palpation,
        186–7
    malignancy, 290–3,
        296
exudates, 87
    seromucinous, 83
    serous, 37
    tympanic membrane
        pathology with, 37
    see also otitis
eye
    disease
        head and face pain
            due to, 233
        thyroid-related, 524
    movements, 29–30,
        63–7
        disorders, 30, 31, 32,
            63–7
        tests for, 62, 63–7
    see also oculoauriculo-
        vertebral dys-
        plasia; orbit; peri-
        ocular hematoma

eyelid
  abscess, **14a**
  swelling, 268–9

F

face, 170–298
  disorders, 203–98
    congenital, 279
    traumatic, 265–78
  investigations, 186–203
  pain, causes, 227,
    228–36
facial nerve (VIIth cranial
    nerve), 3, 18–20,
    163–7
  anatomy, 3, 18–20,
    531–2
  disorders (in general),
    122, 123, 163–7,
    547
    cholesteatoma-
      related, 101
  investigation, 69–71
  neuroma, 133
  paralysis, *see* paralysis
  salivary gland surgery
    preserving, 555–7
familial disposition, oto-
    sclerosis, 115
fascia, cervical, 476–8
fatigue, auditory, patho-
    logic, 50
fatigue nystagmus, 66
feeding, oral/pharyngeal
    aspects, 309–10
Feldmann's classification,
    43
Feldmann's dichotic
    speech test, 56
fetor
  nasal, causes, 219
  oral, causes, 335
fibroma
  nasopharyngeal, **25d**
  ossifying, 289
  see also angiofibroma;
    neurofibroma
fibrosis
  cystic, 244

middle ear (adhesive
    otitis media), 86,
    105, **8b**
fibrous dysplasia, 289
finger–nose pointing test,
    61
first aid procedures, 558
fissured tongue, 336–7,
    339
fistula
  branchial/cervical,
    501–3, **37d**
  congenital/preauricu-
    lar, 82, **2a, b**
  labyrinthine capsule,
    test for, 69
  nasal, 279
  tracheoesophageal,
    471–2
fixation nystagmus, 63,
    65–6
flaps, skin, in head/neck
    reconstructive pro-
    cedures, 285–9
fluids, inner ear, 11–12
follicular carcinoma, thy-
    roid, 527, 528
follicular tonsillitis, 344
folliculitis, nasal vestibu-
    lar, 204
food, oral/pharyngeal
    aspects of eating
    of, 309–10
foreign bodies
  aural, 3, 77–8
  emergency/first aid pro-
    cedures, 558
  esophageal, 465–6,
    35b
  laryngeal, 414
  nasal, 211, **12d**
  oral/pharyngeal,
    370–1, 432, **35a**
  tracheobronchial,
    452–3, **34c**
fossa, cranial, anterior,
    frontobasal injury
    to, 275–8, **16a, b**
Fowler's loudness
    balance test, 48–9
fractures, *see* injury *and
    specific bones*
Freiburg speech test, 52

Frenzel's diagram/chart,
    62, 63
Frenzel's spectacles, 63
frequency-specific
    cochlear ampli-
    fier, 23
Frey's syndrome, 547–8
frontal lobe abscess, rhino-
    genic, 249
frontal sinus
  anatomy, 176
  lavage, 200–1
  pyomucocele, **15c**
  radiography, 198
frontal sinusitis, 226,
    240–2, **14c**
frontobasal injury to ante-
    rior cranial fossa,
    275–8, **16a, b**
frostbite
  aural, 76
  nasal, 204–5
fungal infections/mycoses
  aural, 74–5
  esophageal, 469
  nasal, 221
  oral/pharyngeal, 329,
    341, 349, **18b**
  *see also specific condi-
    tions/pathogens
    and* infections
furuncle
  aural, 73
  cervical, 494
  nasal, 204, **10a**
fusospirochetal (Plaut–
    Vincent) angina,
    349, **23a**

G

gait
  blindfold, 60
  normal, maintenance,
    26
galvanic test, 68
ganglion
  cervical, 489–90
  stellate, *see* stellate gan-
    glion
gaze-evoked nystagmus,
    64–5, 69

gaze-paretic nystagmus,
  64–5, 69
Gellé's test, 42
  otosclerosis, 42, 115
genetic disease
  deafness due to, 152
  tracheobronchial, 454
genetic factors in oto-
  sclerosis, 115
geniculate ganglion
  neuralgia, 231
geographic tongue, 336,
  18a
gingivitis, 324, 328
glanders, 219, 221
glaucoma, acute and
  chronic, 233
gliomas, nasal, 279
globus hystericus, 368–9
globus symptom, 310
glomus tumor, 127–9, **9d**
glossitis, 335–7, **19b**
glossopharyngeal neural-
  gia, 231, 365–8
glottis, 388
  carcinoma, 424, 425,
    431, **33b**
  opening/closing, 391
goiter, 475, 523
Goldenhar syndrome, 504
Gradenigo's sign, 113
grafts
  nerve, with facial nerve
    lesions, 166, 167
  skin, in head/neck
    reconstructive pro-
    cedures, 285, 288,
    289
granuloma
  eosinophilic
    aural, 134
    nasal, 293
  lethal midline, 222
  vocal process, intuba-
    tion-related, 411,
    29b
granulomatosis
  reticuloendothelial, see
    histiocytosis
  Wegener's, 221–2
granulomatous thyroid-
  itis, de Quer-
  vain's, 525

grey smooth tongue, 339
gunfire, aural acoustic
  trauma due to,
  124, 125
gustation/gustometry, see
  taste
gustatory sweating, 547–8

H

hair cells, 12, 13, 14, 15,
  22, 23
  function, 22, 23, 28
  inner, 15, 23
  outer, 15, 23
Hand–Schueller–Chris-
  tian disease, 134
Hashimoto's disease, 525,
  526
head
  lymph nodes, see
    lymph nodes
  plastic–reconstructive
    procedures, 285–9
headache
  nasal and sinus origin,
    228
  otogenic, 234
  pharyngeal, 233
  vasomotor, 229
  vertebral origin, 233
hearing, 10–18, 20–6,
  136–59
  afferent pathways, 16
  disorders, 41–60,
    136–59
    inflammatory, 138–9
    pathophysiological
      basis, 25–6
    tests, 41–60
    toxin-induced,
      136–8
  see also deafness
  loss, see deafness; dis-
    orders (subhead-
    ing above)
  peripheral, 10–18
  physiology, 20–4
  protection from noise,
    127
  range, 45, 46

suprathreshold determi-
  nations, 48, 49–50
  tests, 51–60
    audiometric, see
      audiometry
    non-audiometric,
      41–3
  threshold
    determinations, 41,
      43–5, 47
    Ménière's disease,
      141
    noise-induced shifts,
      126
hearing aids, pediatric/
  congenital condi-
  tions requiring,
  136, 157–9
Heerefordt syndrome, 544
hemangiomas
  cervical, 505
  laryngeal, 401–2
  nasal, 290
  oral, 376–7
hemangiopericytoma, cer-
  vical, 506
hematologic disease, see
  blood disorders
hematoma
  auricular, 3, 76, **2c, d,
    6a**
  nasal septal, 261–2,
    11b
  periocular, 276, **16a**
hemorrhage, see bleeding
hemotympanum, 117, **6d**
heredity, see entries
  under genetic
hernia, hiatus, 468, 472
herpangina, 346
herpes labialis, 324
herpes simplex stomatitis,
  328, **10a**
herpes zoster
  aural, 73, 138, **3c**
  oral, 329–30
hiatus hernia, 468, 472
histiocytosis (reticuloendothelial granulo-
  matosis)
  aural, 134
  nasal, 293
Hitselberger's sign, 3

HIV syndrome, *see* AIDS
hoarseness, cause, 393
Hodgkin's disease,
    510–11
hormones
    disorders, otosclerosis
        due to, 115
    thyroid, 522
horn, cutaneous, 79
humidity, nasal inspira-
        tion and, 183
hump nose, 281, 282, 283
Hunt's neuralgia, 231
Hunter's glossitis, 338,
    19b
hydrocephalus, otitic,
    110–11
hygroma, cystic, 505
hyoid arch development,
    502
hyoid bone, removal, 504
hypergeusia, 312
hyperkeratosis, oral/
        pharyngeal,
        332–3, 349
hyperostosis, meatal, 78
hyperplasia
    pharyngeal wall
        mucosal, 362
    tonsillar, 314, 322–4,
        22a
        pharyngeal (=ade-
            noids), 320–2,
            24c, 25a–c
hyperthyroidism, 524–5
hypertrophy, nasal turbi-
        nate, 215, **25a**
hypogeusia, 312
hypoglossal–facial nerve
        anastomosis, 167
hypopharyngoscopy, 318
hypopharynx, 432–4
    anatomy, 305–6
    diverticulum
        (Zenker's), 306,
        310, 372–3, 467,
        36a
    foreign body, 432, **35a**
    malignancy, 379,
        432–4, **33d, 34a**
    physical examination,
        318
    radiography, 319

stenosis, 440
hyposomia, 182, 196
hypothyroidism, 522, 524
hypotympanic recess, 6

I

imaging, *see* radiography
        and specific
        methods
immune system
    mucosal
        middle ear, 83–4
        nasal, 184
        Waldeyer's ring and,
            312–15
impedance, acoustic, 47
impedance audiometry,
        21, 50–2
    otosclerosis, 115
implants, cochlear, in
        deaf children, 157
incus, 1
    see also ossicles
infants
    hearing tests, 59–60
    nasal patency, assess-
        ment, 194
    newborn, choanal atre-
        sia, 280, **26b**
    osteomyelitis of upper
        jaw, 253
    otitis media, 90–1
    otoscopy, 34
infections
    allergy and, 209
    cervical soft tissue,
        493–500, **37a**
    ear, 87–96, 106–9
        complications,
            106–9
        external, 3, 4, 71–4,
            76
        internal, 138–9
        middle, 4, 87–96,
            106–9
    esophagus, 469
    larynx, 414–17
    maternal, prenatal
        acquired deafness
        with, 153

mouth/pharynx,
        324–8, 329–30,
        331–2, 336–43,
        344–8, 349, 350,
        351
    nose, 219–21, 224,
        224–53
        complications,
            245–53
        external, 204,
            205–6, 206–8
    salivary gland,
        539–42, 544
    thyroid, 525–6
    tracheobronchial,
        453–4
    see also specific condi-
        tions and (types
        of) pathogens and
        sepsis
inflammatory complica-
        tions of sinus
        infections, 245
inflammatory disorders
    cervical soft tissue,
        493–500
    external ear, 71–6
        chronic, 75–6
        non-specific forms,
            71–2
        specific forms, 73–6
    facial nerve, 163
    internal ear, 138–9
    larynx, 414–34
    middle ear, 85–6,
        87–114
        non-specific forms,
            87–113
        specific forms,
            113–14
    mouth/pharynx,
        324–69
    nose/paranasal sinus,
        203–53
    salivary gland, 539–45
        acute, 539–42
        chronic, 542–5
    see also specific dis-
        orders e.g. epitym-
        panitis; mastoid-
        itis; otitis
inflammatory otitis, 74, 88,
        91, **7d**

infratentorial tumors,
    balance disorders
    with, 161
inhalational therapy, 223
inhalational trauma by
    chemical toxins,
    413
inheritance, *see entries
    under* genetic
injury, traumatic
    cervical soft tissue,
    500–1
    cervical syndrome
    after, 147
    cholesteatoma after, 105
    endotracheal intubation-
    related, 410–11,
    448
    esophageal, 463–7
    external ear, 75–6
    facial nerve, 122, 123,
    165, 547
    paralysis due to, 165
    laryngeal, 409–14,
    448, 500, **29b, c,
    30a, 31a**
    middle/internal ear, 37,
    117–27
    nasal, 260, 262, 263–78
    bleeding from, 254
    oral/pharyngeal,
    369–71
    salivary gland, 547–8
    tracheobronchial, 448,
    453
inner ear, *see* internal ear
innervation
    cervical, 487–90
    external ear, 3
    laryngeal, 391–2
    middle ear, 8
    nasal, 171, 179–80
    oral cavity, 303–4
    pharyngeal, 488
    salivary gland, 531, 532
insect bites, oral/pharyn-
    geal, 371
inspection
    external ear, 33
    laryngeal, 395, **27a**
    maxillary fracture, 267
    neck, 490–1

oral/pharyngeal,
    315–16
inspiration
    nose and, 182, 183
    stridor on, 440
internal ear, 10–18,
    20–3, 82–169
    anatomy, 10–18
    pathology/pathophysi-
    ology, 30–3,
    82–169
    *see also specific
    (types of) condi-
    tions/disorders*
    physiology, 20–3
intracranial problems, *see*
    cranium
intubation, endotracheal,
    447, 450–1
    complications,
    410–11, 448, **29b**
irrigation, *see* lavage;
    syringing
isophon curves, 27, 46

J

Jansen–Ritter frontal
    sinus operation,
    241
jaw
    cleft, 279, 374–6
    fracture, 265–71
    locked (trismus), 356
    lower, *see* mandible
    malignancy, 297
    osteomyelitis, 252–3
    upper, *see* maxilla
jugular veins, 481
    injury, 500–1
jugulosubclavian angles,
    right and left,
    485, 486
jugulosubclavian venous
    angles, greater
    and lesser, 482

K

Kaposi's sarcoma, 330,
    20b

Kartagener's triad, 244,
    454
Keil classification, non-
    Hodgkin's lym-
    phoma, 512–13
keratosis
    oral/pharyngeal,
    332–3, 349
    senile, 79
Kiesselbach's plexus,
    178, 253, **11c, d**
Killian's frontal sinus
    operation, 241
Killian's position in
    indirect laryngo-
    scopy, 395, 396
Killian's submucous
    resection of nasal
    septum, 261
Killian's triangle, 306, 373
Klippel–Feil syndrome,
    504
Kuettner's tumor, 542

L

labia, oral, *see* lip
labyrinth of ethmoid, *see*
    ethmoidal laby-
    rinth; ethmoidal
    sinus
labyrinth of inner ear,
    10–18
    anatomy, 10–18
    bony (labyrinthine cap-
    sule), 1, 7, 10–11
    fistula, test for, 69
    non-inflammatory
    disease, 114–17
    concussion, 121–2
    functional assessment,
    67–8
    membranous, 1, 11–12
labyrinthitis, 107
    serous, 139
lacrimal system, injury,
    278
lacunar tonsillitis, 344,
    22a
lamina propria, tympanic
    membrane, 7

laryngeal nerves, inferior, paralysis, 405
laryngeal nerves, recurrent, 405–6
　anatomy, 392, 488, 522
　paralysis, 390–1, 402, 403, 405–6, 407–8
　　bilateral, 406
　　unilateral, 406
laryngeal nerves, superior, 407–8
　anatomy, 391–2
　neuralgia, 368, 408
　paralysis, 405, 407–8
　　unilateral and bilateral, 407
laryngectomy, 426–32
　rehabilitation after, 431–2
laryngitis, 414–20
　acute, 414–17, **28a**
　chronic, 417–20, **28c**
　subglottic, 415–16, 454
laryngoceles, 401, **29a**
laryngography, 399
laryngomalacia, 399–400
laryngoscopy, 318, 395–9, 523
　direct, 397–8
　indirect, 395–9
　micro-, 397–8
　telescopic, 397
laryngotomy, 448–50
laryngotracheobronchitis, 454
larynx, 388–434
　anatomy, 388–93
　disorders, 399–434, 500
　　dysphagia due to, 366
　embryology, 388
　investigation, 318, 395, **27a**
　physiology, 393–4
lavage, paranasal sinus, diagnostic and therapeutic, 199–201
Lee's speech delay test, 57
Le Fort class I-III fractures, 266–7

leiomyoma, cervical, 509
leiomyosarcoma, cervical, 509
leprosy, nasal, 207
Letterer–Siwe disease, 134
leukoplakia, 332–3, **21a**
　hairy, 330, **20a**
　laryngeal, 422–3
lichen planus, 334–5, 339
ligaments, laryngeal, 390
limen nasi, 172, 182
linear movement/acceleration, 28
lingua, see tongue
lingual tonsil, 300, 307
　hyperplasia, 324
　infection, 345
lip
　cleft, 279, 374–6
　inflammatory conditions, 324–35
　malignancy, 377, 378, 381
lipoma, cervical (and Madelung's neck), 508–9, **39d**
liposarcoma, cervical, 509
lockjaw (trismus), 356
loudness, 46
　see also Fowler's loudness balance test
Ludwig's angina, **20c**
Luescher's classification, 43
Luescher's tone intensity-difference threshold, 49
Lukes and Collins classification, non-Hodgkin's lymphoma, 512–13
lung, see alveolar respiratory insufficiency; bronchi; trachea
lupus vulgaris, nasal, 205–6
lye, see alkali
lyme disease, 500
lymphadenitis, 496–7
lymphangiography, cervical, 493

lymphangiomas
　cervical, 505
　nasal, 290
lymphatic system
　cervical, 484–6, 496–500, 510–15
　　inflammatory disorders, 496–50
　　neoplastic disorders, 510–15, 516
　external ear, 3
　laryngeal, 392
　nasal, 179
　oral cavity, 303
　pharyngeal, 307
　salivary gland, 532
　tracheobronchial, 435
lymph nodes
　biopsy, 517
　head and neck, 484–6, 510–15
　　inflammatory disorders, 496–500
　　neoplastic disorders, 510–15, 516
　　palpation, 318, 492, 515
　see also cervical lymph nodes
　metastases, 503, 511–15, 516
　　from laryngeal carcinoma, 424, 426, 431, 433, 434
　　management, 517–21
　　from oral malignancy, 382, 383, 384, 387
　　from salivary glands, 552, 555
lymphoepithelial lesion, benign (Sjögren's syndrome), 339, 363, 543, **38a, c**
lymphoepithelial system, pharyngeal, 307–9, 312–15
　anatomy, 307–9
　disorders, 314–15, 320–4
　function, 312–15

lymphoma, 510–11,
　512–13
　AIDS, 496, **38d**
　benign, 510
　cervical, 510–11
　Hodgkin's, 510–11
　non-Hodgkin's, 511,
　　512–13
　tonsillar, **23c**
　see also cystadenolym-
　　phoma

M

maculae (semicircular
　　canal), 14
　saccular, 28
　static, 12
maculoocular reflex, 28
maculospinal reflex, 28
Madelung's neck, **39d**
magnetic resonance imag-
　　ing
　ear, 38–9
　larynx, 399
　nose and paranasal
　　sinus, 198
malignancy/cancer
　AIDS-related, **20b,
　　38d**
　branchiogenic, 503
　cervical soft tissue, 506
　ear
　　external, 78–81, **3d,
　　　4a–d, 5a, b**
　　middle, 96
　esophageal, 473, **36c**
　laryngeal, 423–32, **32c,
　　33a–c**
　metastatic, see
　　metastases
　nasal, 290–8, **10d,
　　11d, 12d, 17c, d**
　oral/pharyngeal, 330,
　　377–85, 432–4,
　　**18c , 21c, 23c,
　　24a, 26c, 33d**
　salivary gland, 533,
　　538, 550–7, **39c**
　surgery, 557
　thyroid, 526–8

tracheobronchial,
　455–6
see also precancer and
　specific histologic
　forms
malignant exophthalmos,
　248
malignant otitis externa,
　3, 73, 74
malleus, 1
　see also ossicles
Mallory–Weiss syn-
　drome, 466–7
mandible
　anatomy, 301–2
　facial pain in region of,
　233
　fractures/injuries, 278
　swelling in region of,
　270
mandibular arch develop-
　ment, 502
mandibulectomy, 382–3
manometry
　esophageal, 462–3
　intranasal, 193–4
masticatory muscles,
　303–4
masticatory spasm
　(trismus), 356
mastoid antrum/cavity,
　see antritis;
　antrotomy; antrum
mastoidectomy, 93–4,
　96, 102
mastoiditis, 4, 89–90,
　91–4, 113–14,
　8a
　acute, 94
　　facial nerve paraly-
　　sis in, 163
　chronic, 94
　see also pseudomastoid-
　　itis
mastoid process, pneu-
　matization and
　the, 8, 9, 10
maxilla (upper jaw)
　cleft, 374–6
　fracture, 265–71
　function, 180
　malignancy, 297
　osteomyelitis, 252–3

maxillary sinus/antrum
　anatomy, 174–5, 180
　cysts, 244, 245
　lavage, 199–200
　malignancy, 297,
　　17c, d
　physiology, 180
　radiography, 198
maxillary sinusitis, 226,
　237–8
measles otitis, 91
meatus, auditory/acoustic
　cholesteatoma, 105
　external, 1, 3
　　bony, 3
　　function, 20
　　infections, 3
　　tumors, 78, 81
meatus, nasal, 172–3
　anatomy, 172–3
　inferior, 172–3
　　maxillary antral la-
　　　vage via, 199–200
　middle, 173
　　maxillary antral la-
　　　vage via, 200
　superior, 173
mechanoreceptors
　cervical spine and neck
　　muscle, 30
　semi-circular canal, 13,
　　14
mediastinitis, 494
mediastinoscopy, 518, 519
medullary carcinoma, thy-
　roid, 527, 528
melanoma
　external ear, 80, 81, **3d**
　external nose, 291–3
　head and neck, **17a, b**
Melkersson–Rosenthal
　syndrome, 165,
　324, 339
Ménière's disease, 12,
　139–44
meningitis
　otogenic, 108–9, 120
　rhinogenic, 251
　serous, 138
meningoencephalocele,
　nasal, 279–80
Merseburger's triad, 524

mesenchymal nasal
    tumors, 293
mesotympanum, 5–6
metabolic disorders, oto-
    sclerosis due to,
    115
metal stomatitis, 328–9
metaplasia, middle ear
    mucosal, 83–4
metastases, 503, 512–15,
    516
    from laryngeal carci-
        noma, 424, 426,
        431, 433, 434
    lymph node, see lymph
        node
    from mouth/pharynx,
        382, 383, 384, 387
    from salivary glands,
        552, 552–3, 555
microbiology, mouth/
    pharynx condi-
    tions, 319
    see also specific condi-
        tions and patho-
        gens
microlaryngoscopy,
    397–8
microscopy, ear, 36
microtia, 82
middle ear, 4–10, 20–3,
    82–136
    anatomy, 4–10
    disorders, 4, 25, 51,
        82–136, 149, 163
        see also specific
            (types of) dis-
            orders
    physiology, 20–3
    pressure, see pressure
Miescher's disease, 324
migraine, 229
Mikulicz syndrome, 544
mirror (examination by)
    laryngeal, 395–7
    oral/pharyngeal,
        315–16, 318
Moeller–Hunter glossitis,
    341
moistening of air by nose,
    183
moniliasis, see candidiasis

mononucleosis, infec-
    tious, 348, 440,
    22c
motility disorders,
    esophageal,
    469–70
    see also peristalsis
motor nerves
    vagal, 488
    VIIth cranial, 18
mouth, 299–387
    anatomy, 299–309
    disease, clinical
        aspects, 320–87
    floor of, 301
        abscess, 337–43,
            20c
        carcinoma, 380, **21c**
    investigation, 315–20
    physiology and
        pathophysiology,
        309–15
    see also oral cavity
mouthwashes, 369
movement
    balance and, 28–30
    eye, see eye
mucoceles, 244, **15a**
mucociliary apparatus,
    nasal, 183–4
mucoepidermoid tumor,
    salivary, 551–2
mucosa
    laryngeal, 393
        precancer, 422–3
    middle ear, 7–8
        chronic inflamma-
            tion, 37, 94–5
        metaplasia/hyperac-
            tivity, 83–4
    nasal
        anatomy, 173, 177
        drug-related dis-
            orders, 217
        injury, 370–1
        physiology, 183–4
    oral/pharyngeal, inflam-
        matory condi-
        tions, 324–35, 364
mucotomy, nasal, 216
mucoviscidosis, 244, 343
multiple sclerosis

balance problems in,
    162
optokinetic dysfunc-
    tion in, 69, 162
mumps virus
    inner ear infection, 139
    parotid infection,
        540–1, **39b**
muscles
    esophageal, 457–8
    laryngeal, 390, 391
    lingual, 301
    masticatory, 303–4
    neck, 475
    pharyngeal, 301, 305–6
    spasm, see spasm
    see also fascia and
        entries under myo-
musculocutaneous flaps
    in head/neck
    reconstructive pro-
    cedures, 288
musculoskeletal defects,
    cervical, 504–5
mutism, 154
mycoses, see fungal infec-
    tions
myoepithelial sialadenitis
    (Sjögren's syn-
    drome), 339, 363,
    543, **38a, c**
myogenic tumors, 509–10
myringitis, bullous, 74
myringoplasty, 104

N

Naffziger syndrome,
    504–5
nasal anatomy/physiology/
    conditions, see
    nose and specific
    structures/condi-
    tions
nasociliary neuralgia, 231
nasopetal reflex, 184
nasopharyngitis, 345
nasopharynx
    anatomy, 304–5
    examination, 318, **24b**
        endoscopic, 192,
            202, 215, 318

nasopharynx, obstruction,
causes, 216,
320–1
tumors, 385–7
benign, 385–6, **25d**
malignant, 379,
386–7, **26c**
neck, 474–528
dissection, for lymph
node metastases,
519–21
lymph nodes, *see* cervical lymph nodes;
lymph nodes
Madelung's, **39d**
plastic–reconstructive
procedures, 285–9
soft tissues, 474–528
anatomy/physiology,
474–90
disorders, 493–528
embryology, 501
investigations,
490–3
neonates, choanal atresia,
280, **26b**
neoplasms, *see* malignancy; tumors
and specific histologic forms
nerve(s)
excitability test, with
facial nerve
lesions, 71
grafts, with facial
nerve lesions,
166, 167
motor and sensory, see
motor nerves;
sensory nerves
supply, *see* innervation
see also specific nerves
nervous system, *see* autonomic nervous
system; central
nervous system
neuralgias, head/neck/
facial, 231,
365–6, 408
neurapraxia, facial, 70,
163
neuritis, optic, rhinogenic
retrobulbar, 247

neurofibromas, cervical,
507
neurogenic disorders
cervical neoplastic,
507–8
laryngeal, 400, 402
oral/pharyngeal, 367,
371–2
neurogenic potentials,
middle, 57
neuroma
acoustic, 130–3, 142,
146
facial nerve, 133
see also schwannoma
neuronitis, vestibular (vestibular paralysis),
142, 144–5
neurosurgery
brain abscess, 112
tumors, 132–3
neurotmesis, facial, 70
newborn, choanal atresia,
280, **26b**
niacin deficiency, 343
nodes, lymph, *see* lymph
nodes
nodules
thyroid, 526
vocal cord, 409, **30b**
noise
aural damage/hearing
loss caused by,
54, 55, 125–6
definitions, 47
nose, 170–298
anatomy, 170–80
disorders, 182, 185,
203–98, 321
investigations, 186–203
patency, assessment,
193–4
physiology/pathophysiology, 180–6
nosebleeds (epistaxis),
253–60
nostrils
eczema, 227
obstruction, causes, 216
stenosis/atresia, 280
nystagmus, 30, 31, 32,
63–7
adjustment, 66

end-point, 65
fatigue, 66
fixation/congenital/
hereditary pendular, 63, 65–6
gaze-evoked, 64–5, 69
paretic, 64–5, 69
positional
dynamic, 66–7
paroxysmal, 67, 146
static, 66
provoked, 66
spontaneous, 63, 63–4,
65
classification, 62
tests, 63–7

O

obstruction
nasopharynx, causes,
216, 320–1
nose and nasal sinus,
185, 186, 195,
216, 227
causes, 216, 227
tracheobronchial, 442,
446, 447
see also occlusion; stenosis
obstructive respiratory
insufficiency,
442, 447
occlusion
eustachian tube, *see*
eustachian tube
ostial (nasal sinus),
185, 186
see also obstruction;
stenosis
oculoauriculovertebral
dysplasia (Goldenhar syndrome),
504
oculomotor system, *see*
eye
olfaction, 180–2, 194–6
disorders, 182, 196
cause, 195
in sinusitis, 227
tests, 194–6

olfactory epithelium/ mucosa, 173
olfactory nerve, substances stimulating, 194
olfactory receptors, lesions, 195
omoclavicular triangle, 475
ophthalmology, *see* eye *and specific structures/conditions*
optic neuritis, rhinogenic retrobulbar, 247
optokinetics, *see* eye
oral cavity
anatomy, 299–304
diseases, 320–87
see also mouth
orbit
fracture, 272–4
sinus infection affecting, 246–8, **13a–c**, **14a**
orbitopathy, thyroid, 524
organ of Corti, *see* Corti
orientation, spatial
loss/disorders, 30, 31
maintenance, 26
oropharynx
anatomy, 305
dysphagia due to disorders of, 366
malignancy, 378, 380, **24a**
stenosis, 440
Osler(–Weber–Rendu) disease, epistaxis in, 255, 260, **16c, d**
ossicles, auditory, 1
function, 21
ossifying fibroma, 289
osteoma, nasal sinus, 289
osteomyelitis of skull, 251–3, **14c**
osteoplasty frontal operation, 241, 242
ostiomeatal unit, 177, 178
ostium, nasal sinus, 177
occlusion/obstruction, 185, 186
otalgia, 168, 235

otitis
herpes zoster (herpes zoster oticus), 73, 138, **3c**
influenzal, 74, 88, 91, **7d**
otitis externa, 71–6, 88, 93
diffuse, 73
exudative, 71
malignant, 3, 73, 74
otitis media, 73, 85–6, 87–91, 94–105
acute, 87–91, 106, **7c–d**
facial nerve paralysis in, 163
adhesive, 86, 105, **8b**
chronic, 94–105, 106–7
hydrocephalus associated with, 110–11
latent, 89, 89–90
seromucinous (=serous effusions), 51, 85–6, **7a**
chronic, 85–6
otoacoustic emissions, evoked, 20, 23, 59
otoliths, 12, 28
otomycosis, 74–5
otorrhea, 168
otosclerosis, 42, 47, 48, 114–16
otoscopy, 33–6, 36–7
glomus tumor, 128
normal appearance, 36–7
otitis media, 88, 95
trauma to middle ear, 122
wax/foreign bodies, 77
ototoxins, 136–8, 162
outer ear, *see* external ear
ozena, 218–19

P

packing, nasal, with epistaxis, 257–9
anterior, 257–8

posterior, 258–9
pain
ear, 168
facial, 231, 365–6
nasal sinus, 226, 227
referred, 227, 228–36
palate
cleft, 279, 374–6
injuries, 371
Kaposi's sarcoma, **20b**
retraction, 192
palatine tonsil, 307, 308
palpation
external ear, 33
external nose, 186–7
larynx, 395
lymph nodes, head and neck, 318, 492, 515
maxillary fracture, 267–71
mouth/pharynx, 316–18
neck, 491–2
salivary gland, 537
palsies, *see* paralysis
pansinusitis, 225, 243
papillary carcinoma, thyroid, 526–7, 528
papillomas
laryngeal, 421–2, **31c**
nasal, 289–90
oral, 377
paracentesis in otitis media, 85, 86, 89, 91
paraganglioma, non-chromaffin, 127–9, **9d**
parageusia, 312
paralysis/palsy
facial nerve, 69–70, 123, 163–7
central, 69
parotid malignancy causing, 551
peripheral, 69–70, 122, 163–7
reconstructive surgery after, 165–6

paralysis/palsy, laryngeal
    nerve, *see* laryn-
    geal nerves
  pharyngeal, 371–2
  vestibular, 142, 144–5
  vocal cord, 390–1,
    402, 402–8,
    32a, b
  see also paretic nystag-
    mus
parasympathetic nervous
    system, nasal,
    180, 210
  surgical division,
    210–11
paretic nystagmus, 64–5,
    69
parosmia, 196
parotid duct, 531
parotidectomy, 539,
    555–7
parotid gland
  anatomy/physiology,
    531, 531–2
  tumor, 548–9, 550,
    551, 552, **39a–c**
parotitis
  chronic recurrent,
    542–3
  epidemic, virus of, *see*
    mumps virus
paroxysmal positional nys-
    tagmus, 67, 146
pars ampullaris of semi-
    circular canal, 13
pars flaccida of tympanic
    membrane, 6, 7
pars tensa of tympanic
    membrane, 6
Patterson–Brown–Kelly
    syndrome, 341,
    364
pediatrics, *see* children;
    infants; newborn
Pellagra, 343
pemphigoid vesicles, 419
pemphigus, 334
  vulgaris, 419
Pendred's syndrome, 152
perception, auditory, dis-
    orders, 25, 151
perforation (and tearing)
  esophageal, 464–5, 467

nasal septal, 262
  tympanic membrane,
    37, 117, 118,
    6b, c
perichondritis
  aural, 73, 76, **3a**
  laryngeal, 419–20,
    28b
perilymph, 11
perilymphatic system of
    inner ear, 11
periocular hematoma,
    276, **16a**
periostitis, orbital,
    246–7, **13c**
  see also subperiosteal
    abscess
peristalsis, esophageal,
    310, 458
  see also motility dis-
    orders
petrositis, 113
pharyngeal tonsils, *see*
    adenoids
pharyngitis, 345, 381–3
  acute catarrhal, 361–2
  chronic, 362–3
pharyng(oesophag)eal
    pouch (Zenker's
    diverticulum),
    306, 310, 372–3,
    467, **36a**
pharyngoplasty, 376
pharynx, 299–387, 432–4
  anatomy, 299, 301,
    304–9, 488
  disorders, 320–87,
    432–4, 440
  clinical aspects,
    320–87
  headache due to, 233
  investigation, 315–20
  physiology and
    pathophysiology,
    309–15
  see also hypopharynx;
    nasopharynx;
    oropharynx
phlegmon, orbital, 247
phonation, *see* sound;
    voice
photoelectronystagmogra-
    phy, 63

pigmentation disorders,
    325–6
pinna, *see* auricle
Piringer–Kuckinka syn-
    drome, 499
plastic surgery
  cleft lip/jaw/palate,
    375–6
  nasal septum, 261
  nasal shape deformi-
    ties, 282–9
  nasal sinus, 242
  tracheal, 445
Plaut–Vincent angina,
    349, **23a**
Plummer–Vinson syn-
    drome, 341, 364
pneumatic system of
    middle ear, 8–10
pneumococcal tonsillitis,
    344
Politzer's test, 40
polyps
  nasal, 215, 217–18,
    11a, 12c, 26a
  bleeding, 253, 254
  vocal cord, 420, **30c**
polysinusitis, 225
positional nystagmus, *see*
    nystagmus
positional tests, 61
posture, upright, main-
    tenance, 26
potassium–sodium
    exchange pump,
    inner ear, 11–12
precancers
  external ear, 78, 79
  laryngeal mucosal,
    422–3
  oral, 332–3
pregnancy rhinitis, 217
prenatal deafness, 153
presbycusis, 147–8
presbyesophagus, 458
prescalene node biopsy,
    517
pressure
  esophageal, measure-
    ment, 462–3

intracranial, increased, otic tumors associated with, 130, 132
intranasal, measurement, 193–4
middle ear, decreased, 51
pathological effects, 123–4
see also barotrauma protection
of lower airway/respiratory tract, structures involved, 394
by nasal mucosa, 183–4
by saliva, 533, 534
Prussak's space, 7–8
pseudocroup, 415, 416
pseudofistula symptoms, 69
pseudomastoiditis, 71, 93
pterygopalatine (sphenopalatine) ganglion, 180
neuralgia, 231
ptyalismus, 536
pulmonary system, see alveolar respiratory insufficiency; bronchi; trachea
pulpitis, face pain in, 231
pure-tone audiometry, 43–52, 55–7
deaf children, 159
labyrinthine concussion, 121
otosclerosis, 115
purifying of air by nose, 183
pursuit tracking, 68–9
pyo(muco)celes, 244, **15c**
pyramid, nasal, fracture, 2265
pyramidal axis, temporal bone fracture along, 118–19, 120

Q

quinine, ototoxicity, 137

R

radiation sialadenitis, 545
radiography
cervical soft tissues, 493
cholesteatoma, 100
ear (in general), 38–40
esophagus, 459, 473
larynx, 399
mastoiditis, 93
maxillary fracture, 271
mouth/pharynx, 318
nose and paranasal sinuses, 192, 196–9
otitis media, 95
salivary gland, 537–9
sinus thrombosis, 110
trauma to middle/inner ear, 122
see also specific radiographic techniques
radiotherapy
laryngeal cancer, 426
nasal tumors, 298
oral tumors, 384, 387
Ramsay Hunt syndrome (herpes zoster oticus), 73, 138, **3c**
ranula, 533, **21a**
Rappaport classification, non-Hodgkin's lymphoma, 512–13
reactance in sound conduction, 47
receptors
cervical spine and neck muscle, 30
semi-circular canal, 13, 14
recruitment, hearing disorders and, 26, 48–50
recurrent nerve, see laryngeal nerve

red tongue, 338
redundance, central hearing disorders and, 56
reflexes, nasal, 184
see also specific reflexes
reflux esophagitis, 468–9
Refsum's syndrome, 152
Reinke's edema, 393, 420–1
Reinke's space, 393
Rendu–Osler(–Weber) disease, epistaxis in, 255, 260, **16c, d**
resistance in sound conduction, 47
respiration, 393–4, 436
laryngeal/pharyngeal role in, 393–4
nasal role in, 182–3
see also breathing; expiration; inspiration
respiratory epithelium, nasal, 173
respiratory insufficiency
alveolar, 447
cardiac, 442
extrathoracic, 442
obstructive, 442, 447
respiratory, 442
respiratory tract, see airway
retention cyst
laryngeal, 422
sublingual (ranula), 533, **21a**
reticular formation, movement/balance and the, 30
reticuloendothelial granulomatosis, see histiocytosis
retrobulbar optic neuritis, rhinogenic, 247
retrocochlear analysis of acoustic information, 23–4
retrocochlear deafness, 50, 56

retropharyngeal abscess,
360–1
rhabdomyosarcoma,
nasal, 293
rhagades of labial com-
missures, 324
rheobase determination
with facial nerve
lesions, 70
rheumatoid arthritis, cricoarytenoid joint
in, 419
rhinitis, 207–11, 211–17
acute, 207–8, 212
allergic, 208–10, 213,
228
atrophic, 218–19
chronic, 214–16
pregnancy, 217
purulent, 219
vasomotor, 210–11,
213, 228
rhinitis medicamentosa,
217
rhinitis sicca anterior,
211, 254
rhinomanometry, 193–4
rhinophyma, 205, **10b**
rhinoplasty, 282, 283, 284
rhinorrhea, CSF, 276
rhinoscleroma, 206–7
rhinoscopy, 187–92
anterior, 187–9
posterior, 189–92
rhinosporidiosis, 221
rhinovirus, 208
rib, cervical, 504–5
Riedel's frontal sinus
operation, 241
Riedel's thyroiditis, 525,
526
Rinne's test, 42, 43
rodent ulcer, see basal
cell carcinoma
Romberg's test, 60
rubella infection, mater-
nal, congenital
deafness due to,
153
rudiments, auricular, **1d**

S

saccule, 12, 28
saddlenose, 262, 281,
282–4
salicylates, ototoxicity,
137
saliva, formation and function, 533–6
salivary ducts, 531, 532
injuries, 547
salivary glands, 529–57
accessory, 530
disorders, 533, 535–6,
536
age-related, 536
embryology, 529–31
function, 530, 531–6
investigations, 536–9
minor, 533
tumors, 549
structure/anatomy,
529–33
sarcoid(osis) (Boeck's disease)
Besnier–Boeck–
Schaumann, 206
cervical soft tissue, 498
laryngeal, 418
sarcomas
cervical, 506, 509
Kaposi's, 330, **20b**
middle ear, 129
nasal, 293
scalds
emergency/first aid pro-
cedures, 558
oral/pharyngeal,
369–70
scalenus anterior (Naff-
ziger) syndrome,
504–5
scarlet fever
otitis following, 91
strawberry tongue in,
338, **19c**
tonsillar/pharyngeal
inflammation fol-
lowing, 346
scar tissue stenosis,
esophageal, 469
Schirmer's test, 70
Schueller's view, 38

cholesteatoma, 100
mastoiditis, 93
otitis media, 95
sinus thrombosis, 110
Schwabach's test, 42
schwannoma
acoustic (acoustic neu-
roma), 130–3,
142, 146
cervical, 508
scleroma, laryngeal, 419
sclerosing sialadenitis of
submandibular
gland, chronic, 542
sclerosis, see multiple
sclerosis; oto-
sclerosis; tympa-
nosclerosis
screamer's nodules, 409,
30b
sebaceous cervical cysts,
494
secretions
nasal, see discharge
salivary, 533, 534, 535,
535–6
disturbed, 535–6
semicircular canals,
13–14, 29–30
anatomy, 13–14
fistula, test for, 69
function, 29–30
senile keratosis, 79
sensorineural deafness,
25, 26, 55, 136–54
trauma-related, 122
sensory nerves/nervous
systems
cervical, 487–8, 488
external ear (from
VIIth cranial
nerve), 18, 18–20
internal ear, 12, 13,
14–16, 22, 23
balance and, 12, 13,
28
nasal, 179
sepsis, tonsillogenic, 359
septoplasty, 261, 284
septorhinoplasty, 282
septum, nasal, 260–2
anatomy, 171, 172
disease, 260–2

sphenoid sinus surgical
approach via, 242
seromucinous otitis
media, *see* otitis
media
serotympanum, 84–5
serous exudates, *see* exudates
serous labyrinthitis, 139
serous meningitis, 138
short esophagus, 471
short increment sensitivity index (SISI),
49–50
sialadenitis, 539–45
electrolyte, 545
epithelial cell, 544
myoepithelial (Sjögren's syndrome),
339, 363, 543,
38a, c
radiation, 545
submandibular, chronic
sclerosing, 542
sialadenosis, 547
sialography, 537, 538
sialolithiasis, 545–6
sialopenia, 535
sialorrhea, 535
Siegle's speculum/otoscope, 34, 37
singer's nodules, 409,
30b
sinobronchial syndrome,
243–4
sinus(es), carotid, 481
sinus(es), cervical, 501
sinus(es), nasal/paranasal,
170–298
anatomy, 174–9
complications of infection, 245–53
disorders, 203–98, 321
inflammatory, *see*
sinusitis
neoplastic, 289–90,
293–8, **17c, d**
traumatic, 265–78
function, 185–6
investigations, 186–203
lavage, diagnostic and
therapeutic,
199–201

pathophysiological relationships to rest
of body, 243–4
spread of lesions from,
192
see also specific sinuses
sinusitis, 224–53, **14c**
acute, 226, 237, 240,
12b
chronic, 237, 237–8,
240, **12c**
polypous, **26a**
purulent, 219
specific types, 243
subacute, 237
treatment, 238,
239–40, 240–2,
242–3, 243
basic principles, 237
vacuum, 186
sinus thrombosis
otogenic, 109–10
rhinogenic, 250
tonsillogenic, 360
Sjögren's syndrome, 339,
363, 543, **38a, c**
skeletal disorders, otologic manifestations, 117
see also bone; cartilage
and entries under
chondro-; osteo-
skin
disorders
dysphagia due to,
367
oral mucosal lesions
in, 325–7, 334–5
flaps and grafts, in
head/neck reconstructive procedures, 285–9
skull, *see* cranium
Sluder's neuralgia, 231
smell
bad, *see* fetor
sense of, *see* olfaction
sound (waves)
conduction,
audiometry with
disorders of, 45–8
formation (phonation),
393, **27b**

disorders, 393, 402
oral cavity/pharynx
contribution to,
315
see also voice
frequency coding, 24
intensity, 46
coding, 24
perception disorders,
25, 151
stimulus of, *see*
stimulus
volume, 46
see also loudness; noise
sound pressure level
(SPL),
audiometry and,
44, 45
spasm
esophageal, 469–70
masticatory (trismus),
356
pharyngeal, 372
spa treatment, 223
speech
audiometry employing,
52–7
in deaf children, 159
cleft lip/jaw/palate
surgery
improving, 375–6
deafness causing disorders of, 156–7
discomfort threshold
for, hearing aids
and, 159
nasal influence, 185
oral cavity/pharynx
contribution to,
315
post-laryngectomy
rehabilitation,
431–2
whispered and conventional, hearing
threshold, 41, 43
sphenoid sinus
anatomy, 176–7
irrigation, 201
radiography, 198
sphenoid sinusitis (sphenoiditis), 226,
242–3

sphenopalatine ganglion, *see* pterygo-palatine ganglion

sphincters, esophageal, 458

spine, cervical, radiography, 493
see also vertebra

spontaneous deviation reaction, 61

spontaneous nystagmus, *see* nystagmus

spontaneous tone reaction in the arms, 61

spur, nasal septal, 260, **11e**

squamous cell carcinoma
ear
external, 80, 81, **5a, b**
middle, 129
esophagus, 473, **36c**
laryngx, 423, 424, **33b**
mouth/pharynx, 377, 381, 383
nose, 293, **11d**
external, 291
salivary, 554

stapedectomy, 116

stapedius reflex, 50, 51–2, 70

stapes, 1
function, 21
see also ossicles

statoconia (otoliths), 12, 28

steam inhalation, 223

stellate ganglion, 489–90
anatomy, 489
blockage technique, 489–90

Stenger's test, 56

stenosis/strictures
bronchial, 437–52
esophageal, 469, **35c**
congenital, 471
laryngeal, 440–1
nostrils, 280
subglottic, 401
tracheal, 411, 437–52
vertebral artery, 483
see also obstruction; occlusion

Stenson's duct, 531

Stenver's view of ear, 38

sternocleidomastoid muscles, 475

steroid therapy
esophageal chemical burns, 464
upper airway/digestive tract conditions, 224

stimulus (of sound waves)
distribution, 21–3
transformation, 23
transport, 20–1

stomatitis, 324, 327–9, 341

stones, *see* cupulolithiasis; otolith; sialolithiasis

straining, 490

strawberry tongue, 338, **19c**

streptococcal infection, external ear, 73

strictures, *see* stenosis

stridor, inspiratory, 440

styloid process syndrome (stylalgia), 364–5

stylo(kerato)hyoid syndrome, 365

subclavian steal syndrome, 483

subdural abscess, 249

subglottis
anatomy, 388, 389, 392
carcinoma, 425, 431
laryngitis, 415–16, 454
stenosis, 401

sublingual gland, 532–3
tumors, 549

submandibular duct, 532

submandibular gland, 532
sclerosing sialadenitis, chronic, 542
tumors, 549
surgery, 557

submandibular triangle, 475

submental triangle, 475

subperiosteal abscess, 247, **14c**

supraglottis
anatomy, 388, 389, 392

carcinoma, 425, 431

suprahyoid triangle, 475

surgery, *see specific conditions and procedures*

swallowing
disorders, 310, 366–7, 472
physiology, 309–10, 458

swallowing reflex, 394

sweating, gustatory, 547–8

swelling
cervical, 491
facial, 267, 268–70
nasal mucosal, 217
see also edema

swimmer's otitis externa and interna, 73

sycosis, nasal vestibular, 204

sympathetic nervous system
cervical, 488
nasal, 180
salivary gland, 532

synechiae, laryngotracheal, 411

syphilis
aural, 113–14
congenital, 153
cervical soft tissue, 496
laryngeal, 419
nasal, 206, 219, 220
oral/pharyngeal, 324, 347

syringing of ear, 36, 77

T

taste, 311–12, 319
disorders, 312, 313
with facial nerve lesions, 70
tests (gustometry), 310, 319
see also gustatory sweating

T cell lymphoma, 512, 513

teeth, upper jaw, 304

telangiectasia, hereditary hemorrhagic (Rendu–Osler disease), epistaxis in, 255, 260, **16c, d**
temporal bones
  cholesteatoma, 105
  fracture, 107, 118–20
  pneumatic system, 8–10
temporal lobe abscess, otogenic, 111
temporomandibular joint
  anatomy, 302, 304
  fracture, 278
tension septum, 260
thermal injury, *see* burns; frostbite
thermal treatment, local, upper airway/digestive tract, 223
thoracic duct, 495
thoracic fixation, 394
Thornwaldt's disease, 363
thorotrastoma, 510
thrombophlebitis, 250
thrombosis, sinus, *see* sinus thrombosis
thrush, *see* candidiasis
thyrocervical trunk, 481
thyroglossal duct cysts, 504
thyrohyoid membrane, 390
thyroid (gland), 521–8
  anatomy, 521–2
  disorders, 523–8
    diagnosis, 522–3
  ectopic, 523
  function, 522
thyroid artery, 522
thyroid cartilage, 390
thyroiditis, 525–6
thyrotoxicosis, 522
timbre, 47
tinnitus, 169
TNM system, 514
  laryngeal cancer, 425, 431
  nasal cancer, 295, 296–7
  oral/pharyngeal cancer, 378–9, 432

tomography
  computed, *see* computed tomography
  conventional, cervical soft tissues, 493
tone (muscle), in arms, spontaneous reaction, 61
tone (sound)
  decay test, 50
  intensity-difference threshold, 49
  definition, 47
tongue (lingua), 335–43
  anatomy, 301, 302
  bites, 371
  depressor, 316, 317
  disorders, 335–43
  malignancy, 378, 380, 381–5, **18c**
tonotopy, 24
tonsil(s), 307–9, 312–15, 320–4, 344–60
  anatomy, 307–9
  disorders, 314–15, 320–4, 344–60, **22a–24a**
  function, 312–15
  lingual, *see* lingual tonsil
tonsillectomy, 323, 352–4
  abscess, 357
tonsillitis, 344–8, 350–61
  acute, 344–8, **22b, c**
  chronic, 315, 350–4
  complications during/after, 354–61
torticollis, 508, 509
toxins
  hearing and balance disorders due to, 136–8, 163
  inhalational trauma due to, 413
toxoplasmosis, 499–500
Toynbee's test, 40
trachea
  anatomy, 434, 435
  intubation, *see* intubation
  resection, 445
  stenosis, 411, 437–52
  synechiae, 411

tracheitis, 453–4
  diphtheritic, 454
tracheitis sicca, 454
tracheobronchial tree, 434–56
  anatomy, 434–5
  disorders, 437–55
  investigation, 436–7
  physiology, 436
tracheoesophageal fistula, 471–2
tracheomalacia, 439
tracheopathica osteoplastica, 443, **34b**
tracheopexy, 444
tracheoplasty, 445
tracheostomy, 451–2
  nursing care, 451–2
  post-laryngectomy, 432
  tubes, 449
tracheotomy, 446–8
transglottic carcinoma, 424, 425, 431, **33b**
transglottic space, 389
trauma, *see* injury
trigeminal nerve, substances stimulating, 194
trigeminal neuralgia, 231
trismus, 356
trisomy 13, deafness in, 152
trisomy 18, deafness in, 152
Troeltsch's pouch, 7–8
tubal tonsil, 307
tuberculosis
  cervical lymph node, 496–8, **37a**
  laryngeal, 418
  middle ear, 95, 113
  nasal, 205–6, 219, 220
  oral/pharyngeal, 324, 331–2, 347
  salivary gland, 544
tubopharyngeal plicae/bands, 307
  infection, 345–6
Tuerck's position in indirect laryngoscopy, 395, 396
tularemia, 498–9

tumors, 78–81, 127–34
  cervical soft tissue,
      505–21
    surgery, 517–21
  esophageal, 472–3
  external ear, 78–81,
      3d, 4a–d, 5a–b
  infratentorial, balance
      disorders with, 161
  Kuettner's, 542
  laryngeal, 401–2,
      420–32
  malignant, *see* malig-
      nancy
  middle/internal ear, 96,
      127–34
  nasal, 219, 279,
      289–98, **10d,
      12d, 17c, d, 26a**
    bleeding with, 254
  oral/pharyngeal, 330,
      376–87, **18c, 21c,
      23c, 24a, 25d,
      26c, 33d**
  salivary gland, 533,
      538, 539,
      548–57, **39a–c**
    treatment, 554–7
  thyroid, 526–8
  tracheobronchial,
      455–6
  *see also specific histo-
      logic forms*
tuning fork tests, 41
turbinates, nasal
  hypertrophy, 215, **25a**
  surgery, 215–16
turbinectomy, 216
Turning test, 67
tympanic cavity, hemor-
      rhage into
      (hemotympanum),
      117, **6d**
tympanic membrane (ear-
      drum), 6
  anatomy, 6
  blue, 37, 85
  compliance, 47
    increased, 51
  development, 1
  function, 21
  otoscopy

  normal appearance,
      36–7, **5c**
  pathological appear-
      ance, 37
  trauma (perforation/
      tears etc.), 37,
      117, 118, 122,
      122–3, **6b, c**
tympanometry and tym-
      panograms, 50,
      50–1
tympanoplasty, 96, 101,
      102, 103, 104
tympanosclerosis, 84, 86,
      8d
tympanotomy, 123–4

U

ulcer
  contact, laryngeal, 410,
      29c
  rodent, *see* basal cell
      carcinoma
ulcerative esophagitis, 468
ulceromembranous
      angina/tonsillitis,
      349, **23a**
ulceromembranous sto-
      matitis, 327–8
ultrasonography, para-
      nasal sinus, 198
ultrasound, cervical ves-
      sels, 493
Unterberger's stepping
      test, 60
Usher's syndrome, 152
utricle, 12, 13, 28, 29
uveoparotid fever, 544

V

vacuum sinusitis, 186
vagus (nerve), 488
  anatomy, 488
  lesions, 404
    laryngeal effects
      of/vocal cord pal-
      sies due to, 402,
      404
    neuralgia, 231, 368

Valsalva maneuver/test,
      490
  of eustachian tube open-
      ing, 40
valve, nasal, 172, 182
varices, esophageal,
      470–1, **36b**
vascular ligation with
      epistaxis, 256,
      259–60
vascular system
  cervical, 479–83
    disorders, 482
    radiography, 493,
      507
  laryngeal, 392
  middle ear, 8
  nasal, 170–1, 177–8
  oral cavity, 302–3
  pharyngeal, 306–7, 309
  salivary gland, 532
  tracheobronchial, 435
  see also arterial
      supply; lymphatic
      system; venous
      system *and
      specific vessels*
vascular tumors
  cervical, 505–7
  laryngeal, 401–2
  nasal, 290
  oral, 376–7
vasoactive substances for
      upper airway/
      digestive tract con-
      ditions, 224
vasomotor cephalgia, 229
vasomotor headache, 229
vasomotor rhinitis,
      210–11, 213, 228
venous catheterization,
      central, 481
venous system/drainage
  cervical, 481–2
  laryngeal, 392
  middle ear, 8
  nasal, 171, 178
  oral cavity, 302–3
  pharyngeal, 306, 309
ventilation
  of middle ear spaces,
      disorders, 82–7
  nasal role in, 182–3

vertebra, as origin of headache, 233
see also oculoauriculovertebral dysplasia
vertebral arteries, 481
stenosis, 483
vertebral veins, 481
vertebrobasilar insufficiency, 147, 161, 483
vertigo (dizziness), 30, 31, 160, 169
emergency/first aid procedures, 558
vestibular compensation, central, 33
vestibule of ear (vestibular system), 12–14, 26–8, 30–3, 60–9, 136–54, 160–2
anatomy, 12–14
dysfunction, 30–3, 60–9, 136–54, 160–2
clinical aspects, 136–54, 160–2
function, 26–8, 60–9
functional tests, 60–9
with cholesteatoma, 101
vestibule of mouth, anatomy, 299
vestibule of nose
anatomy, 171
carcinoma, **11d**
folliculitis, 204
vestibulocochlear nerve (auditory nerve; VIIIth cranial nerve), 1
balance and the, 18
hearing and the, 17
tumors, 127–34
vestibuloocular reflex, 29, 30
vestibulospinal reflexes, 60–2
Vincent's angina, 349, **23a**

viral infections
external ear, 73, 74
internal ear, 138–9
maternal, congenital deafness due to, 153
middle ear, 91
salivary gland, 540–2
see also specific conditions/viruses and infections
Virchow's node, 515
vocal cord(s)
anatomy, 388, 392
carcinomas, 424, **32c, 33a**
surgery, 426
nodules, 409, **30b**
paralysis/palsy, 390–1, 402, 402–8, **32a, b**
polyps, 420, **30c**
vocal cordectomy, 426, 427
vocal cordotomy, 406
vocal processes
contact ulcer, laryngeal, 410, **29c**
granuloma, intubation-related, 411, **29b**
voice
disorders, 409
deafness causing, 156–7
post-tonsillectomy, 354
post-laryngectomy rehabilitation, 431–2
von Recklinghausen's disease, 507

W

Waardenburg's syndrome, 152
Waldeyer's ring, 344–61
anatomy, 307, 308

disorders, 344–61
function, 312–15
tonsils of, see tonsils
walking a straight line, 60
Wallenberg's syndrome, 483
warming of inspired air, 183
Warthin's tumor, 550
wax, aural, 77–8
web, laryngeal, 401, **27c**
Weber's test, 41–2, 43
Wegener's granulomatosis, 221–2
Wharton's duct, 532
Willis, circle of, 481, 482

X

xeroradiography, cervical soft tissues, 493
xerostomia, 535
X-ray examination, see radiography and techniques employing X-rays

Y

yeast infections, nasal, 221

Z

Zenker's diverticulum, 306, 310, 372–3, 467, 36a
Z-plasty in head/neck reconstructive procedures, 285, 286
zygomatic fracture, 272–3

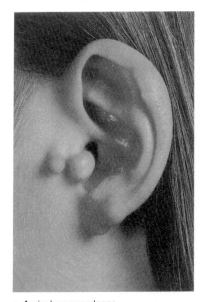

a Auricular appendages

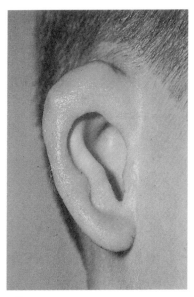

b Cup ear

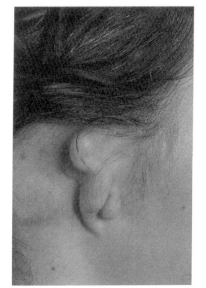

c Auricular dysplasia

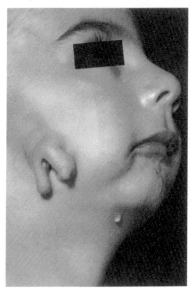

d Caudally displaced auricular rudiment

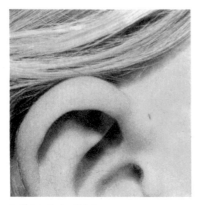

a Preauricular fistula

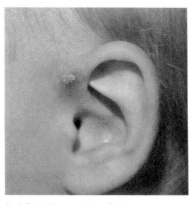

b Infected preauricular fistula

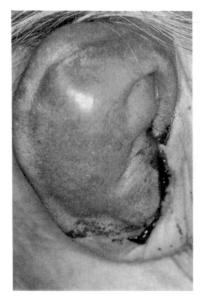

c Fresh auricular hematoma

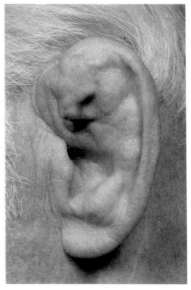

d Cauliflower ear (sclerosis secondary to auricular hematoma)

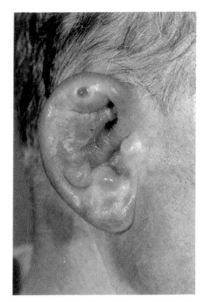

a Perichondritis

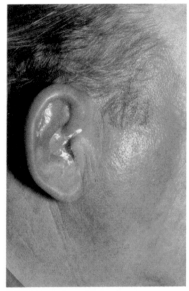

b Bullous erysipelas

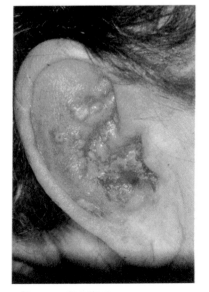

c Herpes zoster oticus

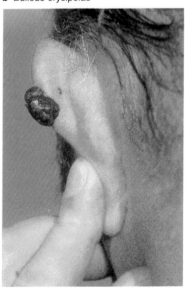

d Nodular melanoma with a small cutaneous metastasis

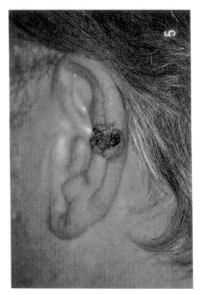

a Nodular basal cell carcinoma

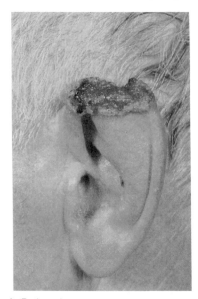

b Rodent ulcer

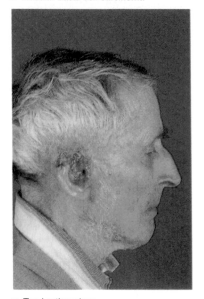

c Terebrating ulcer

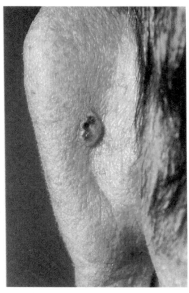

d Pigmented basal cell carcinoma

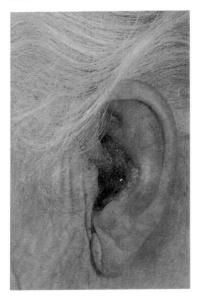

a Auricular carcinoma with invasion of the ear canal

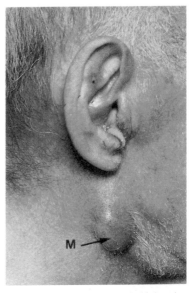

b Carcinoma of the ear canal with lymph node metastasis (M)

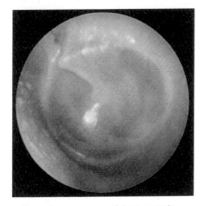

c Normal appearance of the tympanic membrane

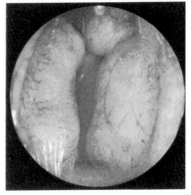

d Sessile, osteoma-like exostoses of the ear canal

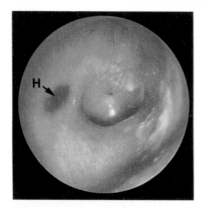

a Subepithelial hematoma (H) and cerumen on the tympanic membrane caused by attempted self-cleaning of the ear

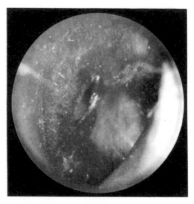

b Right tympanic membrane perforation following a blow to the ear

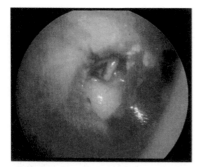

c Extensive tympanic membrane perforation (angular edges) exposing the tympanic cavity and incudostapedial joint

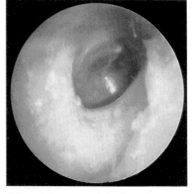

d Hematotympanum following a transverse petrous bone fracture

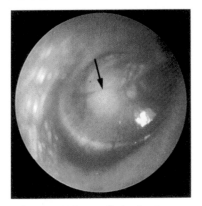

a Serous middle ear effusion (acute serous otitia media) with a fluid level (arrow) and retraction of the tympanic membrane

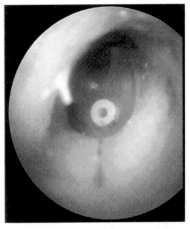

b Transtympanic drainage of the middle ear (myringotomy tube)

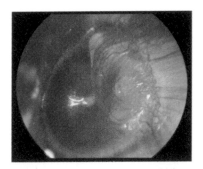

c Incipient acute otitis media with radial vascular congestion

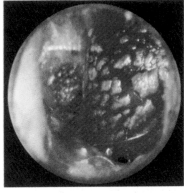

d Acute hemorrhagic otitis media (influenzal otitis) with loss of differentiation of the tympanic membrane

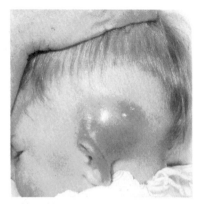

a Mastoiditis with subperiosal abscess

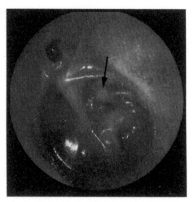

b Adhesive process with atelectasis of the middle ear cleft, a retraction pocket, and destruction of the long process of the incus (arrow) (spontaneous type III)

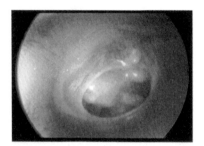

c Chronic mucosal suppuration with a central perforation

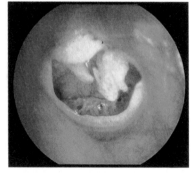

d Tympanosclerosis with central perforation and calcified deposits

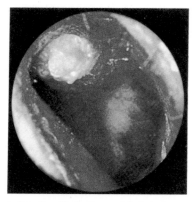

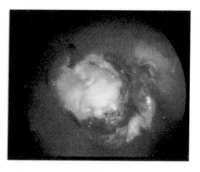

b Extensive, destructive cholesteatoma involving the entire middle ear

a Pars flaccida (epitympanic) cholesteatoma with a marginal perforation

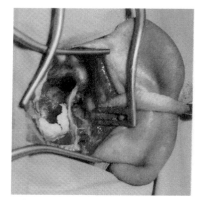

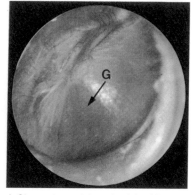

c Cholesteatoma extending to the tip of the mastoid (intraoperative view)

d Glomus tumor (g) on the right side arising from the hypotympanum

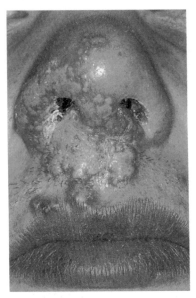

a Herpes simplex

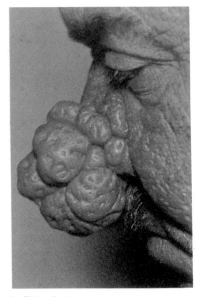

b Rhinophyma

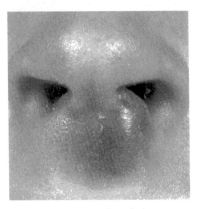

c Furuncle of the nasal vestibule

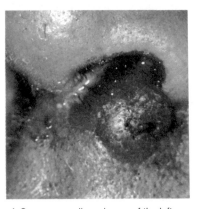

d Squamous cell carcinoma of the left nasal vestibule

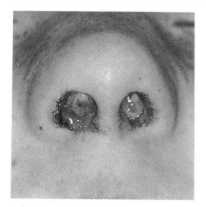

a Bilateral nasal polyps

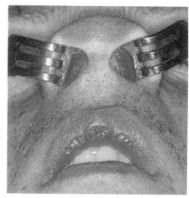

b Septal hematoma

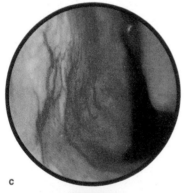

c

d Kiesselbach's area (K)

c Vascular plexus in Kiesselbach's area on the left side

e

e Septal spur (x) impinging on the inferior turbinate (xx)

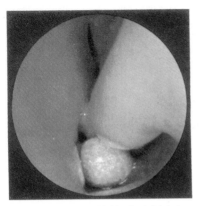

a Foreign body (marble) in the left inferior meatus of a child

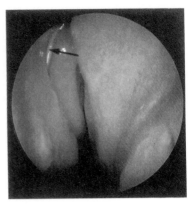

b Purulent secretion in the middle meatus in acute sinusitis (arrow)

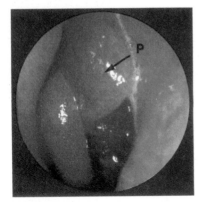

c Polyposis (P) of the middle meatus in chronic sinusitis

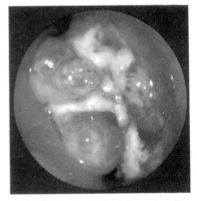

d Malignant tumor in the left nasal cavity

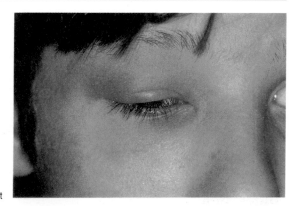

a Periostitis of the orbit

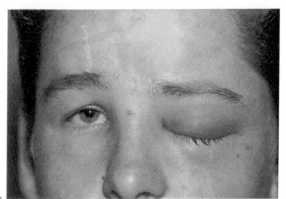

b Subperiosteal abscess

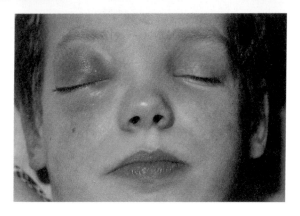

c Orbital cellulitis

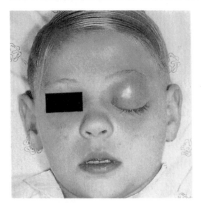

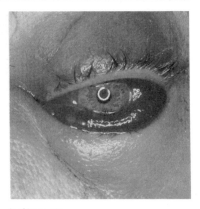

a Orbital cellulitis and abscess of the upper eyelid

b Chemosis

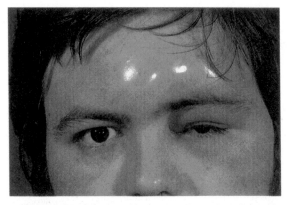

c Osteomyelitis of the frontal bone secondary to frontal sinusitis, with associated subperiosteal abscessation in the frontal region

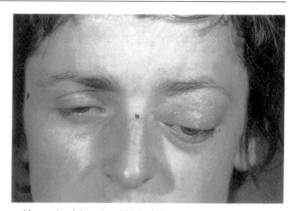

a Mucocele of the ethmoid labyrinth

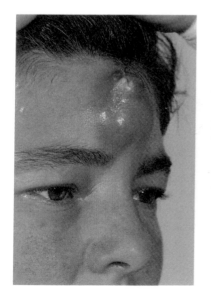

b External eruption of a frontal-sinus pyomucocele

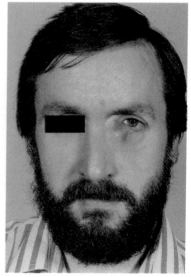

c Dacryocystitis

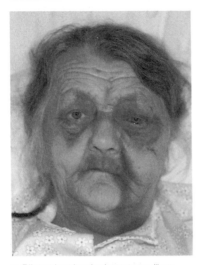

a Bilateral periocular hematoma ("eye-glass" hematoma) following a frontobasal fracture

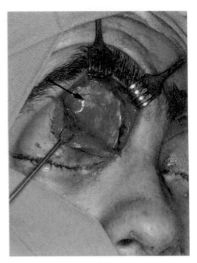

b Frontal lobe prolapse (arrow) into the frontal sinus through a dural tear caused by a frontobasal fracture

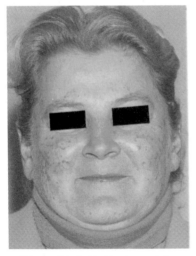

c Ectasia of facil-skin blood vessels in Rendu-Osler disease

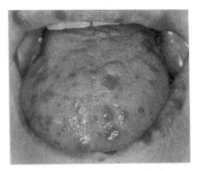

d Ectasia of lingual blood vessels in Rendu-Osler disease

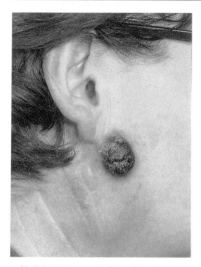

a Nodular melanoma of the cheek

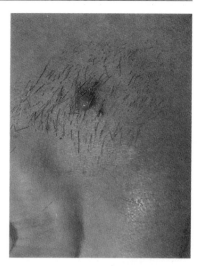

b Nodular melanoma of the scalp (retroauricular) with satellite lesions

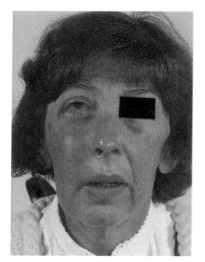

c Carcinoma of the right maxillary sinus causing ocular displacement

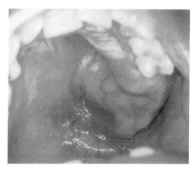

d Maxillary carcinoma on the left side

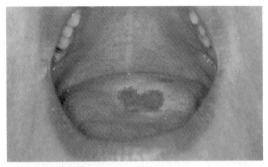

a Geographic tongue

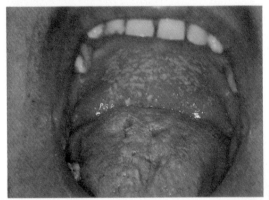

b Candidiasis

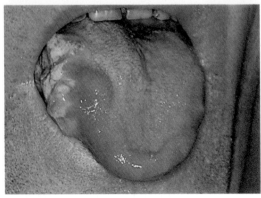

c Carcinoma of the tongue

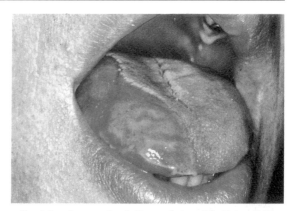

a Exudative drug reaction (with permission of Dr. Braun-Falco, Munich)

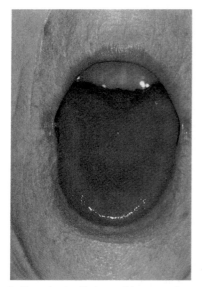

b Hunter's glossitis in pernicious anemia

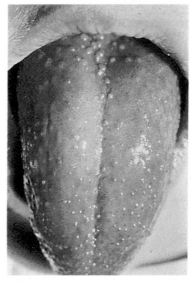

c Strawberry tongue in scarlet fever

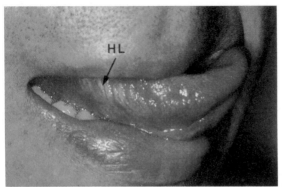

a Hairy leukoplekia (HL) in AIDS

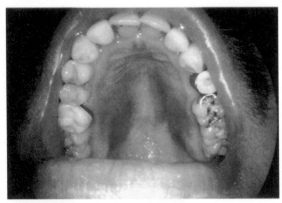

b Kaposi's sarcoma of the palate

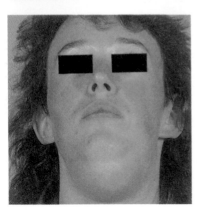

c Oral floor cellulitis (Ludwig's angina)

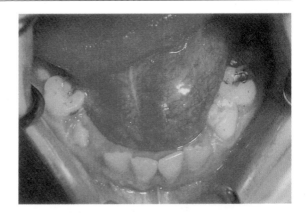

a Ranula

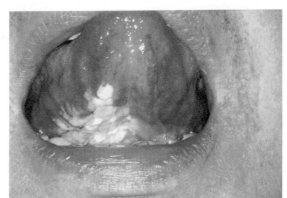

b Leukoplakia of the oral floor

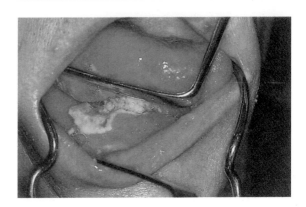

c Carcinoma of the oral floor

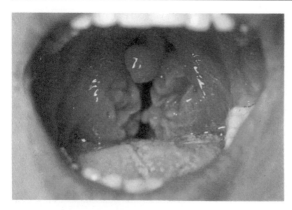

a Pronounced tonsillar hyperplasia

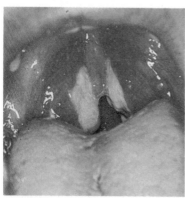

b Tonsillitis in infectious mononucleosis

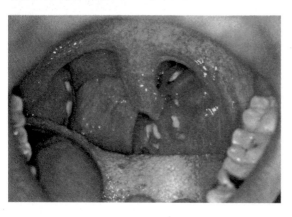

c Lacunar tonsillitis

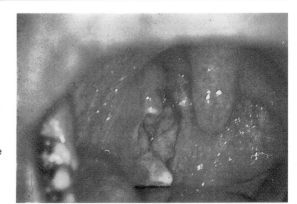

a Plaut–Vincent angina (fusospirochetal infection) on the right side with typical unilateral ulceromembranous tonsillitis in a 21-year-old man

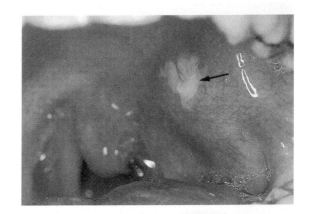

b Peritonsillar abscess with spontaneous perforation (arrow)

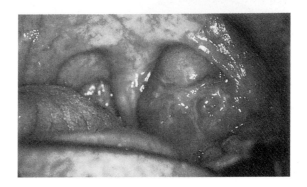

c Malignant lymphoma of the left tonsil

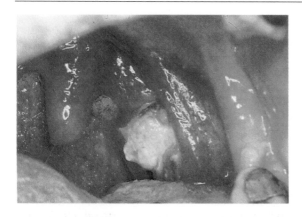

a Tonsillar (oro-pharyngeal) carcinoma

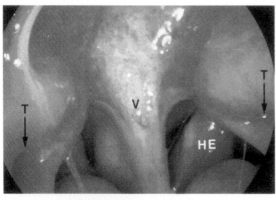

b General view of the nasopharynx (V = edge of vomer, HE = posterior end of nasal turbinate, T = orifice of eustachian tube)

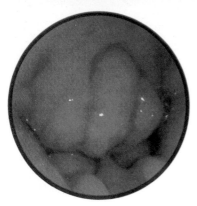

c Hyperplastic adenoids with typical furrows, causing almost complete obstruction of the choanae

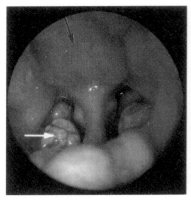

a Adenoids (arrow), hyperplastic posterior ends of the inferior turbinates (open arrow)

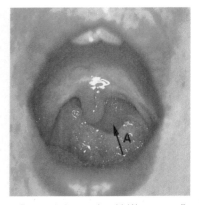

b Extremely large adenoid (A) post-tonsillectomy, with scar tissue bands in the area of the left faucial pillar

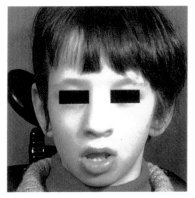

c "Adenoid facies" and oral breathing in a child with large adenosis causing obstruction of nasal respiration

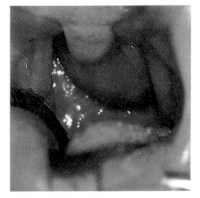

d Nasopharyngeal fibroma presenting as a globular mass behind the soft palate

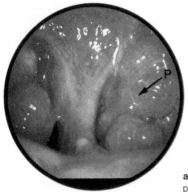

a Bilateral ethmoid polyps (P) in chronic polypous sinusitis, visible in the choanae

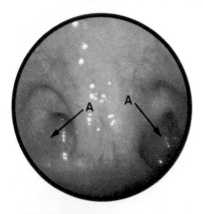

b Bilateral choanal atresia (A) with expansion of the posterior end of the vomer in a newborn

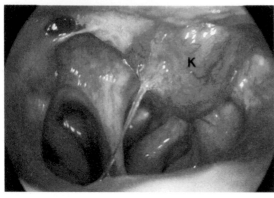

c Lymphepithelial carcinoma (K) of the nasopharynx

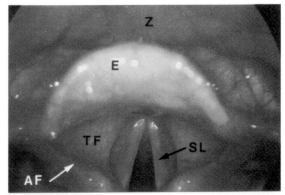

a Normal appearance of the larynx during inspiration (E = epiglottis, SL = vocal cord, TF = vestibular fold, Z = base of tongue, AF = aryepiglottic fold)

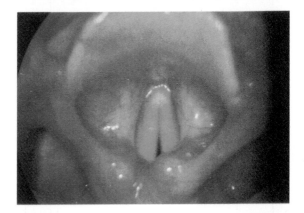

b Phonation

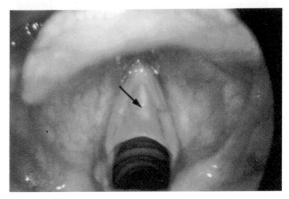

c Partial atresia (webbing) of the larynx in a child

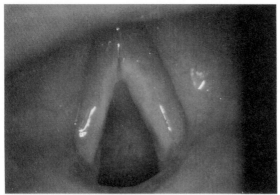

a Acute laryngitis

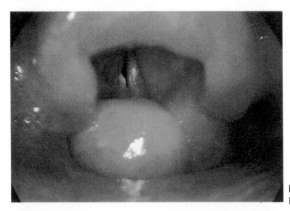

b Perichondritis of the larynx

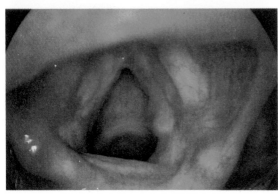

c Chronic laryngitis

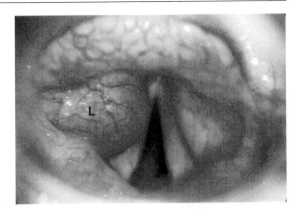

a Internal laryngocele (L) (left side of picture)

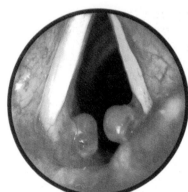

b Bilateral intubation granulomas on the vocal processes

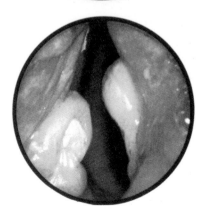

c Contact ulcers occurring at typical sites over the vocal processes on both sides

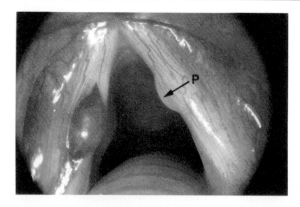

a Subepithelial hematoma secondary to intubation. Note the small polyp (P) on the right side

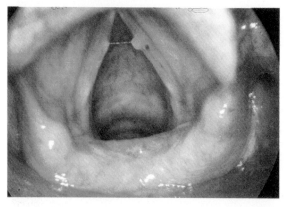

b Bilateral vocal cord nodules "connected" by mucous strand

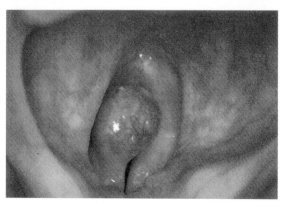

c Sessile vocal cord polyp showing partial cystic degeneration

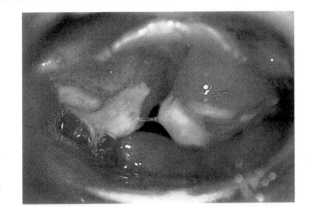

a Laryngeal fracture with mucosal hematoma and a dislocated arytenoid cartilage

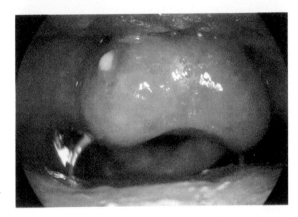

b Hyperacute epiglottitis with abscessation

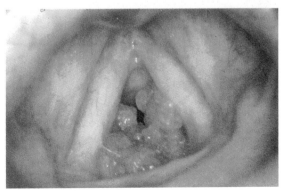

c Laryngeal papillomas

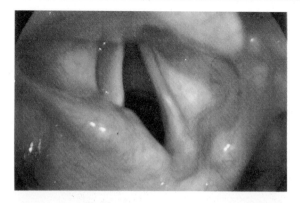

a Vocal cord palsy with atrophy of the vocal fold (right side of picture)

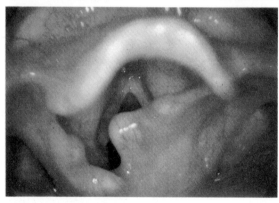

b Prolapse of the arytenoid cartilage in recurrent palsy (right side of picture)

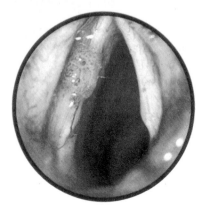

c Carcinoma at the center of the vocal cord extending to the ventricle

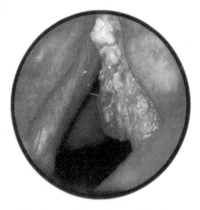

a Carcinoma of the entire vocal cord, ventricle, and anterior commissure. The affected cord is immobile

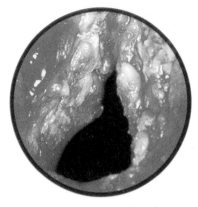

b Transglottic squamous cell carcinoma

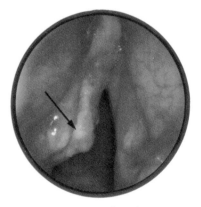

c Laryngeal carcinoma (arrow)

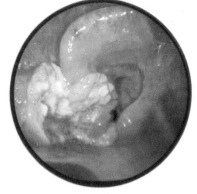

d Carcinoma of the hypopharynx with invasion of the ipsilateral hemilarynx

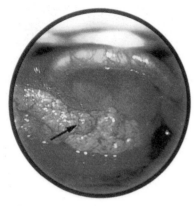

a Postcricoid squamous cell carcinoma

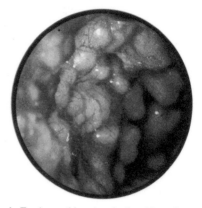

b Tracheopathia osteoplastica. View of the left tracheal wall on direct tracheoscopy

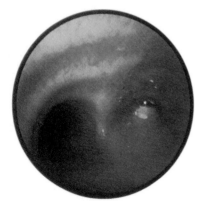

c Peanut lodged in the right main bronchus, partly covered by mucus, in a 2-year-old child. The carina is at the center of the field

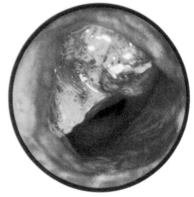

d Bronchial carcinoma in the left main bronchus

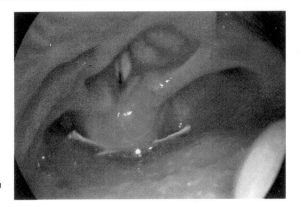

a Bony foreign body in the postcricoid region

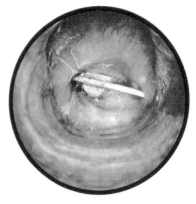

b Key of a toy lodged in the first esopha-geal constriction of a 2-year-old child

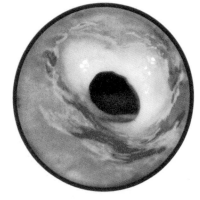

c Esophageal stricture following lye ingestion

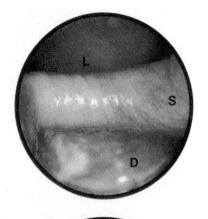

a Zenker's diverticulum. The rim of the diverticulum (S) is at the center, the esophageal lumen (L) above, and the diverticular sac (D) below

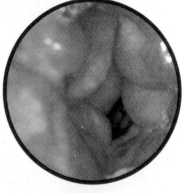

b Multiple esophageal varices

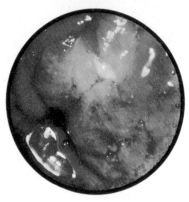

c Esophageal carcinoma (residual lumen is on the left)

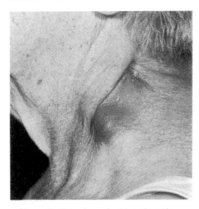

a Exacerbation of cervical lymph node tuberculosis in a 75-year-old-woman. Above the lesion is an old retracted scar

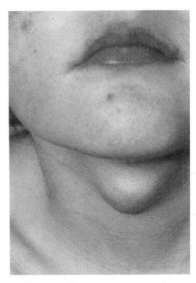

b Midline cervical cyst

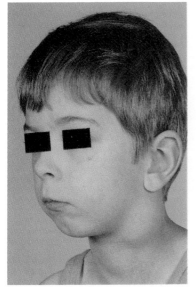

c "Lateral cervical cyst" due to cystic lymphadenopathy

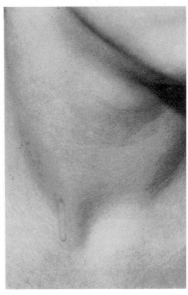

d Lateral right-sided cervical fistula with purulent discharge

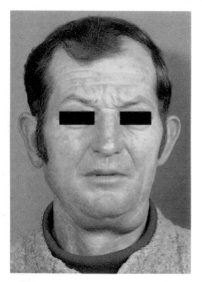

a Sjögren's syndrome (bilateral swelling of the submandibular glands and bilateral keratoconjunctivitis)

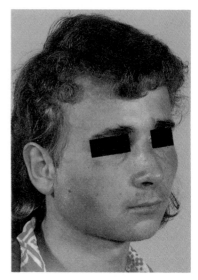

b Acute parotitis

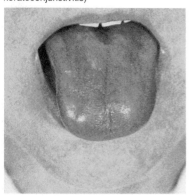

c Appearance of the tongue in myoepithelial sialadenitis (Sjögren's disease)

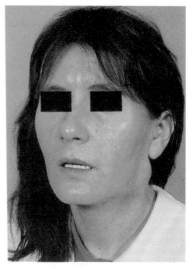

d Lymphoma in an AIDS patient

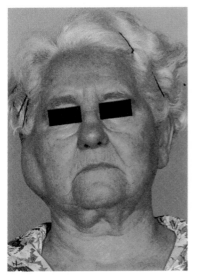

a Tumor of the parotid gland (requires differentiation from pleomorphic adenoma, cystadenoma, and lymphoma)

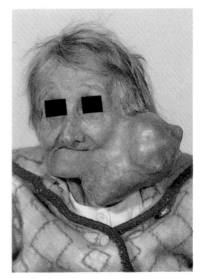

b Large pleomorphic adenoma of the parotid gland

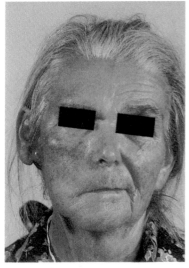

c Carcinoma of the right parotid gland with facial nerve palsy signifying infiltration of the nerve by malignant tumor

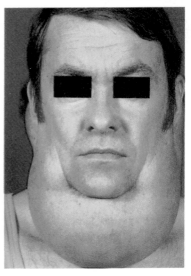

d Madelung's neck